P9-DII-562

✦STEDMAN'S®

MEDICAL TERMINOLOGY

Steps to Success in Medical Language

Charlotte Creason, RHIA

Editor

PROGRAM CHAIR
HEALTH INFORMATION TECHNOLOGY
TYLER JUNIOR COLLEGE
TYLER, TEXAS

◼. Wolters Kluwer | Lippincott Williams & Wilkins
Health
Philadelphia · Baltimore · New York · London
Buenos Aires · Hong Kong · Sydney · Tokyo

Senior Publisher: Julie K. Stegman
Acquisitions Editor: David B. Troy
Senior Managing Editor: Heather A. Rybacki
Developmental Editor: Rose Foltz
Marketing Manager: Allison Powell
Manufacturing Coordinator: Margie Orzech-Zeranko
Cover Design: Itzhack Shelomi Design House
Compositor: Aptara, Inc.
Printer: RRD-Shenzhen

Copyright © 2011 Lippincott Williams & Wilkins, a Wolters Kluwer business.

351 West Camden Street   Two Commerce Square
Baltimore, MD 21201   2001 Market Street
                                Philadelphia, PA 19103

All rights reserved. This book is protected by copyright. No part of this book may be reproduced or transmitted in any form or by any means, including as photocopies or scanned-in or other electronic copies, or utilized by any information storage and retrieval system without written permission from the copyright owner, except for brief quotations embodied in critical articles and reviews. Materials appearing in this book prepared by individuals as part of their official duties as U.S. government employees are not covered by the above-mentioned copyright. To request permission, please contact Lippincott Williams & Wilkins at Two Commerce Square, 2001 Market Street, Philadelphia, PA 19103, via email at permission@lww.com or via our website at lww.com (products and services).

DISCLAIMER
Care has been taken to confirm the accuracy of the information presented and to describe generally accepted practices. However, the authors, editors, and publisher are not responsible for errors or omissions or for any consequences from application of the information in this book and make no warranty, expressed or implied, with respect to the currency, completeness, or accuracy of the contents of the publication. Application of this information in a particular situation remains the professional responsibility of the practitioner; the clinical treatments described and recommended may not be considered absolute and universal recommendations.

Library of Congress Cataloging-in-Publication Data

Stedman's medical terminology : steps to success in medical language / Charlotte Creason, editor.
    p. ; cm.
  Other title: Medical terminology
  Includes bibliographical references and index.
  ISBN 978-1-58255-816-5 (alk. paper)
1. Medicine—Terminology. I. Creason, Charlotte. II. Title: Medical terminology.
  [DNLM: 1. Terminology as Topic—Problems and Exercises. W 18.2 S812 2011]
  R123.S713 2011
  610.1'4—dc22   2010025884

The publishers have made every effort to trace the copyright holders for borrowed material. If they have inadvertently overlooked any, they will be pleased to make the necessary arrangements at the first opportunity.

To purchase additional copies of this book, call our customer service department at (800) 638-3030 or fax orders to (301) 223-2400. International customers should call (301) 223-2300.

Visit Lippincott Williams & Wilkins on the Internet: http://www.LWW.com. Lippincott Williams & Wilkins customer service representatives are available from 8:30 am to 5:00 pm, EST.

                                                    10
                          1 2 3 4 5 6 7 8 9 10

RRS1009

■ PUBLISHER'S PREFACE

For 100 years, STEDMAN'S has been synonymous with quality, accuracy, and comprehensive medical word information. As we cross the century mark, we are proud to present *STEDMAN'S Medical Terminology: Steps to Success in Medical Language,* a textbook that teaches medical terminology in a work text approach, with the care and tradition of excellence you have come to expect from STEDMAN'S.

As the foundation for successful communication and understanding in any health care setting (educational or professional), medical terminology is the backbone of all medical disciplines. In a medical terminology course, students are typically taught word parts—prefixes, suffixes, combining forms, and roots—which allow them to piece words together and understand their meaning. A key aspect of medical terminology is the pronunciation of the words themselves, since learning medical terminology, which is drawn primarily from Latin and Greek, is like learning a different language. Depending upon the course and the approach, students may learn medical terminology in context, via medical records, or by focusing on the terminology associated with certain professions. Medical terminology courses can also cover, either concisely or comprehensively, anatomy and physiology.

Stedman's Medical Terminology provides students and instructors with a straightforward solution for a medical terminology course, including moderate coverage of anatomy and physiology. Recognizing that learning is facilitated by application, *Stedman's Medical Terminology* uses a work text approach that features tables with essential terms organized into clear, relevant categories for easy learning and comprehension, followed by ample exercises for learners to apply what they have learned. Special attention has been paid to ensure that each chapter presents a variety of exercise types that progress in difficulty. Extensive use of case-based scenarios and authentic medical records allow students to connect what they are learning to true-to-life situations.

Representing the Best Words in Medicine, we have worked with our customers to ensure that terminology occasionally missing in other medical terminology textbooks is included: medications and drug therapies are included in each of the body systems chapters; blood is covered in a separate chapter with immunity; and oncology and cancer terms are presented in a separate comprehensive chapter. In addition, we have continued to recognize a "picture is worth a thousand words" and have worked diligently to feature a robust art program which aids in comprehension without being gratuitous.

Finally, continuing Stedman's electronic tradition, we have included substantial learning resources for the reader and instructor. Readers can find hundreds of interactive activities, animations and videos, a comprehensive audio glossary/dictionary, a flash card builder, and other valuable materials in the electronic student resources. Instructors who choose STEDMAN'S are supported by easy-to-use lesson plans, PowerPoint slides, an image bank, test generator, classroom handouts, and more.

The development of *Stedman's Medical Terminology* has greatly benefited from the experience and expertise of our contributors, each of whom painstakingly worked with us to make certain each chapter is comprehensive and relevant for students. Charlotte Creason, our Editor-in-Chief, provided the perspective of our audience, both students and instructors, reviewing and editing all manuscript as well as selecting and critiquing the art and working with us on the design of the book; in the process, she has become a valued member of the Stedman's family and we thank her heartily. Working with Charlotte were our team of authors and consultants who created and reviewed every chapter's content and helped us refine and execute our vision based on their medical terminology teaching experience, and their experience in health care. Our contributors and review can be found on page xvi. Rose Foltz, our development editor, patiently and with dedication, ensured we maintained our vision of a consistent, thorough approach. Much gratitude is also given to Tom Lochhaas, who worked with the STEDMAN'S team to craft the vision for the textbook and guide its safe passage. We are also indebted to Heather Rybacki, Senior Product Manager, who has worked with STEDMAN'S for over 10 years and knows the importance of this undertaking and delivered with her customary excellence. Finally, as with any Stedman's publication, we must thank you, our reader. We appreciate all of the input and suggestions we have received in the past, including the suggestion of making this book, and thank you for your continued support of STEDMAN'S.

Your Medical Word Resource Publisher

We strive to provide our readers—students, educators, and practitioners—with the most up-to-date and accurate medical language resources. We, as always, welcome any suggestions you may have for improvements, changes, corrections, and additions—whatever makes it possible for this Stedman's product to serve you better.

Julie K. Stegman
Senior Publisher

David Troy
Editor, Medical Terminology

Stedman's Medical Terminology: Steps to Success in Medical Language
Lippincott Williams & Wilkins
Baltimore, Maryland

■ EDITOR'S PREFACE

Welcome to the first edition of *Stedman's Medical Terminology: Steps to Success in Medical Language*! This work text is the result of the contributions of a number of authors who have a tremendous amount of experience teaching medical terminology. This text and its ancillary materials introduce the beginning medical terminology student to a large variety of word parts and medical terms necessary to succeed in today's health care settings. It is a perfect match for a medical terminology course that seeks to provide students with a thorough understanding of medical terminology through the use of term tables and an abundance of exercises, and is also appropriate for the independent learner who wants to learn medical language through repetition and application.

Stedman's Medical Terminology uses a hands-on "work text" approach in which sections of related terms are immediately followed by a series of exercises. This method allows the student to immediately recall and apply what he or she has learned. To gain the most from this approach, the student should study the term tables and work the exercises until each word part or medical term is set in his or her memory.

Organization of the Book

Learning medical terminology is the key to successful communication in the health care environment, and each of the book's 16 chapters are geared towards preparing the student for fluency in medical language. Chapters 1 through 3 introduce medical terminology by explaining word structure and how medical terms are formed, then present common word parts and terms related to the body as a whole. Chapters 4 through 15 cover each body system in detail, including moderate coverage of the anatomy and physiology terms needed to understand the content later in the chapter. The book finishes with a chapter devoted to oncology and cancer terms that draws on the terminology presented in each of the preceding chapters. Appendices serve as a quick reference for word parts and their meanings, abbreviations, and other essential medical information.

Features

Thoughtful care has been put into incorporating the elements that will effectively help students gain a solid understanding of the language of health care. Seeking to move beyond simple rote memorization, *Stedman's Medical Terminology* steps up the work text approach with the following features:

- ■ **Logical Grouping of Terms.** Throughout the text, terms are grouped in clearly defined categories (tables) to promote ease of use and student understanding. These distinct categories include: anatomy and physiology, word parts (prefixes, suffixes, and combining forms), adjectives and other related terms, symptoms and medical conditions, laboratory tests and diagnostic procedures, surgical interventions and therapeutic procedures; medications and drug therapies, specialties and specialists, and abbreviations.

■ **Meaningful Progression of Exercises.** Each chapter contains a variety of engaging and effective student exercises to appeal to all learners. As the student moves through each new set of terms, the exercises progress in a meaningful way through five steps of learning:

Simple Recall: promotes commitment to memory through simple term-and-definition type exercises

Advanced Recall: builds upon the Simple Recall exercises by presenting similar content in a different way

Term Construction and Deconstruction: draws on the core method of learning medical terminology and allows the student to practice building and understanding terms based on the meaning of the word parts

Comprehension: requires the student to make connections and demonstrate a deeper understanding of the terminology in the chapter

Application and Analysis: prepares the student for life beyond the classroom by demonstrating how terms are used in the "real world" and building critical thinking skills

Each chapter culminates in a Chapter Review that encompasses terms from throughout the chapter. Illustration activities, pronunciation reviews, and spelling exercises round out the available exercises.

■ **Real-world Application.** Case-based exercises, case studies, and authentic medical records allow students to associate what they are learning with its application in the real world. Medical records scenarios place the medical student in an allied health profession for a "real-life" connection.

■ **Robust Art Program.** Vibrant photos and illustrations bring key concepts to life and further students' understanding of difficult concepts. A stunning 16-page Stedman's Anatomy Atlas serves as a comprehensive reference for the structures of each of the body systems.

■ **Coverage of Key Content.** In response to feedback from instructors, *Stedman's Medical Terminology* includes pharmacology terms within each of the body systems chapters. In addition, blood and immunity are covered in their own chapter (Chapter 8) to ensure comprehensive coverage of these two important topics, and an entire chapter is devoted to Oncology and Cancer Terms.

■ **Additional Features.** Study Tips and Extra Extra! boxes scattered throughout the text include additional information to aid in student learning.

Electronic Student Resources at www.thepoint.lww.com/StedmansMedTerm1e

Use of the student ancillaries is highly encouraged and can be fun! They have been carefully thought out and provide students with different ways of learning this vast amount of medical terms. The electronic student resources are referenced directly in the textbook and include a variety of exercises, games, and additional information for each chapter. Engage with:

■ Electronic flash cards
■ Interactive activities such as Concentration, Roboterms (Hangman), Word Builder, Quiz Show, Complete the Case, Medical Records Review, Look and Label, Image Matching, Spelling Bee, and more!
■ Chapter Quizzes and a Final Exam

- Animations and videos that build upon the content in the text
- Flash card builder that allows students to create and print their own cards
- Audio Glossary/Dictionary
- Additional Appendices and descriptions of various Health Professions Careers
- *LiveAdvise Medical Terminology,* an online tutoring service

Premium Online Course

Also available for adoption, the *Stedman's Medical Terminology* **Premium Online Course** is a complete, ready-to-go course designed to be used in conjunction with the textbook. The course is customized to the text by chapter, and features content and activities that are unique to the online course. Contact your Lippincott Williams & Wilkins Sales Representative for more information.

Instructor Resources

Visit thePoint at **www.thepoint.lww.com/StedmansMedTerm1e** to access resources designed specifically to help instructors teach more effectively and save time. There you will find:

- *Instructor's test generator,* encompassing individual chapter tests and a comprehensive exam
- *PowerPoint slides*, with lecture notes, for each chapter
- *Lesson plans* for each chapter that are easy to follow
- *Classroom hand-outs*
- *Image bank*
- *Animations and videos*
- *Medical record library*
- And more!

A solid understanding of medical terminology provides an essential foundation for any career in health care. The *Stedman's Medical Terminology* product suite makes learning and teaching medical terminology a rewarding and exciting process.

Steps to Success:
How to Use Stedman's Medical Terminology

Stedman's Medical Terminology: Steps to Success in Medical Terminology offers an engaging and hands-on way to learn the language of health care. Using a work text approach and a meaningful progression of exercises, it will provide you with the knowledge you need to communicate successfully in the health care world. Along the way, you'll encounter special features and tools that will help you navigate and understand the material presented. This section explains how to get the most out of each chapter so you can take your new language with you into your chosen health care profession!

Chapter Outline presents a concise overview of the chapter content. Read it to understand what is covered in the chapter, and then use it as roadmap to help you easily navigate the material.

Objectives list fundamental learning goals for the chapter. Review these before beginning the chapter to identify the learning tasks you will need to complete so that you know what to study. When you have finished the chapter exercises and the activities with the Student Resources, review the Objectives to assess your level of mastery.

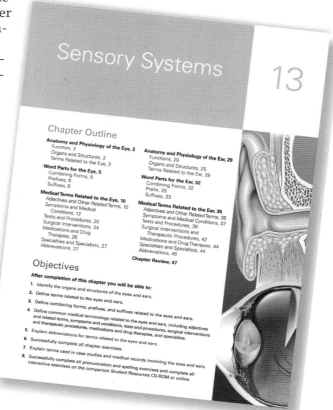

Sensory Systems

13

Chapter Outline

Anatomy and Physiology of the Eye, 2
Function, 2
Organs and Structures, 2
Terms Related to the Eye, 2

Word Parts for the Eye, 5
Combining Forms, 5
Prefixes, 6
Suffixes, 6

Medical Terms Related to the Eye, 10
Adjectives and Other Related Terms, 10
Symptoms and Medical Conditions, 12
Tests and Procedures, 20
Surgical Interventions, 24
Medications and Drug Therapies, 26
Specialties and Specialists, 27
Abbreviations, 27

Anatomy and Physiology of the Ear, 29
Functions, 29
Organs and Structures, 29
Terms Related to the Ear, 29

Word Parts for the Ear, 32
Combining Forms, 32
Prefix, 33
Suffixes, 33

Medical Terms Related to the Ear, 35
Adjectives and Other Related Terms, 35
Symptoms and Medical Conditions, 37
Tests and Procedures, 39
Surgical Interventions and Therapeutic Procedures, 42
Medications and Drug Therapies, 44
Specialties and Specialists, 44
Abbreviations, 45

Chapter Review, 47

Objectives

After completion of this chapter you will be able to:
1. Identify the organs and structures of the eyes and ears.
2. Define terms related to the eyes and ears.
3. Define combining forms, prefixes, and suffixes related to the eyes and ears.
4. Define common medical terminology related to the eyes and ears, including adjectives and related terms, symptoms and conditions, tests and procedures, surgical interventions and therapeutic procedures, medications and drug therapies, and specialties.
5. Explain abbreviations for terms related to the eyes and ears.
6. Successfully complete all chapter exercises.
7. Explain terms used in case studies and medical records involving the eyes and ears.
8. Successfully complete all pronunciation and spelling exercises and complete all interactive exercises on the companion Student Resources CD-ROM or online.

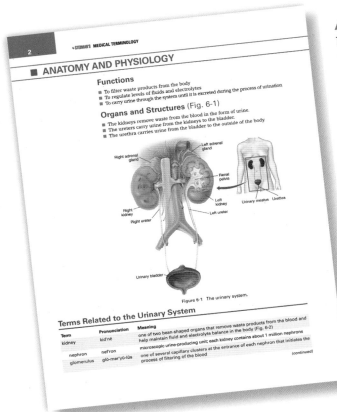

Anatomy and Physiology, the first section of each body system chapter, provides the context for learning the chapter's medical terms. Essential facts and detailed, full-color illustrations showing the body system's key functions, organs, and structures are included. If you have not previously studied Anatomy and Physiology, use this information to familiarize yourself with the specific body system. If you have already studied Anatomy and Physiology, this section can serve as a refresher on key concepts.

Word Parts Tables list the combining forms, prefixes, and suffixes for terms related to the chapter's body system. Study the meanings of these word parts to help you build medical terms and develop your vocabulary. Use your understanding of word parts to help break down unfamiliar terms to figure out their meanings.

Medical Term Tables present need-to-know terms for the specific body system covered. The terms are organized into practical, clearly-defined categories that are relevant across various health care settings. As you review each of the tables, read the terms, practice the pronunciations, and study the meanings. Learn the synonyms listed to expand your vocabulary and understanding. Note that related terms are grouped together, so that you can more easily recognize their connection to specific body structures.

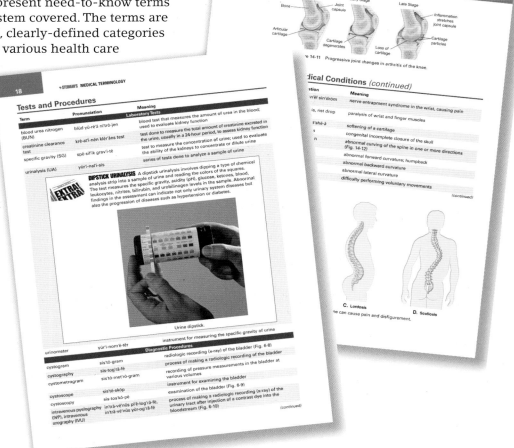

Medications and Drug Therapies are integrated into the chapters and reflect common pharmacologic interventions for disorders related to the chapter's body system. Learning these in context will help you link medical conditions and the drugs used to treat them.

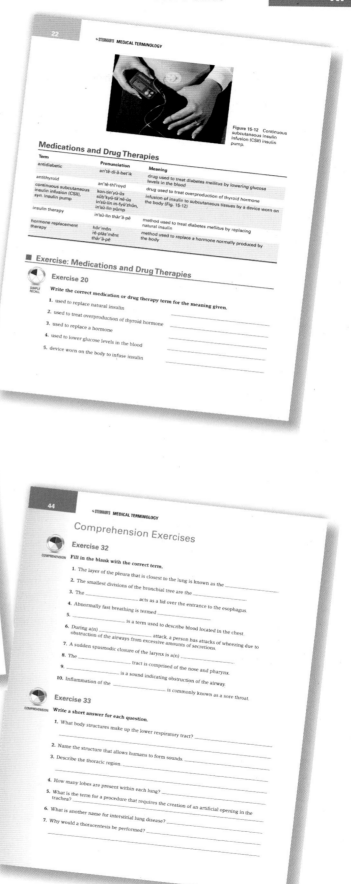

Exercises using varied formats and styles appear throughout this work text, after each chapter section. Questions progress from basic recall to activities involving higher-level critical thinking. Complete each exercise as it is presented, to gain practice and to steadily build your knowledge and reinforce learning. Check your understanding before continuing on to the next section.

Full-Color Illustrations and Photographs offer detailed views of selected medical terms and key concepts. Images of x-rays, CT scans, MRI scans, and other diagnostic tests provide additional real-life examples. Review each of the anatomic drawings and photographs together with the related terms to make visual connections, which can aid memory and comprehension.

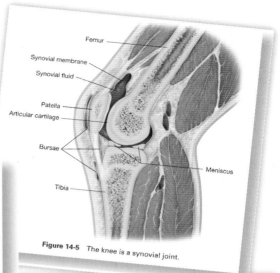

Femur
Synovial membrane
Synovial fluid
Patella
Articular cartilage
Bursae
Tibia
Meniscus

Figure 14-5 The knee is a synovial joint.

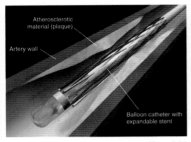

Atherosclerotic material (plaque)
Artery wall
Balloon catheter with expandable stent

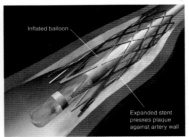

Inflated balloon
Expanded stent presses plaque against artery wall

Figure 7-24 Arterial stent.

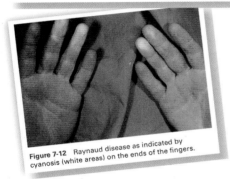

Figure 7-12 Raynaud disease as indicated by cyanosis (white areas) on the ends of the fingers.

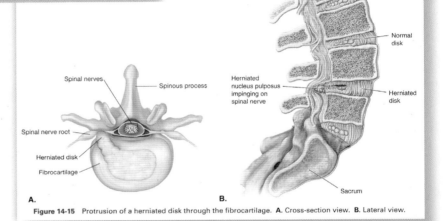

Spinal nerves
Spinous process
Spinal nerve root
Herniated disk
Fibrocartilage

Herniated nucleus pulposus impinging on spinal nerve
Normal disk
Herniated disk
Sacrum

A. B.

Figure 14-15 Protrusion of a herniated disk through the fibrocartilage. **A.** Cross-section view. **B.** Lateral view.

Study Tip

Epispadias and Hypospadias: To avoid confusing the terms epispadias and hypospadias, focus on the prefixes. *Epi-* means on or upon, so epispadias is the urinary meatus on the *upper* side of the penis. *Hypo-* means less than or below, so hypospadias is the urinary meatus on the *under* side of ("below") the penis.

Special Features include Study Tips and Extra! Extra! boxes. Use the Study Tips as memory joggers to help you learn or spell potentially confusing terms. Read the Extra! Extra! boxes to expand your knowledge of topics related to key concepts.

Terms Related to Joints and Joint Movements

Term	Pronunciation	Meaning
meniscus	mĕ-nis'kŭs	cartilage structure in the knee
suture	sū'chŭr	an immovable joint, such as that which joins the bones of the skull

SUTURE When we think of joints, we think of those joints that move. Your skull also has joints, but the joints of the skull do not move. These joints, called sutures, hold the bones of the skull together, just as surgical sutures (or "stitches") hold two surfaces together.

symphysis	sim'fi-sis	a joint that moves only slightly
synovial fluid	si-nō'vē-ăl flū'id	lubricating fluid in a freely moving joint
tendon	ten'dŏn	band of fibrous connective tissue attaching a muscle to a bone
		Joint Movements (Fig. 14-6)
abduction	ab-dŭk'shŭn	moving away from the midline
adduction	ă-dŭk'shŭn	moving toward the midline
circumduction	sir'kŭm-dŭk'shŭn	moving in a circular manner
inversion	in-vĕr'zhŭn	turning inward
eversion	ē-vĕr'zhŭn	turning outward
dorsiflexion	dōr-si-flek'shŭn	bending foot upward
plantar flexion	plan'tahr flek'shŭn	bending foot downward
extension	eks-ten'shŭn	motion that increases the joint angle
flexion	flek'shŭn	motion that decreases the joint angle
pronation	prō-nā'shŭn	turning downward (palm of hand or sole of foot)
supination	sū'pi-nā'shŭn	turning upward (palm of hand or sole of foot)
rotation	rō-tā'shŭn	moving in circular direction around an axis

Study Tip

Adduction, abduction: When distinguishing abduction from adduction, remember the common word abduct, meaning to take away. Adduction has the word "add" meaning to bring to.

▶ View the animation entitled *Muscle Extension and Flexion* for a demonstration of muscles at work.
ANIMATION

DOCUMENTATION INVOLVING THE EYES In a clinical examination, checks the eyes as part of an overall review of the head, eyes, ear throat (abbreviated as *HEENT*). Documentation of the physician's patient's medical record might look something like this:
EYES: Pupils equal, round, and reactive to light and accommodatio are clear. Extraocular movements are intact bilaterally. Sclerae not ic

Case Reports and Medical Records present samples of clinical reports commonly encountered in health care settings. Use these real-world examples to help you learn and remember terminology. Read through each case report and medical record to get a general sense of the clinical situation. Do not stop to decode new terms; underline them and continue reading. Then go back and use context clues to help analyze the meaning of any unfamiliar terms. If necessary, use your medical dictionary.

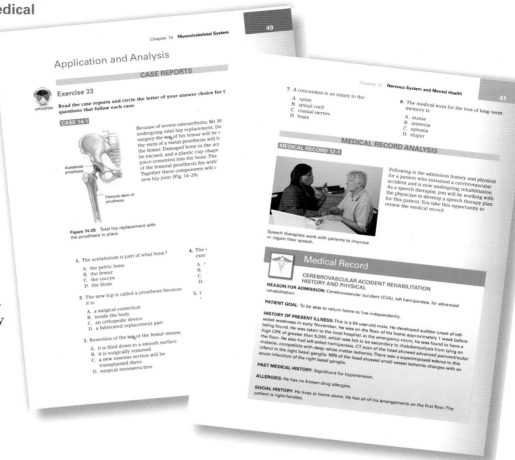

Chapter Review exercises test your knowledge of terminology presented in the chapter. Illustration exercises are also included to help you connect terms to related anatomy, while Pronunciation activities help you practice correct pronunciation. Both visual and auditory learners will be engaged by the diverse activities. Complete all of the exercises to ensure a thorough review of the material, and then check your answers to assess your understanding.

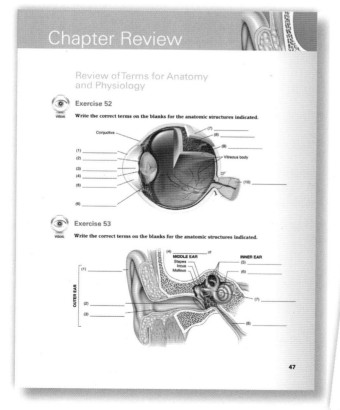

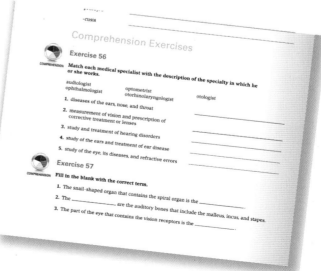

Media Connection is located at the end of each Chapter Review section. It offers a checklist of activities you will find on the electronic Student Resources. Animations and information on relevant health professions careers are also available. Complete the interactive exercises for further practice and to test your learning. View the animations and read about potential careers to expand your knowledge. As a final review, take the Chapter Quiz and record your score.

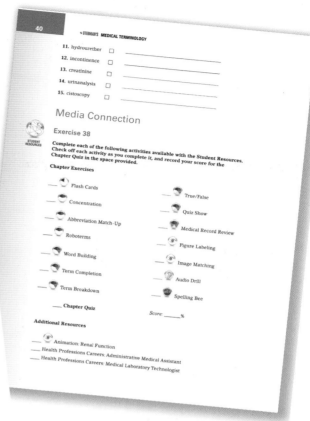

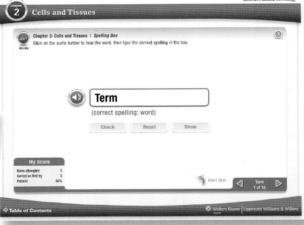

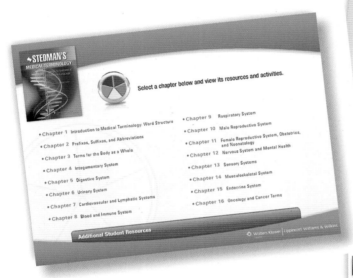

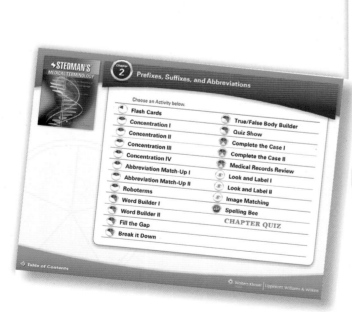

■ ACKNOWLEDGMENTS

Many thanks go out to those who have helped bring this book to fruition. First and foremost are the chapter authors and reviewers; your vast teaching experience, knowledge, and commitment to excellence in medical terminology shows in each and every word. To Julie Stegman, Senior Publisher, thank you for your vision of the book and believing that I could make a contribution by editing this text. To Heather Rybacki, Senior Product Manager, and Rose Foltz, Developmental Editor, your gentle guidance through this process has been invaluable and your genuine concern for content, attention to detail, and student learning made a major impact on this project. To my husband Jody, thank you for encouraging me to take on this new endeavor and for supporting me from beginning to end. To my children, Joe and Rachel, thanks for giving up some of Mom for "the book." Finally, thank you to all the students I have had in the past and will have in the future. You are the reason for this book.

—Charlotte Creason, Editor

■ REVIEWERS AND CONTRIBUTORS

The editor and publisher are extremely grateful to our contributors, who shared their time, wisdom, and love of medical terminology with us by writing chapters or providing other pieces of content for this textbook:

Tammie Bolling, EdD, MBA/HCM, CBCS, CMAA, CHI
Instructor
Business Systems Technology
Tennessee Technology Center at
    Jacksboro
Jacksboro, Tennessee

Diane M. Gilmore, CMT, AHDI-F
Director of Education
Med-Line School of Medical
    Transcription and
Med-Line School of Business and
    Technology
Lake Havasu City, Arizona

Tamra Greco
Former Department Head and
    Instructor
Health Professions
Davenport University
Grand Rapids, Michigan

Debbie Newcomb, MBA, CMM
Assistant Professor
Ventura Community College
Ventura, California

Linda A. Underhill, BS, NCMA
Assistant Professor
Clinical Medical Assistant Technology
New England Institute of Technology
Warwick, Rhode Island

Melinda Wray, BS, CMA (AAMA), RMA
Department Head
Medical Assisting and
    Administration
ECPI College of Technology
Greensboro, North Carolina

We would also like to thank our reviewers, many of whom provided valuable comments and suggestions throughout development of the manuscript, while others supplied feedback on the design of the book:

Diana Alagna, RN, RMA
Medical Assisting Program Director
Medical Assisting
Branford Hall Career Institute
Southington, Conneticut

Emily M. Ambizas, PharmD, CGP
Associate Clinical Professor
Clinical Pharmacy Practice
College of Pharmacy and Allied
    Health Professions, St. John's
    University
Queens, New York

Elaine Appelle
Retired Professor
Office of Technology
Nassau Community College
Garden City, New York

Gerry A. Brasin, AS, CMA (AAMA), CPC
Corporate Education Coordinator
Premier Education Group
Springfield, Massachusetts

Joseph M. Brocavich, PharmD
Associate Clinical Professor/
    Associate Dean for Pharmacy
    Programs
Clinical Pharmacy Practice
College of Pharmacy and Allied
    Health Professions, St. John's
    University
Jamaica, New York

Kathy Carter, MS
Instructor
Life Sciences
Athens Technical College
Athens, Georgia

Michael Covone, MEd, RT(R), CT
Faculty
Health Sciences
Pennsylvania College of Technology
Williamsport, Pennsylvania

Donna Domanke-Nuytten, RN, BSN, MSIMC
Professor, Medical Assisting
Health Science Technology
Macomb Community College
Warren, Michigan

Alycia Dotseth, BS
Medical Terminology GTA
Occupational Therapy
Colorado State University
Fort Collins, Colorado

Marie Fenske, EdD, RRT
Director of Clinical Education/
 Faculty/Coordinator of Health
 Care Core
Respiratory Care and Health Care
 Core
GateWay Community College
Phoenix, Arizona

Cynthia Ferguson, RHIT
Instructor
Allied Health
Texas State Technical College
Sweetwater, Texas

Rebecca Giuliante, MS, RN, LCEP
Director, AHA Training Center and
 Program Development
Our Lady of the Lake Health
 Career Institute
Our Lady of the Lake College
Baton Rouge, Louisiana

Sheila Guillot, CAP/CPS
Instructor IV
Business and Technology
Lamar State College
Port Arthur, Texas

Sharon Harris-Pelliccia, BS, RPAC
Department Chair
Medical Studies
Mildred Elley
Albany, New York

Kathleen Holbrook
Director/Vice President
Andrews & Holbrook Training Corp.
Latham, New York

Susan Horn, AAS, CMA (AAMA)
Medical Program Coordinator
Medical/Education
Indiana Business College
Lafayette, Indiana

Jacqueline M. Johnson, CCMA, BA
Instructor
Office Information Technology
University of Cincinnati/Raymond
 Walters College/Blue Ash
Cincinnati, Ohio

Sandra Johnson, BAAS
Instructor
Health Information Technology
San Juan College
Farmington, New Mexico

Sandy Johnston, MSEd, RHIA, CPC
Educator
Health Information Management
University of Kansas
Kansas City, Kansas

Carrol LaRowe, MBA, RRT, RCP
Director of Clinical Education
Respiratory Care
San Jacinto College
Pasadena, Texas

Tina Lewis, MT (ASCP)(AMT)
Medical Department Co-Director
Spencerian College
Louisville, Kentucy

**Michelle Maguire McDaniel, LPN,
HCC, BA, MA**
Medical Assisting and Health Care
 Support Instructor
Health Sciences
Ivy Tech Community College of
 Indiana
Anderson, Indiana

**Michelle Martin, MEd, MBA,
RHIA, FAHIMA**
Associate Professor
Health Informatics and Information
 Management
Louisiana Tech University
Ruston, LA

Lori McGowan, DPM
Adjuct Professor
Harrisburg Area Community College
Harrisburg, Pennsylvania

Linda L. Miedema, PhD
Provost
Institute of Nursing
Brevard Community College
Titusville, Florida

Pat Moody, RN
RN/Clinical Instructor
Allied Health
Athens Technical College
Athens, Georgia

**Marcia Morse, MBA Health Care,
BS, RMA (AMT)**
Allied Health and Science
Davenport University
Caro, Michigan

Tamra Nasworthy, LPN, PHD, ABD
Nurse/Educator
Allied Health
Athens Technical College
Athens, Georgia

Arlene Normandin, CPC
Instructor, Allied Health
Medical Terminology, Billing and
 Coding
Quinebaug Valley Community College
Danielson, Conneticut

Elaine Olsakovsky, MA
Professor/Coordinator
Health Professions and Related
 Sciences
El Paso Community College
El Paso, Texas

David Peruski, RN, MSA, MSN
Associate Professor
Health and Wellness Division Chair
Delta College
University Center, Michigan

Virginia Przygocki, BS
Health and Wellness Chairperson
Health and Wellness
Delta College
University Center, Michigan

Heather Reinke, BSN
Nursing
Delta College
University Center, Michigan

Carol Ricke, MS
Coordinator of Administrative
 Assistant Program
Lead Business Instructor
Accounting and Business
Pratt Community College
Pratt, Kansas

Betty Rickey, RN, MSN
Professor of Nursing (Emeritus)
Health and Wellness Division
Delta College
University Center, Michigan

Laura Ristrom Goodman, MSSW
Curriculum Coordinator
Corporate Education
Pima Medical Institute
Tucson, Arizona

Patricia A. Sailors
Health Science Instructor
Health Services
West Georgia Technical College
Waco, Georgia

Laura Stoll, BS
Adjunct Instructor
Health and Wellness
Delta College
University Center, Michigan

**Cindy Thompson, RN, RMA,
MA, BS**
Certified Allied Health Instructor/
    Assistant Professor/Allied
    Health Coordinator
Davenport University
Saginaw, Michigan

**Kate Tierney, CPC, CCS-P, CPC-P,
CPhT, CEHRS, CBCS, CMAA, CICS,
COBGC, CGSC, CEMC, CEDC**
Certified Healthcare Instructor
Denver, Colorado

Martha Vigneault, PhD
Associate Professor
Rehabilitative Health
Community College of Rhode Island
Newport, Rhode Island

Donna Walsworth, RN, BSN
Instructor
Adult Education
Genesee Valley Educational
    Partnership
Mt. Morris, New York

Janet E. Warner, RN, MSN
Assistant Professor
Nursing
Southern Utah University
Cedar City, Utah

Kari Williams, BS, DC
Director
Medical Office Technology
Front Range Community College
Longmont, Colorado

■ CONTENTS

Introduction to Medical Terminology: Word Structure

1

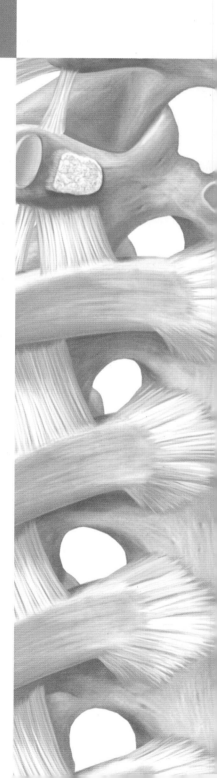

Chapter Outline

Objectives

After completion of this chapter you will be able to:

1. Explain why understanding medical terms is important.

2. Define each of the four basic word parts.

3. Describe how word parts are put together to make a term and give an example.

4. Use the pronunciation key to learn how to pronounce medical terms.

5. Understand medical terms by analyzing their parts.

6. Successfully complete all chapter exercises.

7. Successfully complete all interactive exercises included with the companion Student Resources.

■ WHY USE MEDICAL TERMS?

Every profession has a range of special terms used by practitioners in that field. As someone who may work in a health-related field, you will need to read, write, speak, and understand medical language. Understanding medical terms is also a gateway to learning about the human body, about health care generally, and even about your own health. When learning medical language you are learning much more than just *words*—you are learning fundamental concepts about the body in health and disease and about common health problems.

People often wonder why medical terms have to be used at all. Why not just say it in "plain English"? For example, why not say *stomachache* instead of *gastritis*? As will soon become clear, medical language is not like a foreign language where an everyday word can be translated directly to or from a medical word. Medical terms are much more precise than everyday words. What you call stomachache *might* be the pain caused by gastritis, but you might also be feeling the symptoms of a peptic ulcer, ulcerative colitis, or peritonitis. These medical terms mean very different things to workers in health care (and would to you if you had one of these conditions!). And there is no simple, word-for-word "plain English" translation of any of these terms that carries their full medical meaning. So you have to learn the medical terms to understand these conditions.

The good news, however, is that medical terminology is not nearly as difficult to learn as it may seem at first. Did you notice that three of these medical terms for conditions causing stomach pain all end in *-itis*? Once you know what *-itis* means, you are halfway to understanding the meaning of three different terms. In fact, many common medical terms end in *-itis*, so learning that one word ending gets you halfway to understanding dozens of terms! Although you do need to memorize many word parts to understand medical terminology, after you learn how the meanings of terms are built from common parts, you will likely be surprised at how quickly your understanding will grow. That is what you will be doing as you work through this text.

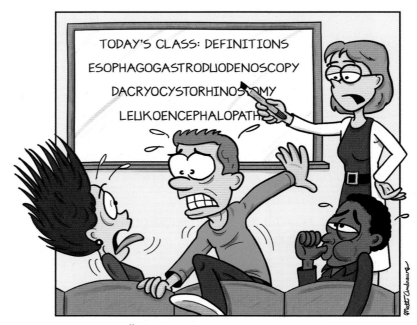

"WHO CAN DEFINE THE TERM
'ESOPHAGOGASTRODUODENOSCOPY?'"

Figure 1-1

■ DERIVATION OF MEDICAL TERMS

It's easier to learn medical terms when you understand where the basic word parts come from and how medical terms were derived. The earliest medical practitioners generally wrote, spoke, and read Greek and Latin, because these were the languages of science and education for more than two thousand years. Although very few in health care today study Greek or Latin, they continue to use medical language based on these ancient tongues because, as just noted, these terms are more precise than most everyday words.

In almost all cases, you will learn not the original Greek or Latin word but a *word root* (think of that as the most basic part of a term) that derives from a Greek or Latin word. For example, the word root *gastr* comes from the Greek word for stomach, *gaster*. A few of the medical terms built from this word root are gastritis, gastrointestinal, gastroenteritis, gastroesophageal, and gastrostomy. Soon you will find it easy to understand these terms as you learn additional roots and word parts. Most medical terms are built from word parts.

In addition, some medical terms are not built from word parts but have their origins in modern languages (which may or may not be indirectly derived from ancient languages). Other terms derive from the name of the person who first identified a condition or developed a procedure. Kaposi sarcoma, for example, is a skin cancer named for a Hungarian dermatologist.

■ UNDERSTANDING TERMS THROUGH THEIR PARTS

As you have already learned, most medical terms are built by combining different word parts. Basic word parts include the root, a prefix, and a suffix; these components are discussed in detail later in this chapter. When you put these parts together to build a medical term, the term's meaning will come from the meaning of its parts. The first medical practitioner to study and write about stomach inflammation, for example, may have been the first one to coin the term *gastritis*. *Gastr-* refers to the stomach, and *-itis* refers to inflammation—gastritis means inflammation of the stomach.

Just as terms are built from word parts, you can understand their meaning by dissecting them into their parts. Suppose that you have never seen the term *gastrotomy* before. You already know that *gastr* refers to the stomach. If you also know that *-tomy* refers to an incision into something, you can easily figure out that a *gastrotomy* must be an incision made into the stomach.

And after you know that *crani* refers to the skull (cranium), can you guess what a craniotomy is? (A craniotomy is an incision into the skull.)

Word Roots

A **word root** is the core or main part of the word. All medical terms have a word root. In this way, word roots are different from the other word parts you will learn about in a moment.

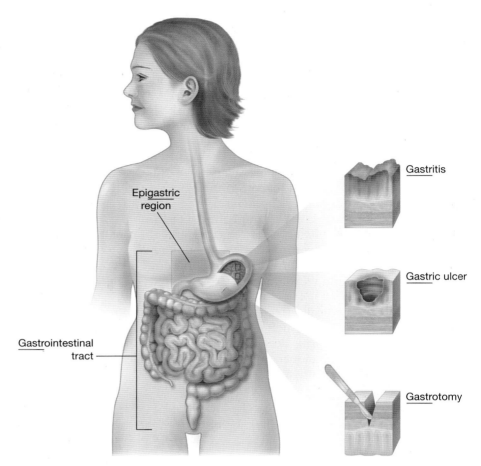

Gastritis

Gastric ulcer

Gastrotomy

Epigastric region

Gastrointestinal tract

Figure 1-2 From one word root comes many different medical terms.

In many cases you will have to memorize the meaning of word roots. You will probably already know many common word roots because some everyday words also are derived from them. Sometimes there are two or more word roots with the same meaning. Memorize the meanings of the following common word roots, then complete the exercises that follow.

Word Root	Meaning
cardi	heart
cerebr	brain, cerebrum
col, colon	colon (section of large intestine)
crani	cranium, skull
dermat	skin
disk	disk (as in disk of spine)
gastr	stomach
nephr, ren	kidney
oste	bone
pulmon	lung

Exercises: Word Roots

Exercise 1

SIMPLE
RECALL

Write the meaning of the word root given.

1. oste _____

2. disk _____

3. cerebr _____

4. pulmon _____

5. dermat _____

Exercise 2

SIMPLE
RECALL

Write the correct word root for the meaning given.

1. skull _____

2. heart _____

3. stomach _____

4. colon _____

5. kidney _____

Prefixes

Prefixes are a second type of word part. *Pre-* means before, and a **prefix** is the word part that comes *before the word root* in a medical term. For example, the term *natal* refers generally to childbirth. What then would the term *prenatal* mean? The term *prenatal* refers to the period of time in pregnancy *before* birth occurs. A health care provider may prescribe prenatal vitamins for a pregnant woman, for example. If so, when would she take these vitamins? (A pregnant woman would take prenatal vitamins before childbirth.)

Many medical terms are built with prefixes. Prefixes always contribute to the meaning of the term, usually by simply adding the meaning of the prefix to the meaning of the word root.

Here is another example. The prefix *post-* means the opposite of *pre-*. *Post-* means after. Thus the term *postsurgical* refers to something that happens after surgery. It may refer to the general postsurgical period of time, or it may refer to something done during that time, such as giving postsurgical medications.

Sometimes prefixes may have somewhat different meanings depending on the word roots to which they are added. Memorize the meanings of the following common prefixes before completing the exercises. Note that, in this text, a prefix is always spelled with a hyphen at the end, indicating that it is not a word in itself but is a word part that is attached to another word part coming after it.

Prefix	Meaning
pre-	before
post-	after, behind
peri-	around, surrounding
intra-	within
inter-	between
sub-, infra-	below, beneath
supra-, super-	above
a-, an-	without, not
poly-	many, much
dys-	painful, difficult, abnormal

■ Exercises: Prefixes

Exercise 3

SIMPLE RECALL

Write the meaning of the prefix given.

1. dys- _____

2. intra- _____

3. peri- _____

4. post- _____

5. poly- _____

Exercise 4

SIMPLE RECALL

Write the correct prefix for the meaning given.

1. before _____

2. between _____

3. without, not _____

4. above _____

5. below _____

Suffixes

Suffixes are a third type of word part. Like prefixes, **suffixes** are attached to a word root, but they come after the root. For example, the suffix -*ac* means "pertaining to." Therefore *cardiac* simply means "pertaining to the heart." The suffix -al also means "pertaining to," so what do you think *cranial* means? (Cranial means pertaining to the skull.)

Almost all medical terms are built with suffixes. Suffixes always contribute to the meaning of the term, usually by simply adding the meaning of the suffix to the meaning of the word root (and prefix when one is present).

Memorize the meanings of the following common suffixes. Note that a suffix always begins with a hyphen, indicating that it is not a word in itself but is a word part that is attached to another word part coming before it.

Suffix	Meaning
-ac, -al, -ary, -ic, -ous	pertaining to
-algia	pain
-ectomy	excision, surgical removal
-gram	record, recording
-ism, -ia	condition of
-itis	inflammation
-ium	tissue, structure
-logy	study of
-oma	tumor
-tomy	incision

■ Exercise: Suffixes

ADVANCED RECALL

Exercise 5

Match each suffix with its meaning.

| -tomy | -ism | -oma | -ectomy | -al |
| -ium | -gram | -algia | -itis | -logy |

Meaning	Suffix
1. incision	_____
2. tissue	_____
3. record, recording	_____
4. pertaining to	_____
5. study of	_____
6. pain	_____
7. inflammation	_____
8. surgical removal	_____
9. condition of	_____
10. tumor	_____

Combining Vowels Added to Roots

There is one more part of medical terms you need to understand, even though, unlike the other three types of word parts, it does not carry a meaning. A **combining vowel** is a vowel (usually "o," and sometimes "i" or "e") that is added to the word root to make it easier to pronounce the term. For example, if you add the suffix -*logy* (study of) directly to the word root *dermat* (skin), you would get "dermatlogy"—something that would sound very odd when you tried to say it. Compare that with how you pronounce "dermatology." Thus in the origins of medical terms, a vowel was often inserted at the end of the word root before joining it to another root or to a suffix.

Because the combining vowel is best learned along with the word root to which it may be added, we call the result a **combining form**. This text will use combining forms rather than word roots. Instead of learning just the word root *cardi,* therefore, you will learn the combining form *cardi/o*. The slash is used to indicate that depending on the other word part following the combining form, the combining vowel may or may not be used. Note the difference here:

> peri- + cardi/o + -ium = pericardium (tissue around the heart)—the "o" is not used
>
> cardi/o + -logy = cardiology (study of the heart)—the "o" is used

If you tried to put in the combining vowel when it is not needed, you would see the problem when you tried to pronounce the word (pericardioum—too many vowels!). Similarly, if you left out the vowel when it is needed, you would hear the problem when you tried to pronounce it (cardilogy—too few vowels!).

You may have noticed something about the first example above: the formation of the term *pericardium*. The combining form in this word is *cardi/o*, and the suffix is -*ium*. If we were to ignore the combining vowel "o" when we joined the two, we would have two "i"s in the middle, since the combining form ends with "i" and the suffix begins with "i". The result would be "pericardiium"—but how would that be pronounced? In cases like this, the rules of language favor common sense and help us pronounce the terms. The rule in this case is simple: If a combining form (without the optional vowel) ends with the same vowel that the suffix begins with, then the vowel is dropped to prevent repetition.

Fortunately, there are only a few rules to learn about how terms are spelled when word parts are put together. We will look at those rules in the next section.

Memorize the spellings of the following common combining forms. Remember that the slash before the combining vowel is used to indicate that the vowel may or may not be used when the combining form is joined to a following word part.

Combining Form	Meaning
cardi/o	heart
cerebr/o	brain, cerebrum
col/o, colon/o	colon (section of large intestine)
crani/o	cranium, skull
dermat/o	skin
disk/o	disk (as in disk of spine)
gastr/o	stomach
nephr/o, ren/o	kidney
oste/o	bone
pulmon/o	lung

■ Exercise: Combining Forms

Exercise 6

SIMPLE
RECALL

Write the correct combining form(s) for the meaning given.

1. disk _____

2. stomach _____

3. kidney _____

4. heart _____

5. skull _____

6. bone _____

7. lung _____

8. brain _____

9. skin _____

10. colon _____

Putting the Parts Together

Medical terms are made up of combining forms usually together with prefixes and/or suffixes. The rules for when to include the combining vowel in forming a term are usually simple:

1. Use the combining vowel when a combining form is joined to a suffix that does not begin with a vowel:

   nephr/o (kidney) + -logy (study of) = nephrology (study of the kidneys)

2. Do not use the combining vowel when a combining form is joined to a suffix that does begin with a vowel:

   arthr/o (joint) + -itis (inflammation) = arthritis (no o) (inflammation of joint)

   And if the suffix begins with the *same* vowel as the combining form ends with, do not repeat it:

   cardi/o + -itis = carditis

3. Use the combining vowel when two combining forms are joined together:

   my/o (muscle) + cardi/o (heart) + -al = myocardial (pertaining to the heart muscle)

   Note that this rule holds true usually even if the second combining form already begins with a vowel:

   oste/o (bone) + arthr/o (joint) + -itis = osteoarthritis (inflammation of bone and joint)

There are a few other special cases where the rule may vary slightly, but these are individual exceptions you will learn later on. Because these rules are generally based on how terms are spelled so that they can be pronounced more easily, get in the habit of saying terms aloud (or at least *think* them aloud to yourself) as you see them in this text. Very soon you will naturally know whether to use the combining vowel or not by how a term *sounds*.

■ Exercise: Putting the Parts Together

TERM
CONSTRUCTION

Exercise 7

With the word parts given, write the medical term (spelled correctly) that matches the given meaning.

1. intra- + crani/o + -al = _____ (pertaining to within the skull)

2. sub- + pulmon/o + -ary = _____ (pertaining to below the lungs)

3. cardi/o + -gram = _____ (record of heart activity)

4. oste/o + -algia = _____ (pain in a bone)

5. gastr/o + -tomy = _____ (incision into the stomach)

■ PLURAL ENDINGS

Most nouns in the English language become plural by adding an -s (or -es) at the end: student, students. Some medical terms also add an -s (or -es) to make a plural, but many do not. They have special endings related to their origins in Greek or Latin.

> **Example:** If the singular ends in *a* (vertebra—one bone in the spine), then the plural ends in *ae* (vertebrae—the bones in the spine).

The following table shows some of the special plural endings common in medical terms. Note that these special plurals do not occur with *all* terms ending in those letters. For example, the plural of sinus is sinuses. In most cases, you have to learn the plural form when you learn the term.

Common Plural Endings for Medical Terms

Singular Ending	Plural Ending	Examples
a	ae	vertebra (a spinal bone), vertebrae
en	ina	lumen (interior space of a vessel), lumina
ex, ix, yx	ices	index (alphabetic list or directory), indices
is	es	ankylosis (stiff joint), ankyloses; testis (male reproductive gland), testes
on	a	phenomenon (occurrence or object perceived), phenomena; spermatozoon (male sex cell), spermatozoa
um	a	diverticulum (pouch or sac within an organ), diverticula; atrium (upper heart chamber), atria
us	i	nucleus (structure within a cell), nuclei; glomerulus (capillary cluster at the entrance of each nephron), glomeruli
x, nx	ges, nges	phalanx (finger bone), phalanges

In addition to these, a few other rare plural forms occur in medical terms. You will learn these when you encounter terms using those special forms.

■ Exercise: Plural Endings

Exercise 8

SIMPLE RECALL

Write the correct plural form of the singular term given.

1. embolus (clot) _____

2. varicosis (swollen vein) _____

3. aorta (vessel of heart) _____

4. larynx (voice box) _____

5. ulcer _____

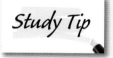

Spelling: Spelling medical terms correctly in health care is vital. Misspelling a term in a patient's record, for example, could cause confusion or even a dangerous situation if another health care worker misunderstands what you have written. Many terms look nearly alike and may even be pronounced the same. For example, *ileum* and *ilium* look similar and sound alike but designate two very different parts of the body. Therefore, take the time to learn correct spellings. Complete the spelling exercises in these chapters—being sure to write out the terms in all exercises.

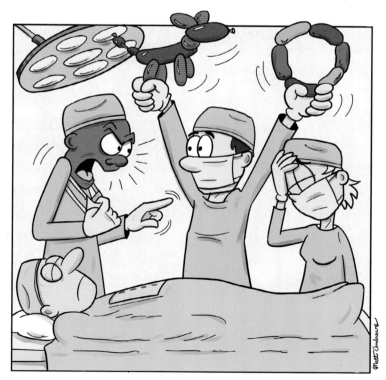

"JENKINS, YOU FOOL! I SAID
'BALLOON STENT', NOT 'BALLOON STUNT!'"

Figure 1-3

■ PRONUNCIATION KEY

Pronunciations are provided for medical terms throughout this text. It is best to learn the pronunciation at the same time you learn the term: Saying it will help you remember its meaning and spelling.

The pronunciation is indicated with letters of the alphabet and stress marks (') that indicate which syllable (or syllables) should be accented. Following is a typical example:

nucleus   nū′klē-ŭs

If you are unfamiliar with stress marks, think of them as the guide to which syllable to say more forcefully when you pronounce the word. Like this: NU-cle-us. *Not like this:* nu-cle-US.

Following is the key to the different sounds of vowels as used in pronunciations:

Symbol	Sound as in:	Symbol	Sound as in:
ā	day	ĭ	pencil
a	mat, far	ō	go, form
ă	about	o	got
ah	father	ŏ	oven, motor
aw	raw, fall	ow	cow
ē	beet, here	oy	boy, oil
e	bed	ū	prune
ě	system	yū	cube
ī	island	u	put
i	hip	ŭ	up, tough

Following is a key to the sounds of consonants used in pronunciations:

Symbol	Sound as in:	Symbol	Sound as in:
b	bad, tab	n	no, run
ch	child, itch	ng	ring
d	dog, good	p	pain, top
dh	this	r	rot, tar
f	fit, defect, phase	s	so, mess, center
g	got, bag	sh	show, wish
h	hit, behold	t	ten, put
j	jade, gender, rigid, edge	th	thin, with
k	cut, tic	v	vote, nerve
ks	extra, tax	w	we, tow
kw	quick, aqua	y	yes
l	law, kill	z	zero, disease, xiphoid
m	me, bum	zh	vision, measure

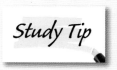

Read, Write, Speak, Listen: Scientists have discovered that using your senses (sight, hearing, touch) reinforces learning and assists in memory. Do not just passively read the terms on the page as you use this text. Practice saying them aloud, listen to their correct pronunciations using the Audio Glossary in the electronic Student Resources, and write them (or their meanings) in the spaces provided in the exercises.

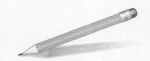
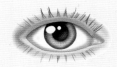
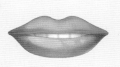
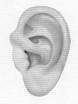

Use your senses as learning tools.

The following exercise provides some practice in using the pronunciation key to learn how to pronounce unfamiliar words.

■ Exercise: Pronunciation

AUDITORY

Exercise 9

Listen to the pronunciations of the following terms using the Dictionary/Audio Glossary included with the electronic Student Resources and practice pronouncing each, referring to the pronunciation guide as needed.

1. varicosis	var'i-kō'sis
2. diverticulum	dī'vĕr-tik'yū-lŭm
3. ankylosis	ang'ki-lō'sis
4. pulmonary	pul'mŏ-nār-ē
5. arthralgia	ahr-thral'jē-ă
6. osteoma	os-tē-ō'mă
7. nephritis	nĕ-frī'tis
8. craniopathy	krā'nē-op'ă-thē
9. gastrectomy	gas-trek'tŏ-mē
10. cardiopulmonary	kahr'dē-ō-pul'mŏ-nār-ē

■ UNDERSTANDING TERMS THROUGH ANALYSIS

As you already have seen, the meaning of a medical term comes from the meaning of the different word parts that together make that term. There is little value in trying to memorize each and every medical term separately. It is much easier to learn the meanings of the parts and then apply those meanings to understand many terms that use the same parts.

Analyzing word parts to understand the larger meaning is also useful when you encounter a medical term for the first time and do not have a dictionary or your textbook available. Quite often you can figure out the meaning of a new term if you know the meaning of its separate word parts.

For example, you already know that the suffix -*itis* refers to inflammation. Earlier you saw the word *diverticulum*, which is a pouch or sac within an organ—such as diverticula that may occur within the large intestine. Its combining form is *diverticul/o*. From this information, can you make an educated guess what *diverticulitis* means?

Diverticulitis is, in fact, the inflammation of a diverticulum.

To define a term based on its word parts:

1. Begin by analyzing the meaning of the suffix.
2. Then analyze the meaning of the prefix (if a prefix is present).
3. Then analyze the meaning of the root or roots.

For example:

$$intra\text{-}\ (within) + cerebr/o\ (brain) + \text{-}al\ (pertaining\ to)$$

$$2 \qquad\qquad\qquad 3 \qquad\qquad\qquad 1$$

pertaining to within the brain

The following exercise will give you more practice understanding terms by analyzing their word parts. As you learn more and more word parts through the chapters of this text, you will find that this becomes a natural process.

■ Exercise: Term Analysis

Exercise 10

TERM CONSTRUCTION

Break the given medical term into its word parts and define each. Then define the medical term.

For example:
nephrectomy	*word parts:*	nephr/o / -ectomy
	meanings:	kidney / excision, surgical removal
	term meaning:	surgical removal of kidney

1. arthritis   *word parts:*   _____ / _____

      meanings: _____ / _____

      term meaning: _____

2. pulmonary   *word parts:*   _____ / _____

      meanings: _____ / _____

      term meaning: _____

3. colonitis   *word parts:*   _____ / _____

      meanings: _____ / _____

      term meaning: _____

4. osteal   *word parts:*   _____ / _____

                    meanings: _____ / _____

                    term meaning: _____

5. cardiotomy   *word parts:*   _____ / _____

                    meanings: _____ / _____

                    term meaning: _____

■ BUILDING TERMS

Just as you can learn terms by breaking them apart and analyzing the meaning of their parts, it helps to learn how to put word parts together too—to build terms. In the real world, these medical terms almost always already exist, but building them on your own will help you learn more efficiently.

For example, you learned earlier that *cardi/o* is the combining form that means heart. Let's say you wanted to build a medical term that means inflammation of the heart. From what you have learned already, you should be able to build this term and write it here:

_____

The answer, of course, is *carditis*. (Did you remember not to repeat the "i"?) If you look in your medical dictionary, you will find that it is a real medical term. And you shouldn't be surprised to learn that it means inflammation of the heart.

The following exercise will give you more practice building terms.

■ Exercise: Term Building

TERM CONSTRUCTION

Exercise 11

Using word parts found anywhere in this chapter, try to construct medical terms for the meanings given. Then check your medical dictionary to see whether you are correct and have spelled the term correctly.

1. inflammation of the skin   _____

2. pertaining to the area around the heart   _____

3. surgical removal of a disk   _____

4. tumor of bone   _____

5. pertaining to the kidney   _____

Summary

■ Medical terms include the following basic parts:
   Word root: main part of the word (crani)
   Prefix: word part added *before* the root (intra-)
   Suffix: word part added *after* the root (-al)

   intra- + crani + -al = intracranial

■ A combining form is a word root with a combining vowel that makes it easier to pronounce the word when a suffix is added to the word root.

   cardi/o (combining form) + -logy (suffix) = cardiology

■ To understand a medical term, first analyze its parts. You can usually figure out what the term means from the meanings of its parts.

■ To build medical terms, use your knowledge of the definitions of word roots, prefixes, and suffixes to combine these parts into a word.

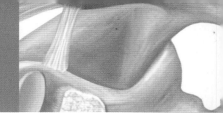

Chapter Review

Review of Terms

In the following exercises you will encounter a few medical terms you have not seen before in this chapter. Nonetheless, you should be able to answer these questions based on the *word parts* used in these terms. Review the earlier tables of word part meanings if needed.

SIMPLE RECALL

Exercise 12

Complete each sentence by writing in the correct term.

1. The cerebral cortex is a part of the brain. A subcortical tumor would therefore be located _____ the cortex.

2. A tumor that grows from bone tissue is called a(n) _____.

3. Given that the suffix *-scopy* means visual examination using an instrument, the term for such an examination of the colon is _____.

4. A dermatologist is a specialist physician who treats _____ disorders.

5. A gastric ulcer seems most likely to cause bleeding inside the _____.

6. An intervertebral disk is located _____ two vertebrae (bones of spine).

7. The term *cardiac* means pertaining to the _____.

8. A physician specializing in cardiopulmonary diseases might often require x-rays of a patient's heart and _____.

9. The prefix *an-* means _____.

10. A tumor in lymph tissue (combining form: *lymph/o*) is called a(n) _____.

COMPREHENSION

Exercise 13

Circle the letter of the best answer in the following questions.

1. Which term refers to surgical removal of the stomach?

   A. gastrotomy
   B. gastrostomy
   C. gastrology
   D. gastrectomy

2. Given that the combining form *my/o* means muscle, which of the following refers to muscle pain?

   A. myogram
   B. myalgia
   C. myocardium
   D. myoma

3. The term *renal* means:

   A. pertaining to the kidney
   B. pertaining to the skull
   C. pertaining to the lung
   D. pertaining to the skin

4. A patient who is having difficulty breathing may have what kind of problem?

   A. cerebral
   B. gastric
   C. cardiac
   D. pulmonary

5. Referring to surgery, an intraoperative procedure is carried out:

   A. before the surgery begins
   B. during the surgery
   C. after the surgery
   D. at any time

6. Which of the following best defines the term *abacterial*?

   A. full of bacteria
   B. not pertaining to bacteria
   C. eaten by bacteria
   D. resulting from bacterial presence

7. The medical term *dysuria* is most likely to mean:

   A. painful urination
   B. frequent urination
   C. infrequent urination
   D. normal urination

8. The medical term *polyuria* is most likely to mean:

   A. painful urination
   B. frequent urination
   C. infrequent urination
   D. normal urination

9. A patient with a cerebral hemorrhage is experiencing bleeding inside the:

   A. kidney
   B. lungs
   C. skull
   D. heart

10. Even if you have never seen the term *angiogram* (an x-ray record of blood vessels), you can assume the combining form used to make this term is:

    A. ang/i
    B. angi/o
    C. angiogr/a
    D. angiogra/o

Spelling

SPELLING

Exercise 14

Circle the correct spelling of each term.

1.	cardioitis	cardiitis	carditis
2.	phenomena	phenomenons	phenomeni
3.	pericardial	perocardial	pericardiol
4.	gastroctomy	gastrectomy	gastroectomy
5.	nucleuses	nuclae	nuclei
6.	ostearthritis	osteoarthritis	ostarthritis
7.	cardigraphy	cardography	cardiography
8.	vertebrae	vertebraes	vertebriae

9. dermatitis   dermatoitis   dermatotis

10. cardipulmonary   cardiopulmonary   cardopulmonary

Additional spelling exercises for this and all chapters in the text are included as Spelling Bee activities in the electronic Student Resources.

STUDENT
RESOURCES

Media Connection

STUDENT
RESOURCES

Exercise 15

Complete each of the following activities available with the Student Resources. Check off each activity as you complete it, and record your score for the Chapter Quiz in the space provided.

Chapter Exercises

____ Flash Cards

____ Concentration

____ Roboterms

____ Word Builder

____ True/False Body Building

____ Quiz Show

____ Complete the Case

____ Spelling Bee

____ **Chapter Quiz**   *Score:* _____%

Additional Resources

____ Dictionary/Audio Glossary

Prefixes, Suffixes, and Abbreviations

2

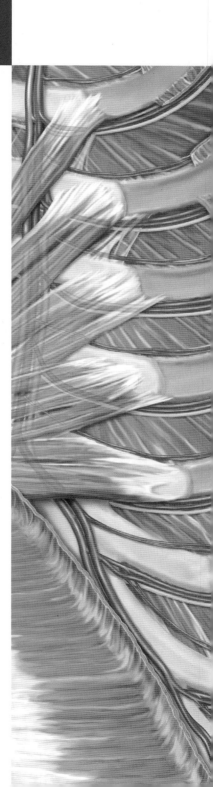

Chapter Outline

Objectives

After completion of this chapter you will be able to:

1. Define common prefixes used in medical terms.

2. Define common suffixes used in medical terms.

3. Understand medical terms by analyzing their prefixes and suffixes.

4. Spell and pronounce medical terms built with common prefixes and suffixes correctly.

5. Understand common abbreviations used in health care.

6. Successfully complete all chapter exercises.

7. Successfully complete all interactive exercises included with the companion Student Resources.

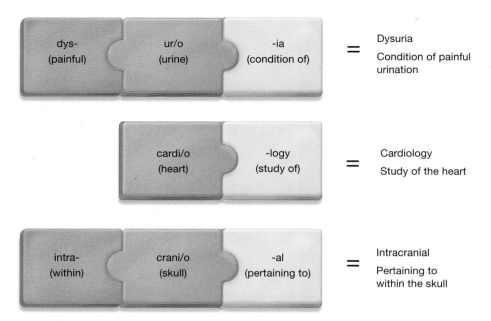

Figure 2-1   Word parts fit together like jigsaw puzzle pieces to form medical terms.

As you learned in Chapter 1, prefixes and suffixes are basic word parts used in most medical terms. This chapter includes the most common prefixes and suffixes. Learning these now will pave the way for learning medical terms related to all body systems in later chapters.

■ COMMON PREFIXES

Prefixes modify the meaning of the combining form to which they are joined. They can be learned in groups based on similar (or opposite) meanings, as seen in the following tables.

Prefixes Involving Number

Prefix	Meaning	Example
uni-	one	unilateral (related to only one side, as of the body)
mono-		mononeural (supplied by one nerve)
bi-	two, twice	bilateral (related to both sides)
di-		diarthric (related to two joints)
tri-	three	trimester (3 months; one-third of pregnancy)
quad-, quadri-	four	quadruplets (four infants born together)
hemi-	half	hemiplegia (paralysis of one side of the body)
semi-		semirecumbent (position of half sitting up in bed)
multi-	many	multidisciplinary (involving people from several fields of study)
poly-	many, much	polyarteritis (inflammation of several arteries)

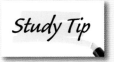

Prefixes with the Same Meaning: Several prefixes have the same basic meaning and yet are not interchangeable with the same word root. For instance, bi- and di- both mean two, twice, but it would be incorrect to use the prefix di- with the word lateral to indicate both sides. The correct term would be bilateral. Unfortunately there are no rules on the usage of prefixes with the same meaning; however, you will learn which prefix goes with each word root as you encounter the actual medical terms in later chapters.

■ Exercises: Common Prefixes

SIMPLE
RECALL

Exercise 1

Write the correct prefix(es) for the meaning given.

1. one   _____ or _____

2. two   _____ or _____

3. three   _____

4. four   _____ or _____

5. many   _____ or _____

Exercise 2

SIMPLE
RECALL

Write the meaning of the prefix given.

1. semi-   _____

2. hemi-   _____

3. poly-   _____

4. uni-   _____

5. quadr-   _____

Prefixes Involving Negation

Prefix	Meaning	Example
a-, an-	without, not	abacterial (not caused by bacteria), anaerobic (without oxygen)
in-, im-	not	incompetent (not capable), impure (not pure)
non-		noninvasive (a procedure that does not involve entering the body)
dis-	separate, remove	disinfect (remove germs by destroying them)
anti-	opposing, against	antisepsis (prevention of infection by opposing growth of pathogens)
contra-		contraception (prevention of conception or impregnation)
de-	away from, cessation, without	deodorant (elimination of an odor)

SIMPLE
RECALL

Exercise 3

Write the meaning of the prefix given.

1. contra- _____

2. im- _____

3. de- _____

4. an- _____

5. dis- _____

Prefixes Involving Position, Time, or Direction

Prefix	Meaning	Example
ex-	out of, away from	exhale (to breathe out)
ecto-, exo-	outer, outside	ectoderm (outer layer of cells in embryo), exocrine (gland that secretes in an outward direction)
en-, end-, endo-	in, within	endemic (present within a region or group), endocrine (gland that secretes internally)
sym-, syn-	together, with	symphysis (type of joint where bones come together), synapse (where one nerve cell meets another)
inter-	between	intercostal (between the ribs)
intra-	within	intraoperative (occurring during surgery)
sub-	below, beneath	subcutaneous (beneath the skin)
infra-		infrasplenic (below the spleen)
supra-, super-	above	suprarenal (above the kidney)
pre-	before (in time or space)	precancerous (lesion that has not yet become cancerous)
post-	after, behind	postmortem (occurring after death)
peri-	around, surrounding	pericarditis (inflammation of the membrane around the heart)
ab-	away from	abnormal (deviating from the normal)
ad-	to, toward	adduct (move toward the midline)
per-	through	percutaneous (passage of substance through unbroken skin)
trans-	across, through	transection (cutting across)

SIMPLE
RECALL

Exercise 4

Write the correct prefix(es) for the meaning given.

1. between _____

2. after, behind _____

3. through _____ or _____

4. above _____ or _____

5. within _____ or _____

Exercise 5

SIMPLE RECALL

Write the meaning of the prefix given.

1. ecto- _____

2. ab- _____

3. pre- _____

4. sub- _____

5. syn- _____

Prefixes Involving Relative Characteristics

Many prefixes express a characteristic that is relative to something else. Relative means there is at least an implied comparison. We have already seen some relative prefixes in the preceding categories—such as prefixes involving time (this happened *before* that) or space (this is located *beneath* that).

Often these prefixes describe a quality or characteristic of something compared with the normal situation.

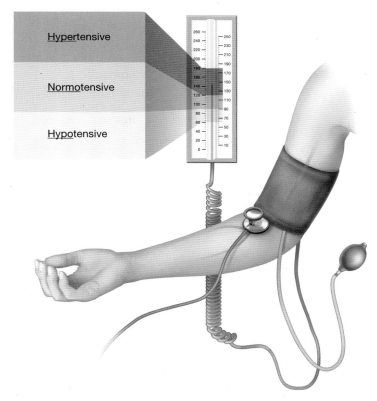

Figure 2-2   Different prefixes used with the same word root and suffix can change the word meaning, and the patient's care, dramatically.

Prefix	Meaning	Example
normo-	normal	normotensive (having normal blood pressure; compare with hypertensive)
hyper-	above, excessive	hypertension (high blood pressure)
hypo-	below, deficient	hypoglycemia (abnormally low blood sugar)
mega-, megalo-	large, oversize	megadose (larger-than-normal dose), megalosplenia (enlarged spleen)
ultra-	excess, beyond	ultrasonography (diagnostic instrument using very high sound frequencies)
macro-	large, long	macrosomia (abnormally large body)
micro-	small	microcardia (abnormally small heart)
pan-	all, entire	panlobar (pertaining to all of the lung lobe)
eu-	good, normal	eupeptic (having good digestion)
dys-	painful, difficult, abnormal	dyspeptic (having impaired gastric function)
iso-	equal, alike	isomorphous (having the same form or shape)
homo-, homeo-	same, alike	homogeneous (of uniform structure throughout)
hetero-	other, different	heterogeneous (made up of elements with differing properties)

Exercise 6

SIMPLE RECALL

Write the correct prefix(es) for the meaning given.

1. other, different _____

2. normal _____

3. large _____ or _____ or _____

4. good, normal _____

5. alike _____ or _____

6. small _____ or _____

Exercise 7

ADVANCED RECALL

Match each prefix with its meaning.

hypo-   iso-   eu-
dys-   hyper-   pan-

Meaning   **Prefix**

1. painful, difficult, abnormal _____

2. good, normal _____

3. above, excessive _____

4. all, entire _____

5. equal, alike _____

6. below, deficient _____

Other Prefixes

Prefix	Meaning	Example
pseudo-	false	pseudomalignancy (benign tumor that appears to be malignant)
neo-	new	neonate (a newborn infant)
re-	again, backward	reactivate (to activate again)
brady-	slow	bradycardia (a slow heartbeat)
tachy-	rapid, fast	tachycardia (a rapid heartbeat)

SIMPLE
RECALL

Exercise 8

Write the meaning of the prefix given.

1. tachy- _____

2. neo- _____

3. brady- _____

4. re- _____

5. pseudo- _____

■ COMMON SUFFIXES

Like prefixes, suffixes modify the meaning of the combining form to which they are joined. They can be learned in groups based on similar (or opposite) meanings, as seen in the following tables. Almost all medical terms have a suffix. Suffixes and a combining form usually form a noun or adjective.

Suffixes Related to Condition or Disease

Suffix	Meaning	Example
-ism	condition of	albinism (genetic disorder causing lack of pigmentation in skin)
-ia		pneumonia (condition involving inflammation in the lung)
-y		atony (condition involving lack of muscle tone)
-algia	pain	myalgia (pain in one or more muscles)

(continued)

Suffixes Related to Condition or Disease *(continued)*

Suffix	Meaning	Example
-emia	blood (condition of)	hypoxemia (condition of abnormally low oxygen in arterial blood)
-itis	inflammation	gastritis (inflammation of the stomach)
-megaly	enlargement	cardiomegaly (enlargement of the heart)
-oma	tumor	osteoma (tumor in bone)
-osis	abnormal condition	diverticulosis (abnormal condition of having diverticula in the intestine)
-pathy	disease	craniopathy (disease involving the cranial bones)
-rrhea	flow, discharge	diarrhea (frequent discharge of poorly formed or fluid fecal matter)

■ Exercises: Common Suffixes

SIMPLE
RECALL

Exercise 9

Write the meaning of the suffix given.

1. -megaly _____

2. -osis _____

3. -ism _____

4. -ia _____

5. -y _____

ADVANCED
RECALL

Exercise 10

Match each suffix with its meaning.

-itis   -emia   -pathy
-algia   -oma   -rrhea

Meaning   **Suffix**

1. pain _____

2. inflammation _____

3. flow, discharge _____

4. blood (condition of) _____

5. tumor _____

6. disease _____

Suffixes Related to Surgery

Suffix	Meaning	Example
-centesis	puncture to aspirate	amniocentesis (needle puncture of amniotic sac in a pregnant woman to remove fluid for diagnosis)
-ectomy	excision, surgical removal	appendectomy (surgical removal of the appendix)
-plasty	surgical repair, reconstruction	abdominoplasty (surgical repair of the abdominal wall)
-rrhaphy	suture	cystorrhaphy (suture of a wound in the urinary bladder)
-stomy	surgical opening	colostomy (surgical creation of an outside opening into the colon)
-tomy	incision	gastrotomy (incision into the stomach)

SIMPLE
RECALL

Exercise 11

Write the meaning of the suffix given.

1. -centesis _____

2. -ectomy _____

3. -stomy _____

4. -plasty _____

SIMPLE
RECALL

Exercise 12

Write the correct suffix for the meaning given.

1. incision _____

2. suture _____

3. opening _____

4. surgical removal _____

Other Suffixes

Suffix	Meaning	Example
-ic, -ac	pertaining to	cardiac (pertaining to the heart)
-al		cranial (pertaining to the skull)
-ar		articular (pertaining to a joint)
-ary		pulmonary (pertaining to the lungs)
-ous		edematous (marked by edema, which is a type of swelling)
-genic, -genesis	originating, producing	osteogenesis (the formation of bone)

(continued)

Other Suffixes (continued)

Suffix	Meaning	Example
-gram	record, recording	cystogram (x-ray of the bladder)
-graphy	process of recording	radiography (x-ray studies)
-ium	tissue, structure	myocardium (heart muscle tissue)
-logist, -ist	one who specializes in	dermatologist (physician who treats skin conditions)
-logy	study of	dermatology (study of skin conditions)
-meter	instrument for measuring	thermometer (instrument to measure heat)
-oid	resembling	lymphoid (resembling lymph)
-ole	small	arteriole (a very small artery)
-scope	instrument for examination	microscope (instrument for examining very small things)
-scopy	process of examining, examination	endoscopy (examination of the interior of a structure by means of a special instrument)

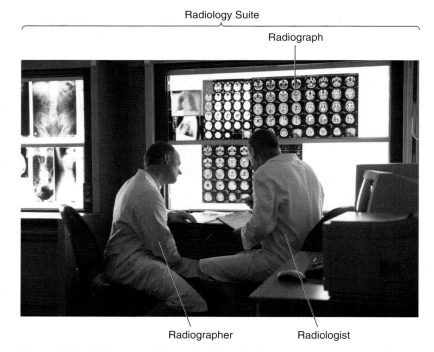

Figure 2-3 Different suffixes combined with the same root word help distinguish terms within the same specialty.

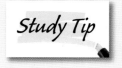

Study Tip

-scope and -scopy: Some suffixes are very closely related and easily confused. For instance, -scope means instrument for examination whereas -scopy means process of examination. A gastroscope is an instrument used for examination of the stomach. A gastroscopy refers to the actual examination using the gastroscope. There are many medical terms with these suffixes so a good understanding of them now will lead to less confusion and easier memorization as you learn them in later chapters.

SIMPLE
RECALL

Exercise 13

Write the meaning of the suffix given.

1. -meter _____

2. -graphy _____

3. -al _____

4. -ous _____

5. -gram _____

6. -ary _____

7. -logy _____

8. -ic _____

ADVANCED
RECALL

Exercise 14

Match each suffix with its meaning.

-genic   -scope   -oid
-ole   -logist   -ium

Meaning	**Suffix**
1. specialist	_____
2. resembling	_____
3. tissue	_____
4. small	_____
5. originating	_____
6. examination instrument	_____

■ COMMON ABBREVIATIONS

Abbreviations are commonly used in health care, particularly in handwritten notes where they save time by allowing busy practitioners to skip writing out a full term or expression. You will learn commonly used abbreviations throughout this text. Following are a few examples of common abbreviations. Appendix D contains a fuller listing of medical abbreviations.

Although using abbreviations is convenient, keep in mind that some abbreviations are prone to misinterpretation, which can lead to dangerous medical errors. To avoid this problem, the Joint Commission has developed an Official "Do Not Use" List of abbreviations that health care workers must never use. These are given in Appendix D. Of course, your health care facility may have its own list of abbreviations that should be avoided or that are acceptable to use; review this information carefully and follow the guidelines in your daily practice.

Abbreviation	Meaning
Diagnosis and Treatment	
pt	patient
H&P	history and physical (examination)
Hx	history
Sx	symptom
Dx	diagnosis
Px	prognosis
Tx, Tr	treatment
Rx	prescription
Practice Areas and Specialists	
MD	doctor of medicine
DC	doctor of chiropractic medicine
DDS	doctor of dental surgery
OD	doctor of optometry
OB/GYN	obstetrics/gynecology
ENT	ears, nose, throat
Peds	pediatrics
PA	physician's assistant
ICU	intensive care unit
ER, ED	emergency room, emergency department
PT	physical therapy
CAM	complementary and alternative medicine
Units of Measurement	
m, cm, mm	meter, centimeter, millimeter
L, mL	liter, milliliter
g or gm, mg, kg	gram, milligram, kilogram
cc	cubic centimeter
oz	ounce
C	Celsius, centigrade (temperature)
F	Fahrenheit (temperature)

(continued)

Abbreviation	Meaning
Prescriptions	
b.i.d.	twice a day
q.i.d.	four times a day
noc	night
p.c.	after meals
p.r.n.	as needed
Other Abbreviations	
NPO	nothing by mouth (don't eat or drink)
RBC	red blood cell
WBC	white blood cell
ADL	activities of daily living
STAT	immediately
AP	anteroposterior (from front to back)
lab	laboratory
CT	computed tomography (type of x-ray)
MRI	magnetic resonance imaging
Ht	height
Wt	weight
preop, pre-op	preoperative (before surgery)
postop, post-op	postoperative (after surgery)
VS	vital signs
BP	blood pressure
T	temperature
P	pulse rate
R	respiratory rate

■ Exercises: Common Abbreviations

Exercise 15

SIMPLE
RECALL

Write the meaning of each abbreviation.

1. ICU _____

2. RBC _____

3. P _____

4. H&P _____

5. ADL _____

6. ED _____

7. L _____

8. Tx _____

9. ENT _____

10. lab _____

Exercise 16

ADVANCED
RECALL

Match each abbreviation with its meaning.

Rx	R	STAT	VS
PT	Sx	Hx	BP
p.r.n.	noc	Ht	Dx

Meaning	**Abbreviation**
1. symptom	_____
2. vital signs	_____
3. diagnosis	_____
4. height	_____
5. immediately	_____
6. as needed	_____
7. respiratory rate	_____
8. blood pressure	_____
9. prescription	_____
10. night	_____
11. physical therapy	_____
12. history	_____

In the following exercises you will encounter a few medical terms you have not seen in this chapter. Nonetheless, you should be able to answer these questions based on the *word parts* used in these terms. Review the earlier tables of word part meanings if needed.

Review of Prefixes and Suffixes

ADVANCED RECALL

Exercise 17

Match each prefix with its meaning.

hypo-	hetero-	dys-	im-	intra-
hemi-	ad-	exo-	per-	poly-

Meaning	Prefix
1. not	_____
2. toward	_____
3. many	_____
4. through	_____
5. within	_____
6. outside	_____
7. half	_____
8. different	_____
9. below	_____
10. painful	_____

ADVANCED RECALL

Exercise 18

Match each suffix with its meaning.

-plasty	-pathy	-ium	-emia	-gram
-graphy	-ar	-osis	-tomy	-rrhaphy

Meaning	Suffix
1. condition of	_____
2. suture	_____

3. record, recording _____

4. incision _____

5. blood (condition of) _____

6. disease _____

7. pertaining to _____

8. surgical repair _____

9. recording process _____

10. tissue _____

Meaning Recognition

TERM
CONSTRUCTION

Exercise 19

Match each word with its meaning. Because you have not yet learned some of the combining forms used in some of these terms, you may have to guess the meaning based on the meaning of the prefix or suffix in the term.

| bisect | polyarthritis | semiconscious | submandibular | panarthritis |
| cardiotomy | endoscope | cavitary | psychology | thrombosis |

Meaning   **Term**

1. cut in two parts _____

2. beneath the mandible (lower jaw) _____

3. pertaining to a cavity _____

4. incision of heart wall _____

5. study of mental processes _____

6. instrument for examining inside an organ _____

7. inflammation of several joints _____

8. condition of having a blood clot _____

9. inflammation of all the joints in body _____

10. drowsy, partially conscious _____

Term Building

TERM
CONSTRUCTION

Exercise 20

Using the given combining form and a prefix or suffix (and sometimes both) from this chapter, try to build a medical term for the meaning given. Check your answer in a medical dictionary.

Use combining form	Meaning of medical term	Medical term
myos/o + suffix	inflammation of muscle	1. _____
lob/o + suffix	surgical removal of lobe	2. _____
cardi/o + suffix	disease of the heart	3. _____
prefix + cost/o (rib) + suffix	pertaining to between the ribs	4. _____
prefix + nas/o (nose) + suffix	pertaining to behind the nose	5. _____
prefix + bi/o + suffix	one specialized in study of very small life forms	6. _____
lymph/o + suffix	tumor of lymph tissue	7. _____
dermat/o + suffix	resembling skin	8. _____
crani/o + suffix	surgical repair of skull	9. _____
ten/o (tendon) + suffix	suture of a tendon	10. _____

Spelling and Pronunciation

SPELLING

Exercise 21

Circle the correct spelling of each term.

1. mononeural   monaneura   mononueral

2. hemoplegia   hemaplegia   hemiplegia

3. ectiderm   ectoderm   ectaderm

4. infrisonic   infrosonic   infrasonic

5. pericarditis   perocarditis   perecarditis

6. megalaspenia   megalesplenia   megalosplenia

7. hetrogeneous   heterogeneous   hetarogeneous

8. bradycardia	bradcardia	braydcardia
9. diarhea	diarrhea	diareah
10. hetrogenic	hetarogenic	heterogenic
11. mylagia	myolgia	myalgia
12. cystorhraphy	cystorrhaphy	cystorhaphry
13. osteogenesis	osteogenisis	osteoginesis
14. edematuos	edematous	edematus
15. gastrotomy	gastrotomomy	gastrotommy

Additional spelling exercises for this and all chapters in the text are included as Spelling Bee activities in the electronic Student Resources.

STUDENT
RESOURCES

Exercise 22

AUDITORY

Listen to the pronunciations of the following terms in the Dictionary/Audio Glossary on the Student Resources and practice pronouncing each, referring to the pronunciation guide as needed.

1. quadruplets	kwahd-rūp′letz	**11.** edematous	e-dēm′ă-tŭs
2. abacterial	ā′bak-tēr′ē-ăl	**12.** antisepsis	an′ti-sep′sis
3. suprarenal	sū′pră-rē′năl	**13.** bradycardia	brad′ē-kahr′dē-ă
4. hypoglycemia	hī′pō-glī-sē′mē-ă	**14.** myocardium	mī′ō-kahr′dē-ŭm
5. diarthric	dī-ahr′thrik	**15.** amniocentesis	am′nē-ō-sen-tē′sis
6. dyspeptic	dis-pep′tik	**16.** tachycardia	tak′i-kahr′dē-ă
7. neonate	nē′ō-nāt	**17.** polyarteritis	pol′ē-ahr-tĕr-ī′tis
8. osteoma	os-tē-ō′mă	**18.** symphysis	sim′fi-sis
9. cardiomegaly	kahr′dē-ō-meg′ă-lē	**19.** gastrotomy	gas-trot′ŏ-mē
10. articular	ahr-tik′yū-lăr	**20.** subcutaneous	sŭb′kyū-tā′nē-ŭs

Study the correct punctuation of terms in this and all chapters with the Dictionary/Audio Glossary in the electronic Student Resources.

STUDENT
RESOURCES

Media Connection

STUDENT
RESOURCES

Exercise 23

Complete each of the following activities available with the Student Resources. Check off each activity as you complete it, and record your score for the Chapter Quiz in the space provided.

Chapter Exercises

____ Flash Cards   ____ Break It Down

____ Concentration   ____ True/False Body Building

____ Abbreviation Match-Up   ____ Quiz Show

____ Roboterms   ____ Complete the Case

____ Word Builder   ____ Spelling Bee

____ Fill the Gap

____ **Chapter Quiz**   *Score:* _____%

Additional Resources

____ Dictionary/Audio Glossary

Terms Involving the Body as a Whole

3

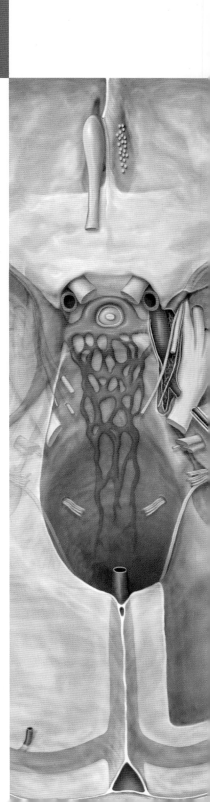

Chapter Outline

Objectives

After completion of this chapter you will be able to:

1. Describe key body structures, regions, and cavities.

2. Define terms related to body structures and regions, directions and positions, and colors.

3. Spell and pronounce medical terms built with common combining forms, prefixes, and suffixes related to the body as a whole correctly.

4. Describe the common types of medical records used in the health care setting.

5. Explain what a body system is and why it is useful to learn medical terminology by body system.

6. Successfully complete all chapter exercises.

7. Successfully complete all pronunciation and spelling exercises, and complete all interactive exercises included with the companion Student Resources.

This chapter continues to build on word parts learned in Chapters 1 and 2. The focus now expands to include common terms used in relationship to the body as a whole, rather than a specific body system as will be covered in later chapters.

■ BODY STRUCTURES IN HEALTH AND DISEASE

Word Parts Related to Body Structures in Health and Disease

Combining Form	Meaning
aden/o	gland
blast/o	immature cell
cyt/o	cell
epitheli/o	epithelium (type of tissue)
fibr/o	fiber
gluc/o, glyc/o	glucose, sugar
hem/o, hemat/o	blood
hist/o	tissue
hydr/o	water, fluid
lei/o	smooth
lip/o	fat
morph/o	form, shape
my/o, myos/o	muscle
necr/o	death
neur/o	nerve
nucle/o	nucleus
oste/o	bone
path/o	disease
sarc/o	flesh
troph/o	nourishment
viscer/o	internal organs

Suffix	Meaning
-cyte	cell
-oma	tumor
-osis	abnormal condition
-pathy	disease
-plasia	formation, growth
-sis	condition, process
-stasis	stopped, standing still

Exercises: Word Parts Related to Body Structures

Exercise 1

SIMPLE RECALL

Write the meaning of the word part given.

1. -sis _____
2. necr/o _____
3. my/o _____
4. -oma _____
5. hydr/o _____
6. path/o _____
7. neur/o _____
8. hem/o _____
9. lei/o _____
10. morph/o _____

Exercise 2

ADVANCED RECALL

Match each word part with its meaning.

oste/o   hist/o   -osis   lip/o   -cyte
blast/o   -pathy   viscer/o   gluc/o   aden/o

Definition   **Word Part**

1. glucose _____
2. immature cell _____
3. internal organs _____
4. tissue _____
5. disease _____
6. abnormal condition _____
7. bone _____
8. fat _____
9. cell _____
10. gland _____

Terms Related to Body Structures in Health and Disease (Fig. 3-1)

Term	Pronunciation	Meaning
body system	bod′ē sis′tĕm	group of organs with related structure or function
cell	sel	smallest independent unit of living structure
chromosome	krō′mŏ-sōm	structure in cell nucleus bearing genes
cytoplasm	sī′tō-plazm	substance of a cell excluding the nucleus
gene	jēn	functional unit of heredity occupying a specific place on a chromosome
nucleus	nū′klē-ŭs	central structure in cells containing chromosomes
cytology	sī-tol′ŏ-jē	study of cells
histology	his-tol′ŏ-jē	study of cells and tissues
homeostasis	hō′mē-ō-stā′sis	state of equilibrium
metabolism	mĕ-tab′ŏ-lizm	sum of the normal chemical and physical changes occurring in tissue
organ	ōr′găn	a differentiated structure of similar tissues or cells with a specific function
somatic	sō-mat′ik	pertaining to the body
systemic	sis-tem′ik	pertaining to the body as a whole
tissue	tish′ū	aggregation of similar cells performing a specific function
visceral	vis′ĕr-ăl	pertaining to the internal organs

Terms Related to Conditions and Disease		
acute	ă-kyūt′	referring to a disease of sudden onset and brief course
chronic	kron′ik	referring to a persistent disease or illness
etiology	ē′tē-ol′ŏ-jē	study of cause of disease

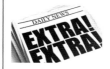 **ETIOLOGY** The term *etiology* is sometimes also used to refer to a specific cause of a disease, such as to say the etiology of an infection is a certain bacteria.

exacerbation	eg-zas′ĕr-bā′shŭn	an increase in the severity of a disease or symptoms
hyperplasia	hī′pĕr-plā′zē-ă	excessive growth of tissue
idiopathic	id′ē-ō-path′ik	related to a disease of unknown cause
inflammation	in′flă-mā′shŭn	cytologic and chemical changes in tissue in response to an injury or disease
lesion	lē′zhŭn	a pathologic change in tissue resulting from disease or injury
necrosis	nĕ-krō′sis	pathologic death of cells or tissue
pathogen	path′ŏ-jĕn	any virus, microorganism, or other substance that causes disease
remission	rē-mish′ŭn	lessening in severity of disease symptoms

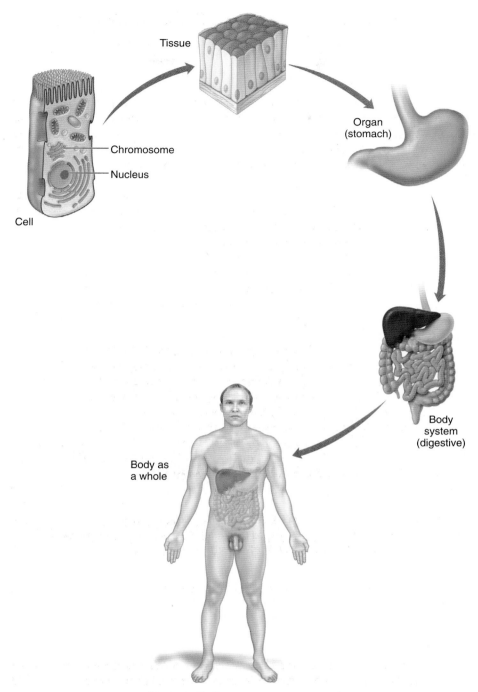

Figure 3-1   Levels of organization in the body.

■ Exercises: Terms Related to Body Structures in Health and Disease

Exercise 3

SIMPLE RECALL

Write the correct medical term for the meaning given.

1. study of cells and tissues _____

2. increase in severity of disease _____

3. pertaining to the body _____

4. injury to or pathologic change in tissue _____

5. referring to persistent disease _____

6. pertaining to disease of unknown cause _____

7. referring to disease of sudden onset _____

8. functional unit of heredity _____

9. pathologic death of cells _____

10. state of equilibrium _____

Exercise 4

SIMPLE RECALL

Write the meaning of the term given.

1. body system _____

2. inflammation _____

3. pathogen _____

4. remission _____

5. visceral _____

6. cytology _____

7. etiology _____

8. organ _____

9. metabolism _____

10. hyperplasia _____

ADVANCED RECALL

Exercise 5

Circle the correct term that is appropriate for the meaning of the sentence.

1. The patient's chronic disease was often well controlled, but he had periods of (*remission, exacerbation, homeostasis*) when his symptoms became much worse.

2. Chromosomes are located within the (*cytology, nucleus, pathogen*) of the cell.

3. Some drugs affect only a specific organ or body area, whereas others may have (*chronic, idiopathic, systemic*) effects causing changes throughout the body.

4. An aggregation of similar cells performing a specific function is termed (*a gene, tissue, a body system*).

5. Because physicians were unable to determine the cause of her symptoms, her disorder was considered (*idiopathic, visceral, systemic*).

6. The substance of a body cell excluding the nucleus is called the (*hyperplasia, chromosome, cytoplasm*).

7. Because the surgeon thought the lesion might be cancerous, he sent a sample of cells to the (*cytology, inflammation, somatic*) lab for analysis.

8. Her physician determined that the lesion on her skin was the result of infection by a (*gene, viscera, pathogen*).

■ BODY AREAS, CAVITIES, AND DIVISIONS OF THE ABDOMEN

Combining Forms Related to Body Areas, Cavities, and Divisions of the Abdomen

Combining Form	Meaning
abdomin/o	abdomen
acr/o	extremity, tip
brachi/o	arm
cervic/o	neck
lumb/o	lumbar region, lower back
ped/o, pod/o	foot
pelv/i	pelvis
thorac/o	thorax, chest

■ Exercises: Combining Forms Related to Body Areas, Cavities, and Divisions of the Abdomen

SIMPLE
RECALL

Exercise 6

Write the meaning of the combining form given.

1. thorac/o _____

2. cervic/o _____

3. lumb/o _____

4. abdomin/o _____

5. pelv/i _____

TERM
CONSTRUCTION

Exercise 7

Using the given combining form and using any of the following suffixes (from earlier in this chapter or Chapter 2), build a medical term for the meaning given.

-meter   -ar   -centesis
-algia   -plasty   -ectomy

Combining Form	Meaning of Medical Term	Medical Term
abdomin/o	removal of abdominal fluid through puncture	**1.** _____
thorac/o	surgical repair of chest wall	**2.** _____
pelv/i	instrument for measuring the pelvis	**3.** _____
lumb/o	pertaining to the lower back	**4.** _____
cervic/o	surgical removal of the cervix	**5.** _____
pod/o	pain in the foot	**6.** _____

Terms Related to Body Areas, Cavities, and Divisions of the Abdomen

Health care professionals use medical terminology to refer to specific areas of the body and to identify precise locations. The term tables below introduce the terms used for different areas of the body, cavities within the body, and clinical divisions of the abdomen.

Term	Pronunciation	Meaning
Body Areas		
abdomen	ab′dŏ-mĕn	the section of the trunk between the pelvis and chest
cranium	krā′nē-ŭm	skull
diaphragm	dī′ă-fram	muscle between the abdominal and thoracic cavities
extremity	eks-trem′i-tē	limb
pelvic region	pel′vik rē′jŭn	area of the pelvis below the abdomen
thorax	thō′raks	chest; upper part of the trunk
Cavities (Fig. 3-2)		
cranial cavity	krā′nē-ăl kav′i-tē	hollow area within the skull occupied by the brain
thoracic cavity	thōr-as′ik kav′i-tē	hollow area within the chest occupied by the lungs, heart, and other organs
abdominal cavity	ab-dom′ĭ-năl kav′i-tē	hollow area within the abdomen occupied by the digestive and other organs
spinal cavity	spī′năl kav′i-tē	hollow area within the spine occupied by the spinal cord
pelvic cavity	pel′vik kav′i-tē	hollow area within the pelvis occupied by certain reproductive, urinary, and digestive organs

(continued)

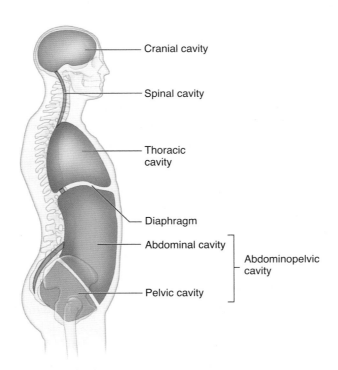

Figure 3-2 The different body cavities shown in the lateral view.

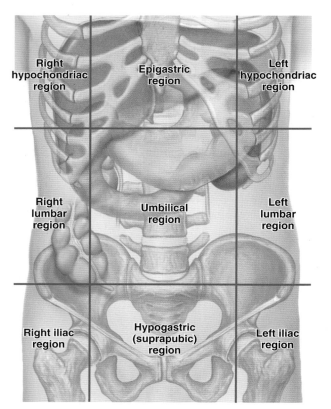

Figure 3-3   The abdominopelvic region is divided into nine regions by two horizontal and two vertical lines.

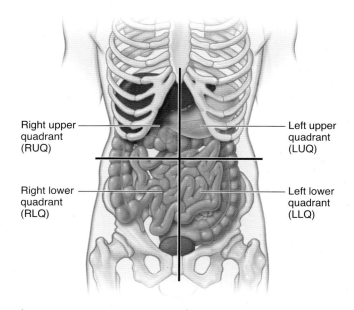

Figure 3-4   The abdominopelvic region can also be divided into four quadrants by one horizontal and one vertical line.

Term	Pronunciation	Meaning
Divisions of the Abdomen		
abdominopelvic regions	ab-dom′i-nō-pel′vik rē′jŭnz	nine specific anatomic areas of the abdominopelvic cavity (Fig. 3-3)
umbilical region	ŭm-bil′i-kăl rē′jŭn	central abdominal region
epigastric region	ep′i-gas′trik rē′jŭn	abdominal region above the umbilical region
hypogastric region	hī′pō-gas′trik rē′jŭn	abdominal region below the umbilical region; also called suprapubic region
lumbar region (left and right)	lŭm′bahr rē′jŭn	abdominal regions to left and right of umbilical region
iliac region (left and right)	il′ē-ak rē′jŭn	abdominal regions to left and right of hypogastric region
hypochondriac region (left and right)	hī′pō-kon′drē-ak rē′jŭn	abdominal region to left and right of epigastric region
abdominopelvic quadrants	ab-dom′i-nō-pel′vik kwahd′rănts	four divisions of the abdominopelvic cavity: left lower quadrant (LLQ), left upper quadrant (LUQ), right lower quadrant (RLQ), and right upper quadrant (RUQ) (Fig. 3-4)

■ Exercises: Terms Related to Body Areas, Cavities, and Divisions of the Abdomen

SIMPLE
RECALL

Exercise 8

Write the correct medical term for the meaning provided.

1. chest   _____

2. hollow area occupied by the spinal cord   _____

3. central abdominal region   _____

4. area between the pelvis and chest   _____

5. skull   _____

SIMPLE
RECALL

Exercise 9

Write the meaning of the term given.

1. extremity   _____

2. epigastric region _____

3. thoracic cavity   _____

4. diaphragm   _____

5. iliac region   _____

ADVANCED
RECALL

Exercise 10

Circle the correct term that is appropriate for the meaning of the sentence.

1. Most digestive organs are located within the (*pelvic, thoracic, abdominal*) cavity.

2. To the left and right of the epigastric region are the (*hypochondriac, iliac, lumbar*) regions.

3. The abdominopelvic quadrants divide the abdominopelvic area of the body into (*four, six, nine*) regions.

4. The brain surgeon operated to remove a bullet lodged within the (*thoracic, cranial, pelvic*) cavity.

5. The diaphragm is located between the abdominal and (*pelvic, thoracic, spinal*) cavities.

■ BODY DIRECTIONS, POSITIONS, AND PLANES

When referring to a position or a direction on the body, it is important that health care professionals use consistent terminology to ensure that the correct meaning is understood. This section introduces word parts and terminology used to visualize the body and talk about specific locations.

Word Parts Related to Body Directions, Positions, and Planes

Combining Forms	Meaning
anter/o	front
caud/o	tail
cephal/o	head
dors/o	back
infer/o	below
later/o	side
medi/o	middle
poster/o	back
proxim/o	near point of origin
super/o	above
ventr/o	belly

Prefixes	Meaning
circum-	around
epi-	on, following
inter-	between
intra-	within
peri-	around, surrounding
retro-	backward, behind
sub-, infra-	below, beneath
supra-	above

■ Exercises: Word Parts Related to Body Positions and Directions

SIMPLE
RECALL

Exercise 11

Write the meaning of the word part given.

1. infer/o _____

2. intra- _____

3. caud/o _____

4. poster/o _____

5. anter/o _____

6. epi- _____

7. later/o _____

8. cephal/o _____

9. circum- _____

10. dors/o _____

TERM
CONSTRUCTION

Exercise 12

Considering the meaning of the word parts from which the medical term is made, write the meaning of the medical term given. (You have not yet learned many of these terms but can build their meaning from the word parts.)

Combining Form	Meaning	Medical Term	Meaning of Term
vertebr/o	vertebra	intervertebral	1. _____
cardi/o	heart	pericardiac	2. _____
cec/o	cecum	retrocecal	3. _____
carp/o	carpal bone	mediocarpal	4. _____
numer/o	number	supernumerary	5. _____

Terms Related to Body Directions, Positions, and Planes

Term	Pronunciation	Meaning
Directional Terms (Fig. 3-5)		
cephalad	sef'ă-lad	toward the head
caudad	kaw'dad	toward the tail (opposite of cephalad)
superior	sŭ-pĕr'ē-ŏr	above or upward
inferior	in-fēr'ē-ŏr	below or downward (opposite of superior)
anterior	an-tēr'ē-ŏr	toward the front of the body
posterior	pos-tēr'ē-ŏr	toward the back of the body (opposite of anterior)
ventral	ven'trăl	pertaining to the belly, front
dorsal	dōr'săl	pertaining to the back (opposite of ventral)
lateral	lat'ĕr-ăl	pertaining to the side
medial	mē'dē-ăl	pertaining to the middle (opposite of lateral)
unilateral	yū'ni-lat'ĕ-răl	pertaining to one side only
bilateral	bī-lat'ĕr-ăl	pertaining to both sides (opposite of unilateral)
proximal	prok'si-măl	nearer the trunk or point of origin
distal	dis'tăl	away from the trunk or point of origin (opposite of proximal)

(continued)

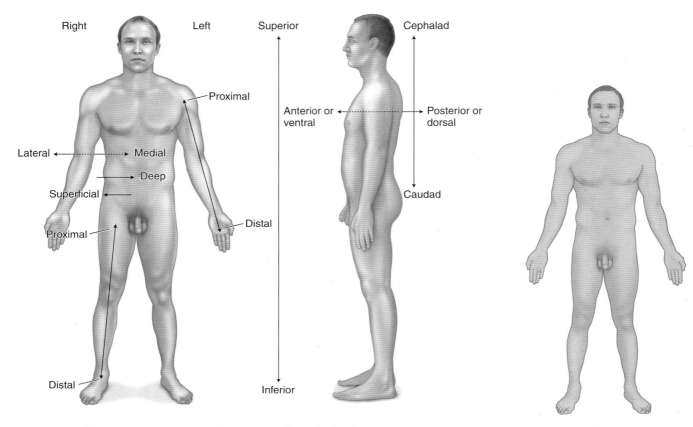

Figure 3-5 Directional terms describe the location of a body part in relationship to another.

Figure 3-6 The anatomic position.

Terms Related to Body Directions, Positions, and Planes (continued)

Term	Pronunciation	Meaning
superficial	sū'pĕr-fish'ăl	near the surface
deep	dēp	far from the surface (opposite of superficial)
anteroposterior	an'tĕr-ō-pos-tĕr'ē-ŏr	from front to back
Positional Terms		
anatomic position	an'ă-tŏm'ik pŏ-zish'ŏn	body in standard reference position: standing erect, arms at the sides, palms facing forward (Fig. 3-6)
decubitus	dē-kyū'bi-tŭs	lying down
dorsal recumbent	dōr'săl rē-kŭm'bĕnt	lying on back with legs bent and feet flat
Fowler position, *syn.* semirecumbent	fowl'ĕr pŏ-zish'ŏn, sem'ē-rē-cŭm'bĕnt	lying on back with head of bed raised 45 degrees
lateral recumbent	lat'ĕr-ăl rĕ-kŭm'bĕnt	lying on the side
prone	prōn	lying face down
supine	sū'pīn	lying face up

(continued)

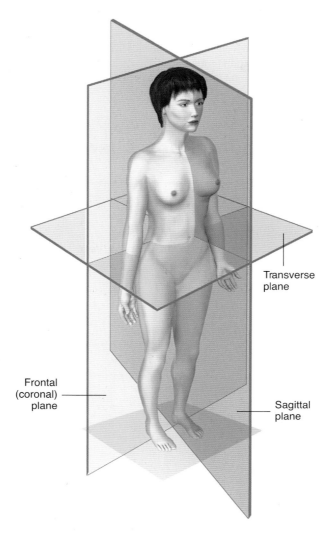

Figure 3-7   Body planes divide the body into halves in different ways for reference purposes. The coronal (frontal) plane divides the body into anterior and posterior halves. The sagittal plane divides the body into left and right halves. The transverse plane divides the body into upper and lower halves.

Terms Related to Body Directions, Positions, and Planes *(continued)*

Term	Pronunciation	Meaning
Body Planes (Fig. 3-7)		
plane	plān	an imaginary surface that extends through two definite points
coronal plane, *syn.* frontal plane	kōr'ŏ-năl plān, frŏn'tăl plān	vertical plane dividing the body into anterior and posterior halves
sagittal plane	saj'i-tăl plān	vertical plane dividing the body into left and right halves
transverse plane	trans-věrs' plān	horizontal plane dividing the body into upper and lower halves

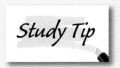

Planes of the Body: Think of a plane as an invisible, flat surface dividing parts of the body. The coronal and sagittal planes are positioned in a vertical (up and down) direction in relation to the body or parts of the body, whereas the transverse plane runs in a horizontal direction across the body.

■ Exercises: Terms Related to Body Directions, Positions, and Planes

SIMPLE
RECALL

Exercise 13

Write the correct medical term for the meaning given.

1. away from the trunk _____

2. lying face up _____

3. above or upward _____

4. near the surface _____

5. pertaining to the side _____

6. toward the front of the body _____

7. from front to back _____

8. pertaining to the belly, front _____

9. toward the head _____

10. lying on back with head of bed raised _____

SIMPLE
RECALL

Exercise 14

Write the meaning of the term given.

1. supine _____

2. inferior _____

3. coronal plane _____

4. proximal _____

5. caudad _____

6. transverse plane _____

7. bilateral _____

8. anatomic position _____

9. medial _____

10. dorsal _____

ADVANCED
RECALL

Exercise 15

Complete each sentence by writing in the correct medical term.

1. A patient in the lateral recumbent position is lying on his or her _____.

2. The _____ plane divides the body vertically into left and right halves.

3. An internal organ that is far from the surface of the body is said to be _____.

4. A disease that affects only one side of the body is _____.

5. The opposite of anterior is _____.

6. The ankle is farther _____ (away from the trunk) than the knee.

7. The palm is the _____ (front) surface of the hand.

8. The stomach is located _____ (above) to the intestine.

9. The general term for lying down (not specifically face up or down) is _____.

10. The knee is located more _____ (toward the trunk) than the ankle.

ANIMATION

View the animation Terms Related to the Body as a Whole *on the Student Resources for an in-depth overview of terminology related to direction and position, planes, positions, regions and cavities.*

■ COLORS

Combining Forms Related to Colors

Combining Form	Meaning
chlor/o	green
chrom/o	color
cyan/o	blue
erythr/o	red
leuk/o	white
melan/o	black, dark
xanth/o	yellow

■ Exercises: Combining Forms Related to Colors

Exercise 16

SIMPLE
RECALL

Write the meaning of the combining form given.

1. melan/o _____

2. cyan/o _____

3. xanth/o _____

4. chlor/o _____

5. leuk/o _____

6. erythr/o _____

7. chrom/o _____

Terms Related to Colors

Term	Pronunciation	Meaning
chloroma	klōr-ō'mă	abnormal mass of green cells
chromaturia	krō'mă-tyūr'ē-ă	abnormal coloration of urine
cyanosis	sī'ă-nō'sis	blue discoloration of the skin and other tissues
erythrocyte	ĕ-rith'rŏ-sīt	red blood cell
leukocyte	lū'kō-sīt	white blood cell
melanoma	mel'ă-nō'mă	tumor characterized by dark appearance
xanthoderma	zan'thō-dĕr'mă	yellow coloration of the skin

■ Exercises: Terms Related to Colors

Exercise 17

SIMPLE
RECALL

Write the correct medical term for the meaning given.

1. red blood cell _____

2. yellow discoloration of skin _____

3. tumor that is dark _____

4. abnormal discoloration of urine _____

5. white blood cell _____

6. cyanosis _____

■ INTRODUCTION TO MEDICAL RECORDS

In health care settings, medical terminology is used in both spoken and written communication. The primary form of written communication is the patient's medical record. Because you will likely encounter different types of medical records in your work, later chapters in this text frequently include medical records so that you can become familiar with the different formats and experience real-life uses of medical terminology.

Following are common types of medical records:

- ■ **Hospital and clinic records**, sometimes simply called the patient's record, typically are a collection of all written documents related to a patient's examination, diagnosis, and care.
- ■ **History and physical (H&P) examination** is a record of the patient's past medical history, which may include forms the patient fills out, and the health care provider's examination of the patient. This is usually a standardized report because the examination is performed in a standard, systematic manner.
- ■ **Consent forms** are signed by the patient to give permission for health care to be provided, including special forms for surgery and other procedures.
- ■ **Health care provider patient care notes** are written into the patient record whenever a physician, nurse, or other health care provider gives the patient any form of care. Generally all diagnostic procedures and treatments are documented, along with observations, test results, consultations with other specialists, and so on.
- ■ **Laboratory and diagnostic test reports** may come from sources outside the primary care team, such as blood test results from an outside laboratory or a pathology report, or from another department within the health care facility.
- ■ **Other specialty reports** include reports from other caregivers (such as a physical therapist or an anesthesiologist during surgery) and discharge reports when the patient leaves a hospital.

Following is a small portion of a typical medical record. This is a section of a consultation note for a patient who has undergone treatment for lung cancer. As you read this record, underline all medical terms that you do not understand.

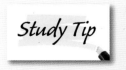

Study Tip

Reading Medical Records: When reading a medical record the first time, do not stop to puzzle out every new term you encounter. Instead, read the record all the way through to gain a general sense of its meaning. You will find it easier to understand specific terms once you are familiar with the overall context. If you are still unsure of some terms, however, consult your medical dictionary.

Medical Record

FOLLOW-UP NOTE

The patient is a 46-year-old white female with a diagnosis of stage IIB (T2, N1, M0) large cell carcinoma of the right upper lobe status post right upper lobectomy. She received a course of postoperative radiation therapy directed to the mediastinum, receiving a total dose of 5,040 rads with completion of treatment on April 13, 20xx. She was last seen in followup on July 28, 20xx, and returns today for a routine 4-month follow-up. She was recently seen by Dr. Smith.

Chest x-ray was obtained on October 14, 20xx. This was compared with previous one of June 15, 20xx. The left lung remains completely clear. There is a slight increase in interstitial markings around the left hilar area. This is within the prior radiation therapy field. This most likely represents radiation-induced scarring.

She is feeling well overall. Her appetite has been good. She has occasional chest discomfort with occasional cough. She denies any pain referable to the thoracotomy site. She has no hemoptysis. She denies any bone pain. She has no bowel or bladder complaints. She remains active and is feeling well overall.

PHYSICAL EXAMINATION: Blood pressure is 110/74, pulse 72, and respirations 20. Weight is 153 pounds, up 4-1/2 pounds since last being seen. Today on HEENT examination, extraocular movements are intact. Pupils are equal, round, and reactive to light and accommodation. Normocephalic. She has no palpable cervical, supraclavicular, axillary, or inguinal lymphadenopathy. The heart beats with a regular rate and rhythm. Lungs are clear to auscultation and percussion. The right thoracotomy incisional site is well healed. There are no palpable abnormalities. The abdomen is soft and nontender, with no mass or organomegaly. Extremities reveal no edema, cyanosis, or clubbing.

ASSESSMENT: We are pleased with the patient's condition with no evidence of recurrent, residual, or metastatic disease.

PLAN: She is scheduled to see Dr. Smith in January. We have asked her to return for routine follow-up in 6 months. We have requested a chest x-ray at that time. We will keep you informed of her progress.

■ Exercise: Medical Records

Exercise 18

APPLICATION

For each of the following medical terms used in this medical record, write the definition. Most of these terms are built from word parts used in this or the preceding chapters (or are provided here). Because a term's meaning may not be precisely the sum of the meaning of its parts, check your answers against your medical dictionary.

Term	Meaning
1. lobectomy (lob/o = lobe [of lung])	_____
2. postoperative	_____
3. thoracotomy	_____

4. supraclavicular (clavicul/o = collar bone) _____

5. lymphadenopathy (lymph/o = lymph) _____

6. organomegaly (organ/o = organ) _____

7. cyanosis _____

■ INTRODUCTION TO BODY SYSTEMS

A **body system** is a group of organs with related structure or function. For example, the respiratory system includes the lungs and the airway passages from the nose and mouth to the lungs. The primary functions are to take in oxygen when we breathe in and move it into the blood to reach all body tissues, and to remove carbon dioxide, a waste product, from the body when we breathe out.

Human anatomy and disease are usually learned in relation to body systems. It helps to learn about different organs that work together with a related body system function rather than simply study every organ by itself. Because many diseases also affect single body systems, understanding health and health care by body system also makes good sense. And because much medical terminology involves anatomy or health care by body systems, it also makes good sense to learn medical terminology by body systems.

The main portion of this text is organized by body systems. Note that because many organs and body functions overlap, body systems can be organized in somewhat different ways. For example, the skeletal system (bones, ligaments) and the muscular system (muscles, tendons) work very closely together to provide body movement. Therefore these are often combined as the musculoskeletal system. Similarly, because the lymph system drains into the cardiovascular system, these are often studied together. Here are the body systems covered in this text:

■ Integumentary system (skin and related structures)
■ Digestive system (sometimes called the gastrointestinal system)
■ Urinary system
■ Cardiovascular and lymph systems (heart and vessels)
■ Blood and immune system
■ Respiratory system
■ Male reproductive system
■ Female reproductive system
■ Nervous system (brain, nerves)
■ Sensory system (eye, ear)
■ Musculoskeletal system
■ Endocrine system (glands and hormones)

Because many diseases involve primarily one system, medical specialties often focus on individual body systems also. Here are a few examples:

■ Dermatologists diagnose and treat skin conditions.
■ Neurologists diagnose and treat conditions of the nervous system.
■ Orthopedists diagnose and treat conditions of the musculoskeletal system.
■ Endocrinologists diagnose and treat conditions of the endocrine system.

You will learn more about these medical specialties, and the health conditions they care for, in the chapters on specific body systems.

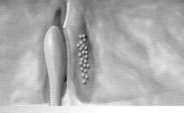

Chapter Review

Review of Terms

VISUAL

Exercise 19

Write the appropriate terms for body cavities on the blanks indicated.

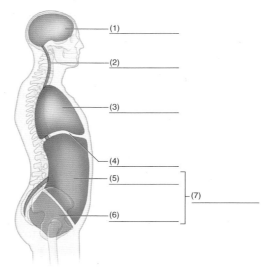

(1) _____

(2) _____

(3) _____

(4) _____

(5) _____

(6) _____

(7) _____

VISUAL

Exercise 20

Write the appropriate terms for abdominopelvic regions on the blanks indicated.

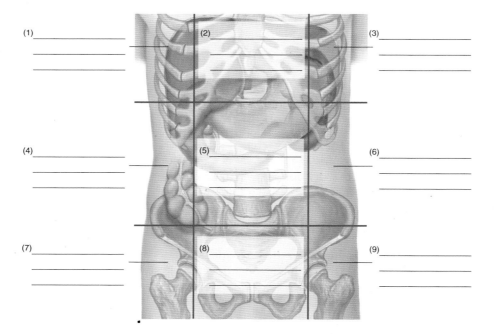

(1) _____
_____
_____

(2) _____
_____
_____

(3) _____
_____
_____

(4) _____
_____
_____

(5) _____
_____
_____

(6) _____
_____
_____

(7) _____
_____
_____

(8) _____
_____
_____

(9) _____
_____
_____

Understanding Term Structure

TERM
CONSTRUCTION

Exercise 21

Break the given medical term into its word parts and define each part. Then define the medical term. (Note: you may need to use word parts from previous chapters.) Check your definition against your medical dictionary.

For example:

arthritis	*word parts:*	arthr/o / -itis
	meanings:	joint / inflammation
	term meaning:	inflammation of a joint

1. fibrosis   *word parts:*   _____ / _____

                  meanings: _____ / _____

                  term meaning: _____

2. pathogenic   *word parts:*   _____ / _____

                  meanings: _____ / _____

                  term meaning: _____

3. hemostasis   *word parts:*   _____ / _____

                  meanings: _____ / _____

                  term meaning: _____

4. neuroblast   *word parts:*   _____ / _____

                  meanings: _____ / _____

                  term meaning: _____

5. osteonecrosis   *word parts:*   _____ / _____ / _____

                  meanings: _____ / _____ / _____

                  term meaning: _____

6. cervicobrachial   *word parts:*   _____ / _____ / _____

                  meanings: _____ / _____ / _____

                  term meaning: _____

7. craniocerebral   *word parts:*   _____ / _____ / _____

                  meanings: _____ / _____ / _____

                  term meaning: _____

8. superolateral   *word parts:*   _____ / _____ / _____

                               meanings: _____ / _____ / _____

                               term meaning: _____

9. visceromegaly   *word parts:*   _____ / _____

                               meanings: _____ / _____

                               term meaning: _____

10. hyperglycemia   *word parts:*   _____ / _____ / _____

                               meanings: _____ / _____ / _____

                               term meaning: _____

Comprehension Exercises

Exercise 22

COMPREHENSION   **Fill in the blank with the correct term or word.**

1. Excessive growth of tissue is termed _____.

2. Even if you do not recognize the term *acidosis*, you can assume that because of the suffix -osis, this term likely refers to a(n) _____ condition.

3. Based on its two word parts, the term *morphology* means

   _____.

4. Based on its word parts, the term *lipemia* likely refers to _____.

5. After weeks of treatment, the patient no longer had symptoms, and although his chronic disease was still present, his physician said the disease was in _____.

6. The patient felt a sharp pain on the side of her abdomen to left of her navel, in the _____ abdominal region.

7. The x-ray unit was positioned in front of the patient such that the x-rays passed through him in a(n) _____ direction.

8. The patient was lying supine in bed until the nurse raised the head of the bed 45 degrees to put the patient in the _____ position.

9. Because of a severe breathing problem, the patient was experiencing cyanosis, and her lips were turning _____.

10. An increase in the severity of a disease or symptoms is called _____.

COMPREHENSION

Exercise 23

Write a short answer for each question.

1. When speaking of a skin lesion on the arm, which is the most proximal edge of the lesion?

2. Describe the appearance of someone in the anatomic position.

3. What is a body system?

4. What part of a body cell is not considered part of the cytoplasm?

5. When is a disease considered chronic?

6. Strictly speaking, what does etiology mean?

7. What is the main characteristic of a body cavity?

8. What is the dorsal surface of the hand?

9. Describe the appearance of someone with xanthoderma.

10. If an illness of the mind is called a psychic condition, what is an illness of the body called?

COMPREHENSION

Exercise 24

Circle the letter of the best answer in the following questions.

1. If the fluid taken into the body equals the fluid lost from the body, this balance can be described as a state of:

   A. hyperplasia
   B. homeostasis
   C. necrosis
   D. inflammation

2. The lungs are located in the:

   A. thoracic cavity
   B. abdominal cavity
   C. pelvic cavity
   D. spinal cavity

3. The abdominal region located below the umbilical region is the:

   A. epigastric region
   B. iliac region
   C. hypochondriac region
   D. hypogastric region

4. After a stroke, the patient had partial paralysis of his left side, a condition said to be:

   A. idiopathic
   B. sagittal
   C. unilateral
   D. metastatic

5. A study of cells and tissues is called:

   A. histology
   B. etiology
   C. cytology
   D. morphology

6. A xanthoma is generally what color?

   A. red
   B. yellow
   C. black
   D. blue

7. An acute illness is most likely to be:

   A. fatal
   B. persistent
   C. malignant
   D. brief

8. A toxin may cause symptoms throughout the body. Thus it can be said to have what kind of effects?

   A. metabolic
   B. idiopathic
   C. systemic
   D. inflammatory

9. Which of these terms may apply to both an injury and a disease?

   A. cytoplasm
   B. hyperplasia
   C. proximal
   D. lesion

10. The diaphragm is a:

   A. cavity
   B. muscle
   C. tumor
   D. quadrant

Application and Analysis

MEDICAL RECORD EXERCISE

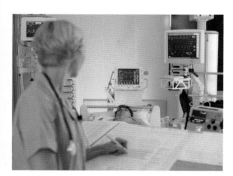

A registered nurse attends to a patient in the Intensive Care Unit.

Following is the operative report for Mr. Stern, who has been diagnosed with bronchogenic carcinoma of the lung. As a registered nurse (RN) specializing in critical care, you are reviewing the patient's medical record to understand the procedure that was performed.

STUDENT
RESOURCES

Learn more about careers in nursing and the other health professions highlighted in this text in the Additional Resources section of the Student Resources.

Medical Record

OPERATIVE REPORT

BRONCHOGENIC CARCINOMA EXCISION

PREOPERATIVE DIAGNOSIS: Solitary pulmonary nodule with bronchogenic carcinoma.

POSTOPERATIVE DIAGNOSIS: Solitary pulmonary nodule with bronchogenic carcinoma.

PROCEDURES PERFORMED
1. Bronchoscopy.
2. Right thoracotomy.
3. Lateral segmentectomy of right middle lobe, followed by completion of right middle lobectomy.
4. Mediastinal lymphadenectomy.

ANESTHESIA: General endotracheal.

DESCRIPTION OF PROCEDURE: After successful induction of general endotracheal anesthesia, the patient was placed in the supine position and bronchoscopy performed via the endotracheal tube. The left upper lingular lobes, right upper and lower lobes were unremarkable. The bronchoscopy tube was well situated within the left main stem bronchus. Then the patient was positioned, prepped, and draped in the usual sterile fashion and underwent a right lateral thoracotomy.

The thorax was entered. The pleura was unremarkable. The lung was explored. There was a nodule present within the lateral segment of the right middle lobe. The dissection was carried down to the artery, which was doubly tied proximally and distally and divided, and this segment was then stapled off and sent for frozen section. The frozen section was consistent with a squamous cell carcinoma. Consequently the lobectomy was completed, and lymph nodes were harvested.

A chest tube was brought out through a separate stab incision. The intercostal membranes were closed. The muscles, subcutaneous tissue, and the skin were closed. A Dermabond dressing was applied. The chest tube was attached to drainage. The sponge, needle, and lap counts were correct x3, and the patient was taken to the recovery room in stable condition.

APPLICATION

Exercise 25

Write the appropriate medical terms used in this medical record on the blanks after their definitions. You should be able to identify these terms based on word parts included in this or the preceding chapters.

1. pertaining to the lungs   _____

2. incision into the thorax   _____

3. surgical removal of lobe   _____

4. pertaining to the side   _____

5. nearer the trunk or point of origin   _____

6. away from the trunk or point of origin   _____

Exercise 26

APPLICATION

Write the appropriate medical terms used in this medical record on the blanks after their definitions. The meaning of new combining forms is provided to help you build these medical terms that may be new to you.

1. originating in the bronchus (bronch/o) _____

2. surgical removal of a segment _____

3. surgical removal of a lymph gland _____

4. pertaining to within the trachea (trache/o) _____

5. examination by instrument inside the bronchus (bronch/o) _____

6. pertaining to between ribs (cost/o) _____

7. pertaining to beneath the skin (cutane/o) _____

Pronunciation and Spelling

Exercise 27

AUDITORY

Review the Chapter 3 terms in the Dictionary/Audio Glossary in the Student Resources and practice pronouncing each term, referring to the pronunciation guide as needed.

Exercise 28

SPELLING

Circle the correct spelling of each term.

1. chromosome   chromosone   chronosome

2. diafragm   diaphragm   diphragm

3. homostasis   homeostesis   homeostasis

4. cepholad   cephalad   cepadad

5. cytoplasm   cyteplasm   cyteplazm

6. erythrocyte   erthrocyte   erythracyte

7. decubitus   decubetus   decubitous

8. umbilical   umbillical   umobilical

9. pathegen   pathogen   pathagen

10. luekocyte   lukeocyte   leukocyte

11. inflamation   inflammation   enflamation

12. citology   cytology   cytolagy

13. matabolism   matebolism   metabolism

14. cyenosis   cyanosis   cyonasis

15. nuclei   nucli   nuklei

Media Connection

STUDENT
RESOURCES

Exercise 29

Complete each of the following activities available with the Student Resources. Check off each activity as you complete it, and record your score for the Chapter Quiz in the space provided.

Chapter Exercises

____ Flash Cards   ____ Quiz Show

____ Concentration   ____ Complete the Case

____ Roboterms   ____ Medical Record Review

____ Word Builder   ____ Look and Label

____ Fill the Gap   ____ Image Matching

____ Break It Down   ____ Spelling Bee

____ True/False Body Building

      ____ **Chapter Quiz**   *Score:* _____%

Additional Resources

____ Animation: Terms Related to the Body as a Whole

____ Dictionary/Audio Glossary

____ Health Professions Careers: Registered Nurse

Integumentary System

4

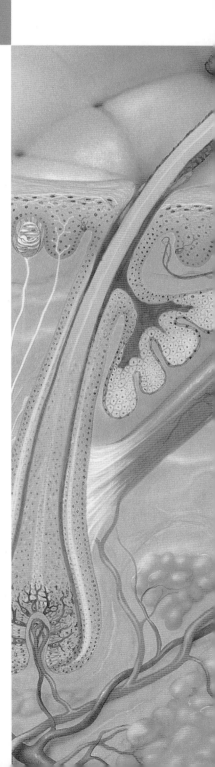

Chapter Outline

Objectives

After completion of this chapter you will be able to:

1. Identify the functions of the skin.

2. Define terms related to the layers and the accessory structures of the skin.

3. Define combining forms, prefixes, and suffixes related to the integumentary system.

4. Define common medical terminology related to the integumentary system, including adjectives and related terms, symptoms and conditions, tests and procedures, surgical interventions and therapeutic procedures, medications and drug therapies, and specialties.

5. Explain abbreviations for terms related to the integumentary system.

6. Successfully complete all chapter exercises.

7. Explain terms used in medical records and case studies involving the integumentary system.

8. Successfully complete all pronunciation and spelling exercises, and complete all interactive exercises included with the companion Student Resources.

■ ANATOMY AND PHYSIOLOGY

Functions

- To protect the body from harmful microorganisms
- To protect the body from the harmful effects of ultraviolet (UV) radiation
- To protect the body from dehydration
- To produce vitamin D
- To assist with temperature regulation
- To communicate sensory information

Organs and Structures

- The largest organ system of the body is the integumentary system.
- All of the skin combined weighs about 6 pounds or 2.72 kg.
- The accessory organs of the integumentary system are the hair, nails, sudoriferous glands (sweat glands), and sebaceous glands (oil glands).

Terms Related to the Integumentary System (Fig. 4-1)

Term	Pronunciation	Meaning
Layers of the Skin		
epidermis	ep'i-dĕrm'is	outer layer of skin; waterproof layer that functions as protection and contains melanocytes
dermis	dĕr'mis	deep layer of skin that contains the sweat and oil glands; also contains tiny muscles attached to the hair follicles
subcutaneous layer	sŭb'kyū-tā'nē-ŭs lā'ĕr	layer of loose connective tissue that connects the skin to the surface muscles; contains the blood vessels and fat
Accessory Structures		
adipocytes	ad'i-pō-sītz	fat cells that make up most of the subcutaneous layer
arrector pili	ă-rek'tŏr pī'lī	tiny muscle that attaches to the hair follicle

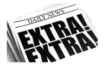 **ARRECTOR PILI** Goose bumps are made by the contraction of the arrector pili muscles, an activity that causes the hair to stand straight up!

Term	Pronunciation	Meaning
hair	hār	keratinized fibers that arise from hair follicles
hair follicle	hār fol'i-kĕl	area from which hair grows; located in the dermal layer of skin (dermis)
keratin	ker'ă-tin	protein found in the hair and nails that promotes hardness
keratinocytes	ke-rat'i-nō-sītz	cells that make up the epidermal layer of skin and assist in waterproofing the body
melanocytes	mel'ă-nō-sītz	cells that give color to skin, eyes, and hair
nail	nāl	translucent plate made of keratin that covers and protects the ends of the fingers and toes
sebaceous glands	sĕ-bā'shŭs	glands that secrete oil (sebum) into the hair follicle and to the epidermal layer of skin (epidermis)
sebum	sē'bŭm	oily secretion of the sebaceous gland
sudoriferous glands	sū'dōr-if'ĕr-ŭs	glands that secrete sweat to the outside of the body; also assist in body temperature regulation

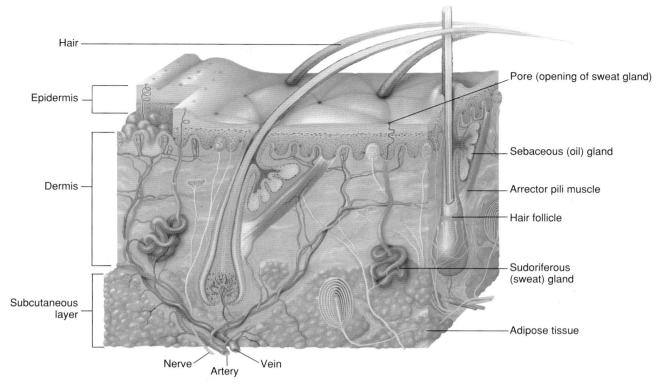

Figure 4-1 Layers of the skin and accessory structures.

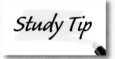

Epidermis Remember that the prefix *epi-* means *on*; therefore, the epidermis is the layer of skin *on top of* the dermis.

■ Exercises: Anatomy and Physiology

Exercise 1

Write the correct anatomic structure or related term for the meaning given.

1. outer layer of skin that contains melanocytes _____

2. sweat glands _____

3. largest organ system of the body _____

4. oil glands _____

5. layer that contains blood vessels _____

6. tiny muscle attached to the hair follicle _____

7. deep layer of the skin _____

8. layer that provides protection _____

9. keratinized fibers   _____

10. oily secretions of the sebaceous gland   _____

Exercise 2

ADVANCED RECALL

Match each medical term with its meaning.

adipocytes	sebaceous glands	keratinocytes	nail
keratin	hair follicle	sudoriferous glands	melanocytes

Meaning   **Term**

1. translucent plate made of keratin   _____

2. area from which hair grows   _____

3. assist in temperature regulation   _____

4. give color to the skin   _____

5. secrete oil to the epidermal layer of skin _____

6. cells that make up the outermost layer of skin _____

7. protein found in the hair and nails that promotes hardness _____

8. fat cells that make up most of the subcutaneous layer _____

■ WORD PARTS

Note that some word parts that have been introduced earlier in the book may not be repeated here.

Combining Forms

Combining Form	Meaning
cry/o	cold
cyan/o	blue
derm/o, dermat/o, cutane/o	skin
electr/o	electric, electricity
erythr/o	red
hidr/o	sweat
kerat/o, scler/o	hard
lip/o, adip/o	fat
melan/o	black, dark
myc/o	fungus

(continued)

Combining Forms *(continued)*

Combining Form	Meaning
necr/o	death
onych/o	nail
pachy/o	thick
py/o	pus
rhytid/o	wrinkle
seb/o	sebum
trich/o	hair
xanth/o	yellow
xer/o	dry

Prefixes

Prefix	Meaning
a-, an-	without, not
bio-	life
epi-	on, following
intra-	within
para-	beside
per-	through
sub-	below, beneath
trans-	across, through

Suffixes

Suffix	Meaning
-derma	skin condition
-ectomy	excision, surgical removal
-genic	originating, producing
-itis	inflammation
-logist	one who specializes in
-logy	study of
-malacia	softening
-pathy	disease
-phagia	to eat
-plasia	formation, growth
-plasty	surgical repair, reconstruction
-rrhea	flow, discharge
-tome	instrument used to cut

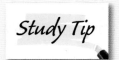

Spelling Remember the difference between *hidr/o* and *hydr/o*. *Hidr/o* is the combining form that means sweat. *Hydr/o* is the combining form that means water.

■ Exercises: Word Parts

Exercise 3

Write the meaning of the combining form given.

1. trich/o _____

2. rhytid/o _____

3. onych/o _____

4. cutane/o _____

5. lip/o _____

6. seb/o _____

7. xer/o _____

8. dermat/o _____

9. scler/o _____

10. erythr/o _____

11. hidr/o _____

12. cry/o _____

Exercise 4

Write the correct combining form(s) for the meaning given.

1. yellow _____

2. sebum _____

3. blue _____

4. skin _____

5. electric _____

6. red _____

7. thick _____

8. pus _____

9. fungus _____

10. black, dark _____

11. death _____

12. sweat _____

13. hard _____

SIMPLE
RECALL

Exercise 5

Write the meaning of the prefix or suffix given.

1. -malacia _____

2. sub- _____

3. -pathy _____

4. -itis _____

5. per- _____

6. para- _____

7. -tome _____

8. -phagia _____

9. intra- _____

10. -rrhea _____

11. trans- _____

12. -plasia _____

13. bio- _____

ADVANCED
RECALL

Exercise 6

Considering the meaning of the combining form from which the medical term is made, write the meaning of the medical term. (You have not yet learned many of these terms but can build their meaning from the word parts.)

Combining Form	Meaning	Medical Term	Meaning of Term
dermat/o	skin	dermatitis	**1.** _____
py/o	pus	pyorrhea	**2.** _____

myc/o	fungus	mycology	3. _____
hidr/o	sweat	hidrosis	4. _____
onych/o	nail	onychectomy	5. _____

TERM CONSTRUCTION

Exercise 7

Build a medical term from an appropriate combining form and suffix, given their meanings.

Use Combining Form for	Use Suffix for	Term
1. dry	skin condition	_____
2. skin	instrument used to cut	_____
3. skin	one who specializes in	_____
4. wrinkle	surgical repair, reconstruction	_____
5. death	abnormal condition	_____
6. nail	softening	_____
7. black, dark	cell	_____

TERM CONSTRUCTION

Exercise 8

Break the given medical term into its word parts and define each part. Then define the medical term.

For example:
dermatitis

word parts: dermat/o / -itis
meanings: skin / inflammation
term meaning: inflammation of the skin

1. anhidrosis

word parts: _____ / _____ / _____

meanings: _____ / _____ / _____

term meaning: _____

2. erythroderma

word parts: _____ / _____

meanings: _____ / _____

term meaning: _____

3. scleroderma

word parts: _____ / _____

meanings: _____ / _____

term meaning: _____

4. seborrhea

word parts: _____ / _____

meanings: _____ / _____

term meaning: _____

5. onychophagia

word parts: _____ / _____

meanings: _____ / _____

term meaning: _____

6. rhytidectomy

word parts: _____ / _____

meanings: _____ / _____

term meaning: _____

7. transdermal

word parts: _____ / _____ / _____

meanings: _____ / _____ / _____

term meaning: _____

8. epidermal

word parts: _____ / _____ / _____

meanings: _____ / _____ / _____

term meaning: _____

9. subcutaneous

word parts: _____ / _____ / _____

meanings: _____ / _____ / _____

term meaning: _____

10. mycosis

word parts: _____ / _____

meanings: _____ / _____

term meaning: _____

11. keratogenic

word parts: _____ / _____

meanings: _____ / _____

term meaning: _____

■ MEDICAL TERMS

Adjectives and Other Related Terms

Term	Pronunciation	Meaning
adipose	ad'i-pōs	fat, fatty
atypical	ā-tip'i-kăl	unusual
circumscribed	sĭr'kŭm-skrībd	contained to a specific area
cyanosis	sī'ă-nō'sis	blue discoloration of the skin and other tissues
diaphoresis	dī'ă-fŏr-ē'sis	profuse sweating
dysplasia	dis-plā'zē-ă	abnormal growth of tissue
erythematous	er'i-them'ă-tŭs	condition of being red
eschar	es'kahr	blackened area of burned tissue
exfoliation	eks'fō-lē-ā'shŭn	shedding of dead skin cells
hyperplasia	hī'pĕr-plā'zē-ă	excessive growth of tissue
indurated	in'dūr-ā-tĕd	pertaining to an area of hardened tissue
integumentary	in-teg'yū-men'tăr-ē	pertaining to the skin and accessory structures
pallor	pal'ŏr	abnormally pale skin coloration
pruritic	prūr-it'ik	pertaining to itching
purulent	pyūr'ū-lĕnt	containing pus
sebaceous	sĕ-bā'shŭs	pertaining to sebum
sudoriferous	sū'dŏr-if'ĕr-ŭs	pertaining to sweat
turgor	tŭr'gŏr	condition of fullness

■ Exercises: Adjectives and Other Related Terms

SIMPLE
RECALL

Exercise 9

Write the correct medical term for the meaning given.

1. excessive growth of tissue _____

2. unusual _____

3. containing pus _____

4. pertaining to an area of hard tissue _____

5. pertaining to the skin and accessory structures _____

6. abnormal growth of tissue _____

7. contained in a specific area _____

8. fat, fatty _____

ADVANCED
RECALL

Exercise 10

Circle the term that is most appropriate for the meaning of the sentence.

1. After working in the bright sun all day without applying sunscreen, Mr. Hughitt noticed his (*eschar, cyanosis, erythematous*) skin.

2. The physician diagnosed Mrs. Diaz with dehydration, which can lead to loss of skin fullness or (*turgor, pallor, hyperplasia*).

3. The patient's (*erythematous, pallor, cyanosis*), a bluish discoloring of the skin, was likely caused by lack of oxygenated blood to the body's peripheral areas.

4. Mrs. Davis was seen in the physician's office for extreme fatigue and (*eschar, pallor, turgor*), which is abnormally pale skin.

5. The dermatologist informed the patient that (*indurated, exfoliation, diaphoresis*) is the process of ridding the skin's surface of dead cells.

6. The deeply burned area on Mr. Botta's arm developed a thick black layer of necrotic tissue known as (*necrosis, eschar, purulent*).

7. The poison ivy patch that Mr. DeCostas stumbled into caused his skin to become (*purulent, pruritic, indurated*).

8. The physician explained that, along with chest pain, nausea, and vomiting, another symptom of a possible heart attack is profuse sweating, known medically as (*atypical, circumscribed, diaphoresis*).

Symptoms and Medical Conditions

Term	Pronunciation	Meaning
abrasion	ă-brā′zhŭn	injury resulting in removal or disturbance of the superficial layers of the skin
abscess	ab′ses	a circumscribed collection of pus caused by a bacterial infection
acne	ak′nē	inflammatory disease of sebaceous glands and hair follicles marked by papules and pustules
albinism	al′bi-nizm	a group of inherited disorders with deficiency of pigment in the skin, hair, and eyes (Fig. 4-2)
burn	bŭrn	injury to the skin caused by heat or other means (Fig. 4-3)
superficial burn	sū′pĕr-fish′ăl bŭrn	a burn involving only the epidermis; causes redness and swelling but no blisters (for example, most cases of sunburn); commonly called a first-degree burn
partial-thickness burn	pahr′shăl-thik′nĕs bŭrn	a burn involving the epidermis and dermis that usually involves blisters; commonly called a second-degree burn
full-thickness burn	ful-thik′nĕs bŭrn	a burn involving destruction of the entire skin; extends into subcutaneous fat, muscle, or bone and often causes severe scarring; commonly called a third-degree burn
carbuncle	kahr′bŭng-kĕl	collection of large localized abscesses seated in groups of hair follicles and connected by channels
cellulitis	sel′yū-lī′tis	inflammation of the subcutaneous layer of the skin (Fig. 4-4)

(continued)

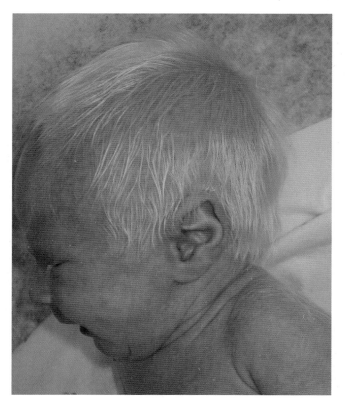

Figure 4-2   Albinism.

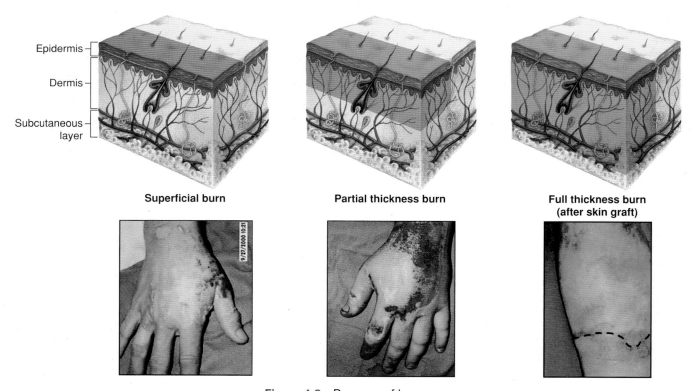

Figure 4-3   Degrees of burns.

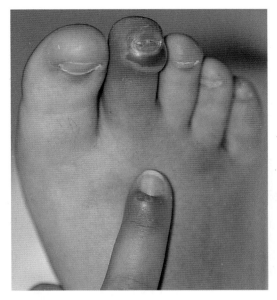

Figure 4-4 Cellulitis.

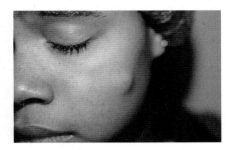

Figure 4-5 Cyst.

Symptoms and Medical Conditions *(continued)*

Term	Pronunciation	Meaning
cicatrix	sik′ă-triks	the fibrous tissue replacing normal tissues destroyed by disease or injury; commonly called a scar
comedo	kom′ĕ-dō	dilated hair follicle filled with bacteria and sebum; commonly called a whitehead or blackhead
contusion	kŏn-tū′zhŭn	injury producing discoloration and swelling without causing a break in the skin; commonly called a bruise
cyst	sist	a closed sac that contains liquid or semiliquid substances (Fig. 4-5)
decubitus ulcer	dē-kyū′bi-tŭs ŭl′sĕr	a pressure sore of the skin and underlying tissues (see Fig. 4-27)
eczema	ek′sĕ-mă	inflammatory condition of the skin causing redness, scaling, blisters, itchiness, and burning (Fig. 4-6)
excoriation	eks-kōr′ē-ā′shŭn	a scratch mark on the skin
fissure	fish′ŭr	a deep furrow, cleft, slit, or tear in the skin (Fig. 4-7)
furuncle	fŭr-ŭng′kĕl	infection of a hair follicle; commonly called a boil
gangrene	gang′-grēn	area of necrosis due to lack of blood flow
herpes simplex	her′pēz sim′pleks	an eruption of blisters on the skin and submucous membranes caused by a local infection of the herpes virus
herpes zoster	hĕr′pēz zos′tĕr	a viral infection that affects the peripheral nerves and causes an eruption of blisters that follows the course of the affected nerves; closely related to varicella; commonly called shingles (Fig. 4-8)
impetigo	im-pĕ-tī′gō	a contagious bacterial skin infection typically occurring on the face of children (Fig. 4-9)
jaundice	jawn′dis	abnormal yellowing of the skin

(continued)

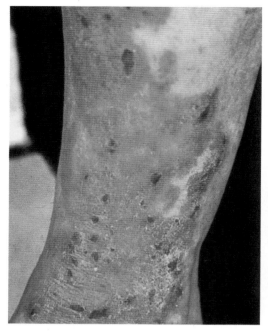

Figure 4-6   Eczema.

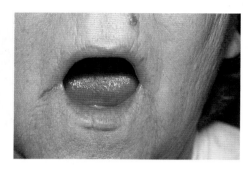

Figure 4-7   Fissure.

Symptoms and Medical Conditions *(continued)*

Term	Pronunciation	Meaning
keloid	kē'loyd	an overgrowth of scar tissue (Fig. 4-10)
lesion	lē'zhŭn	a pathologic change in tissue resulting from disease or injury
macule	mak'yūl	a small flat circumscribed area of the skin different in color than the surrounding skin (see Fig. 4-25)
nevus	nē'vŭs	a circumscribed malformation of the skin, usually a different color than surrounding skin; commonly called a mole

(continued)

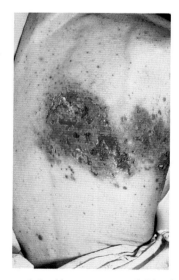

Figure 4-8   Herpes zoster (shingles).

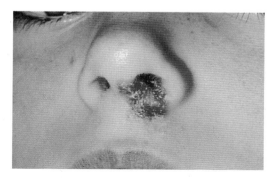

Figure 4-9   Impetigo.

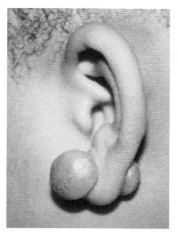

Figure 4-10   Keloid on site of earlobe piercing.

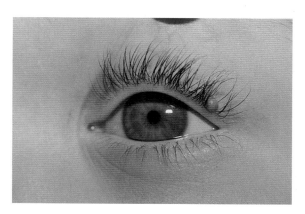

Figure 4-11   Nodule.

Symptoms and Medical Conditions *(continued)*

Term	Pronunciation	Meaning
nodule	nod′jūl	solid raised area located in any layer of the skin (Fig. 4-11)
papule	pap′yūl	a small, raised, solid circumscribed area of the skin (Fig. 4-12)
paronychia	par-ō-nik′ē-ă	inflammation and infection around the nail due to bacteria or fungi (Fig. 4-13)
pediculosis	pĕ-dik-yū-lō′sis	an infestation of lice
psoriasis	sōr-ī′ă-sis	common inherited condition causing silvery discolored areas of rough skin primarily on the scalp, knees, elbows, and trunk (Fig. 4-14)
pustule	pŭs′chūl	a small circumscribed elevation of the skin containing pus (Fig. 4-15)
rosacea	rō-sā′shă	chronic disorder of the skin causing erythematous areas, papules, and pustules and also increased sebum production; usually occurs on the face
scabies	skā′bēz	a dermal eruption (caused by mites) that causes extensive pruritus (itching) (Fig. 4-16)
tinea	tin′ē-ă	fungal infection of the hair, skin, and nails; commonly called ringworm (Fig. 4-17)
tinea capitis	tin′ē-ă kap′i-tis	fungal infection of the scalp

(continued)

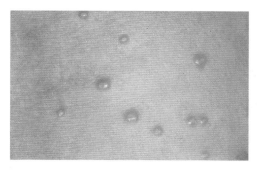

Figure 4-12   Papules.

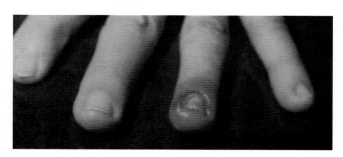

Figure 4-13   Paronychia.

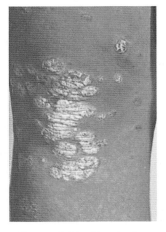

Figure 4-14   Psoriasis.

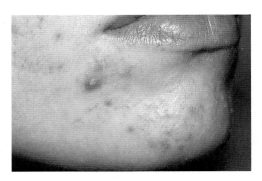

Figure 4-15   Pustule.

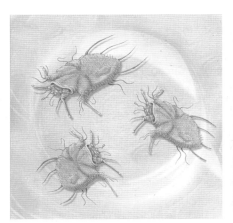

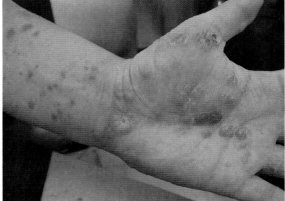

Figure 4-16   Scabies mites and infestation.

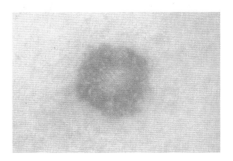

Figure 4-17   Tinea on the arm.

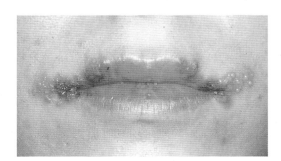

Figure 4-18   Vesicles.

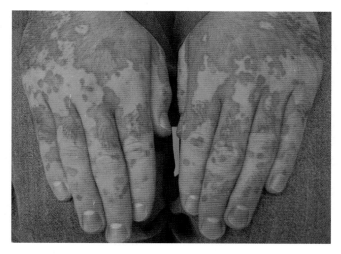

Figure 4-19   Vitiligo.

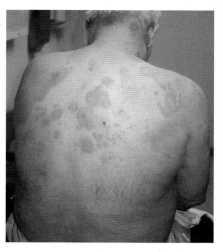

Figure 4-20   Wheals.

Symptoms and Medical Conditions *(continued)*

Term	Pronunciation	Meaning
tinea pedis	tin'ē-ă ped'is	fungal infection of the feet; commonly called athlete's foot
urticaria	ŭr'ti-kar'ē-ă	an eruption of itchy wheals usually related to an allergy; commonly called hives
varicella	var'i-sel'ă	an acute contagious disease caused by the varicella zoster virus and producing various skin eruptions; commonly known as chicken pox
verruca	vĕr-ū'kă	a flesh-colored elevation of skin caused by a virus; commonly called a wart
vesicle	ves'i-kĕl	a clear, fluid-filled, raised lesion; commonly called a blister (Fig. 4-18)
vitiligo	vit'i-lī'gō	areas of skin that have decreased levels of melanocytes causing white patches of varied sizes (Fig. 4-19)
wheal	wēl	a raised reddish lesion that often changes size and shape and extends into adjacent areas; usually associated with an allergen (Fig. 4-20)
xanthoderma	zan'thō-dĕr'mă	any yellow coloration of the skin

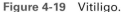

XANTHODERMA   Several conditions can cause yellowing of the skin, including hepatitis, excessive vitamin intake, and eating foods high in carotene. Foods high in carotene include carrots, tomatoes, and sweet potatoes. It is important to determine the difference between xanthoderma caused by a disease process and that caused by dietary intake.

■ Exercises: Symptoms and Medical Conditions

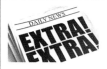

SIMPLE
RECALL

Exercise 11

Write the correct medical term for the meaning given.

1. burn involving destruction of the entire skin   _____

2. small, raised circumscribed area of the skin   _____

3. small elevation of the skin containing pus   _____

4. acute contagious disease causing skin eruptions   _____

5. burn involving only the epidermis   _____

6. inflammation of the subcutaneous layer   _____

7. viral infection affecting peripheral nerves   _____

8. common inherited skin condition   _____

9. inflammatory condition causing redness and scales   _____

10. condition caused by local infection of herpes virus   _____

11. overgrowth of scar tissue   _____

12. abnormal yellowing of the skin   _____

13. pathologic change in tissue   _____

14. injury resulting in removal of superficial skin layer   _____

Exercise 12

ADVANCED
RECALL

Circle the term that is most appropriate for the meaning of the sentence.

1. After examination, the medical assistant noted that the raised, reddish lesion on the anterior side of the patient's forearm could be a (*fissure, wheal, carbuncle*).

2. The physician examined the circumscribed malformation of the skin, or (*nevus, excoriation, furuncle*), for signs of cancer.

3. After lying in the same position for several hours, the patient developed a pressure sore of the skin, called a (*decubitus ulcer, keloid, comedo*), on the posterior aspect of his ankle.

4. Mary felt a solid raised area, called a (*tinea, nodule, paronychia*), while performing her monthly breast self-exam.

5. Several children at the day care center contracted (*psoriasis, scabies, verruca*), a condition that is caused by mites, and were advised not to return to the center until 24 hours after treatment.

6. After cardiac surgery, Mr. Henry developed a scar or (*comedo, cicatrix, wheal*) on his chest where the incision had been made.

7. The patient's erythematous face was diagnosed as (*rosacea, tinea, vitiligo*).

8. Because of a lack of blood flow, an area of (*eczema, gangrene, pediculosis*) developed on the patient's leg.

9. Missy landed on her hip when she fell off her bicycle and developed an area of discoloration and swelling, called a (*contusion, verruca, cyst*).

10. When he was feeling particularly stressed, the teenager's (*acne, boil, abscess*) grew worse, as noted by the development of more papules and pustules.

ADVANCED
RECALL

Exercise 13

Match each medical term with its meaning.

urticaria	pediculosis	impetigo	macule
cyst	comedo	paronychia	vesicle
burn	tinea pedis	verruca	abscess

Meaning   **Term**

1. fluid-filled, raised lesion   _____

2. flat area of skin that is changed in color   _____

3. wart   _____

4. an infestation of lice   _____

5. athlete's foot   _____

6. blackhead   _____

7. hives   _____

8. inflammation around the nail   _____

9. semiliquid substance within a closed sac   _____

10. facial infection most commonly seen in children   _____

11. injury to skin by heat   _____

12. circumscribed collection of pus   _____

Tests and Procedures

Term	Pronunciation	Meaning
biopsy (bx)	bī′op-sē	process of removing tissue from living patients for microscopic examination
culture and sensitivity (C&S)	kŭl′chŭr and sen′si-tiv′i-tē	growing of an organism from a specimen from the body to determine its susceptibility to particular medications
frozen section (FS)	frō′zĕn sek′shŭn	a thin slice of tissue cut from a frozen specimen used for rapid microscopic diagnosis
scratch test	skrach test	type of allergy test in which an antigen is applied through a scratch in the skin
tuberculosis skin test, *syn.* Mantoux test, purified protein derivative (PPD) test	tū-bĕr′kyū-lō′sis skin test, mahn-tū′test, prō′tēn dĕ-riv′ă-tiv test	an intradermal test to determine whether a patient has tuberculosis or has been exposed to the disease

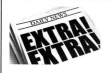

TUBERCULOSIS TESTING An older version of the tuberculosis skin test is the tuberculosis tine test. This test was performed by using a four- or six-pronged device and sticking the skin evenly with all prongs, which were coated with tuberculin antigen. Studies have ultimately proven that the current PPD test, which is given as a single-puncture injection, gives more accurate results than the older tine test, so the tine test is not often used today because of the variation in its results.

■ Exercise: Tests and Procedures

ADVANCED RECALL

Exercise 14

Circle the term that is most appropriate for the meaning of the sentence.

1. Every year, all medical office personnel at Central Hospital undergo a (*tuberculosis skin test, biopsy, scratch test*) to determine whether they have been exposed to the tuberculosis bacterium, *Myobacterium tuberculosis*.

2. To determine the specific triggers for his allergies, Mr. Sabatino had a (*needle biopsy, scratch test, culture and sensitivity*).

3. The young man had a (*biopsy, tuberculosis skin test, scratch test*), which involved the removal of tissue for microscopic examination.

4. The physician ordered a (*biopsy, culture and sensitivity, frozen section*) to determine which medication is needed to treat the patient's infected hand.

5. The surgeon ordered a (*culture and sensitivity, scratch test, frozen section*) of the tissue specimen for rapid microscopic diagnosis.

Surgical Interventions and Therapeutic Procedures

Term	Pronunciation	Meaning
cauterization	kaw'tĕr-īz-ā'shŭn	the use of heat, cold, electric current, or caustic chemicals to destroy tissue
cryosurgery	krī'ō-ser'jer-ē	the use of freezing temperatures to destroy tissue (Fig. 4-21)
débridement	dā-brēd-mōn[h]'	the removal of any necrotic skin or foreign matter from a wound
dermabrasion	dĕrm'ă-brā'zhŭn	the removal of acne scars from the skin with sandpaper, rotating brushes, or other abrasive materials
dermatoautoplasty, *syn.* autograft	dĕr'mă-tō-aw'to-plas-tē, aw'tō-graft	a graft transplanted using the patient's own skin
dermatoheteroplasty, *syn.* allograft	dĕr'mă-tō-het'ĕr-ō-plas-tē, al'ō-graft	a graft transplanted using skin from a source other than the patient

(continued)

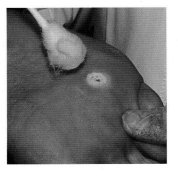

Figure 4-21 Cryosurgery with liquid nitrogen.

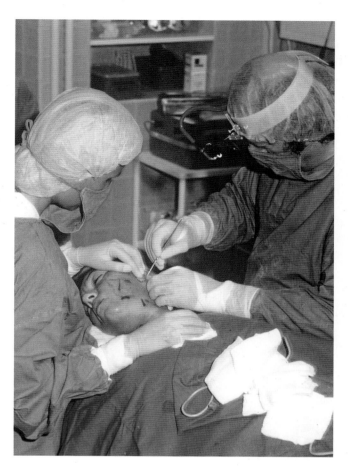

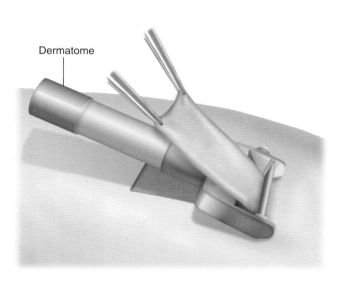

Dermatome

Figure 4-22 Dermatome preparing skin for grafting.

Figure 4-23 Rhytidoplasty.

Surgical Interventions and Therapeutic Procedures *(continued)*

Term	Pronunciation	Meaning
dermatome	dĕr'mă-tōm	instrument used for cutting thin slices of skin for grafting or excising small lesions (Fig. 4-22)
dermatoplasty	dĕr'mă-tō-plas-tē	surgical repair of the skin
electrodesiccation and curettage (ED&C)	ĕ-lek'trō-des-i-kā'shŭn and kūr'ĕ-tahzh'	burning off of skin growths using electrical currents
excision	ek-sizh'ŭn	the act of cutting out
incision	in-sizh'ŭn	the act of cutting into (surgically)
incision and drainage (I&D)	in-sizh'ŭn and drān'ăj	a sterile cut into the skin to release fluid
irrigation	ir'i-gā'shŭn	washing out an area with fluid
rhytidectomy	rit'i-dek'tŏ-mē	surgical removal of wrinkles
rhytidoplasty	rit'i-dō-plas-tē	surgical repair of wrinkles (Fig. 4-23)
suture	sū'chŭr	to unite two surfaces by sewing (Fig. 4-24)

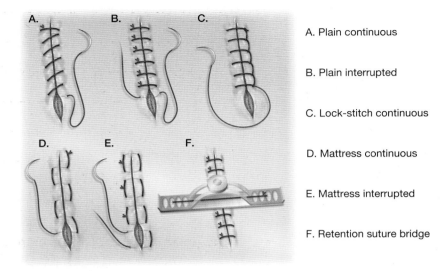

A. Plain continuous

B. Plain interrupted

C. Lock-stitch continuous

D. Mattress continuous

E. Mattress interrupted

F. Retention suture bridge

Figure 4-24   Types of sutures.

■ Exercises: Surgical Interventions and Therapeutic Procedures

SIMPLE
RECALL

Exercise 15

Write the meaning of the term given.

1. dermatoplasty   _____

2. cauterization   _____

3. dermatoheteroplasty   _____

4. excision   _____

ADVANCED
RECALL

Exercise 16

Circle the term that is most appropriate for the meaning of the sentence.

1. The physician diagnosed the infected condition as a furuncle and treated it with (*incision and drainage, punch biopsy, suturing*) to release fluid.

2. The surgeon had to make a(n) (*incision, excision, suture*), or cut, into the patient's skin to remove the bullet lodged there.

3. Saline solution was used for (*cauterization, irrigation, punch biopsy*) to wash out the grass and dirt from the patient's laceration.

4. The child had a long, gaping wound on the back of his leg that needed to be closed, or (*excised, sutured, incised*).

5. When the young man was brought into the emergency department after his motorcycle accident, his wounds had to be (*cauterized, débrided, excised*) to remove foreign matter and debris before other treatment.

6. After suffering severe burns, Mr. Simone had several skin grafts, including (*dermatoautoplasty, dermatoheteroplasty, dermatoplasty*), which involved a graft using his own skin.

TERM
CONSTRUCTION

Exercise 17

Write the combining form used in the medical term, followed by the meaning of the combining form.

Term	Combining Form	Combining Form Meaning
1. rhytidoplasty	_____	_____
2. dermabrasion	_____	_____
3. cryosurgery	_____	_____
4. electrodesiccation	_____	_____
5. rhytidectomy	_____	_____
6. dermatome	_____	_____

Medications and Drug Therapies

Term	Pronunciation	Meaning
antifungal	an'tē-fŭng'găl	drug used to kill fungi
antiinfective	an'tē-in-fek'tiv	drug used to decrease or remove infection
antiinflammatory	an'tē-in-flam'ă-tōr-ē	drug used to decrease inflammation
antipruritic	an'tē-prūr-it'ik	drug used to relieve itching
intralesional injection	intra-lē'zhŭn-al in-jek'shŭn	injecting medications into a lesion or scar
liquid nitrogen	lik'wid nī'trŏ-jĕn	gas used in cryosurgery to remove a verruca or other lesion
pediculicide	pĕ-dik'yū-li-sīd	medication used to kill lice
scabicide	skā'bi-sīd	medication used to kill mites associated with scabies
steroid	ster'oyd	drug used to treat many inflammatory skin conditions

■ Exercise: Medications and Drug Therapies

SIMPLE
RECALL

Exercise 18

Write the correct medication or drug therapy term for the meaning given.

1. treats inflammatory skin conditions _____

2. decreases or removes infection

3. kills fungi

4. kills lice

5. decreases inflammation

6. gas used in cryosurgery for verruca or other lesions

7. relieves itching

8. injecting medications into a lesion

9. kills mites that cause scabies

Specialties and Specialists

Term	Pronunciation	Meaning
dermatology	dĕr′mă-tol′ŏ-jē	a medical specialty focusing on the study and treatment of disorders of the skin
dermatologist	dĕr′mă-tol′ŏ-jist	physician who specializes in dermatology
medical esthetician	med′i-kăl es-thet′i-shun	licensed professional in the field of cosmetic beauty

■ Exercise: Specialties and Specialists

SIMPLE
RECALL

Exercise 19

Write the correct medical term for the meaning given.

1. a professional in the field of cosmetic beauty

2. specialist in the study of skin

3. specialty focusing on the study and treatment of skin

Abbreviations

Abbreviation	Meaning
Bx	biopsy
C&S	culture and sensitivity
ED&C	electrodesiccation and curettage
FS	frozen section
I&D	incision and drainage
PPD	purified protein derivative

■ Exercises: Abbreviations

SIMPLE
RECALL

Exercise 20

Write the meaning of each abbreviation.

1. PPD _____

2 C&S _____

3. I&D _____

ADVANCED
RECALL

Exercise 21

Match each abbreviation with the appropriate description.

ED&C   bx   FS

Meaning   **Abbreviation**

1. slice of tissue from a frozen specimen   _____

2. removing tissue for microscopic examination   _____

3. burning off of skin growths   _____

Review of Terms for Anatomy and Physiology

VISUAL

Exercise 22

Write the correct terms on the blanks for the anatomic structures indicated.

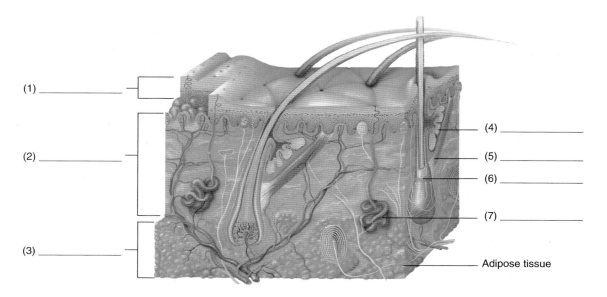

(1) _____

(2) _____

(3) _____

(4) _____

(5) _____

(6) _____

(7) _____

Adipose tissue

Understanding Term Structure

TERM
CONSTRUCTION

Exercise 23

Write the combining form(s) used in the medical term, followed by the meaning of the combining form(s).

Term	Combining Form(s)	Combining Form Meaning(s)
1. hidrosis	_____	_____
2. keratosis	_____	_____
3. cryosurgery	_____	_____
4. dermatology	_____	_____
5. scleroderma	_____	_____

6. onychomycosis _____   _____

7. rhytidectomy _____   _____

8. pyosis _____   _____

9. lipectomy _____   _____

10. seborrhea _____   _____

11. dermatomycosis _____   _____

12. subcutaneous _____   _____

TERM
CONSTRUCTION

Exercise 24

Break the given medical term into its word parts and define each part. Then define the medical term.

For example:
dermatitis   *word parts:*   dermat/o / -itis
                              meanings: skin / inflammation of
                              term meaning: inflammation of the skin

1. anhidrosis   *word parts:*   _____ / _____ / _____

                              meanings: _____ / _____ / _____

                              term meaning: _____

2. erythrocyanosis   *word parts:*   _____ / _____ / _____

                              meanings: _____ / _____ / _____

                              term meaning: _____

3. trichopathy   *word parts:*   _____ / _____

                              meanings: _____ / _____

                              term meaning: _____

4. pyoderma   *word parts:*   _____ / _____

                              meanings: _____ / _____

                              term meaning: _____

5. paronychia

word parts: _____ / _____ / _____

meanings: _____ / _____ / _____

term meaning: _____

6. dermatologist

word parts: _____ / _____

meanings: _____ / _____

term meaning: _____

7. transdermal

word parts: _____ / _____ / _____

meanings: _____ / _____ / _____

term meaning: _____

8. dermatoheteroplasty

word parts: _____ / _____ / _____

meanings: _____ / _____ / _____

term meaning: _____

9. pachyderma

word parts: _____ / _____

meanings: _____ / _____

term meaning: _____

10. onychomalacia

word parts: _____ / _____

meanings: _____ / _____

term meaning: _____

11. cyanosis

word parts: _____ / _____

meanings: _____ / _____

term meaning: _____

12. onychophagia

word parts: _____ / _____

meanings: _____ / _____

term meaning: _____

13. intradermal

word parts: _____ / _____ / _____

meanings: _____ / _____ / _____

term meaning: _____

14. xeroderma   *word parts:*   _____ / _____

                       meanings: _____ / _____

                       term meaning: _____

Comprehension Exercises

Exercise 25

COMPREHENSION

Fill in the blank with the correct term.

1. The three layers of skin are the _____, the _____, and the _____.

2. Contraction of the _____ muscles causes hairs to stand up straight.

3. The filling of a dilated hair follicle with bacteria and sebum causes a(n) _____.

4. The _____ glands assist in body temperature regulation.

5. A licensed professional in the field of cosmetic beauty is called a(n) _____.

6. A bacterial infection that includes a collection of pus is called a(n) _____.

7. A facelift is the surgical repair of wrinkles, also known as _____.

8. _____ and blood vessels make up the subcutaneous layer of the skin.

9. When reading the tuberculin skin test, the medical assistant determines the amount of _____ (or hardened) tissue around the site of the injection.

10. White patches of various sizes on the skin caused from a decrease in melanocytes indicate a condition called _____.

11. _____, a fungal infection of the hair, skin, and nails, causes ringlike lesions on the skin.

12. A(n) _____ develops when the skin surface is scratched.

13. A(n) _____ is caused by infection of a hair follicle.

14. Gangrene results from the _____ of tissue due to lack of blood flow.

15. Athlete's foot is a type of fungal infection called _____.

16. A child born without pigment in the skin, eyes, and hair would be diagnosed with _____.

17. A(n) _____ occurs when a tear extends deep into the dermis.

Exercise 26

COMPREHENSION

Circle the letter of the best answer in the following questions.

1. The type of burn that involves the dermis and epidermis is a:

   A. superficial burn
   B. partial-thickness burn
   C. full-thickness burn
   D. subcutaneous burn

2. What is the medical term for a flesh-colored elevation that is caused by a virus?

   A. papule
   B. purpura
   C. verruca
   D. comedo

3. When normal tissue is replaced by fibrous tissue it is called a(n):

   A. contusion
   B. cicatrix
   C. abscess
   D. fissure

4. Which term involves secretions from the sudoriferous glands?

   A. keratosis
   B. alopecia
   C. diaphoresis
   D. pruritus

5. What is the medical term for what may form after a partial-thickness burn occurs?

   A. piloerections
   B. nodules
   C. melanocytes
   D. vesicles

6. Which layer of skin is affected in a superficial burn?

   A. dermis
   B. subdermis
   C. dermal layer
   D. epidermis

7. Which combining form refers to the secretions that come from the sebaceous gland?

   A. seb/o
   B. sudor/o
   C. hidr/o
   D. hydr/o

8. The medical term for a mole is a:

   A. sarcoma
   B. carbuncle
   C. nevus
   D. cyst

9. A raised reddish lesion that may be caused by an allergen is called a:

   A. macule
   B. wheal
   C. keratin
   D. dermatome

Exercise 27

COMPREHENSION

Fill in the blank with the correct term.

1. A treatment for acne scars that involves the use of abrasive material is known as _____.

2. A lesion that is contained within a certain area is said to be _____.

3. A surgical procedure that is used to remove gangrenous tissue is called _____.

4. A(n) _____ is a collection of abscesses in a group of hair follicles.

5. The fungal infection that can affect various areas of the body is called _____.

6. An infection that is more commonly found in children and involves the face is known as

 _____.

7. Itchy wheals related to an allergy are known as hives or _____.

8. The condition that involves fungi around the nail is called _____.

9. The physician who performs an allergy test on the skin may call it a(n) _____

 test.

10. An instrument called a(n) _____ is used as a part of a skin graft procedure.

Application and Analysis

Exercise 28

APPLICATION **Read the case reports and circle the letter of your answer choice for the questions that follow.**

CASE 4-1

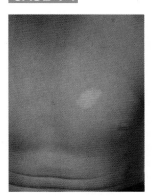

A young man visited his dermatologist because he noticed a macular rash on his chest (Fig. 4-25). The rash had been present for several weeks and was pruritic.

Figure 4-25 Macular rash on chest.

1. The term *macular* means that the rash is:

    A. flat
    B. raised
    C. purulent
    D. the same color as the surrounding skin

2. Because the rash was pruritic, what type of medication do you think the physician prescribed?

    A. scabicide
    B. antiitch

    C. steroid
    D. antiinfective

3. The suffix *-logist* means:

    A. study of
    B. softening
    C. disease
    D. one who specializes in

CASE 4-2

A class of preschool students experienced a scabies outbreak. All afflicted children presented with erythematous areas on their hands and on other areas where clothing was tight. All the affected areas also showed excoriations due to the extreme pruritus.

4. The excoriations are known in layman's terms as:

    A. bruises
    B. scabs
    C. scratches
    D. warts

5. Scabies is caused by:

    A. a fungus
    B. poison ivy

    C. lice
    D. mites

6. Treatment for scabies is through the use of a(n):

    A. scabicide
    B. antimite tablet
    C. antipruritic medication
    D. antifungal

CASE 4-3

When the patient arrived in the clinic, the medical assistant noticed a group of verrucae on the lateral aspect of the patient's ankle. She informed the physician and they prepared to remove the verrucae with electrodesiccation and curettage.

7. Verrucae is the plural form of the medical term more commonly known as:

    A. hives
    B. warts
    C. comedos
    D. papules

8. As the medical assistant prepared the patient for the procedure, she informed him that the physician would:

    A. use cryosurgery to remove the verrucae
    B. use ultraviolet radiation to remove the verrucae
    C. give the patient an antifungal to use when he got home
    D. use electrical current to remove the verrucae

MEDICAL RECORD ANALYSIS

MEDICAL RECORD 4-1

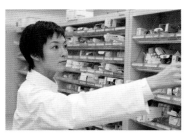

A patient was seen in the emergency room this afternoon for an accidental burn. You, as a pharmacy technician, are assisting the pharmacist in dispensing a prescription for acetaminophen with codeine as prescribed by the emergency room physician.

A pharmacy technician helps dispense prescriptions to patients.

Medical Record

SUPERFICIAL AND PARTIAL THICKNESS BURNS

SUBJECTIVE: This is an emergency visit for a 20-year-old man who accidentally knocked over a pot of boiling water onto his left leg and foot. He is complaining of extreme pain. He stated that he used some aloe on his leg and foot immediately after the accident occurred. Because of the continued pain, he presented to the office to ensure that the burn was nothing more than superficial.

OBJECTIVE: BP 130/76; P 98; T 98.6°F. This is a well-developed, well-nourished young man who presents with a reddened and blistered area on the anterior aspect of his left leg and on the dorsum of the left foot. Some of the blisters have broken and are weeping.

ASSESSMENT: Superficial and partial-thickness burns on the anterior aspect of the left lower leg and dorsum of the left foot.

PLAN: The patient was prescribed acetaminophen with codeine to take one every 4 hours p.r.n. for pain. The area was treated with silver sulfadiazine for possible infection. The patient was instructed to change the dressing daily and was given supplies to do this. He was instructed to return in 3 days for a recheck.

Exercise 29

APPLICATION

Read the medical report and circle the letter of your answer choice for the following questions.

1. What type of medication is silver sulfadiazine?

   A. antipruritic
   B. antifungal
   C. antiinfective
   D. antibiotic

2. A superficial burn involves the:

   A. dermis and the epidermis
   B. dermis and subcutaneous layer
   C. dermis, epidermis, and subcutaneous layer
   D. epidermis

3. A partial-thickness burn involves the:

   A. dermis and the epidermis

   B. dermis and subcutaneous layer

   C. dermis, epidermis, and subcutaneous layer

   D. epidermis

Bonus Question

4. Recalling the meaning of the word part *dors/o*, where is the dorsum of the foot?

_____

MEDICAL RECORD 4-2

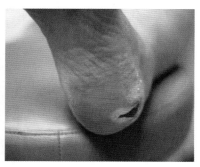

You are a nursing assistant (NA) in a long-term care facility. One of your assignments is to reposition patients who are unable to move properly on their own. As you are moving a patient from the supine position onto her right side, you notice an area on her heel that you report to the physician (Fig. 4-27). The physician examined the patient and wrote the following note.

Figure 4-27 Stage II decubitus ulcer on heel.

Medical Record

DECUBITUS ULCER

SUBJECTIVE: Nursing assistant noticed an area of broken skin on the right heel of the patient.

OBJECTIVE: This 83-year-old female is cachetic from her long-standing Alzheimer's disease and refusal to take in sufficient nutrition. She is fed by way of nasogastric tube, which she has been known to pull out. Her weight is 110 pounds.

Her skin turgor is poor, and the area of broken skin is erythematous and shiny. Some areas of blackness are noted around the edges.

ASSESSMENT: C&S will be performed on a swab from the area in question. It appears to be a stage II starting into stage III decubitus ulcer. At this point, it has not developed to the point where there is any necrotic tissue that needs to be débrided.

PLAN: The patient will be turned on a more frequent basis. The timeframe will be increased from every 2 hours to every hour. Her tube feedings will have increased calories and protein to promote wound healing. The wound will be cleaned with normal saline. If the C&S comes back positive, the patient will be started on antibiotics. The heel area will be placed on an egg crate mattress when she is in the supine position.

Exercise 30

APPLICATION **Read the medical report and circle the letter of your answer choice for the following questions.**

1. The area of broken skin on the right heel of the patient appears to be a(n):

   A. fissure
   B. decubitus ulcer
   C. excoriation
   D. necrosis

2. C&S is the abbreviation used when the physician wants:

   A. to find out if there is infection
   B. to perform a surgical procedure

   C. to bill for more tests
   D. to increase tube feeding times

3. Necrotic tissue is:

   A. red and full of turgor
   B. red but has no turgor
   C. black due to lack of blood flow
   D. black and is full of turgor

Bonus Question

4. The combining form *nas/o* means *nose*. Based on this meaning and the word parts learned in previous chapters, define the term *nasogastric*.

_____

Pronunciation and Spelling

Exercise 31

AUDITORY **Review the Chapter 4 terms in the Dictionary/Audio Glossary in the Student Resources and practice pronouncing each term, referring to the pronunciation guide as needed.**

Exercise 32

SPELLING **Circle the correct spelling of each term.**

1. anhydrosis   anhidrosis   enhydrosis

2. sicatricks   cixatrix   cicatrix

3. dermatomycosis   dermotamycosis   dermatomicosis

4. onychofagia   unicoophagia   onychophagia

5. erticareia   urtycaria   urticaria

6. soriasis	psoriasis	psoryasis
7. gangreen	ganrene	gangrene
8. tinyea	tinia	tinea
9. dysplasia	displazia	dysplasai
10. puritic	pureitic	pruritic
11. keritogenic	kerratagenic	keratogenic
12. zeraderma	xeraderma	xeroderma
13. jawndice	jaundice	jandice
14. erythematous	erathematus	eryathematous
15. arrector pili	arector pili	erector pili

Media Connection

STUDENT
RESOURCES

Exercise 33

Complete each of the following activities available with the Student Resources. Check off each activity as you complete it, and record your score for the Chapter Quiz in the space provided.

____ Flash Cards   ____ Break It Down

____ Concentration   ____ True/False Body Building

____ Abbreviation Match-Up   ____ Quiz Show

____ Roboterms   ____ Complete the Case

____ Word Builder   ____ Medical Record Review

____ Fill the Gap

____ Look and Label   ____ Spelling Bee

____ Image Matching

____ **Chapter Quiz**   *Score:* _____%

Additional Resources

____ Dictionary/Audio Glossary

____ Health Professions Careers: Pharmacy Technician

____ Health Professions Careers: Nursing Assistant

Digestive System

5

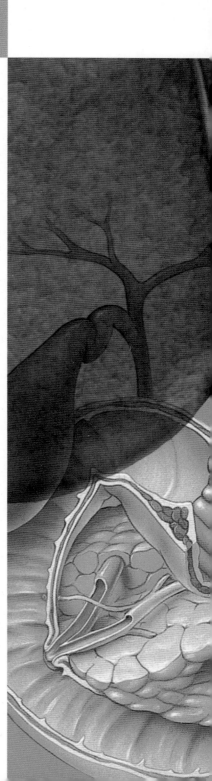

Chapter Outline

Objectives

After completion of this chapter you will be able to:

1. Identify the functions of the digestive system and its major and accessory structures.

2. Define terms related to the digestive system.

3. Define combining forms, prefixes, and suffixes related to the digestive system.

4. Define common medical terminology related to the digestive system, including adjectives and related terms, symptoms and conditions, tests and procedures, surgical interventions and therapeutic procedures, medications and drug therapies, and specialties.

5. Explain abbreviations for terms related to the digestive system.

6. Successfully complete all chapter exercises.

7. Explain terms used in case studies and medical records involving the digestive system.

8. Successfully complete all pronunciation and spelling exercises, and complete all interactive exercises included with the companion Student Resources.

■ ANATOMY AND PHYSIOLOGY

Functions

■ To intake food to provide nutrients to the body
■ To break down food into usable nutrients
■ To absorb nutrients from the breakdown of food
■ To eliminate the solid waste products not used by the body

Organs and Structures

■ The digestive system is composed of the digestive tract and its associated glands and organs.
■ The digestive tract leads from the mouth to the anus through the pharynx, esophagus, stomach, and intestines.
■ The digestive tract is also known as the gastrointestinal (GI) tract or the alimentary canal.

Terms Related to the Digestive System

Term	Pronunciation	Meaning
Primary Digestive Structures and Organs (Fig. 5-1)		
mouth, *syn.* oral cavity	mowth, ōr'ăl kav'i-tē	opening where food enters the body and undergoes the first process of digestion
palate	pal'ăt	the roof of the mouth; separates the oral cavity from the nasal cavity
uvula	yū'vyū-lă	small piece of tissue that hangs in the posterior portion of the oral cavity
tongue	tŭng	muscular organ at the floor of the mouth; assists in swallowing and speaking
teeth	tēth	structures that provide the hard surfaces needed for mastication
salivary glands	sal'i-var-ē glandz	saliva-secreting glands in the oral cavity; include the parotid, sublingual, and submandibular glands
saliva	să-lī'vă	clear, tasteless, odorless fluid that helps to lubricate food in the mouth
pharynx, *syn.* throat	far'ingks, thrōt	space behind the mouth that serves as a passage for food from the mouth to the esophagus and for air from the nose and mouth to the larynx
esophagus	ĕ-sof'ă-gŭs	muscular tube that moves food from the pharynx to the stomach
stomach	stŏm'ăk	saclike organ in which the chemical part of digestion begins (Fig. 5-2)
cardia	kahr'dē-ă	area where the esophagus connects to the stomach

(continued)

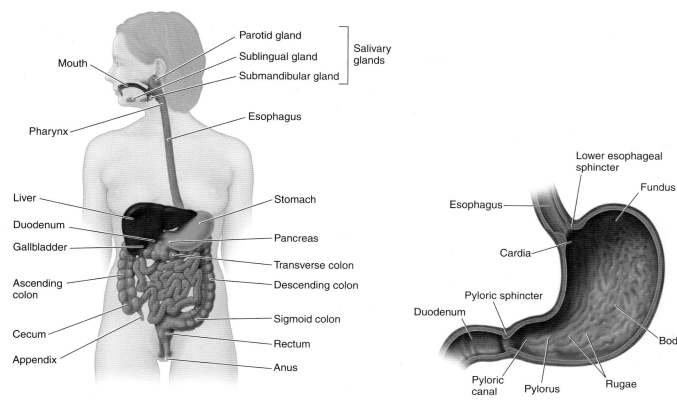

Figure 5-1 The digestive system.

Figure 5-2 The stomach and its sections.

Terms Related to the Digestive System *(continued)*

Term	Pronunciation	Meaning
fundus	fŭn′dŭs	superior domed portion of the stomach
body	bod′ē	largest part of the stomach, between the fundus and pylorus
pylorus	pī-lōr′ŭs	lower part of the stomach that connects to the small intestine
rugae	rū′gē	folds in the stomach lining that increase the surface area for absorption of nutrients
small intestine	smawl in-tes′tin	long hollow tube where most absorption of nutrients occurs (Fig. 5-3)
duodenum	dū′ō-dē′nŭm	first section of the small intestine
jejunum	je-jū′nŭm	the middle section of the small intestine
ileum	il′ē-ŭm	the terminal part of the small intestine that connects to the large intestine
large intestine	lahrj in-tes′tin	large tube where water is reabsorbed and solid waste products are produced (Fig. 5-3)
cecum	sē′kŭm	first portion of the large intestine
appendix, *syn.* vermiform appendix	ă-pen′diks, vĕr′mi-fōrm ă-pen′diks	fingerlike projection off the cecum of the large intestine

(continued)

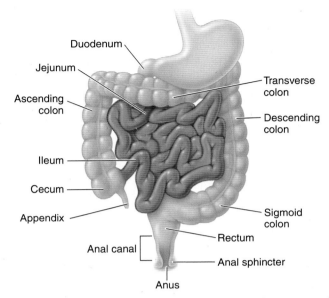

Figure 5-3 The small and large intestines.

Terms Related to the Digestive System *(continued)*

Term	Pronunciation	Meaning
colon	kō′lŏn	portion of the large intestine that extends from the cecum to the rectum
ascending colon	ă-send′ing kō′lŏn	the portion of the large intestine that lies on the right side arising from the cecum and joins to the transverse colon
transverse colon	trans-vĕrs′ kō′lŏn	area of large intestine between the ascending colon and descending colon
descending colon	dĕ-send′ing kō′lŏn	section of the large intestine that follows the transverse colon
sigmoid colon	sig′moyd kō′lŏn	terminal portion of the large intestine that joins with the rectum
rectum	rek′tŭm	extension of the large intestine that is a pouch that holds solid waste material before elimination from the body
anus	ā′nŭs	exit from the large intestine to the outside of the body
Accessory Digestive Organs (Fig. 5-4)		
liver	liv′ĕr	large organ that produces and secretes bile into the gallbladder
bile	bīl	fluid that is secreted by the liver into the duodenum and aids in digestion
gallbladder	gawl′blad-ĕr	organ located behind the liver that stores bile and sends it to the duodenum
pancreas	pan′krē-ăs	organ that secretes pancreatic juices into the small intestine that assist in digestion

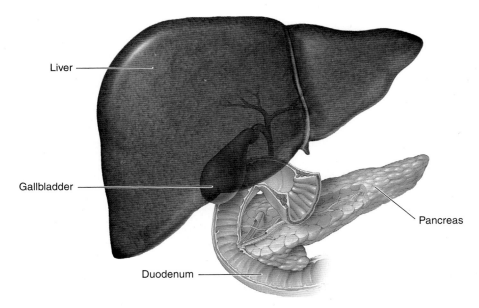

Figure 5-4   Accessory organs of the digestive system.

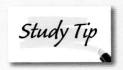 **Study Tip**

Spelling homonyms—ilium and ileum *Ilium* and *ileum* are homonyms; that is, they are spelled differently but sound alike. Here is an easy way to remember the difference in meaning—and spelling. *Ilium* is the upper section of the hip bone, and both *hip* and *ilium* contain the letter "i." For *ileum*, remember that it is part of the small intestine and that both *intestine* and its combining form *enter/o* contain the letter "e."

ANIMATION

Learn more about digestion and the organs involved in the digestion process by viewing the animation General Digestion *on the Student Resources.*

■ Exercises: Anatomy and Physiology

SIMPLE
RECALL

Exercise 1

Write the correct anatomic structure for the meaning given.

1. middle section of the small intestine   _____

2. fingerlike projection located on the large intestine   _____

3. organ that stores bile   _____

4. site where food enters the body   _____

5. the roof of the mouth   _____

6. medical term for throat   _____

7. superior portion of stomach   _____

8. organ that secretes bile   _____

9. portion of small intestine that connects with large intestine   _____

10. structure through which solid wastes pass to exterior of body _____

11. structures that secrete saliva   _____

12. fluid secreted by the liver   _____

ADVANCED
RECALL

Exercise 2

Match each medical term with its meaning.

rugae   esophagus   rectum   cecum   sigmoid colon
duodenum   pancreas   descending colon   uvula   pylorus

Meaning   **Term**

1. first section of the small intestine   _____

2. organ that secretes juices that aid in digestion   _____

3. muscular tube that moves food to the stomach   _____

4. portion of colon between the rectum and the descending colon   _____

5. section of stomach that connects to the small intestine _____

6. area where solid waste is temporarily stored   _____

7. first section of the large intestine   _____

8. portion of the colon following the transverse colon   _____

9. structure that hangs in the oral cavity   _____

10. folds in the stomach lining   _____

ADVANCED
RECALL

Exercise 3

Circle the term that is most appropriate for the meaning of the sentence.

1. The (*duodenum, stomach, large intestine*) is where chemical digestion begins.

2. Located in the mouth, the (*uvula, pharynx, teeth*) provide the hard surfaces
   for mastication.

3. The (*transverse, ascending, sigmoid*) colon is the second portion of the colon.

4. The muscular organ on the floor of the mouth is called the (*palate, tongue, uvula*).

5. The large intestine reabsorbs (*food, waste, water*) and produces solid waste products.

6. The area of the stomach where the esophagus connects is called the (*fundus, cardia, body*).

7. The small intestine is made up of (*two, three, four*) parts.

8. The fluid that helps lubricate food in the mouth is called (*bile, saliva, rugae*).

9. The largest part of the stomach is called the (*body, fundus, pylorus*).

10. The (*ascending, descending, sigmoid*) colon arises from the cecum and joins the transverse colon.

■ WORD PARTS

Note that some word parts that have been introduced earlier in the book may not be repeated here.

Combining Forms

Combining Form	Meaning
aliment/o	nutrition
an/o	anus
appendic/o	appendix
bil/o	bile
bucc/o	cheek
cec/o	cecum
chol/e	gall, bile
cholecyst/o	gallbladder
col/o, colon/o	colon
duoden/o	duodenum
enter/o	small intestine
esophag/o	esophagus
diverticul/o	diverticulum
gastr/o	stomach
hemat/o, hem/o	blood
hepat/o	liver
herni/o	hernia
ile/o	ileum

(continued)

Combining Forms (continued)

Combining Form	Meaning
jejun/o	jejunum
labi/o, cheil/o	lip
lapar/o, abdomin/o	abdomen
lingu/o	tongue
lith/o	stone, calculus
odont/o, dent/o	tooth
or/o, stomat/o	mouth
palat/o	palate
pancreat/o	pancreas
peps/o	digestion
phag/o	eat, swallow
pharyng/o	pharynx
polyp/o	polyp
proct/o	rectum and anus
pylor/o	pylorus
rect/o	rectum
sial/o	saliva
sigmoid/o	sigmoid colon

Prefixes

Prefix	Meaning
endo-	in, within
hyper-	above, excessive
peri-	around, surrounding
post-	after, behind
retro-	backward, behind

Suffixes

Suffix	Meaning
-algia, -dynia	pain
-ase	enzyme
-cele	herniation, protrusion
-centesis	puncture to aspirate
-emesis	vomiting
-gen	origin, production
-gram	record, recording
-graphy	process of recording

(continued)

Suffixes *(continued)*

Suffix	Meaning
-iasis	condition of
-logist	one who specializes in
-logy	study of
-malacia	softening
-megaly	enlargement
-prandial	meal
-ptosis	prolapse, drooping, sagging
-rrhaphy	suture
-scope	instrument for examination
-scopy	process of examining, examination
-stenosis	stricture, narrowing
-stomy	surgical opening
-tomy	incision
-tripsy	crushing

■ Exercises: Word Parts

SIMPLE
RECALL

Exercise 4

Write the meaning of the combining form given.

1. duoden/o _____

2. stomat/o _____

3. pancreat/o _____

4. enter/o _____

5. cheil/o _____

6. sial/o _____

7. hepat/o _____

8. bucc/o _____

9. an/o _____

10. peps/o _____

11. pharyng/o _____

12. proct/o _____

13. pylor/o _____

14. col/o _____

15. sigmoid/o _____

16. odont/o _____

17. lapar/o _____

Exercise 5

SIMPLE
RECALL

Write the correct combining form(s) for the meaning given.

1. jejunum _____

2. appendix _____

3. swallow _____

4. blood _____

5. stomach _____

6. esophagus _____

7. cheek _____

8. rectum _____

9. polyp _____

10. gallbladder _____

11. cecum _____

12. tongue _____

13. ileum _____

14. tooth _____

15. colon _____

16. stone, calculus _____

17. palate _____

18. bile _____

19. hernia _____

20. abdomen _____

21. nutrition _____

Exercise 6

SIMPLE RECALL

Write the meaning of the prefix or suffix given.

1. endo- _____

2. -tripsy _____

3. -ase _____

4. peri- _____

5. -stomy _____

6. -iasis _____

7. -logist _____

8. -cele _____

9. -gen _____

10. -megaly _____

11. retro- _____

12. -ptosis _____

13. -scopy _____

14. -prandial _____

15. post- _____

16. hyper- _____

17. -dynia _____

18. -malacia _____

19. -graphy _____

20. -emesis _____

21. -scope _____

22. -centesis _____

23. -stenosis _____

24. -gram   _____

25. -rrhaphy   _____

26. -algia   _____

27. -tomy   _____

ADVANCED
RECALL

Exercise 7

Considering the meaning of the combining form from which the medical term is made, write the meaning of the medical term. (You have not yet learned many of these terms but can build their meanings from the word parts.)

Combining Form	Meaning	Medical Term	Meaning of Term
pancreat/o	pancreas	pancreatitis	1. _____
sigmoid/o	sigmoid colon	sigmoidoscope	2. _____
aliment/o	nutrition	alimentary	3. _____
col/o	colon	colostomy	4. _____
cholecyst/o	gallbladder	cholecystectomy	5. _____
diverticul/o	diverticulum	diverticulitis	6. _____

TERM
CONSTRUCTION

Exercise 8

Build a medical term for each meaning using one of the listed combining forms and one of the listed suffixes.

Combining Forms		Suffixes	
gastr/o	lith/o	-logist	-al
abdomin/o	hepat/o	-itis	-centesis
an/o	proct/o	-scopy	-ectomy
bucc/o	colon/o	-tripsy	-plasty

1. one who specializes in disorders of the rectum and anus   _____

2. inflammation of the liver   _____

3. pertaining to the cheek   _____

4. crushing of stones   _____

5. puncture to aspirate (fluid) from the abdomen   _____

6. surgical repair of the anus   _____

7. surgical removal of the stomach _____

8. process of examining the colon _____

Exercise 9

TERM CONSTRUCTION

Build a medical term from an appropriate combining form and suffix, given their meanings.

Use Combining Form for	Use Suffix for	Term
1. esophagus	inflammation	_____
2. appendix	surgical removal	_____
3. stomach	examination	_____
4. colon	surgical opening	_____
5. lip	suture	_____
6. abdomen	incision	_____
7. gallbladder	record, recording	_____
8. mouth	pertaining to	_____
9. nutrition	pertaining to	_____
10. liver	inflammation	_____
11. pancreas	disease	_____

Exercise 10

TERM CONSTRUCTION

Break the given medical term into its word parts and define each part. Then define the medical term.

For example:

appendicitis	*word parts:*	appendic/o / -itis
	meanings:	appendix / inflammation of
	term meaning:	inflammation of the appendix

1. gastroenterologist   *word parts:*   _____ / _____ / _____

meanings: _____ / _____ / _____

term meaning: _____

2. dyspepsia   *word parts:*   _____ / _____ / _____

meanings: _____ / _____ / _____

term meaning: _____

3. hyperemesis   *word parts:*   _____ / _____

                               meanings: _____ / _____

                               term meaning: _____

4. colectomy   *word parts:*   _____ / _____

                               meanings: _____ / _____

                               term meaning: _____

5. herniorrhaphy   *word parts:*   _____ / _____

                               meanings: _____ / _____

                               term meaning: _____

6. dysphagia   *word parts:*   _____ / _____ / _____

                               meanings: _____ / _____ / _____

                               term meaning: _____

7. cholelithiasis   *word parts:*   _____ / _____ / _____

                               meanings: _____ / _____ / _____

                               term meaning: _____

8. hematemesis   *word parts:*   _____ / _____

                               meanings: _____ / _____

                               term meaning: _____

9. rectocele   *word parts:*   _____ / _____

                               meanings: _____ / _____

                               term meaning: _____

10. palatoplasty   *word parts:*   _____ / _____

                               meanings: _____ / _____

                               term meaning: _____

11. ileostomy   *word parts:*   _____ / _____

                               meanings: _____ / _____

                               term meaning: _____

12. sublingual   *word parts:*   _____ / _____ / _____

                         meanings: _____ / _____ / _____

                         term meaning: _____

■ MEDICAL TERMS

Adjectives and Other Related Terms

Term	Pronunciation	Meaning
anorexia	an'ŏ-rek'sē-ă	decreased appetite
bolus	bō'lŭs	a moistened bit of food that is ready for deglutition/swallowing
chyme	kīm	partially digested food that passes into the duodenum
defecation, *syn.* bowel movement (BM)	def-ĕ-kā'shun, bow'ĕl mūv'mĕnt	passage of solid waste products through the rectum and anus
deglutition	dē-glū-tish'ŭn	the act of swallowing
digestion	di-jes'chŭn	the process of converting food into usable energy and waste products
eructation	ē-rŭk-tā'shŭn	the voiding of gas or acid fluid from the stomach through the mouth; commonly called a burp or belch
feces	fē'sēz	solid waste products
flatus	flā'tŭs	gas that passes through the anus
halitosis	hal-i-tō'sis	bad breath
hematochezia	hē'mă-tō-kē'zē-ă	the passage of bloody stools
inguinal	ing'gwi-năl	relating to the groin
mastication	mas'ti-kā'shŭn	chewing
melena	mĕ-lē'nă	black, tarry stools due to the presence of occult blood
nausea	naw'zē-ă	the urge to vomit
occult blood	ŏ-kŭlt' blŭd	blood in the feces in amounts that are too small to be seen by the naked eye

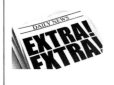 **FECAL OCCULT BLOOD TEST** The easiest and first screening test performed to check for colon cancer involves checking the feces for hidden blood. This test, called the fecal occult blood test (or FOBT) can also be used to check for bleeding in the digestive tract, which can be a cause of anemia. The FOBT can be done at home by the patient or in the office by the physician during a routine physical exam.

peristalsis	per'i-stal'sis	wavelike motion that moves substances through an open lumen such as the intestines (Fig. 5-5)
vomit, *syn.* regurgitate	vom'it, rē-gŭr'ji-tāt	to eject matter from the stomach through the mouth

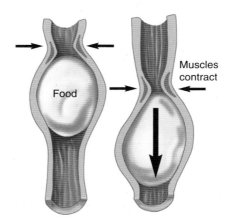

Figure 5-5 Peristalsis. The muscles in the esophagus contract to move food toward the stomach.

■ Exercises: Adjectives and Other Related Terms

Exercise 11

SIMPLE RECALL

Circle the term that is most appropriate for the meaning of the sentence.

1. To remove gas from the body through the oral cavity is called (*flatus, vomit, eructation*).

2. Blood that is hidden in the stools is known as (*halitosis, occult, chyme*).

3. The solid waste products that are removed from the body are known as (*vomitus, melena, feces*).

4. Moving food through the digestive system using wavelike motions is known as (*peristalsis, regurgitation, retroflexed*).

5. The first step in the digestion of food is called (*regurgitation, mastication, eructation*).

6. Someone who has forgotten to brush her or his teeth may have a condition known as (*eructation, halitosis, flatus*).

7. The process of converting food into usable energy is (*peristalsis, digestion, mastication*).

8. A moistened bit of food that is ready for swallowing is called a (*bolus, chyme, feces*).

9. Another term that means having a bowel movement is (*mastication, defecation, peristalsis*).

10. The term hematochezia means the passing of (*vomit, bloody stools, chyme*).

ADVANCED RECALL

Exercise 12

Match each medical term with its meaning.

melena	nausea	deglutition	flatus
inguinal	chyme	vomit	anorexia

Meaning   **Term**

1. swallowing   _____

2. black, tarry stools   _____

3. relating to the groin   _____

4. the urge to vomit   _____

5. gas that passes through the anus   _____

6. partially digested food   _____

7. to eject matter from the stomach   _____

8. decreased appetite   _____

Symptoms and Medical Conditions

Term	Pronunciation	Meaning
anorexia nervosa	an-ō-rek′sē-ă něr-vō′să	eating disorder characterized by an extreme fear of becoming obese and by an aversion to eating
ascites	ă-sī′tēz	accumulation of fluid in the abdominal/peritoneal cavity (Fig. 5-6)
cholecystitis	kō′lě-sis-tī′tis	inflammation of the gallbladder
cholelithiasis	kō′le-li-thī′ă-sis	condition involving the presence of stones in the gallbladder (Fig. 5-7)
cirrhosis	sir-ō′sis	chronic liver disease characterized by gradual failure of liver cells and loss of blood flow in the liver
constipation	kon′sti-pā′shŭn	decreased number of bowel movements often associated with hard stools
Crohn disease, *syn.* regional enteritis	krōn di-zēz′, rē′jŭn-ăl en′těr-ī′tis	chronic enteritis of unknown cause characterized by deep ulcers and thickening of the intestine
diarrhea	dī′ă-rē′ă	abnormally frequent discharge of semi-solid or liquid feces
diverticulitis	dī′věr-tik′yū-lī′tis	inflammation of a diverticulum
diverticulum	dī′věr-tik′yū-lŭm	an abnormal pouch on the wall of a hollow organ that protrudes outward (Fig. 5-8)
dysentery	dis′ěn-ter′ē	a disease marked by frequent watery stools containing blood and mucus
gastric ulcer	gas′trik ŭl′sěr	an ulcer in the stomach
gastroenteritis	gas′trō-en-těr-ī′tis	inflammation of the stomach and intestines

(continued)

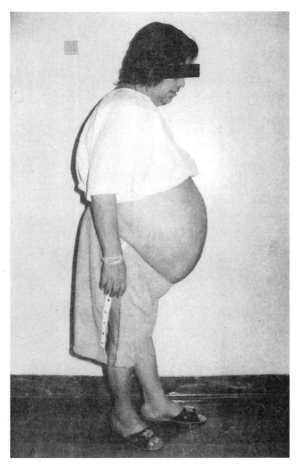

Figure 5-6   Patient with ascites as indicated by protruding abdomen.

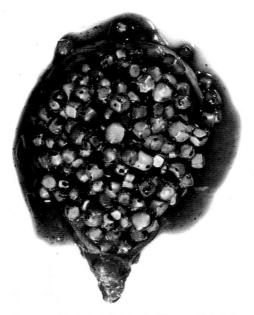

Figure 5-7   Cholelithiasis. The gallbladder has been opened to reveal numerous yellow cholesterol gallstones.

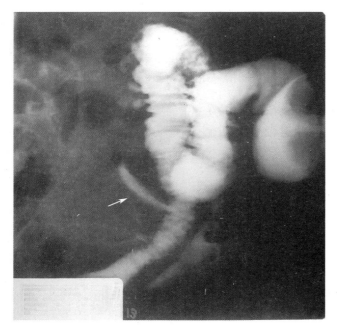

Figure 5-8   Barium enema showing ruptured diverticulum, which is the elongated extension off the intestine.

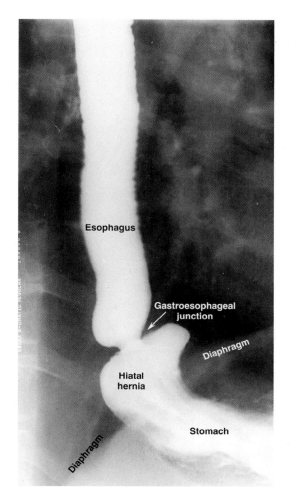

Figure 5-9   **X-ray of hiatal hernia.**

Symptoms and Medical Conditions *(continued)*

Term	Pronunciation	Meaning
gastroesophageal reflux disease (GERD)	gas′trō-ĕ-sŏ-fā′jē-ăl rē′flŭks di-zēz′	backward flow of stomach acid into the esophagus
hemorrhoids	hem′ŏr-oydz	varicose veins in the anal region; may be internal or external
hepatomegaly	hep′ă-tō-meg′ă-lē	enlargement of the liver
hiatal hernia	hī-ā′tăl hĕr′nē-ă	protrusion of a part of the stomach through the esophageal opening in the diaphragm (Fig. 5-9)
ileus	il′ē-ŭs	an obstruction of the intestine
incontinence	in-kon′ti-nĕns	inability to prevent the discharge of feces or urine
intussusception	in′tŭ-sŭ-sep′shŭn	the sliding (enfolding) of one section of the intestine into an adjacent section; much like the parts of a collapsible telescope (Fig. 5-10)
irritable bowel syndrome (IBS), *syn.* spastic colon	ir′i-tă-bĕl bow′ĕl sin′drōm, spas′tik kō′lŏn	painful intestinal disease characterized by alternating constipation with diarrhea
pancreatitis	pan′krē-ă-tī′tis	inflammation of the pancreas

(continued)

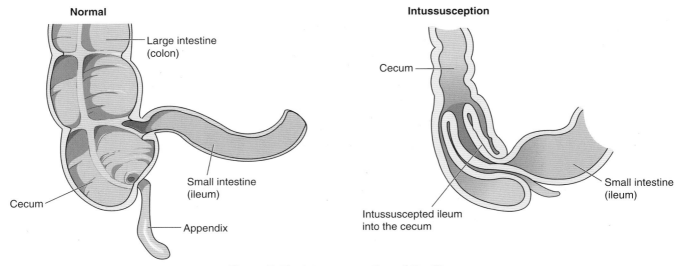

Normal

Intussusception

Large intestine (colon)

Cecum

Small intestine (ileum)

Appendix

Cecum

Small intestine (ileum)

Intussuscepted ileum into the cecum

Figure 5-10   Intussusception of the ilium.

Symptoms and Medical Conditions *(continued)*

Term	Pronunciation	Meaning
peptic ulcer, *syn.* peptic ulcer disease (PUD)	pep'tik ŭl'ser, pep'tik ŭl'ser di-zēz'	ulcer of the stomach or duodenum that is caused by gastric acid
peritonitis	per'i-tō-nī'tis	inflammation of the peritoneal cavity
polyp	pol'ip	section of tissue that grows abnormally and protrudes from a surface (Fig. 5-11)
polyposis	pol'i-pō'sis	condition of polyps
pruritus ani	prŭr-ī'tŭs ā'nī	itching around the opening of the anus
ulcerative colitis	ŭl'sĕr-ă-tiv kō-lī'tis	painful condition in which ulcers form in the colon and rectum (Fig. 5-12)
volvulus	vol'vyū-lŭs	a twisting of the intestine that can cause obstruction

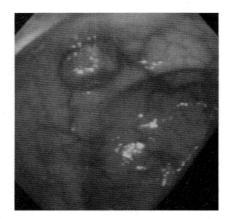

Figure 5-11   Polyp as seen through an endoscopic camera.

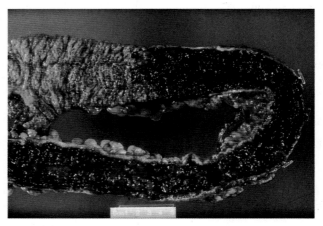

Figure 5-12   Ulcerative colitis of the ascending colon and rectosigmoid area.

■ Exercises: Symptoms and Medical Conditions

Exercise 13

SIMPLE RECALL

Write the correct medical term for the meaning given.

1. fluid in the abdominal cavity _____

2. eating disorder involving an aversion to eating _____

3. a twisting of the intestine _____

4. backward flow of stomach acids into the esophagus _____

5. chronic enteritis _____

6. an obstruction of the intestine _____

7. inability to prevent the discharge of feces or urine _____

8. anal itching _____

9. ulcer of the stomach _____

10. protrusion of the stomach through the diaphragm _____

Exercise 14

ADVANCED RECALL

Circle the term that is most appropriate for the meaning of the sentence.

1. During the sigmoidoscopy, Ms. Heller was found to have several abnormal pouches in her colon known as (*volvulus, intussusception, diverticula*).

2. After three treatments of peritoneal dialysis inflamed her peritoneum, Mrs. Jonas developed an infection that was diagnosed as (*cholecystitis, gastritis, peritonitis*).

3. Ms. Amity was constantly straining with bowel movements and subsequently began to have irregular bowel movements with hard and small stools. This is known as (*pancreatitis, constipation, polyposis*).

4. The medical assistant noticed that Ms. LaRocca had lost weight during her last four visits and asked Ms. LaRocca about her appetite. The patient stated she had lost interest in food and was not eating a normal amount each day. The physician is concerned that Ms. LaRocca has (*pruritus ani, ulcerative colitis, anorexia nervosa*).

5. Mr. Hernandez has a chronic disease with frequent watery, bloody diarrhea, which is called (*Crohn disease, gastroenteritis, dysentery*).

6. When the patient complained of extreme pain in the stomach, the physician ran tests for (*incontinence, peptic ulcer disease, hemorrhoids*).

7. The physician diagnosed Mr. Smith with the chronic liver disease called (*cholelithiasis, cholecystitis, cirrhosis*).

8. Mr. Hansen complained of abdominal pain, constipation and diarrhea and was found to have (*intussusception, irritable bowel syndrome, ulcerative colitis*).

9. During an endoscopic examination, Mrs. Reyes was found to have a (*pruritus ani, spastic colon, polyp*), which is a section of tissue that grows abnormally and protrudes from a surface.

10. After surgery, Ms. Adams was told that part of her intestine had folded inside itself, a condition known as (*intussusception, ileus, incontinence*).

TERM
CONSTRUCTION

Exercise 15

Using the given suffix, build a medical term for the meaning given.

Suffix	Meaning of Medical Term	Medical Term
-itis	inflammation of the pancreas	1. _____
-algia	pain in the stomach	2. _____
-osis	abnormal condition of polyps	3. _____
-itis	inflammation of the stomach and small intestine	4. _____
-megaly	enlargement of the liver	5. _____
-iasis	condition of gallstones	6. _____
-itis	inflammation of the gallbladder	7. _____

TERM
CONSTRUCTION

Exercise 16

Write the combining form used in the medical term, followed by the meaning of the combining form.

Term	Combining Form	Combining Form Meaning
1. polyposis	_____	_____
2. hepatomegaly	_____	_____
3. diverticulitis	_____	_____
4. esophageal	_____	_____
5. cholecystitis	_____	_____
6. stomatitis	_____	_____
7. hematemesis	_____	_____
8. appendicitis	_____	_____
9. dysphagia	_____	_____
10. cheilosis	_____	_____

Tests and Procedures

Term	Pronunciation	Meaning
Laboratory Tests		
Hemoccult test	hēm'ō-kŭlt' test	screening test used to determine the presence of hidden blood in feces
stool culture	stūl kŭl'chŭr	microscopic examination of feces for identification of possible pathogens
Diagnostic Procedures		
abdominal ultrasound	ab-dom'ĭ-năl ŭl'tră-sownd	use of sound waves to view digestive system organs/structures (Fig. 5-13)
abdominocentesis, *syn.* paracentesis	ab-dom'i-nō-sen-tē'sis, par'ă-sen-tē'sis	puncture into the abdomen to obtain fluid for culture or to relieve pressure
barium enema (BE)	bar'ē-ŭm en'ĕ-mă	use of contrast medium to view the lower gastrointestinal tract (Fig. 5-14)
cholecystogram	kō'lĕ-sis'tŏ-gram	x-ray record of the gallbladder
colonoscopy	kō'lŏn-os'kŏ-pē	process of examining the colon using an endoscope
endoscopy	en-dos'kŏ-pē	use of an endoscope to examine the inside of organs (Fig. 5-15)
esophagogastroduodenoscopy (EGD)	ĕ-sof'ă-gō-gas'trō-dū'ō-den-os'kŏ-pē	process of examining the esophagus, stomach, and duodenum, usually using a fiberoptic endoscope
flexible sigmoidoscopy	fleks'i-bĕl sig'moy-dos'kŏ-pē	examination using a fiberoptic endoscope to visualize the sigmoid colon and the descending colon (Fig. 5-16)
laparoscopy	lap'ă-ros'kŏ-pē	process of examining the abdominal area with a type of endoscope called a laparoscope (Fig. 5-17)
proctoscopy	prok-tos'kŏ-pē	process of examining the rectal and anal area with an endoscope
upper gastrointestinal series (UGI), *syn.* barium swallow	ŭp'ĕr gas'trō-in-tes'ti-năl sēr'ēz, bar'ē-ŭm swahl'ō	viewing of the stomach and the duodenum with the use of contrast medium

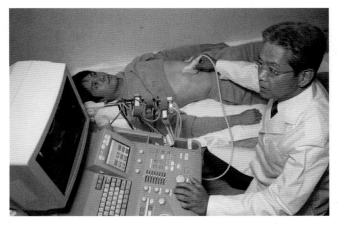

Figure 5-13 Abdominal ultrasound.

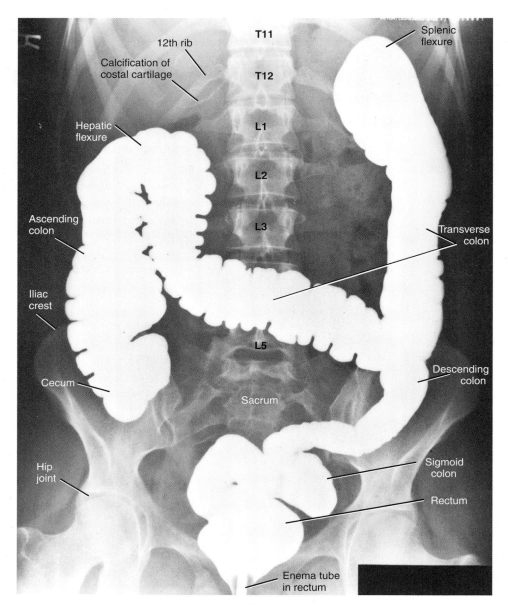

Figure 5-14   Barium enema.

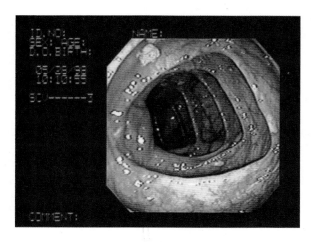

Figure 5-15   Endoscopic view of cecum.

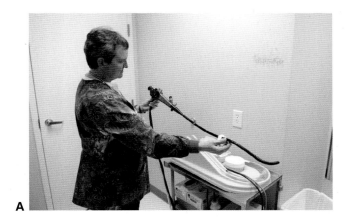

A

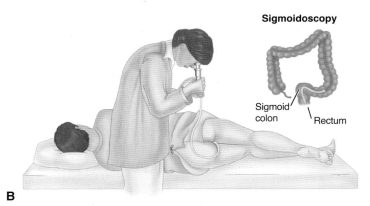

B

Sigmoidoscopy

Sigmoid colon

Rectum

Figure 5-16   A. Medical assistant prepares a flexible sigmoidoscope. B. Flexible sigmoidoscopy.

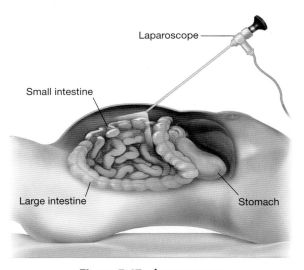

Laparoscope

Small intestine

Large intestine

Stomach

Figure 5-17   Laparoscopy.

■ Exercises: Tests and Procedures

SIMPLE
RECALL

Exercise 17

Circle the term that is most appropriate for the meaning of the sentence.

1. A microscopic examination of feces for identification of possible pathogens is called a (*Hemoccult test, proctoscopy, stool culture*).

2. A (*barium enema, barium swallow, colonoscopy*) is the viewing of the stomach and the duodenum with the use of contrast medium.

3. The use of an endoscope to examine the inside of organs is called (*endoscopy, colonoscopy, proctoscopy*).

4. Another name for abdominocentesis is (*barium enema, barium swallow, paracentesis*).

5. A (*Hemoccult test, stool culture, proctoscopy*) is a type of test used to locate hidden blood in the feces.

Exercise 18

ADVANCED RECALL

Complete each sentence by writing in the correct medical term.

1. The process of examining the rectal and anal area with an endoscope is called

   _____ .

2. Examination of the sigmoid and descending colon using a fiberoptic endoscope is called a(n)

   _____ .

3. The process of examining the colon is called _____ .

4. The use of sound waves to view the digestive system is called _____ .

5. The use of contrast medium to view the lower gastrointestinal tract is called a(n)

   _____ .

6. An x-ray record of the gallbladder is called a(n) _____ .

7. The process of examining the esophagus, the stomach, and the duodenum is called

   _____ .

Exercise 19

TERM CONSTRUCTION

Write the combining form used in the medical term, followed by the meaning of the combining form.

Term	Combining Form	Combining Form Meaning
1. abdominocentesis	_____	_____
2. cholecystogram	_____	_____
3. laparoscopy	_____	_____
4. sigmoidoscopy	_____	_____
5. colonoscopy	_____	_____
5. proctoscopy	_____	_____

Surgical Interventions and Therapeutic Procedures

Term	Pronunciation	Meaning
abdominoperineal (A&P) resection	ab-dom'i-nō-per-i-nē'ăl rē-sek'shŭn	surgical removal of the colon and rectum by both abdominal and perineal approaches; includes a colostomy and is performed to treat severe lower intestinal diseases including cancer
abdominoplasty	ab-dom'i-nō-plas-tē	surgical repair of the abdominal area

(continued)

Surgical Interventions and Therapeutic Procedures *(continued)*

Term	Pronunciation	Meaning
anastomosis	ă-nas'tŏ-mō'sis	an operative union of two hollow or tubular structures
appendectomy	ap'pĕn-dek'tŏ-mē	removal of the appendix
bariatric surgery	bar'ē-at'rik sŭr'jĕr-ē	any operation performed for the management of obesity

> **OBESITY** Bariatric surgery is used for treatment of obesity. Obesity is defined as a body mass index of greater than 30 kg/m^2. Normal body mass index is between 18 and 24 kg/m^2.

Term	Pronunciation	Meaning
gastric bypass	gas'trik bī'pas	type of bariatric surgery that involves stomach stapling to bypass a large area of the stomach and anastomosis of its upper part to the small intestine (Fig. 5-18)
cholecystectomy	kō'lĕ-sis-tek'tŏ-mē	removal of the gallbladder
cholelithotripsy	kō'lĕ-lith'ō-trip-sē	crushing of gallstones
colostomy	kō-los'tŏ-mē	artificial opening into the colon (Fig. 5-19)

(continued)

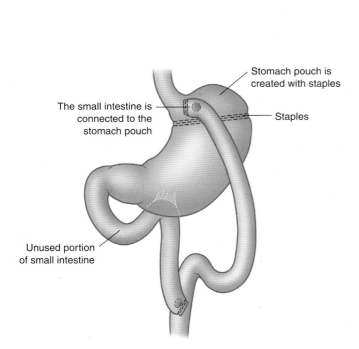

Figure 5-18   Gastric bypass. The most common type, called Roux-en-Y, is shown here.

The small intestine is connected to the stomach pouch

Stomach pouch is created with staples

Staples

Unused portion of small intestine

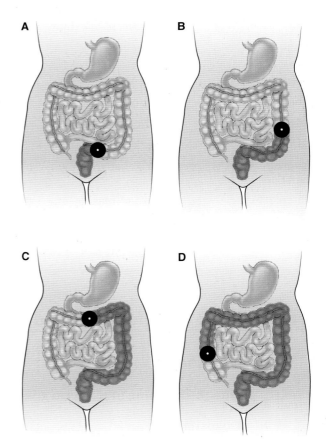

Figure 5-19   Colostomy sites.

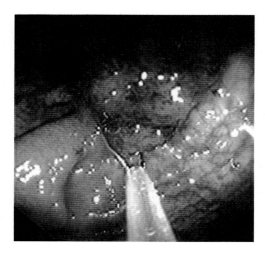

Figure 5-20   Endoscopic colon polypectomy.

Surgical Interventions and Therapeutic Procedures *(continued)*

Term	Pronunciation	Meaning
gastrectomy	gas-trek'tŏ-mē	removal of the stomach
gastric lavage	gas'trik lă-vahzh'	insertion of a tube from the mouth into the stomach to wash and suction out its contents for examination and treatment; usually done to remove blood clots or monitor bleeding.
gastric resection	gas'trik rē-sek'shŭn	removal of a section of the stomach
gavage	gă-vahzh'	process of feeding a patient through nasogastric intubation
glossorrhaphy	glos-ōr'ă-fē	suturing of the tongue
herniorrhaphy	hĕr'nē-ōr'ă-fē	suturing of a hernia
ileostomy	il'ē-os'tŏ-mē	artificial opening into the ileum of the small intestine
laparotomy	lap'ă-rot'ŏ-mē	incision into the abdominal area
nasogastric (NG) intubation	nā'zō-gas'trik in'tū-bā'shŭn	insertion of a tube from the nose into the stomach for feeding or suctioning stomach contents
palatoplasty	pal'ă-tō-plas-tē	surgical repair of the roof of the mouth
polypectomy	pol'i-pek'tŏ-mē	surgical removal of polyps (Fig. 5-20)
total parenteral nutrition (TPN)	tō'tăl pă-ren'tĕr-ăl nū-trish'ŭn	feeding maintained entirely by intravenous injection or other nongastrointestinal route

■ Exercises: Surgical Interventions and Therapeutic Procedures

SIMPLE RECALL

Exercise 20

Write the meaning of the term given.

1. laparotomy _____

2. glossorrhaphy _____

3. gastrectomy _____

4. gavage _____

5. palatoplasty _____

6. gastric resection _____

7. anastomosis _____

8. cholelithotripsy _____

9. appendectomy _____

10. ileostomy _____

Exercise 21

ADVANCED
RECALL

Circle the term that is most appropriate for the meaning of the sentence.

1. Mr. Juno was morbidly obese, so his physician suggested (*abdominoperineal resection, bariatric surgery, gastric lavage*) to manage his condition.

2. Due to severe intestinal disease, Mrs. Wainwright underwent a(n) (*gavage, gastrectomy, abdominoperineal resection*) which included a colostomy.

3. After the car accident, the patient was unable to eat due to his comatose state and had to be fed by a process known as (*anoscopy, gavage, laparotomy*).

4. To correct the condition of cleft palate, the patient underwent a (*glossorrhaphy, lingulectomy, palatoplasty*).

5. Mr. Ruiz underwent an ileocolostomy, which is an (*anastomosis, oligodontia, effusion*) between the large intestine and the ileum.

6. Because Mr. Taylor had been diagnosed with multiple gallstones, the physician suggested that he have a (*colotomy, appendectomy, cholecystectomy*) to treat the condition.

7. Mr. Gray had a large amount of blood in his stomach, so the physician ordered (*gastric lavage, total parenteral nutrition, gastric bypass*).

8. A patient who has a tube inserted through the nose and into the stomach has had (*herniorrhaphy, gastric lavage, nasogastric intubation*).

9. The physician ordered (*TPN, NG, GL*), which is feeding maintained entirely by intravenous injection or other nongastrointestinal route.

10. Mrs. Anderson had a(n) (*gastric lavage, gastric bypass, abdominoperineal resection*), which included a stomach stapling and anastomosis to the jejunum.

Exercise 22

TERM
CONSTRUCTION

Build the correct medical term for the meaning given. Write the term in the blank indicating the word parts (P = prefix, CF = combining form, S = suffix).

1. surgical opening into the colon   _____ / _____
                                              CF   S

2. process of recording the pancreas   _____ / _____
                                              CF   S

3. pertaining to surrounding the tooth _____ / _____ / _____
                                              P   CF   S

4. suture of the lip   _____ / _____
                                              CF   S

5. surgical incision into the ileum   _____ / _____
                                              CF   S

6. crushing of stones in the gallbladder _____ / _____ / _____
                                              CF   CF   S

7. surgical removal of polyps   _____ / _____
                                              CF   S

8. surgical removal of half the colon   _____ / _____ / _____
                                              P   CF   S

9. surgical repair of the abdomen   _____ / _____
                                              CF   S

Exercise 23

TERM
CONSTRUCTION

For each term, first write the meaning of the term. Then write the meaning of the word parts in that term.

1. palatoplasty   _____

   palat/o   _____

   -plasty   _____

2. colostomy   _____

   colon/o   _____

   -stomy   _____

3. herniorrhaphy _____

    herni/o _____

    -rrhaphy _____

4. ileotomy _____

    ile/o _____

    -tomy _____

5. appendectomy _____

    appendic/o _____

    -ectomy _____

6. glossorrhaphy _____

    gloss/o _____

    -rrhaphy _____

Medications and Drug Therapies

Term	Pronunciation	Meaning
antacid	ant-as′id	drug used to reduce stomach acid
antidiarrheal	an′tē-dī-ă-rē′ăl	drug used to stop or prevent diarrhea
antiemetic	an′tē-ĕ-met′ik	drug used to stop or prevent nausea and vomiting
emetic	ĕ-met′ik	drug used to induce vomiting
laxative, _syn._ cathartic	lak′să-tiv, kă-thahr′tik	drug used to promote the expulsion of feces

■ Exercise: Medications and Drug Therapies

SIMPLE
RECALL

Exercise 24

Write the correct medication or drug therapy term for the meaning given.

1. used to stop diarrhea _____

2. used to relieve constipation _____

3. used to decrease stomach acid _____

4. used to induce vomiting _____

5. used to stop vomiting _____

Specialties and Specialists

Term	Pronunciation	Meaning
gastroenterology	gas'trō-en-tĕr-ol'ŏ-jē	medical speciality concerned with diagnosis and treatment of disorders of the gastrointestinal tract
gastroenterologist	gas'trō-en-tĕr-ol'ŏ-jist	physician who specializes in gastroenterology
proctology	prok-tol'ŏ-jē	medical speciality concerned with diagnosis and treatment of disorders of the anus and rectum
proctologist	prok-tol'ŏ-jist	physician who specializes in proctology

■ Exercise: Specialties and Specialists

Exercise 25

SIMPLE
RECALL

Write the meaning of the term given.

1. gastroenterology _____

2. proctologist _____

3. proctology _____

4. gastroenterologist _____

Abbreviations

Abbreviation	Meaning
A&P resection	abdominoperineal resection
BE	barium enema
BM	bowel movement
EGD	esophagogastroduodenoscopy
GERD	gastroesophageal reflux disease
GI	gastrointestinal
IBS	irritable bowel syndrome
NG	nasogastric
PUD	peptic ulcer disease
TPN	total parenteral nutrition
UGI	upper gastrointestinal

Exercises: Abbreviations

Exercise 26

SIMPLE
RECALL

Write the meaning of each abbreviation.

1. GI _____

2. BE _____

3. TPN _____

4. EGD _____

5. NG _____

6. UGI _____

7. GERD _____

Exercise 27

ADVANCED
RECALL

Match each abbreviation with the appropriate description.

BE   PUD   IBS
BM   A&P resection

1. intestinal condition with symptoms of gas,   _____
   bloating, diarrhea, constipation, and pain

2. passage of feces   _____

3. condition that affects the stomach   _____

4. surgical removal of the colon and rectum   _____

5. use of contrast medium to view the lower gastrointestinal tract   _____

Review of Terms for Anatomy and Physiology

VISUAL

Exercise 28

Write the correct terms on the blanks for the anatomic structures indicated.

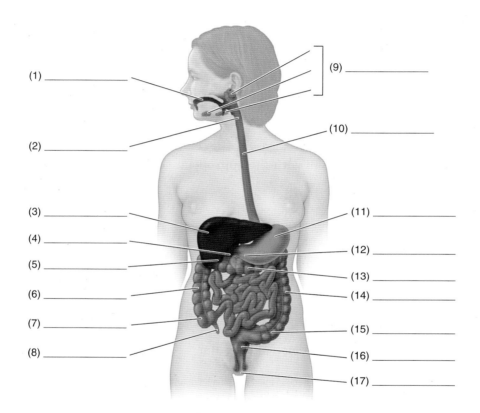

(1) _____

(2) _____

(3) _____

(4) _____

(5) _____

(6) _____

(7) _____

(8) _____

(9) _____

(10) _____

(11) _____

(12) _____

(13) _____

(14) _____

(15) _____

(16) _____

(17) _____

VISUAL

Exercise 29

Write the correct terms on the blanks for the anatomic structures indicated.

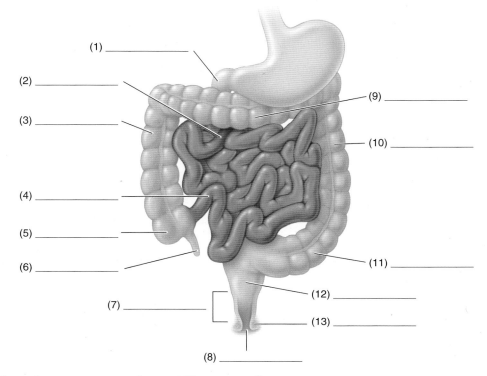

(1) _____

(2) _____

(3) _____

(4) _____

(5) _____

(6) _____

(7) _____

(8) _____

(9) _____

(10) _____

(11) _____

(12) _____

(13) _____

Understanding Term Structure

TERM
CONSTRUCTION

Exercise 30

For each term, first write the meaning of the term. Then write the meaning of the word parts in that term.

1. pyloroplasty   _____

   pylor/o   _____

   -plasty   _____

2. esophagocele   _____

   esophag/o   _____

   -cele   _____

3. gastrodynia   _____

   gastr/o   _____

   -dynia   _____

4. stomatomalacia   _____

    stomat/o   _____

    -malacia   _____

5. hepatomegaly   _____

    hepat/o   _____

    -megaly   _____

6. laparogastroscopy   _____

    lapar/o   _____

    gastr/o   _____

    -scopy   _____

7. anoscope   _____

    an/o   _____

    -scope   _____

8. cheilophagia   _____

    cheil/o   _____

    -phagia   _____

9. sigmoidoproctostomy   _____

    sigmoid/o   _____

    proct/o   _____

    -stomy   _____

10. enterocolitis   _____

    enter/o   _____

    col/o   _____

    -itis   _____

11. rectostenosis   _____

    rect/o   _____

    -stenosis   _____

12. cheilorrhaphy _____

    cheil/o _____

    -rrhaphy _____

13. odontalgia _____

    odont/o _____

    -algia _____

14. appendicopathy _____

    appendic/o _____

    -pathy _____

15. cholelithotomy _____

    chol/e _____

    lith/o _____

    -tomy _____

16. jejunostomy _____

    jejun/o _____

    -stomy _____

17. esophagogastrectomy _____

    esophag/o _____

    gastr/o _____

    -ectomy _____

18. proctoptosis _____

    proct/o _____

    -ptosis _____

Exercise 31

TERM
CONSTRUCTION

Write the combining form(s) used in the medical term, followed by the meaning of the combining form(s).

Term	Combining Form(s)	Combining Form Meaning(s)
1. sialocele	_____	_____
2. alimentary	_____	_____

3. pylorostenosis   _____   _____

4. pharyngospasm   _____   _____

5. duodenorrhaphy   _____   _____

6. gastroenteropathy   _____   _____

7. hepatectomy   _____   _____

8. palatoplasty   _____   _____

9. buccopharyngeal   _____   _____

10. dentofacial   _____   _____

11. cecostomy   _____   _____

12. proctologist   _____   _____

13. polyposis   _____   _____

Comprehension Exercises

Exercise 32

COMPREHENSION **Fill in the blank with the correct term.**

1. Puncture into the abdomen to remove fluid and relieve abdominal pressure is called

   _____ .

2. A specialist whose focus is on disorders of the rectum and anus is called a(n) _____

   _____ .

3. The test used to identify the presence of occult blood is called a(n) _____ .

4. When stomach acids begin to flow backward into the esophagus, this disease is called

   _____ .

5. Excessive vomiting is called _____ .

6. To remove stones from the pancreas, a patient would have a surgery known as

   _____ .

7. An anastomosis between the stomach and the small intestine is called a(n)

   _____ .

Exercise 33

COMPREHENSION   **Circle the letter of the best answer in the following questions.**

1. A patient diagnosed with _____ experiences problems during mastication.

   A. esophagitis
   B. odontitis
   C. hepatitis
   D. laryngitis

2. Which of the following is *not* a primary organ of the digestive system?

   A. liver
   B. stomach
   C. large intestine
   D. pharynx

3. The substance that helps to form a bolus in the mouth is called:

   A. chyme
   B. stoma
   C. saliva
   D. uvula

4. The correct order of the sections of the small intestine is:

   A. duodenum, jejunum, ileum
   B. duodenum, ileum, jejunum
   C. ileum, duodenum, jejunum
   D. jejunum, duodenum, ileum

5. Surgical repair of the rectum is called:

   A. anoplasty
   B. sigmoidoplasty
   C. rectoplasty
   D. hepatoplasty

6. Which condition does not involve the passing of hard stools?

   A. spastic colon
   B. dysentery
   C. constipation
   D. irritable bowel syndrome

7. A gastric lavage is performed for blood clots in the:

   A. stomach
   B. palate
   C. mouth
   D. anus

8. A dangerous twisting of the colon is called:

   A. ileus
   B. ilius
   C. volvulus
   D. intussusception

9. Black, tarry stools contain what substance?

   A. diarrhea
   B. melena
   C. occult blood
   D. flatus

10. Increased fluid in the abdominal area that is not a normal finding is called:

    A. ascites
    B. eructation
    C. cirrhosis
    D. cholestasis

11. Difficulty in the act of deglutition is called:

    A. dyspepsia
    B. dysentery
    C. dysodontiasis
    D. dysphagia

12. Which condition involves the large organ that produces and secretes bile into the gallbladder?

    A. cirrhosis
    B. dysentery
    C. dysodontiasis
    D. pancreatitis

13. The procedure used to treat stones in the gallbladder without removing the gallbladder is called:

A. cholecystectomy
B. cholecystostomy
C. cholelithotripsy
D. cholelithiasis

14. An incision into the duodenum is called a:

A. duodenoscopy
B. duodenostomy
C. duodenotomy
D. duodenorrhaphy

15. The condition known as halitosis occurs in the:

A. stomach
B. rectum
C. anus
D. mouth

Application and Analysis

CASE REPORTS

APPLICATION

Exercise 34

Read the case reports and circle the letter of your answer choice for the questions that follow.

CASE 5-1

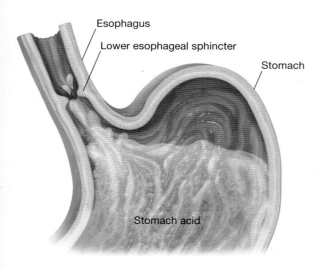

Esophagus
Lower esophageal sphincter
Stomach
Stomach acid

Figure 5-21   Stomach acid flowing back into the esophagus in gastroesophageal reflux disease (GERD).

Mr. Patel complained of dysphagia and dyspepsia. He stated these problems had been occurring for the past 6 months and were increasing in frequency. His physician diagnosed him with GERD (Fig. 5-21) and encouraged him to stay away from chocolate and decrease his caffeine intake.

1. The patient has been diagnosed with:

    A. gastric regurgitation disease
    B. gastroesophageal rectal disease
    C. gastroesophageal reflux disease
    D. gastric reflux disease

2. Because of his dyspepsia, the patient has:

    A. trouble with pepsin production
    B. painful digestion

    C. enlarged liver
    D. decreased stomach acid production

3. Backward flow of stomach acids into the esophagus is known as:

    A. dyspepsia
    B. gastroesophageal reflux disease
    C. dysphagia
    D. esophagitis

CASE 5-2

Mr. Desalvo had been experiencing abdominal pain and anorexia for the past day, but when it became unbearable he went to the ER. This evening, the ER physician determined that Mr. Desalvo had peritonitis resulting from a ruptured appendix.

4. Peritonitis is defined as:

    A. inflammation of the palate
    B. inflammation of the pharynx
    C. inflammation of the peritoneum
    D. inflammation of the polyps

5. To treat the ruptured appendix, the patient would have to undergo emergency:

    A. appendicolith
    B. appendectomy

    C. appendicostomy
    D. appendicopathy

6. Anorexia is a condition characterized by:

    A. decreased flatus
    B. decreased bowel movements
    C. decreased appetite
    D. decreased digestion

MEDICAL RECORD ANALYSIS

MEDICAL RECORD 5-1

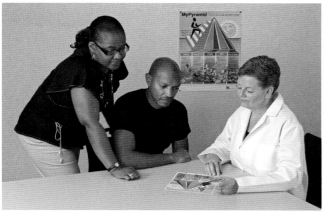

Mr. Riggins was recently seen by his family physician after finding blood in his stool. After Mr. Riggins' clinic visit, he was referred to you, a nutritionist, to answer any questions he and his family might have concerning the addition of fiber to his diet.

A nutritionist meets with a patient and his family to discuss his diet.

Medical Record

ANAL FISSURE

Patient: David Riggins
Chart Number: 00675

Physician: Dr. Henry Preston
Date: March 21, 20—

Patient presented to the clinic today with having had a BM this morning in which he noticed a large amount of bright red blood in the toilet. He denied any pain with the BM. This was the first time this has happened. No associated nausea and vomiting or diarrhea. He did mention that he has been constipated for the past week or so. He stated he had small, hard stools that he had to strain to pass a couple of times during the last week. The patient has no history of peptic ulcers or gastrointestinal cancer.

OBJECTIVE: Wt. 195, BP 160/88, P 88. The patient is a well-developed, well-nourished male in no acute distress. Examination of the rectal area reveals a small tear in the rectal mucosa.

MEDICATIONS: Ibuprofen p.r.n.; metoprolol 50 mg b.i.d.

ASSESSMENT: The patient has a small anal fissure. This is most likely caused from several incidences of constipation with associated straining.

PLAN: The patient was instructed to increase the amount of fiber in his diet as well as to use an OTC laxative to increase the frequency of his BM and to soften the stool. He was advised to not strain as this would increase the likelihood that any hard stools that are passed will worsen the tear. This should resolve on its own. The patient is instructed to call the clinic should he continue to have issues.

APPLICATION

Exercise 35

Write the appropriate medical terms used in this medical record on the blanks after their meanings. Note that not all the terms appear in the chapter, but you should be able to identify these terms based on word parts that are included in this chapter.

1. pertaining to the stomach and intestines   _____

2. abnormally frequent discharge of semi-solid or liquid feces   _____

3. decreased number of bowel movements with passage of hard stools   _____

4. passage of solid waste products (abbreviation)   _____

5. the urge to vomit   _____

6. pertaining to the anus   _____

7. condition of the stomach or duodenum caused by gastric acid   _____

Bonus Question

8. Recalling the meaning of the term *fissure* in Chapter 4, what is the definition of an anal fissure?   _____

MEDICAL RECORD 5-2

As a medical coding specialist, you are responsible for evaluating patient medical records and documentation to accurately bill for services provided. You are reviewing the medical record that follows to determine the codes needed for submission to the insurance company for appropriate reimbursement.

 # Medical Record

GERD

Patient: Adrian Edwards   Physician: Dr. Carter Price
Chart Number: 03151   Date: March 21, 20—

Mr. Edwards came to the clinic today with complaints of heartburn and postprandial regurgitation. He states that these symptoms increase in severity soon after he lies down in his recliner after eating to watch TV. He is on no regular medications except that he does take occasional Maalox when his symptoms are "too much to handle." These symptoms have only started to bother him recently, within the past month or so. He also complains of some flatus.

OBJECTIVE: This is an obese, well-developed male. Currently, he is in no distress. Weight today is 295. This is an increase since his last visit 6 months ago when he weighed 256. He has just recently lost his job and has stopped going to the gym because he had let his membership lapse.

ASSESSMENT: GERD with increase in weight and decreased activity.

PLAN: Start proton pump inhibitor b.i.d. Encourage patient to try to get back into routine of exercise. Discussed dietary guidelines to decrease fatty food intake. Discussed the need to abstain from coffee, tea, chocolate, and activities such as lying down or reclining immediately or soon after eating. The patient was encouraged to raise the head of his bed about 2 inches. If symptoms persist, Mr. Edwards is to return to clinic. More aggressive evaluation with endoscopy will then be scheduled.

Exercise 36

APPLICATION

Read the medical report and circle the letter of your answer choice for the following questions.

1. In GERD, the backward flow of acid into the esophagus comes from the:

   A. small intestine
   B. pharynx
   C. stomach
   D. mouth

2. If the patient is scheduled for an endoscopy, the physician will:

   A. use an endoscope to examine the inside of the upper gastrointestinal tract
   B. obtain an x-ray examination of the esophagus
   C. view the condition of the mouth
   D. obtain a recording of the large intestine

3. When does the patient experience regurgitation?

   A. after meals
   B. after defecating
   C. after waking
   D. before leaving for work

4. Flatus is:

   A. bile
   B. feces
   C. gas
   D. urine

Bonus Question

5. Why is the patient encouraged to raise the head of his bed?_____

_____

Pronunciation and Spelling

AUDITORY

Exercise 37

Review the Chapter 5 terms in the Dictionary/Audio Glossary in the Student Resources and practice pronouncing each term, referring to the pronunciation guide as needed.

SPELLING

Exercise 38

Circle the correct spelling of each term.

1. ruggae	rugea	rugae
2. cecum	cekum	secum
3. tonge	tonk	tongue
4. regurgitation	regergatation	regergitashun
5. illeus	ileus	eelius
6. feeces	feces	fesees
7. acult	ocult	occult
8. pieloris	pilorus	pylorus
9. youvyoula	uvule	uvula
10. gavage	gabage	gavach
11. nawsea	nausea	nalsea
12. mastication	mastikashun	mustication
13. polyposias	poliposis	polyposis
14. pilate	palate	palit
15. incontinence	incontinance	incontinense

Media Connection

STUDENT
RESOURCES

Exercise 39

Complete each of the following activities available with the Student Resources. Check off each activity as you complete it.

____ Flash Cards

____ Concentration

____ Abbreviation Match-Up

____ Roboterms

____ Word Builder

____ Fill the Gap

____ Break It Down

____ True/False Body Building

____ Quiz Show

____ Complete the Case

____ Medical Record Review

____ Look and Label

____ Image Matching

____ Spelling Bee

____ **Chapter Quiz**   *Score:* _____%

Additional Resources

____ Animation: General Digestion

____ Dictionary/Audio Glossary

____ Health Professions Careers: Nutritionist

____ Health Professions Careers: Medical Coding Specialist

Urinary System

6

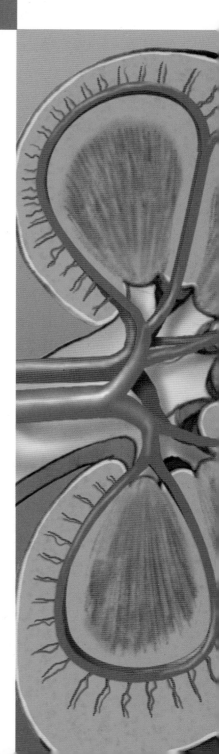

Chapter Outline

Objectives

After completion of this chapter you will be able to:

1. Describe the location of main structures in the urinary system.

2. Define terms related to the urinary system.

3. Define combining forms, prefixes, and suffixes related to the urinary system.

4. Define common medical terminology related to the urinary system, including adjectives and related terms, symptoms and conditions, tests and procedures, surgical interventions and therapeutic procedures, medications and drug therapies, and specialties.

5. Explain abbreviations for terms related to the urinary system.

6. Successfully complete all chapter exercises.

7. Explain terms used in case studies and medical records involving the urinary system.

8. Successfully complete all pronunciation and spelling exercises, and complete all interactive exercises included with the companion Student Resources.

■ ANATOMY AND PHYSIOLOGY

Functions

- ■ To filter waste products from the body
- ■ To regulate levels of fluids and electrolytes
- ■ To carry urine through the system until it is excreted during the process of urination

Organs and Structures (Fig. 6-1)

- ■ The kidneys remove waste from the blood in the form of urine.
- ■ The ureters carry urine from the kidneys to the bladder.
- ■ The urethra carries urine from the bladder to the outside of the body.

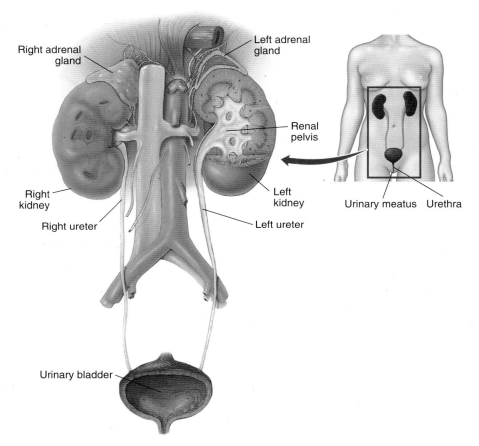

Figure 6-1   The urinary system.

Terms Related to the Urinary System

Term	Pronunciation	Meaning
kidney	kid′nē	one of two bean-shaped organs that remove waste products from the blood and help maintain fluid and electrolyte balance in the body (Fig. 6-2)
nephron	nef′ron	microscopic urine-producing unit; each kidney contains about 1 million nephrons
glomerulus	glō-mer′yū-lŭs	one of several capillary clusters at the entrance of each nephron that initiates the process of filtering of the blood

(continued)

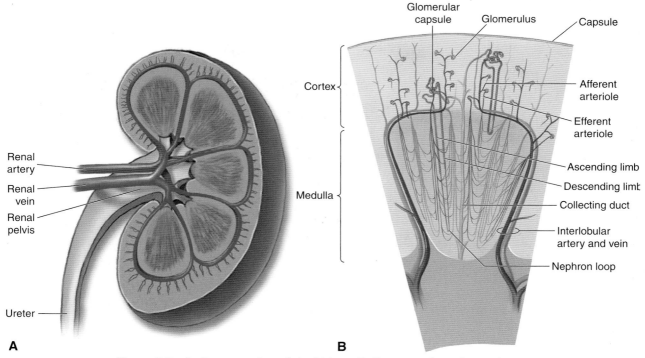

Figure 6-2 **A.** Cross section of the kidney. **B.** Cross section of a nephron.

Terms Related to the Urinary System *(continued)*

Term	Pronunciation	Meaning
renal pelvis	rē'năl pel'vis	a reservoir in each kidney that collects urine
ureter	yū're-tur	one of two narrow tubes that carry urine from the kidneys to the bladder
urethra	yū-rē'thră	tubular structure through which urine passes from the urinary bladder to the outside of the body
urinary bladder*	yūr'i-nār'ē blad'er	muscular organ that holds the urine until it is released (Fig. 6-3)
urinary meatus	yūr'i-nār'ē mē-ā'tŭs	opening that carries urine from the urethra to the outside of the body
urine	yūr'in	water, waste products, and other substances excreted by the kidneys

*The term *bladder* will refer to the urinary bladder in this chapter.

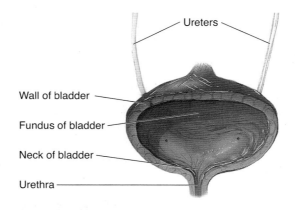

Figure 6-3 The bladder.

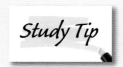

Study Tip   **Ureters vs. Urethra:** Here is an easy way to remember the difference between the ureters and the urethra: There are two ureters in the body, and the word *ureter* has two "e"s. There is only one urethra in the body, and the word *urethra* has only one "e."

ANIMATION

To learn more about the function of the kidneys, view the animation Renal Function *on the Student Resources.*

■ Exercises: Anatomy and Physiology

SIMPLE
RECALL

Exercise 1

Write the meaning of the anatomic structure given.

1. urinary meatus   _____

2. ureter   _____

3. kidney   _____

4. nephron   _____

5. renal pelvis   _____

ADVANCED
RECALL

Exercise 2

Match each medical term with its meaning.

| urinary meatus | kidney | glomerulus | urine |
| renal pelvis | urethra | urinary bladder | |

Meaning   **Term**

1. capillary cluster at entrance to nephrons   _____

2. opening carrying urine to outside of body   _____

3. removes waste products from the blood   _____

4. tube carrying urine from bladder to outside of body   _____

5. muscular organ that holds urine until it is released   _____

6. reservoir in the kidney that collects urine   _____

7. fluid excreted by the kidneys   _____

■ WORD PARTS

Note that some word parts that have been introduced earlier in the book may not be repeated here.

Combining Forms

Combining Form	Meaning
albumin/o	albumin
bacteri/o	bacteria
cyst/o*, vesicul/o, vesic/o	fluid-filled sac (urinary bladder)
enur/o	to urinate in
glomerul/o	glomerulus
glycos/o, glyc/o	glucose, sugar
hemat/o	blood
hydr/o	water, fluid
lith/o	stone, calculus
meat/o	meatus
nephr/o, ren/o	kidney
noct/i	night
olig/o	scanty, few
py/o	pus
pyel/o	renal pelvis
son/o	sound, sound waves
ureter/o	ureter
urethr/o	urethra
ur/o, urin/o	urine, urinary system/tract

*The combining form *cyst/o* may also refer to a cyst but will refer to the urinary bladder in this chapter unless otherwise specified.

Prefixes

Prefix	Meaning
dys-	painful, difficult, abnormal
poly-	many, much

Suffixes

Suffix	Meaning
-cele	herniation, protrusion
-emia	blood (condition of)
-iasis, -esis	condition of
-lith	stone, calculus

(continued)

Suffixes *(continued)*

Suffix	Meaning
-lysis	destruction, breakdown, separation
-ptosis	prolapse, drooping, sagging
-scopy	process of examining, examination
-stenosis	stricture, narrowing
-stomy	surgical opening
-tripsy	crushing
-uria	urine, urination

■ Exercises: Word Parts

Exercise 3

SIMPLE RECALL

Write the correct combining form(s) for the meaning given.

1. meatus   _____

2. scanty   _____

3. urine   _____

4. kidney   _____

5. water, fluid   _____

6. renal pelvis   _____

7. night   _____

8. stone   _____

9. to urinate in   _____

Exercise 4

SIMPLE RECALL

Write the correct suffix(es) for the meaning given.

1. surgical opening   _____

2. stone   _____

3. herniation   _____

4. process of examining   _____

5. drooping, sagging   _____

6. blood (condition of) _____

7. condition of _____

8. stricture, narrowing _____

Exercise 5

ADVANCED
RECALL

Match each word part with its meaning.

| py/o | hydr/o | son/o | nephr/o |
| urethr/o | ureter/o | vesic/o | |

Meaning	Word Part
1. kidney	_____
2. pus	_____
3. urethra	_____
4. sound, sound waves	_____
5. urinary bladder	_____
6. ureter	_____
7. water, fluid	

Exercise 6

TERM
CONSTRUCTION

Build a medical term from an appropriate combining form and suffix, given their meanings.

Use Combining Form for	Use Suffix for	Term
1. blood	urine, urination	_____
2. ureter	stricture, narrowing	_____
3. stone, calculus	crushing	_____
4. urine	blood (condition of)	_____
5. glomerulus	inflammation	_____
6. ureter	stone, calculus	_____
7. sound, sound waves	record	_____
8. renal pelvis	process of recording	_____

Exercise 7

TERM CONSTRUCTION

Using the given suffix, build a medical term for the meaning given.

Suffix	Meaning of Medical Term	Medical Term
-uria	pus in the urine	1. _____
-uria	blood in the urine	2. _____
-uria	albumin in the urine	3. _____
-uria	glucose in the urine	4. _____
-uria	scanty amounts of urine	5. _____
-uria	bacteria in the urine	6. _____
-uria	much urination	7. _____
-uria	painful urination	8. _____

Exercise 8

TERM CONSTRUCTION

Break the given medical term into its word parts and define each part. Then define the medical term.

For example:
urethritis   *word parts:*   urethr/o / -itis
                 meanings: urethra / inflammation
                 term meaning: inflammation of the urethra

1. nephromegaly   *word parts:*   _____ / _____

                     meanings: _____ / _____

                     term meaning: _____

2. cystoscope   *word parts:*   _____ / _____

                     meanings: _____ / _____

                     term meaning: _____

3. nocturia   *word parts:*   _____ / _____

                     meanings: _____ / _____

                     term meaning: _____

4. ureterostomy   *word parts:*   _____ / _____

                       meanings: _____ / _____

                       term meaning: _____

5. renogram   *word parts:*   _____ / _____

                       meanings: _____ / _____

                       term meaning: _____

6. nephrolysis   *word parts:*   _____ / _____

                       meanings: _____ / _____

                       term meaning: _____

7. vesicular   *word parts:*   _____ / _____

                       meanings: _____ / _____

                       term meaning: _____

8. nephrorrhaphy   *word parts:*   _____ / _____

                       meanings: _____ / _____

                       term meaning: _____

■ MEDICAL TERMS

Adjectives and Other Related Terms

Term	Pronunciation	Meaning
cystic, *syn.* vesical	sis'tik, ves'i-kăl	pertaining to the urinary bladder
genitourinary (GU)	jen'i-tō-yūr'i-nar-ē	pertaining to the organs of reproduction and urination
meatal	mē-ā'tăl	pertaining to the meatus
micturition	mik'chū-rish'ŭn	process of releasing urine from the bladder
nephric, *syn.* renal	nef'rik, rē'năl	pertaining to the kidney
ureteral	yū-rē'tĕr-ăl	pertaining to the ureter
urethral	yū-rē'thrăl	pertaining to the urethra
urinary	yūr'i-nār'ē	pertaining to urine
urinate, *syn.* micturate, void	yūr'i-nāt, mik'chū-rāt, voyd	to release urine from the bladder

■ Exercises: Adjectives and Other Related Terms

Exercise 9

SIMPLE RECALL

Write the meaning of the term given.

1. void _____

2. renal _____

3. cystic _____

4. micturate _____

5. urethral _____

6. urinary _____

Exercise 10

ADVANCED RECALL

Match each medical term with its meaning.

| urinate | vesical | nephric | genitourinary |
| meatal | ureteral | micturition | |

Meaning   **Term**

1. process of releasing urine from the bladder   _____

2. pertaining to the bladder   _____

3. pertaining to the meatus   _____

4. pertaining to the organs of reproduction and urination   _____

5. pertaining to the kidney   _____

6. to release urine from the bladder   _____

7. pertaining to a ureter   _____

Exercise 11

TERM CONSTRUCTION

Break the given medical term into its word parts and define each part. Then define the medical term.

For example:

meatal   *word parts:*   meat/o / -al
                     meanings: meatus / pertaining to
                     term meaning: pertaining to the meatus

1. urinary   *word parts:*   _____ / _____

                    meanings: _____ / _____

                    term meaning: _____

2. renal   *word parts:*   _____ / _____

                    meanings: _____ / _____

                    term meaning: _____

3. cystic   *word parts:*   _____ / _____

                    meanings: _____ / _____

                    term meaning: _____

4. urethral   *word parts:*   _____ / _____

                    meanings: _____ / _____

                    term meaning: _____

5. ureteral   *word parts:*   _____ / _____

                    meanings: _____ / _____

                    term meaning: _____

Symptoms and Medical Conditions

Term	Pronunciation	Meaning
albuminuria	al-bū-min-yū′rē-ă	albumin in the urine
anuria	an-yū′rē-ă	absence of urine formation
bacteriuria	bak-tēr′ē-yū′rē-ă	bacteria in the urine
cystitis	sis-tī′tis	inflammation of the bladder
cystocele	sis′tō-sēl	protrusion of the bladder
cystolith	sis′tō-lith	stone in the bladder
diuresis	dī′yū-rē′sis	condition of excreting increased amounts of urine
dysuria	dis-yū′rē-ă	difficulty urinating; painful urination
end-stage renal disease (ESRD)	end-stāj rē′năl diz-ēz′	the final phase of chronic kidney disease
enuresis	en′yū-rē′sis	involuntary discharge of urine
epispadias	ep′i-spā′dē-ăs	congenital defect in which the urinary meatus is on the upper surface of the penis (Fig. 6-4B)

(continued)

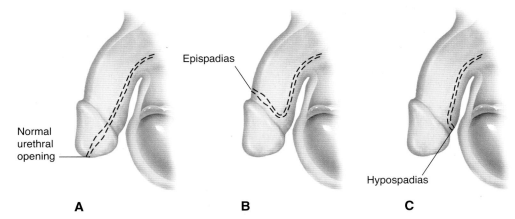

Figure 6-4 **A.** Normal urethral opening. **B.** Epispadias. **C.** Hypospadias.

Symptoms and Medical Conditions *(continued)*

Term	Pronunciation	Meaning
glomerulonephritis	glō-mer′yū-lō-ne-frī′tis	inflammation of the glomeruli of the kidney
glycosuria	glī′kō-syū′rē-ă	glucose in the urine
hematuria	hē′mă-tyū′rē-ă	blood in the urine
hydronephrosis	hī′drō-ne-frō′sis	condition of fluid in the kidney(s); a buildup of urine caused by obstruction of urine flow usually due to a stone or stricture (Fig. 6-5)
hydroureter	hī′drō-yūr′ē- tĕr	condition of fluid in the ureter(s); a buildup of urine caused by obstruction of urine flow usually due to a stone or stricture (Fig. 6-5)

(continued)

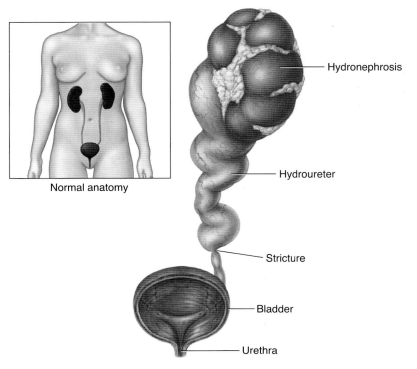

Normal anatomy

Figure 6-5 Hydronephrosis and hydroureter from a stricture.

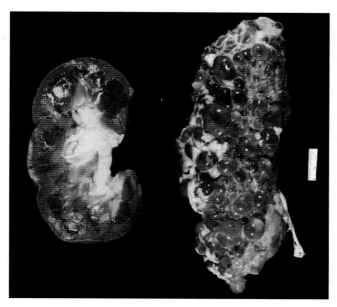

Figure 6-6   Normal kidney (**left**). Polycystic kidney (**right**).

Symptoms and Medical Conditions *(continued)*

Term	Pronunciation	Meaning
hypospadias	hĭ′pō-spā′dē-ăs	congenital defect in which the urinary meatus is on the underside of the penis (Fig. 6-4C)
nephritis	ne-frī′tis	inflammation of the kidney
nephrolithiasis	nef′rō-li-thī′ă-sis	condition of stones in the kidney
nephromegaly	nef′rō-meg′ă-lē	enlargement of the kidney
nephroptosis	nef′rop-tō′sis	drooping of the kidney
nocturia	nokt-yū′rē-ă	excessive urination at night
nocturnal enuresis	nok-ter′năl en′yū-rē′sis	involuntary discharge of urine at night; bed-wetting
oliguria	ol′i-gyū′rē-ă	scanty amount of urine
polycystic kidney disease	pol′ē-sis′tik kid′nē diz-ēz′	condition in which many cysts occur within and upon the kidneys, resulting in the loss of functional tissue (Fig. 6-6)
polyuria	pol′ē-yū′rē-ă	excessive and frequent urination
proteinuria	prō′tē-nūr′ē-ă	protein in the urine
pyelitis	pī′ĕ-lī′tis	inflammation of the renal pelvis
pyelonephritis	pī′ĕ-lō-ne-frī′tis	inflammation of the renal pelvis and kidney
pyuria	pī-yūr′ē-ă	pus in the urine
renal calculus, *syn.* nephrolith	rē′năl kal′kyū-lŭs	stone in the kidney (Fig. 6-7)
renal failure	rē′năl fāl′yŭr	an acute (ARF) or chronic (CRF) condition in which the kidney fails to excrete urine
renal hypertension	rē′năl hī′pĕr-ten′shŭn	elevated blood pressure resulting from kidney disease

(continued)

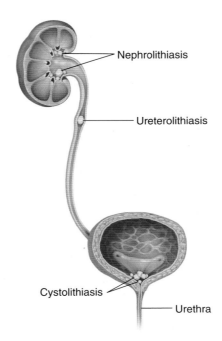

Figure 6-7 Calculi throughout the urinary system.

Symptoms and Medical Conditions *(continued)*

Term	Pronunciation	Meaning
stress urinary incontinence (SUI)	stres yūr'i-nār'ē in-kon'ti-nens	involuntary discharge of urine during coughing, straining, or sudden movements
stricture	strik'chŭr	narrowing of an organ
uremia	yū-rē'mē-ă	urine components in the blood
ureteritis	yū'rē-tĕr-ī'tis	inflammation of the ureter
ureterocele	yū-rē'tĕr-ō-sēl'	protrusion of the ureter
ureterolith	yū-rē'tĕr-ō-lith	stone in the ureter
ureterostenosis	yū-rē'tĕr-ō-ste-nō'sis	narrowing of the ureter
urethral stenosis	yū-rē'thrăl ste-nō'sis	narrowing of the urethra
urethritis	yū'rĕ-thrī'tis	inflammation of the urethra
ureterolith	yūr-ē'tĕr-ō-lith	stone in the ureter
urinary retention	yūr'i-nār'ē rē-ten'shŭn	abnormal accumulation of urine in the bladder, due to inability to empty the bladder
urinary suppression	yūr'i-nār'ē sŭ-presh'ŭn	suppression of urine formation
urinary tract infection (UTI)	yūr'i-nār'ē trakt in-fek'shŭn	infection in one or more organs of the urinary system
urge incontinence	ŭrj in-kon'ti-nens	involuntary leakage of urine with a sudden, strong desire to urinate

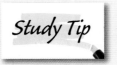

Study Tip

Epispadias and Hypospadias: To avoid confusing the terms epispadias and hypospadias, focus on the prefixes. *Epi-* means on or upon, so epispadias is the urinary meatus on the *upper* side of the penis. *Hypo-* means less than or below, so hypospadias is the urinary meatus on the *under* side of ("below") the penis.

■ Exercises: Symptoms and Medical Conditions

Exercise 12

Write the correct medical term for the definition given.

1. narrowing of an organ _____

2. involuntary discharge of urine _____

3. kidney stone _____

4. condition of stones in the kidney _____

5. condition in which the kidney fails to excrete urine _____

6. narrowing of the urethra _____

7. infection in urinary system organ(s) _____

8. urine components in the blood _____

9. urinary meatus on underside of penis _____

10. absence of urine formation _____

11. buildup of fluid (urine) in the kidney _____

12. excessive urination _____

Exercise 13

Circle the term that is most appropriate for the meaning of the sentence.

1. Mrs. Canter's urine leakage when she coughs is due to (*hypospadias, glycosuria, stress urinary incontinence*).

2. The medication caused (*epispadias, diuresis, pyuria*), so Mr. Samuels had to urinate frequently.

3. A stone in the patient's ureter caused a backup of urine, a condition that the physician called (*hydroureter, hematuria, ureterocele*).

4. Mr. Gill complained of fatigue from having to get up so many times at night because of his (*hypospadias, nocturia, nephroma*).

5. Laboratory testing showed that the patient was not urinating enough owing to (*nocturnal enuresis, uremia, urinary suppression*).

6. Mr. Horvath was diagnosed with (*ureteritis, polycystic kidney disease, anuria*) because his right kidney contained cysts.

7. The patient's prostate enlargement had caused him to develop (*diuresis, urinary retention, nephroptosis*) because he was having trouble emptying his bladder.

8. The physician explained to Mrs. Marianas that the medical term for her drooping kidney was (*nephroptosis, oliguria, urethral stenosis*).

9. A urinalysis revealed (*ureterocele, cystolith, hematuria*) because it was positive for the presence of blood in the urine sample.

10. Mrs. Katz had difficulty traveling because she had leaking of urine with a strong desire to urinate, which the physician called (*urethritis, anuria, urge incontinence*).

11. The newborn's examination revealed (*hypospadias, epispadias, enuresis*) when the physician noticed that the urinary meatus was on the upper surface of the penis.

12. Dr. Delgado told Mr. Peterson that his dysuria was due to (*proteinuria, urethritis, urethral stenosis*), which caused the urine to flow through a narrow urethra.

13. Mr. Berger's kidney disease led to elevated blood pressure called (*renal hypertension, hydroureter, enuresis*).

14. The parents expressed concern to Dr. Dodge about their son's (*oliguria, nephritis, nocturnal enuresis*) because the bed-wetting was affecting him socially.

15. Mr. Segel had (*chronic renal failure, end-stage renal disease, acute renal failure*), which is the final phase of chronic renal disease.

Exercise 14

TERM CONSTRUCTION

Build the correct medical term for the meaning given. Write the term in the blank indicating the word parts (CF, combining form; S, suffix).

1. stone in the ureter

   _____ / _____
   CF   S

2. protein in the urine

   _____ / _____
   CF   S

3. albumin in the urine

   _____ / _____
   CF   S

4. urine components in the blood

   _____ / _____
   CF   S

5. inflammation of the urethra

   _____ / _____
   CF   S

6. glucose in the urine

   _____ / _____
   CF   S

7. inflammation of the ureter

_____ / _____
                                    CF   S

8. inflammation of the renal pelvis and kidney

_____ / _____ / _____
                          CF   CF   S

9. condition of stones in the kidney

_____ / _____ / _____
                          CF   CF   S

10. inflammation of the glomeruli of the kidney

_____ / _____ / _____
                          CF   CF   S

TERM
CONSTRUCTION

Exercise 15

Write the remainder of the term for the meaning given.

1. stone in the ureter   uretero _____

2. pus in the urine   _____uria

3. inflammation of the bladder   cyst _____

4. drooping of the kidney   nephro _____

5. protrusion of the bladder   _____cele

6. difficulty urinating   _____uria

7. excessive amounts of urine   poly_____

8. inflammation of the renal pelvis   _____ itis

9. scanty amounts of urine   _____ uria

10. protrusion of the ureter   uretero_____

11. inflammation of the kidney   _____itis

12. stone in the bladder   cysto_____

13. bacteria in the urine   _____uria

14. enlargement of the kidney   nephro_____

15. narrowing of the ureter   uretero_____

Tests and Procedures

Term	Pronunciation	Meaning
Laboratory Tests		
blood urea nitrogen (BUN)	blŭd yū-rē′ă nĭ′trō-jen	blood test that measures the amount of urea in the blood; used to evaluate kidney function
creatinine clearance test	krē-at′i-nĕn klĕr′ăns test	test done to measure the total amount of creatinine excreted in the urine, usually in a 24-hour period, to assess kidney function
specific gravity (SG)	spĕ-sif′ik grav′i-tē	test to measure the concentration of urine; used to evaluate the ability of the kidneys to concentrate or dilute urine
urinalysis (UA)	yūr′i-nal′i-sis	series of tests done to analyze a sample of urine

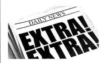

DIPSTICK URINALYSIS A dipstick urinalysis involves dipping a type of chemical analysis strip into a sample of urine and reading the colors of the squares. The test measures the specific gravity, acidity (pH), glucose, ketones, blood, leukocytes, nitrites, bilirubin, and urobilinogen levels in the sample. Abnormal findings in the assessment can indicate not only urinary system diseases but also the progression of diseases such as hypertension or diabetes.

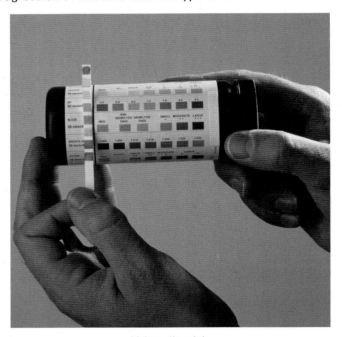

Urine dipstick.

Term	Pronunciation	Meaning
urinometer	yūr′i-nom′ĕ-tĕr	instrument for measuring the specific gravity of urine
Diagnostic Procedures		
cystogram	sis′tō-gram	radiologic recording (x-ray) of the bladder (Fig. 6-8)
cystography	sis-tog′ră-fē	process of making a radiologic recording of the bladder
cystometrogram	sis′tō-met′rō-gram	recording of pressure measurements in the bladder at various volumes
cystoscope	sis′tō-skōp	instrument for examining the bladder
cystoscopy	sis-tos′kŏ-pē	examination of the bladder (Fig. 6-9)
intravenous pyelography (IVP), intravenous urography (IVU)	in′tră-vē′nŭs pī′ĕ-log′ră-fē, in′tră-vē′nŭs yūr-og′ră-fē	process of making a radiologic recording (x-ray) of the urinary tract after injection of a contrast dye into the bloodstream (Fig. 6-10)

(continued)

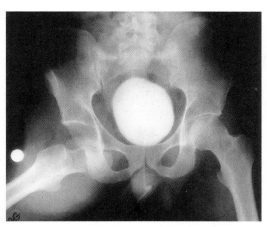

Figure 6-8 Normal cystogram showing contrast-filled bladder for a patient with a dislocated hip.

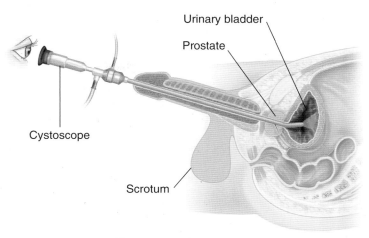

Figure 6-9 Cystoscopy.

Tests and Procedures *(continued)*

Term	Pronunciation	Meaning
kidneys, ureters, and bladder (KUB) x-ray	kid'nēz, yūr'ĕ-tĕrz, and blad'ĕr	x-ray of the kidneys, ureters, and bladder (Fig. 6-11)
nephrogram	nef'rō-gram	radiologic recording (x-ray) of the kidney
nephrography	ne-frog'ră-fē	process of making a radiologic recording (x-ray) of the kidney
nephroscope	nef'rō-skōp	instrument used to examine the kidney
nephroscopy	nef-ros'kŏ-pē	examination of the kidney(s)
nephrosonography	nef'rō-sŏ-nog'ră-fē	process of making a recording of the kidneys using sound waves (ultrasound)
nephrotomogram	nef'rō-tō'mō-gram	recording of cuts or sections of the kidney; a computed tomograph of the kidneys
renogram	rē'nō-gram	recording of kidney function after injection of a radioactive substance into the bloodstream; note that this is not an x-ray view
retrograde pyelogram	ret'rō-grād pī'el-ō-gram'	recording of the renal pelvis and kidneys taken after injection of a contrast dye into the ureters; retrograde means to go opposite to the normal direction
urethroscope	yū-rē'thrō-skōp	instrument used for examination of the urethra
urethroscopy	yū'rē-thros'kŏ-pē	examination of the urethra
urodynamics	yūr'ō-dī-nam'iks	recording of the force and flow of urine
voiding cystourethrography (VCUG)	voy'ding sis'tō-yū-rē-throg'ră-fē	process of making a radiologic recording (x-ray) of the bladder and urethra during urination after instillation of a contrast dye into the bladder

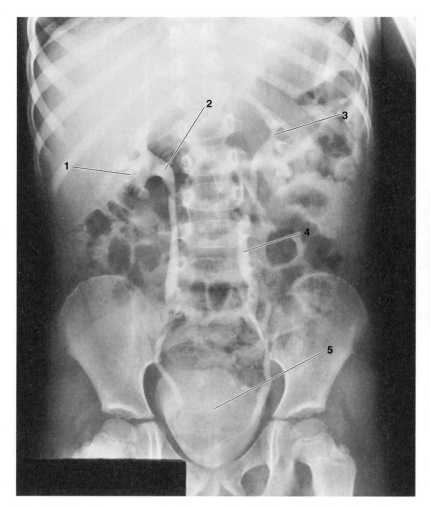

Figure 6-10 Intravenous pyelogram 20 minutes after injection of contrast material. Numbered lines show right kidney **(1)**, renal pelvis **(2)**, left kidney **(3)**, left ureter **(4)**, and urinary bladder **(5)**.

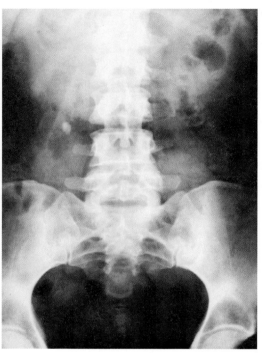

Figure 6-11 Kidney-ureter-bladder radiograph of a patient with acute right renal colic, demonstrating a 9- by 14-mm calculus between L3 and L4.

■ Exercises: Tests and Procedures

Exercise 16

SIMPLE
RECALL

Write the correct medical term for the meaning given.

1. test for measuring creatinine in urine   _____

2. instrument for examining the bladder   _____

3. x-ray of kidneys, ureters, and bladder   _____

4. recording of kidney function after injection
   of radioactive substance   _____

5. tests that analyze a urine sample   _____

6. test of the concentration of urine   _____

7. examination of the urethra   _____

8. process of taking an x-ray of the urinary
   tract after injecting dye   _____

9. x-ray of kidney   _____

10. blood test for measuring urea in the blood   _____

Exercise 17

ADVANCED
RECALL

Match each medical term with its meaning.

| urinometer | retrograde pyelogram | voiding cystourethrogram | urodynamics |
| cystometrogram | nephrosonography | nephrotomogram | urinalysis |

Meaning   **Term**

1. recording of pressure measurements in the bladder   _____

2. recording of renal pelvis and kidneys after dye injection   _____

3. recording of the force and flow of urine   _____

4. process of recording of kidneys using sound waves   _____

5. process of taking an x-ray of the bladder and urethra
   during urination   _____

6. recording of cuts or sections of the kidney   _____

7. instrument for measuring the specific gravity of urine   _____

8. series of tests that analyze a sample of urine   _____

Exercise 18

TERM
CONSTRUCTION

Using the given suffix, build a medical term for the meaning given.

Suffix	Meaning of Medical Term	Medical Term
-scopy	examination of the kidney	**1.** _____
-gram	x-ray of the bladder	**2.** _____

-graphy	process of x-raying the kidney	3. _____
-scope	instrument for examining the urethra	4. _____
-scopy	examination of the bladder	5. _____
-gram	recording of kidney function	6. _____
-graphy	process of x-raying the bladder	7. _____
-scope	instrument for examining the kidney	8. _____

Surgical Interventions and Therapeutic Procedures

Term	Pronunciation	Meaning
catheterization (cath)	kath'ĕ-ter-ī-zā'shŭn	procedure of inserting a tube through the urethra into the bladder to drain it of urine (Fig. 6-12)
cystectomy	sis-tek'tō-mē	excision of the bladder
cystolithotomy	sis'tō-li-thot'ō-mē	incision into the bladder to remove a stone
cystoplasty	sis'tō-plas'tē	repair of the bladder
cystorrhaphy	sis-tōr'ă-fē	suturing of the bladder
cystostomy	sis-tos'tō-mē	creating a surgical opening into the bladder
extracorporeal shock wave lithotripsy (ESWL)	eks'tră-kōr-pōr'ē-ăl shok wāv lith'ō-trip'sē	breaking up of renal or ureteral calculi by focused ultrasound energy
hemodialysis	hē'mō-dī-al'i-sis	removal of waste products from the blood by pumping the blood through a machine that works as an artificial kidney (Fig. 6-13)

(continued)

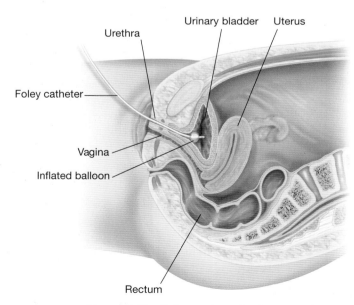

Figure 6-12 Foley catheterization.

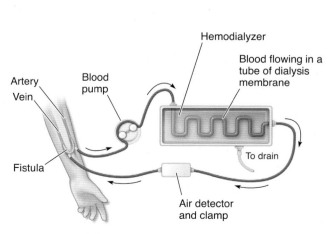

Figure 6-13 Hemodialysis.

Surgical Interventions and Therapeutic Procedures (continued)

Term	Pronunciation	Meaning
lithotomy	li-thot′ŏ-mē	incision made to remove a stone surgically
lithotripsy	lith′ō-trip′sē	crushing of a stone
meatotomy	mē′ă-tot′ŏ-mē	incision into a meatus
nephrectomy	ne-frek′tō-mē	excision of a kidney
nephrolithotomy	nef′rō-li-thot′ŏ-mē	incision into a kidney to remove a stone
nephrolysis	ne-frol′i-sis	separation of the kidney from adhesions
nephropexy	nef′rō-pek′sē	surgical fixation of a drooping kidney
nephrotomy	ne-frot′ŏ-mē	incision into a kidney
peritoneal dialysis	per′i-tō-nē′ăl dī-al′i-sis	removal of waste products in the blood or impurities from the body by using the peritoneum of the abdominal cavity as a filter (Fig. 6-14)
pyelolithotomy	pī′ĕ-lō-li-thot′ŏ-mē	incision into a renal pelvis to remove a stone
pyeloplasty	pī′ĕ-lō-plas′tē	repair of a renal pelvis
renal transplant, *syn.* kidney transplant	rē′năl trans′plant	surgical removal of a kidney and replacement with a donor kidney (Fig. 6-15)
ureterectomy	yū′rē-tĕr-ek′tō-mē	excision of a ureter
ureterostomy	yū-rē′tĕr-os′tō-mē	creation of a surgical opening into a ureter
ureterotomy	yū-rē′tĕr-ot′ŏ-mē	incision into a ureter
urethroplasty	yū-rē′thrō-plas′tē	repair of the urethra
urethrotomy	yū′rĕ-throt′ŏ-mē	incision into the urethra
vesicourethral suspension	ves′i-kō-yū-rē′thrăl sŭs-pen′shŭn	surgical suspension of the urethra and bladder for correction of stress urinary incontinence

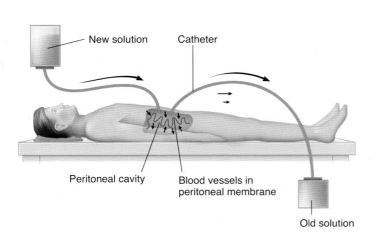

Figure 6-14   Peritoneal dialysis.

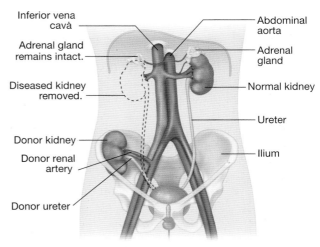

Figure 6-15   Renal transplant.

■ Exercises: Surgical Interventions and Therapeutic Procedures

Exercise 19

SIMPLE
RECALL

Write the meaning of the term given.

1. catheterization _____

2. cystolithotomy _____

3. nephropexy _____

4. cystostomy _____

5. pyelolithotomy _____

6. ureterectomy _____

7. urethroplasty _____

8. cystectomy _____

9. extracorporeal shock wave lithotripsy _____

Exercise 20

ADVANCED
RECALL

Complete each sentence by writing in the correct medical term.

1. The removal of waste products from the blood by pumping through an artificial kidney is called _____.

2. The removal of a kidney and replacement with a donor kidney is called a(n) _____ _____.

3. _____ is an incision made into a kidney to remove a stone.

4. _____ means to create a surgical opening into a ureter.

5. Removing waste products or impurities from the body using the peritoneum as a filter is called _____.

6. _____ means to repair the bladder.

7. A procedure done to suspend and support the bladder and urethra to correct SUI is called a(n) _____.

8. To make an incision into the kidney is called _____.

TERM
CONSTRUCTION

Exercise 21

Break the given medical term into its word parts and define each part. Then define the medical term.

For example:

cystectomy	*word parts:*	cyst/o / -ectomy
	meanings:	urinary bladder / excision, surgical removal
	term meaning:	excision of the bladder

1. lithotomy   *word parts:* _____ / _____

    meanings: _____ / _____

    term meaning: _____

2. cystorrhaphy   *word parts:* _____ / _____

    meanings: _____ / _____

    term meaning: _____

3. ureterotomy   *word parts:* _____ / _____

    meanings: _____ / _____

    term meaning: _____

4. nephrectomy   *word parts:* _____ / _____

    meanings: _____ / _____

    term meaning: _____

5. pyeloplasty   *word parts:* _____ / _____

    meanings: _____ / _____

    term meaning: _____

6. meatotomy   *word parts:* _____ / _____

    meanings: _____ / _____

    term meaning: _____

7. lithotripsy   *word parts:* _____ / _____

    meanings: _____ / _____

    term meaning: _____

8. nephrolysis   *word parts:* _____ / _____

    meanings: _____ / _____

    term meaning: _____

9. urethrotomy   *word parts:*   _____ / _____

                   meanings: _____ / _____

                   term meaning: _____

Medications and Drug Therapies

Term	Pronunciation	Meaning
antibacterial	an'tē-bak-tēr'ē-ăl	drug used to destroy or prevent the growth of bacteria
antibiotic	an'tē-bī-ot'ik	drug that acts against susceptible microorganisms
diuretic	dī-yūr-et'ik	drug that increases the amount of urine secreted
urinary analgesic	yūr'i-nār-ē an'ăl-jē'zik	drug used to relieve pain within the urinary system

■ Exercise: Medications and Drug Therapies

Exercise 22

SIMPLE RECALL

Write the correct medication or drug therapy term for the definition given

1. relieves pain within the urinary system   _____

2. acts against susceptible microorganisms   _____

3. increases the amount of urine secreted   _____

4. destroys or prevents the growth of bacteria   _____

Specialties and Specialists

Term	Pronunciation	Meaning
nephrology	ne-frol'ŏ-jē	medical specialty focusing on the study and treatment of kidney conditions
nephrologist	nef'rol'ŏ-jist	physician who specializes in nephrology
urology	yū-rol'ŏ-jē	medical specialty focusing on the study and treatment of conditions of the urinary system
urologist	yū-rol'ŏ-jist	physician who specializes in urology

■ Exercise: Specialties and Specialists

Exercise 23

SIMPLE RECALL

Write the correct medical term for the definition given.

1. specialist in the study and treatment of kidney conditions   _____

2. specialty focusing on the study and
   treatment of urinary system conditions

   _____

3. specialist in the study and treatment of
   urinary system conditions

   _____

4. specialty focusing on the study and treatment
   of kidney conditions

   _____

Abbreviations

Term	Meaning
ARF	acute renal failure
BUN	blood urea nitrogen
cath	catheter; catheterize; catheterization
CRF	chronic renal failure
ESRD	end-stage renal disease
ESWL	extracorporeal shock wave lithotripsy
GU	genitourinary
IVP	intravenous pyelogram; intravenous pyelography
IVU	intravenous urogram; intravenous urography
KUB	kidneys, ureters, and bladder (x-ray)
SG	specific gravity
SUI	stress urinary incontinence
UA	urinalysis
UTI	urinary tract infection
VCUG	voiding cystourethrogram; voiding cystourethrography

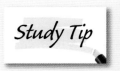

Study Tip

Same Abbreviation, Different Meanings: Some abbreviations can stand for two
(or even more) medical terms, depending on the context in which they are used.
For example, the abbreviation *cath* (see Abbreviations table) can stand for three
variations of the word *catheter*. Also, words that have the same prefix and combining
form but a different suffix (most commonly *-gram* or *-graphy*) can have the same
abbreviation (see IVP, IVU, and VCUG in the Abbreviations table).

■ Exercises: Abbreviations

Exercise 24

ADVANCED
RECALL

Write the meaning(s) for each abbreviation.

1. UTI   _____

2. IVP   _____

3. ESRD _____

4. SG _____

5. cath _____

6. VCUG _____

7. BUN _____

8. ARF _____

9. GU _____

10. IVU _____

ADVANCED
RECALL

Exercise 25

Write the meaning of each abbreviation used in these sentences.

1. The physician told Mrs. Cooper that a **KUB** was needed to look for stones in her urinary system.

_____

2. Dr. Shapiro ordered **ESWL** to try to break up the stones found in the patient's bladder.

_____

3. Mr. Kent's **CRF** was probably due to diabetic nephropathy.

_____

4. A **UA** was ordered to help diagnose the cause of the patient's dysuria.

_____

5. Ms. Stefano's physician told her that her urinary leakage when she coughs is a condition known as **SUI**.

_____

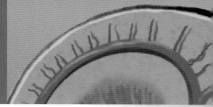

Review of Terms for Anatomy and Physiology

VISUAL

Exercise 26

Write the appropriate combining forms on the blanks for the anatomic structures indicated.

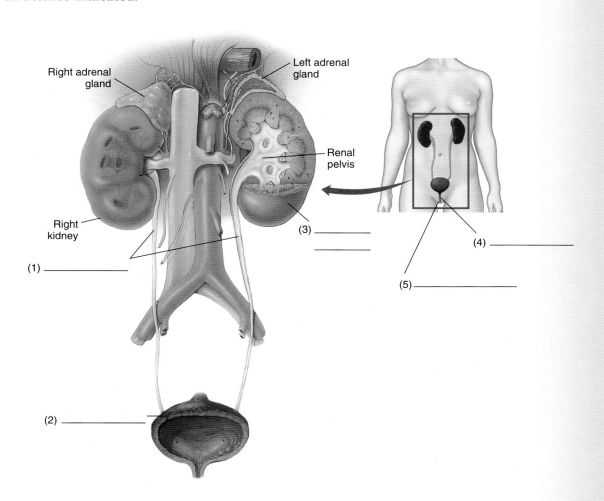

Right adrenal gland

Left adrenal gland

Renal pelvis

Right kidney

(1) _____

(2) _____

(3) _____

_____

(4) _____

(5) _____

Exercise 27

VISUAL

Write the correct terms on the blanks for the anatomic structures indicated.

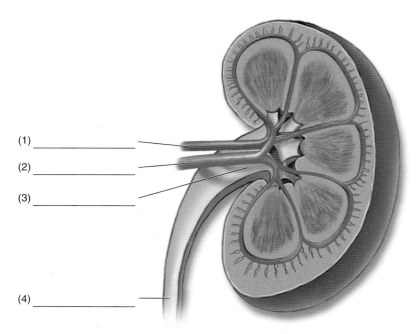

(1) _____

(2) _____

(3) _____

(4) _____

Understanding Terms

Exercise 28

TERM CONSTRUCTION

Write the combining form used in the medical term, followed by the meaning of the combining form.

Term	Combining Form	Combining Form Definition
1. cystorrhaphy	_____	_____
2. meatal	_____	_____
3. urethritis	_____	_____
4. hematuria	_____	_____
5. cystitis	_____	_____
6. renal	_____	_____
7. ureterostenosis	_____	_____
8. pyuria	_____	_____
9. pyelitis	_____	_____

10. urethroscope _____ _____

11. glycosuria _____ _____

12. nephrectomy _____ _____

13. vesical _____ _____

14. nocturia _____ _____

15. uremia _____ _____

16. cystoscopy _____ _____

17. nephrogram _____ _____

18. urethroplasty _____ _____

19. oliguria _____ _____

20. ureterolith _____ _____

TERM
CONSTRUCTION

Exercise 29

Break the given medical term into its word parts and define each part. Then define the medical term.

For example:

cystectomy	*word parts:*	cyst/o / -ectomy
	meanings:	urinary bladder / excision, surgical removal
	term meaning:	excision of the bladder

1. ureterolith *word parts:* _____ / _____

  meanings: _____ / _____

  term meaning: _____

2. glycosuria *word parts:* _____ / _____ / _____

  meanings: _____ / _____ / _____

  term meaning: _____

3. nephroptosis *word parts:* _____ / _____

  meanings: _____ / _____

  term meaning: _____

4. ureterostenosis *word parts:* _____ / _____

  meanings: _____ / _____

  term meaning: _____

5. nephrotomy   *word parts:*   _____ / _____

                     meanings: _____ / _____

                     term meaning: _____

6. uremia   *word parts:*   _____ / _____

                     meanings: _____ / _____

                     term meaning: _____

7. pyelitis   *word parts:*   _____ / _____

                     meanings: _____ / _____

                     term meaning: _____

8. glomerulonephritis   *word parts:*   _____ / _____ / _____

                     meanings: _____ / _____ / _____

                     term meaning: _____

Comprehension Exercises

Exercise 30

COMPREHENSION   **Fill in the blank with the correct term.**

1. _____ is a test that measures the concentration of urine.

2. An x-ray of the kidneys, ureters, and bladder is commonly referred to by its abbreviation _____ .

3. When a stone causes urine to back up in the ureter, the condition is called _____ .

4. The process of inserting a tube into the bladder to drain it is termed _____ .

5. A condition involving protein in the urine is known as _____ .

6. Removing waste products from the blood by pumping the blood through an artificial kidney is called _____ .

7. Involuntary release of urine when coughing or sneezing is called _____ .

8. High blood pressure caused by kidney disease is known as _____ .

9. The procedure for suspending and supporting the bladder and urethra to hold them in the proper position is called _____ .

10. A prolapsed or "drooping" kidney is called _____ .

11. A(n) _____ is a recording of pressure measurements in the bladder.

12. A(n) _____ is a series of tests done to analyze a urine sample.

13. A buildup of urine in the bladder owing to inability to release it is called _____.

14. The term for involuntary release of urine during the night is _____.

15. _____ is a congenital defect in which the urinary meatus is located on the underside of the penis.

Exercise 31

COMPREHENSION **Write a short answer for each question.**

1. What does a BUN test for? _____

2. What organ is removed in a renal transplant? _____

3. What kind of a sample is obtained for a specific gravity test? _____

4. Why might a patient with a renal calculus also have hydronephrosis? _____
   _____

5. Why is voiding an important function of the body? _____
   _____

6. Why would a patient with a cystolith require a lithotripsy? _____
   _____

7. What organ is examined using a nephroscope? _____

8. What type of physician would treat polycystic kidney disease? _____

9. What type of drug would be prescribed to relieve a patient of dysuria? _____
   _____

10. What substance cannot flow properly if a patient has a ureteral stricture? _____

11. What anatomic structures are suspended in the surgical treatment of stress urinary
    incontinence? _____

12. What procedure might be used to treat urinary retention? _____

13. What specialty might involve studying new treatment options for cystitis? _____

14. What does a lithotomy enable a physician to do? _____
    _____

15. What is fixated in a nephropexy? _____

16. What is protruding in a ureterocele? _____

17. What x-ray of a single organ would be used to diagnosis a cystolith? _____

18. What instrument is used to measure specific gravity? _____

19. What two types of drugs might be used to treat bacteriuria? _____

_____

20. What organ is examined in a nephrotomogram? _____

Exercise 32

COMPREHENSION   **Circle the letter of the best answer in the following questions.**

1. In the condition hypospadias, what structure is displaced?

   A. glomerulus
   B. renal pelvis
   C. urethra
   D. meatus

2. A condition that results from nonfunctioning nephrons is:

   A. dysuria
   B. anuria
   C. urinary retention
   D. nephromegaly

3. Which pair of terms indicates the same condition?

   A. cystocele and ureterolith
   B. nephritis and cystitis
   C. epispadias and hypospadias
   D. nephrolith and renal calculus

4. The procedure that produces an ultrasound recording of the kidney is called:

   A. nephrosonography
   B. nephrography
   C. nephrotomography
   D. cystometrography

5. Which of these conditions is a congenital defect?

   A. hydromegaly
   B. epispadias

C. diuresis
D. cystitis

6. Which term indicates that the nephrons are not functioning properly?

   A. urinary suppression
   B. dysuria
   C. renal hypertension
   D. micturition

7. Which test does not involve the testing of urine?

   A. specific gravity
   B. BUN
   C. urinalysis
   D. creatinine clearance

8. The procedure that involves making an incision into the reservoir of the kidney to remove a stone is called:

   A. nephrolithotomy
   B. cystolithotomy
   C. lithotripsy
   D. pyelolithotomy

9. Which condition does not indicate an abnormal substance in the urine?

   A. pyuria
   B. hematuria
   C. dysuria
   D. proteinuria

10. Which procedure involves the use of the patient's own body for the removal of waste products from the blood?

   A. peritoneal dialysis
   B. hemodialysis
   C. nephrosonography
   D. urodynamics

11. Which procedure records the backward flow of dye through the urinary tract?

   A. intravenous pyelogram
   B. cystometrogram
   C. retrograde pyelogram
   D. renogram

12. A patient who is excreting increased amounts of urine has:

   A. diuresis
   B. urge incontinence
   C. stress urinary incontinence
   D. hydronephrosis

13. The procedure that is done during micturition is called a:

   A. nephrogram
   B. cystometrogram
   C. voiding cystourethrogram
   D. retrograde pyelogram

14. Which procedure does not involve fixation or repair?

   A. nephrolysis
   B. nephropexy
   C. cystoplasty
   D. pyeloplasty

15. Narrowing of the structure that carries urine to the outside of the body is known as:

   A. urethritis
   B. ureteritis
   C. ureterostenosis
   D. urethrostenosis

Application and Analysis

CASE REPORTS

Exercise 33

APPLICATION

Read the case report and circle the letter of your answer choice for the questions that follow each case.

CASE 6-1

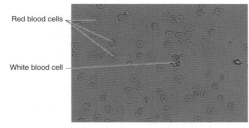

Mrs. Kendall was seen in the office today for complaints of dysuria, polyuria, and hematuria (Fig. 6-16). She has a past history of urge incontinence and polycystic kidneys. A urinalysis was performed, which revealed elevated leukocytes and the presence of some blood. The diagnosis was a urinary tract infection; she was started on antibiotic therapy for this condition.

Figure 6-16   Hematuria. Microscopic view of a urine sample shows a large number of red blood cells (RBCs) accompanied by a single while blood cell near the center.

1. Which term indicates that the patient had excessive urination?

   A. hematuria
   B. polyuria
   C. urge incontinence
   D. dysuria

2. The patient's past history indicates that she sometimes has a sudden and strong urge to urinate. What is the term used in the case for this condition?

   A. urge incontinence
   B. urinary tract infection
   C. hematuria
   D. polycystic kidney disease

3. The term for the presence of blood in the urine is:

   A. dysuria
   B. pyuria
   C. hematuria
   D. proteinuria

4. Which is a test used to analyze a sample of urine?

   A. cystogram
   B. nephrogram
   C. renogram
   D. urinalysis

5. Which is the term for an infection in one or more organs of the urinary system?

   A. urge incontinence
   B. hematuria
   C. urinary tract infection
   D. polycystic kidneys

MEDICAL RECORD ANALYSIS

MEDICAL RECORD 6-1

As the administrative medical assistant working in a physician's office, you have been asked to abstract information from the patient's medical record to obtain a rush authorization from his insurance company for a procedure. The patient's progress note from today's visit is as follows:

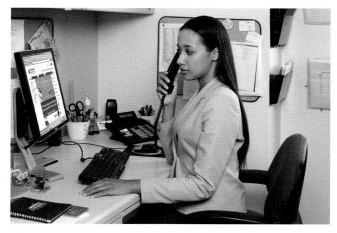

An administrative medical assistant performs critical medical office duties.

Medical Record

PROBLEM WITH URINATION

SUBJECTIVE: The patient presented in the office today with complaints of a feeling of fullness in his pelvic area as well as oliguria for the past 3 days. He feels the need to urinate and "not much comes out." He states that he also had some nocturnal enuresis off and on over the past week. He has a past history of pyelonephritis 1 year ago.

OBJECTIVE: The patient is a 52-year-old underweight male in obvious discomfort. Examination of the abdomen and pelvis was notable for pain on palpation of the pelvic area over the bladder. Percussion of this area revealed a distended bladder. A digital rectal exam was performed and revealed no enlargement of the prostate.

A urinalysis was ordered, but the patient was unable to void so in-and-out catheterization was performed and the bladder was drained. Urinalysis was performed on a sample of the urine and revealed dark color and a high SG.

ASSESSMENT: Diagnosis is urinary retention due to a probable stone in the urinary tract causing hydroureter or hydronephrosis.

PLAN: A stat KUB was ordered. I will call the patient as soon as I have the results of the KUB. Treatment will be determined based on the results of the x-ray.

Exercise 34

APPLICATION   **Write the appropriate medical terms or abbreviations used in this medical record on the blanks after their definitions.**

1. scanty amounts of urine   _____

2. involuntary release of urine at night   _____

3. inflammation of the renal pelvis and kidneys   _____

4. condition of fluid in the kidney(s)   _____

5. series of tests done to analyze a urine sample   _____

6. inserting a tube into the bladder to drain it of urine _____

7. specific gravity (abbreviation)   _____

8. abnormal accumulation of urine in the bladder   _____

9. backing up of urine in the ureter   _____

10. x-ray of the kidney, ureters, and bladder (abbreviation) _____

Bonus Question

11. According to the Assessment section of the report, what does the physician expect the KUB to

    reveal? _____

MEDICAL RECORD 6-2

You are a medical laboratory technologist working in a physician's office. Mrs. Talbot, a patient in your office, was referred to a urologist 1 month ago and is returning for a preoperative clearance. You are to perform the urinalysis in the office laboratory.

Medical Record

UROLOGY CONSULTATION REPORT

I saw Mrs. Talbot today on referral by your office. She presented as a pleasant 45-year-old woman with a history of stress urinary incontinence for the past year. She states that the symptoms have been increasing in severity over the past 2 months and that you referred her for possible surgical correction of the problem.

Past medical history reveals a right nephrectomy due to polycystic kidneys. She has no history of frequent urinary tract infections. The patient is multigravida. She had four vaginal deliveries without complications. She is also an asthmatic and finds the symptoms worse when an asthma exacerbation causes increased coughing.

Examination revealed an overweight female in no acute distress. Pelvic exam revealed a cystocele. Urinalysis done in the office today was normal.

The patient was scheduled for cystoscopy, urodynamics, a pelvic ultrasound, and a voiding cystourethrogram. I informed the patient that her SUI is likely caused by weakness of the pelvic muscles due to multiple childbirths and this has left her with a prolapsed bladder. She may be an excellent candidate for a transvaginal tape procedure. We will discuss this further following her workup, and I will keep you updated as to the results.

Exercise 35

APPLICATION

Read the medical report and circle the letter of your answer choice for the following questions.

1. The urologist indicated that the patient's SUI is likely due to weakness of the pelvic muscles. What does the abbreviation SUI mean?

   A. strong urinary infection
   B. stressing urinary infection
   C. stress urinary incontinence
   D. stress urethral incontinence

2. The pelvic examination revealed a cystocele. What is a cystocele?

   A. protrusion of the rectum
   B. protrusion of the bladder
   C. inflammation of the bladder
   D. stone in the bladder

3. The term that means an x-ray of the bladder and urethra made during urination is:

   A. nephrogram
   B. intravenous pyelogram
   C. retrograde pyelogram
   D. voiding cystourethrogram

4. What procedure was previously performed because of the patient's polycystic kidney?

   A. nephrectomy
   B. renography
   C. nephrolysis
   D. nephrostomy

5. The diagnostic test that will record the force and flow of urine is a:

    A. urethroscopy
    B. cystometrogram
    C. urodynamics
    D. intravenous pyelogram

6. Which test ordered by the urologist will involve examination of the bladder using a scope?

    A. nephroscopy
    B. cystoscopy

    C. urethroscopy
    D. cystography

7. Which of the patient's conditions would result in loss of functioning kidney tissue?

    A. SUI
    B. polycystic kidneys
    C. prolapsed bladder
    D. cystocele

Bonus Question

8. If the term *vaginal* means "pertaining to the vagina," what does the term *transvaginal*

   mean? _____

Pronunciation and Spelling

Exercise 36

AUDITORY

Review the Chapter 6 terms in the Dictionary/Audio Glossary in the Student Resources and practice pronouncing each term, referring to the pronunciation guide as needed.

Exercise 37

SPELLING

Check the spelling of each term. If it is correct, check off the correct box. If incorrect, write the correct spelling on the line.

1. glomarulus ☐ _____

2. meatis ☐ _____

3. cistic ☐ _____

4. vesical ☐ _____

5. micturate ☐ _____

6. nefromegaly ☐ _____

7. oliguria ☐ _____

8. cystosele ☐ _____

9. dieuresis ☐ _____

10. glycosuria ☐ _____

11. hydrourether ☐ _____

12. incontinence ☐ _____

13. creatinine ☐ _____

14. urinanalysis ☐ _____

15. cistoscopy ☐ _____

Media Connection

STUDENT RESOURCES

Exercise 38

Complete each of the following activities available with the Student Resources. Check off each activity as you complete it, and record your score for the Chapter Quiz in the space provided.

Chapter Exercises

____ Flash Cards

____ Concentration

____ Abbreviation Match-Up

____ Roboterms

____ Word Builder

____ Fill the Gap

____ Break It Down

____ True/False Body Building

____ Quiz Show

____ Complete the Case

____ Medical Record Review

____ Look and Label

____ Image Matching

____ Spelling Bee

____ **Chapter Quiz**   *Score:* _____%

Additional Resources

____ Animation: Renal Function

____ Dictionary/Audio Glossary

____ Health Professions Careers: Administrative Medical Assistant

____ Health Professions Careers: Medical Laboratory Technologist

Cardiovascular and Lymphatic Systems

7

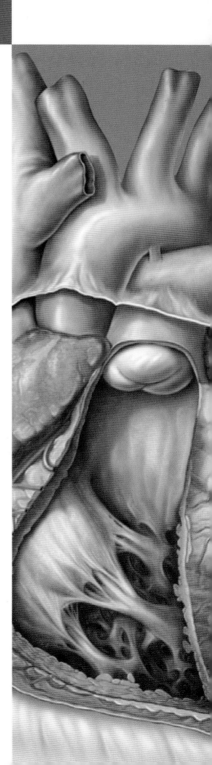

Chapter Outline

Objectives

After completion of this chapter you will be able to:

1. Describe the location of the main cardiovascular and lymphatic structures in the body.

2. Define terms related to the heart, the vascular system, and the lymphatic system.

3. Define combining forms, prefixes, and suffixes related to the cardiovascular and lymphatic systems.

4. Define common medical terminology related to the cardiovascular and lymphatic systems, including adjectives and related terms, symptoms and conditions, tests and procedures, surgical interventions and therapeutic procedures, medications and drug therapies, and specialties.

5. Explain abbreviations for terms related to the cardiovascular and lymphatic systems.

6. Successfully complete all chapter exercises.

7. Explain terms used in medical records and case studies involving the cardiovascular and lymphatic systems.

8. Successfully complete all pronunciation and spelling exercises, and complete all interactive exercises included with the companion Student Resources.

■ ANATOMY AND PHYSIOLOGY

Functions of the Cardiovascular System

■ To transport blood throughout the body (Fig. 7-1)
■ To deliver oxygen and nutrients to body cells through arteries and capillaries
■ To remove waste products from body cells through capillaries and veins
■ To pump blood through the heart with the aid of electrical conduction

Structures of the Cardiovascular System

■ The heart wall consists of three tissue layers.
■ The heart has four chambers aided by four valves to keep blood moving in one direction.
■ The heart has specialized tissue that transmits electrical impulses.
■ The heart muscle contracts in a rhythmic sequence, pushing blood through the chambers and vessels.
■ The arteries carry blood away from the heart.
■ The capillaries allow exchange of gasses, nutrients, and wastes between the blood and body cells.
■ The veins return blood back to the heart.

Functions of the Lymphatic System

■ To return lymph from body tissues to the blood (Fig. 7-1)
■ To protect the body by filtering microorganisms and foreign particles from the lymph
■ To maintain the body's internal fluid level
■ To absorb fats from the small intestines

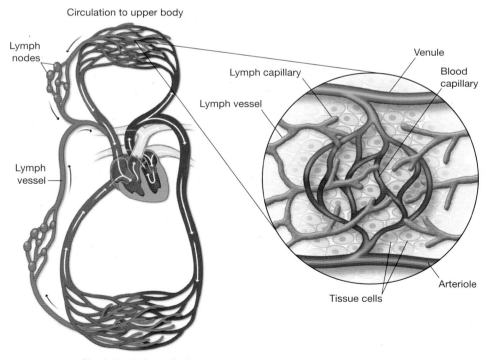

Figure 7-1   Blood and lymph flow in the cervical region.

Structures of the Lymphatic System

- The lymph is clear tissue fluid consisting of white blood cells and a few red blood cells.
- The lymph nodes filter the lymph.
- The lymph nodes are primarily concentrated in the neck, chest, armpits, and groin.
- The lymph vessels transport the lymph from the body tissues to the venous system.
- The lymph vessels have valves that facilitate one-way transport of lymph.

Terms Related to the Cardiovascular and Lymphatic Systems

Term	Pronunciation	Meaning
The Heart (Fig. 7-2)		
cardiovascular system	kahr'dē-ō-vas'kyū-lăr sis'tĕm	heart and blood vessels carrying oxygen and nutrients to the body cells and carrying away waste (Fig. 7-3)
heart	hahrt	muscular organ taking deoxygenated blood from the veins, pumping it to the lungs for oxygen, and returning it to the body through the arteries (Fig. 7-4)

(continued)

ANIMATION

View the animation *Cardiac Cycle* on the Student Resources to learn how blood flows through the heart.

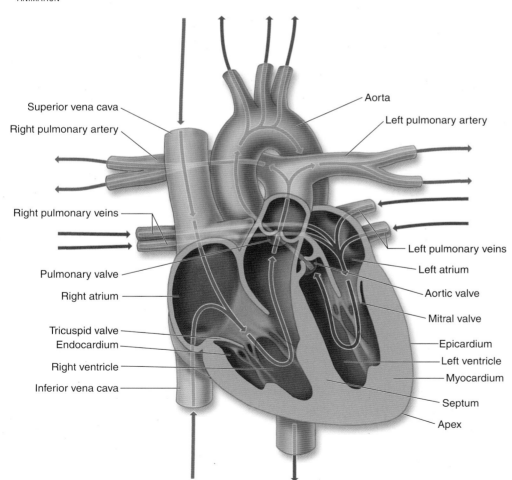

Figure 7-2   Heart and great vessels.

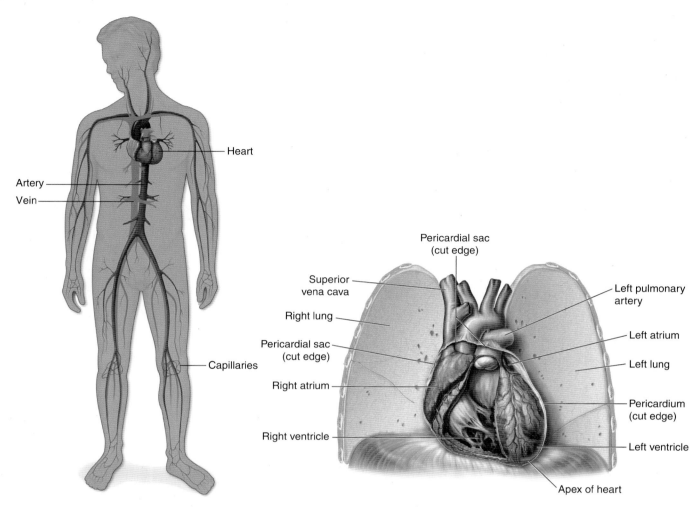

Figure 7-3 The cardiovascular system.   **Figure 7-4** Cross-section of the heart and lungs showing the heart's relative position in the body.

Terms Related to the Cardiovascular and Lymphatic Systems (continued)

Term	Pronunciation	Meaning
apex	ā′peks	the lower pointed end of the heart
septum	sep′tŭm	wall of heart tissue separating the right and left sides
atrium	ā′terē-ŭm	upper receiving chamber of the heart; right and left
ventricle	ven′tri-kĕl	lower pumping chamber of the heart; right and left structures
endocardium	en′dō-kahr′dē-ŭm	inner lining of the heart
myocardium	mī′ō-kahr′dē-ŭm	middle muscular layer of heart tissue
epicardium	ep′i-kahr′dē-ŭm	outer lining of the heart
pericardium	per′i-kahr′dē-ŭm	sac around the heart that facilitates movement of the heart as it beats

(continued)

Terms Related to the Cardiovascular and Lymphatic Systems *(continued)*

Term	Pronunciation	Meaning
aortic valve	ā-ōr′tik valv	heart valve between the left ventricle and aorta
mitral valve	mī′trăl valv	heart valve between the left atrium and left ventricle; also called a bicuspid valve
pulmonary valve	pul′mŏ-nār-ē valv	heart valve between the right ventricle and the pulmonary artery; also called a semilunar valve due to the half-moon shape of its three cusps
tricuspid valve	trī-kŭs′pid valv	heart valve between the right atrium and right ventricle; also called a semilunar valve due to the half-moon shape of its three cusps
The Vascular System		
blood vessels	blŭd ves′ĕlz	structures that carry or transport blood
artery	ar′tĕr-ē	vessel carrying blood away from the heart (Fig. 7-5)
arteriole	ahr-tēr′ē-ōl	small artery

(continued)

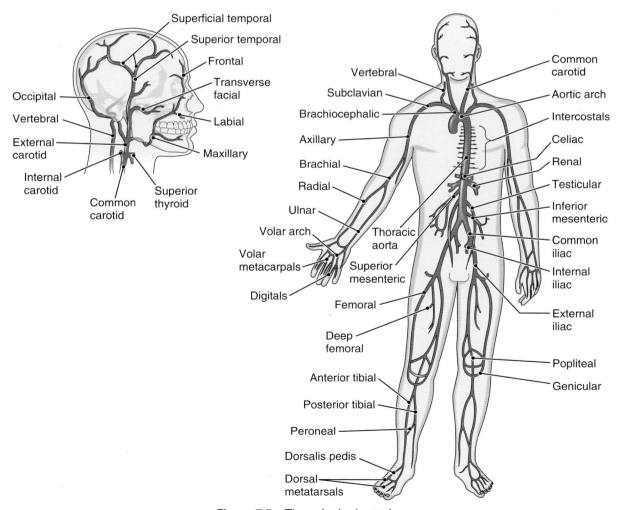

Figure 7-5 The principal arteries.

Terms Related to the Cardiovascular and Lymphatic Systems (continued)

Term	Pronunciation	Meaning
capillary	kap′i-lār-ē	microscopic thin-walled vessel connecting arterioles and venules where gas, nutrient, and waste exchange take place between the blood and cells of the body
lumen	lū′měn	interior space of a vessel
venule	ven′yūl	small vein
vein	vān	vessel carrying blood to the heart
aorta	ā-ōr′tă	largest artery that begins as an arch from the left ventricle then branches and descends through the thoracic and abdominal cavities; carries oxygenated blood away from the heart
inferior vena cava	in-fēr′ē-ŏr vē′nă kā′vă	large vein carrying blood to the heart from the lower part of the body (Fig. 7-6)
superior vena cava	sŭ-pēr′ē-ŏr vē′nă kā′vă	large vein carrying blood to the heart from the upper part of the body (Fig. 7-6)
The Lymphatic System (Fig. 7-7)		
lymph	limf	clear fluid consisting of fluctuating amounts of white blood cells and a few red blood cells that accumulates in tissue and is removed by the lymphatic capillaries
lymph nodes, *syn.* lymph glands	limf nōdz, limf glandz	small bean-shaped masses of lymphatic tissue that filter bacteria and foreign material from the lymph; located on larger lymph vessels in the axillary, cervical, inguinal, and mediastinal areas (Fig. 7-8)
lymph vessels	limf ves′ĕlz	vessels transporting lymph from body tissues to the venous system
lymph capillaries	limf kap′i-lar-ēz	microscopic thin-walled lymph vessels that pick up lymph, proteins, and waste from body tissues
lymph ducts	limf dŭkts	the largest lymph vessels that transport lymph to the venous system

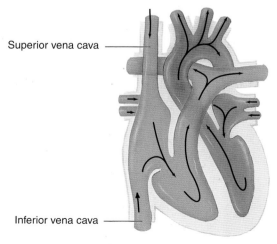

Superior vena cava

Inferior vena cava

Figure 7-6 Anterior view of the coronary arteries.

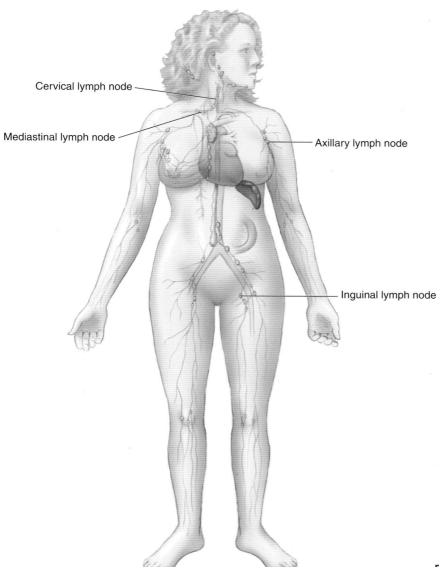

Cervical lymph node

Mediastinal lymph node

Axillary lymph node

Inguinal lymph node

Figure 7-7   Major lymph node locations.

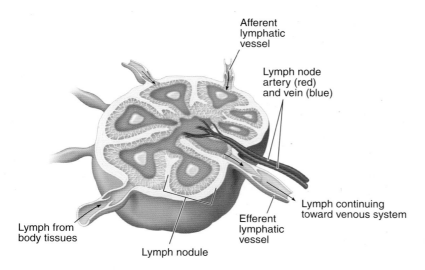

Afferent
lymphatic
vessel

Lymph node
artery (red)
and vein (blue)

Lymph continuing
toward venous system

Efferent
lymphatic
vessel

Lymph nodule

Lymph from
body tissues

Figure 7-8   The interior of a lymph
node.

■ Exercises: Anatomy and Physiology

SIMPLE
RECALL

Exercise 1

Write the correct anatomic structure for the meaning given.

1. upper chamber of the heart _____

2. small vein _____

3. middle muscular layer of heart _____

4. valve between the left ventricle and aorta _____

5. wall of heart tissue _____

6. small artery _____

7. large veins carrying blood to the heart _____

8. muscular pumping organ _____

9. inner lining of the heart _____

10. sac around the heart _____

ADVANCED
RECALL

Exercise 2

Write the meaning or function of the term given.

1. lymph _____

2. artery _____

3. vein _____

4. lymph capillaries _____

5. aorta _____

6. blood vessels _____

7. lymph vessels _____

8. lymph ducts _____

9. lymph nodes _____

10. tricuspid valve _____

ADVANCED RECALL

Exercise 3

Circle the term that is most appropriate for the meaning of the sentence.

1. The two upper receiving chambers of the heart are called the right and left (*aortas, atria, ventricles*).

2. The epicardium is the (*inner, middle, outer*) lining of the heart.

3. The (*endocardium, myocardium, pericardium*) is the inner lining of the heart.

4. Another name for the mitral valve is the (*semilunar, bicuspid, tricuspid*) valve.

5. The largest artery in the body is the (*inferior vena cava, superior vena cava, aorta*).

6. The pulmonary valve is located between the right ventricle and the pulmonary (*vein, artery, vena cava*).

7. The lymph (*nodes, ducts, capillaries*) pick up lymph, proteins, and waste from the body cells.

8. The inferior vena cava is a large (*artery, vein, capillary*).

9. The smallest blood vessel where gas and nutrients are exchanged is a(n) (*arteriole, capillary, venule*).

10. The (*aortic, mitral, tricuspid*) valve is also referred to as a semilunar valve.

11. The mitral valve has (*one, two, three*) cusps or leaflets that open and close.

12. The (*endocardium, myocardium, pericardium*) is the sac around the heart.

13. A small artery is called a(n) (*arteriolo, arteriole, capillary*).

14. The muscular organ pumping blood through the body is the (*circulatory system, pulmonary system, heart*).

ADVANCED RECALL

Exercise 4

Match each medical term with its meaning.

myocardium   septum   lymph
pulmonary valve   lumen   apex

Meaning   **Term**

1. structure between the right ventricle and pulmonary artery   _____

2. middle muscular layer of heart tissue   _____

3. interior space of a vessel   _____

4. clear fluid that accumulates in tissues   _____

5. wall inside the heart   _____

6. the lower pointed end of the heart   _____

Exercise 5

ADVANCED
RECALL

Complete each sentence by writing in the correct medical term.

1. Bacteria and foreign material are filtered out of circulation by the _____ .

2. The bottom chambers of the heart responsible for forcing the blood through the body are the

_____ .

3. The vessels that carry blood away from the heart are _____ .

4. The _____ regulates the flow of blood between the left ventricle and the aorta.

5. The _____ is a sac found around the heart that facilitates movement as it beats.

6. The interior space of a vessel is called a(n) _____ .

7. A microscopic vessel that picks up fluid and proteins from the cells is a lymph

_____ .

8. The lymph _____ are the largest lymph vessels.

9. The clear fluid that accumulates in tissue is called _____ .

10. The _____ vena cava carries blood to the heart from the lower part of the body.

■ WORD PARTS

Note that some word parts that have been introduced earlier in the book may not
be repeated here.

Combining Forms

Combining Form	Meaning
Related to the Cardiovascular System	
angi/o, vas/o, vascul/o	vessel, duct
aort/o	aorta
arteri/o	artery
ather/o	fatty paste
atri/o	atrium

(continued)

Combining Forms *(continued)*

Combining Form	Meaning
cardi/o	heart
coron/o	circle or crown
electr/o	electric, electricity
my/o	muscle
phleb/o, ven/i, ven/o	vein
pulmon/o	lung
scler/o	hard
son/o	sound, sound waves
sphygm/o	pulse
steth/o, thorac/o	thorax, chest
thromb/o	blood clot
valv/o, valvul/o	valve
varic/o	swollen or twisted vein
ventricul/o	ventricle
Related to the Lymphatic System	
aden/o	gland
lymph/o	lymph

Prefixes

Prefix	Meaning
Related to the Cardiovascular System	
brady-	slow
de-	away from, cessation, without
endo-	in, within
epi-	on, following
inter-	between
intra-	within
peri-	around, surrounding
tachy-	rapid, fast
tel-	end
trans-	across, through
tri-	three

Suffixes

Suffix	Meaning
Related to the Cardiovascular System	
-al, -ar, -ary, -ic	pertaining to
-ectasia	dilation, stretching

(continued)

Suffixes *(continued)*

Suffix	Meaning
-gram	record, recording
-graph	instrument for recording
-graphy	process of recording
-icle, -ole, -ule	small
-lytic	pertaining to destruction, breakdown, separation
-ium	tissue, structure
-stenosis	stricture, narrowing
Related to the Lymphatic System	
-oid	resembling

■ Exercises: Word Parts

SIMPLE
RECALL

Exercise 6

Write the meaning of the combining form given.

1. atri/o _____

2. my/o _____

3. vas/o _____

4. angi/o _____

5. ven/o _____

6. electr/o _____

7. arteri/o _____

8. cardi/o _____

9. ventricul/o _____

10. pulmon/o _____

11. coron/o _____

12. phleb/o _____

13. vascul/o _____

14. thorac/o _____

15. valvul/o _____

Exercise 7

SIMPLE RECALL

Write the correct combining form(s) for the meaning given.

1. hard _____

2. pulse _____

3. swollen or twisted vein _____

4. lymph _____

5. valve _____

6. aorta _____

7. artery _____

8. atrium _____

9. heart _____

10. thorax, chest _____

Exercise 8

SIMPLE RECALL

Write the meaning of the prefix or suffix given.

1. -stenosis _____

2. -ule, -icle, -ole _____

3. tachy- _____

4. trans- _____

5. intra- _____

6. inter- _____

7. endo- _____

8. -graph _____

9. brady- _____

10. epi- _____

11. peri- _____

12. -ium _____

13. -al, -ar, -ary, -ic _____

14. tri- _____

15. de- _____

16. -lytic _____

ADVANCED
RECALL

Exercise 9

Considering the meaning of the combining form from which the medical term is made, write the meaning of the medical term. (You have not yet learned many of these terms but can build their meaning from the word parts.)

Combining Form	Meaning	Medical Term	Meaning of Term
phleb/o	vein	phlebitis	**1.** _____
cardi/o	heart	cardiology	**2.** _____
my/o, cardi/o	muscle, heart	myocardium	**3.** _____
thromb/o	blood clot	thrombosis	**4.** _____
ven/o	vein	venogram	**5.** _____
ather/o	fatty paste	atherectomy	**6.** _____
lymph/o	lymph	lymphoid	**7.** _____
aort/o	aorta	aortography	**8.** _____

TERM
CONSTRUCTION

Exercise 10

Using the given combining form, build a medical term for the meaning given.

Combining Form	Meaning of Medical Term	Medical Term
angi/o	surgical repair or reconstruction of a vessel	**1.** _____
thorac/o	pertaining to the chest	**2.** _____
arteri/o	small artery	**3.** _____
ven/o	small vein	**4.** _____
vascul/o	pertaining to vessels, ducts	**5.** _____
aden/o	resembling a gland	**6.** _____
lymph/o	disease of the lymph vessels or nodes	**7.** _____
son/o	process of recording using sound	**8.** _____

■ MEDICAL TERMS

Adjectives and Other Related Terms

Term	Pronunciation	Meaning
arteriovenous (AV)	ahr-tēr′ē-ō-vē′nŭs	pertaining to both arteries and veins
atrioventricular (AV)	ā′trē-ō-ven-trik′yū-lăr	pertaining to the atria and ventricles
cardiovascular	kahr′dē-ō-vas′kyū-lăr	pertaining to the heart and blood vessels
constriction	kŏn-strik′shŭn	process of narrowing or tightening of a structure
cyanotic	sī′ă-not′ik	pertaining to a blue or purple discoloration due to deoxygenated blood
deoxygenation	dē-ok′si-jĕ-nā′shŭn	process of removing or having a lack of oxygen
diastole	dī-as′tŏ-lē	the relaxation phase of the ventricles in the heartbeat cycle
ischemic	is-kē′mik	pertaining to a lack of blood flow
oxygenation	ok′si-jĕ-nā′shŭn	process of adding oxygen
paroxysmal	par-ok-siz′măl	sudden
patent	pā′tĕnt	open or exposed
precordial	prē-kōr′dē-ăl	pertaining to the anterior left chest
sphygmic	sfig′mik	pertaining to the pulse
stenotic	sten-ot′ik	pertaining to the condition of narrowing
supraventricular	sū′pră-ven-trik′yū-lăr	pertaining to above the ventricles
systole	sis′tŏ-lē	the contraction phase of the ventricles in the heartbeat cycle
thoracic	thōr-as′ik	pertaining to the chest
thrombotic	throm-bot′ik	pertaining to a thrombus or blood clot
varicose	var′i-kōs	pertaining to swollen or twisted veins

■ Exercises: Adjectives and Other Related Terms

SIMPLE
RECALL

Exercise 11

Circle the term that is most appropriate for the meaning of the sentence.

1. The term supraventricular refers to (*above, below, beside*) the ventricles.

2. A sudden arrhythmia, such as an atrial tachycardia, is described as (*stenotic, precordial, paroxysmal*).

3. An open coronary artery is referred to as (*patent, stenotic, varicose*).

4. A stenotic vessel is one that is (*widened, narrowed, stretched*).

5. The medical term used to describe a blue or purple discoloration is (*pathologic, varicose, cyanotic*).

6. (*Diastole, Systole, Stenosis*) refers to the contraction phase of the ventricles in the heartbeat cycle.

7. The relaxation phase of the ventricles in the heartbeat cycle is (*diastole, stenosis, systole*).

Exercise 12

ADVANCED
RECALL

Match each medical term with its meaning.

precordial	constriction	cardiovascular	cyanotic	deoxygenation
varicose	oxygenation	atrioventricular	ischemic	thoracic

Meaning   **Term**

1. process of narrowing or tightening   _____

2. pertaining to the heart and blood vessels   _____

3. pertaining to a blue or purple discoloration _____

4. pertaining to the anterior left chest   _____

5. pertaining to twisted, swollen veins   _____

6. process of adding oxygen   _____

7. pertaining to the chest   _____

8. pertaining to lack of blood flow   _____

9. pertaining to atria and ventricles   _____

10. process of removing oxygen   _____

Exercise 13

TERM
CONSTRUCTION

Write the combining form(s) used in the medical term, followed by the meaning of the combining form.

Term	Combining Form(s)	Combining Form Meaning(s)
1. sphygmic	_____	_____
2. cardiovascular	_____	_____
3. varicose	_____	_____
4. arteriovenous	_____	_____
5. thrombosis	_____	_____

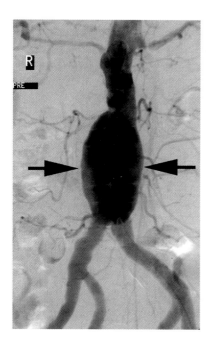

Figure 7-9   Aortic arteriogram in a 68-year-old man demonstrates an infrarenal abdominal aortic aneurysm (*arrows*).

Symptoms and Medical Conditions

Term	Pronunciation	Meaning
Related to the Cardiovascular System		
Disorders of the Heart and Arteries		
acute coronary syndrome (ACS)	ă-kyūt′ kōr′ŏ-năr-ē sin′drōm	chest pain and other signs and symptoms associated with cardiac ischemia
aneurysm	an′yūr-izm	dilation of an artery; usually due to a weakness in the wall of the artery (Fig. 7-9)
angina pectoris	an′ji-nă pek′tō′ris	chest pain or pressure resulting from lack of blood flow to the myocardium
angiostenosis	an′jē-ō-stĕ-nō′sis	narrowing of a blood vessel
aortic stenosis	ă-ŏr′tik stĕ-nō′sis	narrowing of the aortic valve opening (Fig. 7-10)
arteriosclerosis, *syn.* arteriosclerotic heart disease (ASHD)	ahr-tēr′ē-ō-skler-ō′sis, ahr-tēr′ē-ō-skler-ot′ik hahrt diz′ēz	hardening or loss of elasticity of the arteries

(continued)

Normal semilunar valve

Stenotic semilunar valve

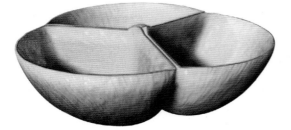
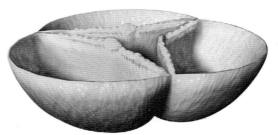

Figure 7-10   Stenosis of a semilunar valve. The aortic and pulmonary valves are semilunar valves.

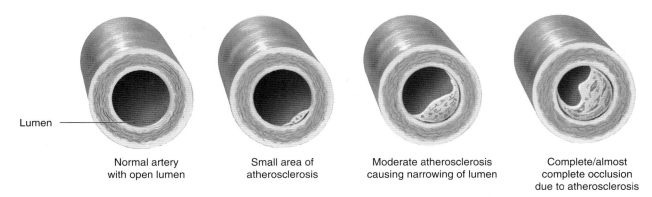

Lumen

| Normal artery with open lumen | Small area of atherosclerosis | Moderate atherosclerosis causing narrowing of lumen | Complete/almost complete occlusion due to atherosclerosis |

Figure 7-11 The progression of atherosclerosis.

Symptoms and Medical Conditions *(continued)*

Term	Pronunciation	Meaning
atherosclerosis	ath′ĕr-ō-skler-ō′sis	buildup of plaque or fatty paste inside arterial walls (Fig. 7-11)
cardiac arrest	kahr′dē-ak ă-rest′	complete, sudden cessation of cardiac activity
cardiac tamponade	kahr′dē-ak tam′pŏ-nahd′	compression of the heart due to an increase of fluid in the pericardium
cardiomegaly	kahr′dē-ō-meg′ă-lē	enlargement of the heart
cardiomyopathy	kahr′dē-ō-mī-op′ă-thē	disease of the heart muscles
cardiopathy	kahr′dē-op′ă-thē	any disease of the heart

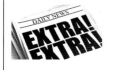

RISK FACTORS FOR CARDIOPATHY Risk factors for heart disease can be placed in two categories: those that are changeable and those that cannot be changed. Risk factors that are changeable include obesity, hypertension, smoking, lack of exercise, and poor diet. Diabetes and stress are also considered changeable risk factors because they can be controlled. Unchangeable risk factors include age, gender, race, and family history.

cardiovalvulitis	kahr′dē-ō-val-vyū-lī′tis	inflammation of the valves of the heart
coarctation of the aorta	kō′ahrk-tā′shŭn ā-ōr′tă	narrowing of the aorta causing hypertension, ventricular strain, and ischemia
congestive heart failure (CHF)	kŏn-jes′tiv hahrt fāl′yŭr	inefficiency of cardiac circulation causing edema and pulmonary congestion
coronary artery disease (CAD)	kōr′ŏ-nār-ē ahr′tĕr-ē di-zēz′	narrowing of coronary arteries causing a decrease of blood flow or ischemia to the myocardium
coronary occlusion	kōr′ŏ-nār-ē ŏ-klū′zhŭn	blockage of a coronary vessel often leading to a myocardial infarction
embolus	em′bō-lŭs	vascular blockage made up of a thrombus, bacteria, air, plaque, and/or other foreign material

(continued)

Symptoms and Medical Conditions *(continued)*

Term	Pronunciation	Meaning
endocarditis	en'dō-kahr-dī'tis	inflammation of the endocardium
hypertension	hī'pĕr-ten'shŭn	persistently elevated blood pressure
hypotension	hī'pō-ten'shŭn	blood pressure that is below normal
intermittent claudication	in'tĕr-mit'ĕnt klaw'di-kā'shŭn	cramping of the lower leg muscles usually caused by lack of blood flow
ischemia	is-kē'mē-ă	lack of blood flow
mitral valve prolapse	mī'trăl valv prō'laps	backward movement of the mitral valve cusps allowing regurgitation
mitral valve stenosis	mī'trăl valv stĕ-nō'sis	narrowing of the mitral valve opening usually caused by scarring from rheumatic fever
murmur	mŭr'mŭr	abnormal heart sound
myocardial infarction (MI)	mī'ō-kahr'dē-ăl in-fahrk'shŭn	death of heart tissue usually due to coronary artery occlusion (Fig. 7-12)
myocarditis	mī'ō-kahr-dī'tis	inflammation of the heart muscle
occlusion	ŏ-klū'zhŭn	blockage or closure
pericarditis	per'i-kahr-dī'tis	inflammation of the pericardial sac around the heart
peripheral arterial disease (PAD)	pĕr-if'ĕr-ăl ahr-tēr'ē-ăl di-zēz'	any disorder of the arteries outside of, or peripheral to, the heart
plaque	plak	fat or lipid deposit on an arterial wall
polyarteritis	pol'ē-ahr-tĕr-ī'tis	inflammation of many arteries
Raynaud disease, *syn.* Raynaud syndrome	rā-nō' diz'ēz, rā-nō' sin'drōm	cyanosis of the fingers or toes due to vascular constriction, usually caused by cold tem peratures or emotional stress (Fig. 7-13)

(continued)

ANIMATION

Learn how elevated blood pressure affects the heart and other organs of the body by viewing the animation *Hypertension* in the electronic Student Resources.

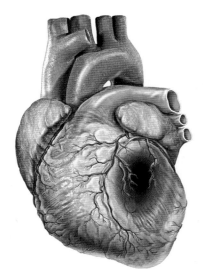

Figure 7-12 Myocardial infarction (MI) (*darkened area*).

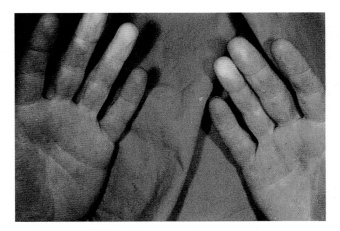

Figure 7-13 Raynaud disease as indicated by cyanosis (white areas) on the ends of the fingers.

Symptoms and Medical Conditions *(continued)*

Term	Pronunciation	Meaning
rheumatic heart disease (RHD)	rū-mat′ik hahrt di-zēz′	valvular disease resulting from rheumatic fever
stenosis	stĕ-nō′sis	narrowing or stricture of a vessel
thrombus	throm′bŭs	blood clot
Heart Rhythm and Conduction Disorders		
arrhythmia	ā-ridh′mē-ă	abnormality or disturbance of heart rhythm (Fig. 7-14)
bradycardia	brad′ē-kahr′dē-ă	slow heart rate
dysrhythmia	dis-ridh′mē-ă	defective heart rhythm
fibrillation	fib′ri-lā′shŭn	rapid irregular muscular contractions of the atria or ventricles
flutter	flŭt′ĕr	rapid regular muscular contractions of the atria or ventricles
palpitation	pal-pi-tā′shŭn	forceful or irregular heart beat felt by the patient
premature ventricular contraction (PVC)	prē′mă-chŭr′ ven-trik′yū-lăr kŏn-trak′shŭn	early contraction of the ventricles
tachycardia	tak′i-kahr′dē-ă	fast heart rate
Disorders of the Veins		
deep venous thrombosis (DVT)	dēp vē′nŭs throm-bō′sis	blood clot formation in a deep vein, usually of the legs or pelvic region
phlebitis	fle-bī′tis	inflammation of a vein
telangiectasia	tel-an′jē-ek-tā′zē-ă	dilation of small or terminal vessels
thrombophlebitis	throm′bō-flĕ-bī′tis	inflammation of a vein with formation of a clot
varicose vein	var′i-kōs vān	swollen and/or twisted veins, usually of the legs (Fig. 7-15)

Related to the Lymphatic System		
edema	ĕ-dē′mă	accumulation of excess fluid in intercellular spaces; can be caused by blockage of lymph vessels
elephantiasis	el′ĕ-fan-tī′ă-sis	enlargement of the lower extremities due to blockage of lymph vessels commonly caused by filarial worms (filariae) (Fig. 7-16)
filariae	fi-lar′ē-ē	small parasitic worms that are transmitted by mosquitoes; the worms invade tissues as embryos and block lymph vessels as they grow
lymphadenitis	lim-fad′ĕ-nī′tis	inflammation of the lymph nodes
lymphadenitis	lim-fad′ĕ-nī′tis	inflammation of the lymph nodes
lymphadenopathy	lim-fad′ĕ-nop′ă-thē	disease of the lymph nodes; usually causes enlargement of the nodes

(continued)

Normal sinus rhythm (NSR)

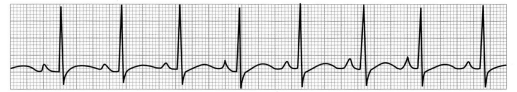

Bradycardia

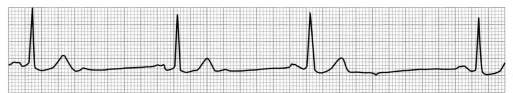

Fibrillation (ventricular)

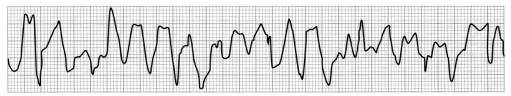

Flutter (atrial)

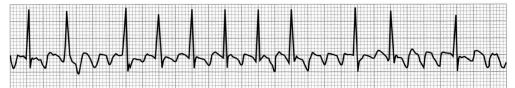

Premature ventricular contraction (PVC)

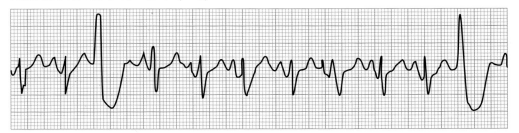

Tachycardia (sinus)

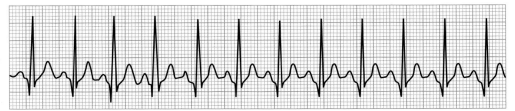

Figure 7-14   Common types of arrhythmias shown through electrocardiogram tracings.

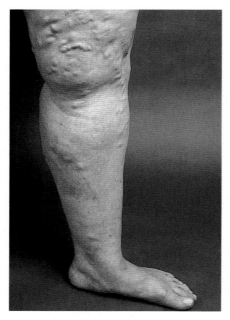

Figure 7-15   Varicose veins.

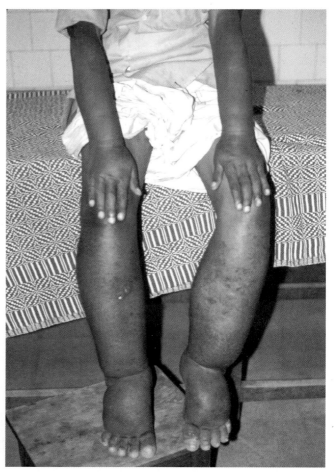

Figure 7-16   Patient with advanced elephantiasis.

Symptoms and Medical Conditions (continued)

Term	Pronunciation	Meaning
lymphangiitis	lim-fan'jē-ī'tis	inflammation of a lymph vessel
lymphedema	lim'fĕ-dē'mă	edema due to a blocked lymph node or lymph vessel
pitting edema	pit'ing ĕ-dē'mă	edema that retains an indentation of a finger that had been pressed firmly on the skin (Fig. 7-17)

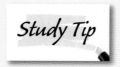

Study Tip

Arteriosclerosis vs. Atherosclerosis: To avoid confusing the meanings of the terms *arteriosclerosis* and *atherosclerosis*, focus on the combining forms. *Arteri/o* means artery, so *arteriosclerosis* refers to hardening of the arteries. *Ather/o* means fatty paste, so *atherosclerosis* refers to buildup of plaque or fatty paste, which hardens the artery walls. Atherosclerosis is actually a type of arteriosclerosis.

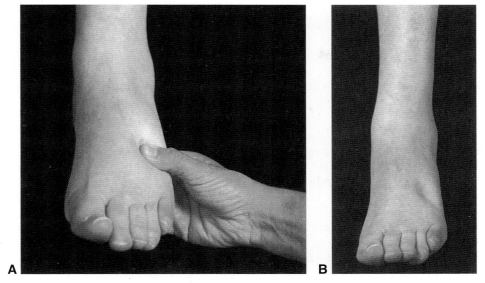

Figure 7-17   A. Palpation of the foot. **B.** Pitting edema.

■ Exercises: Symptoms and Medical Conditions

Exercise 14

SIMPLE
RECALL

Circle the word that best completes the meaning given.

1. aneurysm = (*weakening, rupture*) of an arterial wall

2. atherosclerosis = condition of fatty build-up and (*enlarging, hardening*) of blood vessels

3. hypertension = (*low, high*) blood pressure

4. hypotension = (*low, high*) blood pressure

5. aortic stenosis = (*hardening, narrowing*) of the aortic valve opening

6. myocardial infarction = (*death, pain*) of the myocardium due to lack of blood supply

7. rheumatic heart disease = damage to the heart (*ventricle, valve*) due to rheumatic fever

8. ischemia = (*lack of, increase in*) blood flow

9. fibrillation = rapid (*irregular, regular*) heart contractions

10. flutter = rapid (*irregular, regular*) heart contractions

11. premature ventricular contraction = (*early, late*) contraction of the ventricles

12. murmur = (*normal, abnormal*) heart sounds

13. elephantiasis = (*anemia, edema*) of the lower extremities due to lymph vessel blockage

14. acute coronary syndrome = (*Raynaud disease, chest pain*) and other signs and symptoms associated with cardiac ischemia

15. intermittent claudication = (*cramping, edema*) of the lower legs

16. peripheral artery disease = any disorder of the arteries (*inside, outside*) of, or peripheral to, the heart

SIMPLE
RECALL

Exercise 15

Circle the term that is most appropriate for the meaning of the sentence.

1. Mitral valve prolapse is when the blood flow moves (*backward, forward, circuitously*) through the valve.

2. Edema is the excess accumulation of intracellular (*blood, fluid, lymph*).

3. In coarctation of the aorta, the aorta is (*widened, dilated, narrowed*).

4. Small parasitic worms that invade tissues and cause elephantiasis are called (*telangiectasia, filariae, ringworm*).

5. The death of heart tissue usually due to coronary artery occlusion is called a(n) (*cardiac arrest, myocardial infarction, angina pectoris*).

6. Chest pain or pressure resulting from lack of blood flow to the myocardium is called (*cardiac arrest, myocardial infarction, angina pectoris*).

7. The medical term for when the heart stops beating is (*cardiac arrest, myocardial infarction, angina pectoris*).

8. With Raynaud disease, the fingers and toes become (*cyanotic, diaphoretic, syncopal*) due to vascular constriction.

9. Congestive heart failure is inefficiency of cardiac (*circulation, valves, pressure*) causing edema and pulmonary congestion.

10. A sudden onset of a fast heart rate is called (*tachycardia, palpitation, flutter*).

11. An inflammation of a vein is called (*phlebitis, telangiectasia, varicose vein*).

12. Coronary artery disease is a narrowing of the coronary arteries causing a(n) (*increase, decrease, leakage*) of blood flow to the myocardium.

13. A vascular blockage that is a combination of clotted blood and other foreign materials is a(n) (*regurgitation, embolus, thrombus*).

14. Deep vein thrombosis is (*plaque, fat, blood clot*) formation in a deep vein.

15. Swollen and/or twisted veins are called (*deep, varicose, phlebitis*) veins.

16. Blockage of a coronary vessel often leading to a myocardial infarction is called (*coronary stenosis, coronary occlusion, congestive heart failure*).

Exercise 16

ADVANCED RECALL

Match each medical term with its meaning.

palpitation	lymphedema	angiostenosis	dysrhythmia	cardiomegaly
lymphadenitis	occlusion	plaque	mitral valve stenosis	arrhythmia

Meaning   **Term**

1. narrowing of a blood vessel   _____

2. forceful irregular heart beat felt by the patient   _____

3. abnormality or disturbance of heart rhythm   _____

4. edema due to blocked lymph node   _____

5. blockage or closure   _____

6. fat deposit on an arterial wall   _____

7. narrowing of the mitral valve opening   _____

8. inflammation of the lymph nodes   _____

9. defective heart rhythm   _____

10. enlargement of the heart   _____

Exercise 17

TERM CONSTRUCTION

Build a medical term from an appropriate prefix, combining form, and suffix, given their meanings.

Prefix	Combining Form	Suffix	Term
1. slow	heart	condition of	_____
2. around or surrounding	heart	inflammation	_____
3. in, within	heart	tissue, structure	_____
4. between	ventricles	pertaining to	_____
5. around, surrounding	heart	tissue, structure	_____
6. rapid, fast	heart	condition of	_____
7. many, much	artery	inflammation	_____

TERM
CONSTRUCTION

Exercise 18

Break the given medical term into its word parts and define each part. Then define the medical term. (Note: This exercise uses some suffixes learned previously.)

For example:

pericarditis *word parts:*   peri- /   cardi/o   / -itis
                               meanings: around, surrounding /   heart   / inflammation
                               term meaning: inflammation of the pericardial sac around the heart

1. lymphangiitis   *word parts:* _____ / _____ / _____

                      meanings: _____ / _____ / _____

                      term meaning: _____

2. lymphadenopathy   *word parts:* _____ / _____ / _____

                      meanings: _____ / _____ / _____

                      term meaning: _____

3. thrombophlebitis   *word parts:* _____ / _____ / _____

                      meanings: _____ / _____ / _____

                      term meaning: _____

4. cardiomyopathy   *word parts:* _____ / _____ / _____

                      meanings: _____ / _____ / _____

                      term meaning: _____

5. endocarditis   *word parts:* _____ / _____ / _____

                      meanings: _____ / _____ / _____

                      term meaning: _____

6. cardiovalvulitis   *word parts:* _____ / _____ / _____

                      meanings: _____ / _____ / _____

                      term meaning: _____

7. myocarditis   *word parts:* _____ / _____ / _____

                      meanings: _____ / _____ / _____

                      term meaning: _____

8. telangiectasia   *word parts:* _____ / _____ / _____

                      meanings: _____ / _____ / _____

                      term meaning: _____

Tests and Procedures

Term	Pronunciation	Meaning
Laboratory Tests Related to the Cardiovascular System		
cardiac enzyme tests	kahr'dē-ak en'zīm tests	blood tests used to measure the level of creatine kinase (CK), creatine phosphokinase (CPK), and lactate dehydrogenase (LDH) that, when such levels are increased, may indicate a myocardial infarction
cardiac troponin	kahr'dē-ak trō'pō-nin	blood test used to measure the level of a protein that is released in the blood when myocardial cells die
C-reactive protein (CRP)	sē-rē-ak'tiv prō'tēn	blood test used to measure the level of inflammation in the body; may indicate conditions that lead to cardiovascular disease
electrolyte panel	ĕ-lek'trō-līt pan'ĕl	blood test used to measure the level of sodium (Na), potassium (K), chloride (Cl), and carbon dioxide (CO_2); used to diagnose an acid-base or pH imbalance that may cause arrhythmias, muscle damage, or death
lipid panel, *syn.* lipid profile	lip'id pan'ĕl, lip'id prō'fīl	blood test to measure the level of total cholestrol, high density lipoprotein (HDL), low density lipoprotein (LDL), and triglycerides, all of which may signal an increased risk of cardiovascular disease
Diagnostic Procedures Related to the Cardiovascular System		
Imaging Studies		
angioscopy	an'jē-os'kŏ-pē	insertion of a catheter with an attached camera to visualize a structure or vessel
aortography	ā-ŏr-tog'ră-fē	process of recording the aorta after injection of a dye
arteriography	ahr-ter'ē-og'ră-fē	process of recording an artery after injection of a dye
coronary angiography, *syn.* cardiac catheterization	kŏr'ŏ-nār-ē an'jē-og'ră-fē, kahr'dē-ak kath'ĕ-tĕr-ī-zā'shŭn	process of recording the heart and major vessels after injection of a dye (Fig. 7-18)
magnetic resonance imaging (MRI)	mag-net'ik rez'ŏ-năns im'ăj-ing	imaging technique that uses magnetic fields and radiofrequency waves to visualize anatomic structures
magnetic resonance angiography (MRA)	mag-net'ik rez'ŏ-năns an'jē-og'ră-fē	MRI of the heart and blood vessels with an injection of dye
multiple uptake gated acquisition (MUGA) scan	mŭl'ti-pĕl-gāt'ĕd ak-wi-zi'shŭn skan	nuclear medicine technique used to assess ventricular function by producing an image of a beating heart
sonography, *syn.* ultrasonography	sŏ-nog'ră-fē, ŭl'tră-sŏ-nog'ră-fē	use of ultrasonic sound waves to visualize internal organs
Doppler sonography (DS)	dop'lĕr sŏ-nog'ră-fē	technique used to record velocity of blood flow
echocardiography	ek'ō-kahr-dē-og'ră-fē	process of recording the structure and function of the heart at rest and with exercise (Fig. 7-19)

(continued)

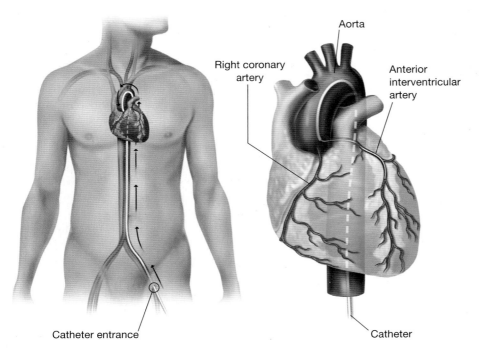

Figure 7-18 Coronary angiography.

Tests and Procedures *(continued)*

Term	Pronunciation	Meaning
transesophageal echocardiography (TEE)	tranz-ē-sō-fā'jē-ăl ek'ō-kahr-dē-og'ră-fē	placement of the ultrasonic transducer inside the patient's esophagus to assess cardiac function and examine cardiac structure
vascular sonography	vas'kyū-lăr sŏ-nog'ră-fē	placement of the ultrasound transducer at the tip of a catheter within a blood vessel to assess blood flow
single photon emission computed tomography (SPECT) scan	sing'gĕl fō'ton ē-mi'shŭn kŏm-pyūt'ĕd tŏ-mog'ră-fē skan	nuclear medicine technique used to assess ventricular function by producing a three-dimensional image of a beating heart

(continued)

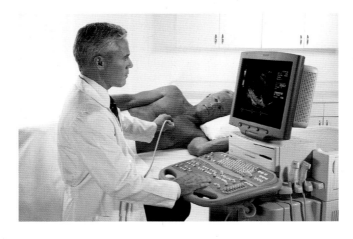

Figure 7-19 Echocardiography.

Tests and Procedures *(continued)*

Term	Pronunciation	Meaning
venography	vē-nog′ră-fē	process of recording a vein after injection of a dye
ventriculography	ven-trik′yū-log′ră-fē	process of recording the heart ventricles after injection of a dye or radioactive substance (radionuclide)
Other Procedures		
auscultation	aws′kŭl-tā′shŭn	listening to body sounds with a stethoscope
blood pressure monitoring (BP)	blŭd presh′ŭr mon′i-tŏr′ing	auscultation of the systolic and diastolic arterial pressure using a stethoscope and a sphygmomanometer
electrocardiography (ECG or EKG)	ĕ-lek′trō-kahr-dē-og′ră-fē	process of recording (in a graphic format) the heart's electrical activity; the waves are labeled with the letters P, Q, R, S, and T (see Fig. 7-14)
graded exercise test (GXT), *syn.* stress electrocardiogram, exercise stress test	grăd′ĕd eks′ĕr-sīz test, stres ĕ-lek′trō-kahr′dē-ō-gram, eks′ĕr-sīz stres test	electrocardiogram performed with controlled stress, usually with a treadmill or bicycle (Fig. 7-20)
Holter monitor (HM)	hōl′tĕr mon′i-tŏr	portable electrocardiographic device usually worn for 24 hours

(continued)

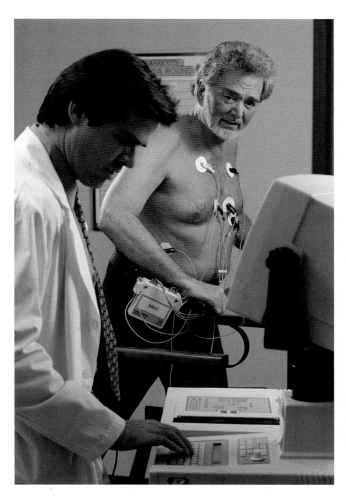

Figure 7-20 Exercise stress test.

Tests and Procedures *(continued)*

Term	Pronunciation	Meaning
percussion	pĕr-kŭsh'ŭn	physical examination method of tapping over the body to elicit vibrations and sounds to estimate the size, border, or fluid content of a cavity
pulse	pŭls	rhythmic dilation of an artery with each heart contraction, usually felt at the wrist or neck
sphygmomanometer	sfig'mō-mă-nom'ĕ-tĕr	device used for measuring blood pressure
stethoscope	steth'ŏ-skōp	instrument used for auscultation of vascular or other sounds in the body

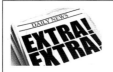 **STETHOSCOPE** Did you know that the first stethoscope was invented by a French physician who rolled paper into the shape of a cylinder to listen to heart sounds? Prior to this, physicians would listen to a patient's chest by placing their ear directly on the chest wall.

	Diagnostic Procedures Related to the Lymphatic System	
lymphangiography	lim-fan'jē-og'ră-fē	process of recording a lymph node or lymph vessel after injection of a dye

■ Exercises: Tests and Procedures

SIMPLE RECALL

Exercise 19

Circle the term that is most appropriate for the meaning of the sentence.

1. A portable ECG monitoring device that can be worn for 24 hours is a (*graded exercise test, Holter monitor, MUGA scan*).

2. The process of recording an artery after injecting a dye or radionuclide is called (*arteriography, angiography, aortography*).

3. The process of recording a lymph vessel after injecting a dye is called (*angiography, vascular sonography, lymphangiography*).

4. Insertion of a catheter with a camera to visually assess a vessel is called (*angioscopy, fine-needle aspiration, cardiac catheterization*).

5. The process of listening to body sounds with a stethoscope is called (*echocardiography, ultrasound, auscultation*).

6. The process of recording the heart's electrical activity is called (*echocardiography, electrocardiography, sonography*).

7. A(n) (*MUGA, MRI, SPECT*) scan produces a three-dimensional image of a beating heart.

8. Doppler (*electrocardiography, venography, sonography*) is used to record the velocity of blood flow.

9. The examination method of tapping over the body to elicit vibrations and sounds is called (*percussion, auscultation, blood pressure*).

10. An MRI of the heart and blood vessels with an injection of dye is called (*magnetic resonance imaging, MUGA, magnetic resonance angiography*).

Exercise 20

ADVANCED RECALL

Complete each sentence by writing in the correct medical term.

1. An ECG performed with controlled stress is a(n) _____.

2. The process of recording the structure and function of the heart using sonography is called

    _____.

3. To perform _____, an ultrasound transducer is placed inside the patient's esophagus.

4. Two examples of nuclear medicine studies that assess ventricular function are

    _____ and _____.

5. The process of recording the heart and major vessels after injection of a dye is called

    _____ or _____.

6. An echocardiogram assesses structure and function of the heart at rest and with

    _____.

7. A ventriculography records the _____ after injection with dye.

8. Magnetic resonance imaging uses magnetic fields and _____ to visual anatomic structures.

9. Measurement of blood pressure requires a(n) _____.

10. A stethoscope is used to _____ to body sounds.

Exercise 21

ADVANCED RECALL

Match each type of lab test with the description of the test.

cardiac troponin   electrolyte panel   C-reactive protein
lipid panel   cardiac enzyme tests

Description	Term
1. evaluation of Na, K, Cl, and CO_2	_____
2. evaluation of CK, CPK, and LDH	_____

3. evaluation of protein released when myocardial cells die _____

4. evaluation of cholesterol, HDL, LDL, and triglycerides _____

5. measurement of inflammation in the body _____

Exercise 22

TERM CONSTRUCTION

Using the given suffix, build a medical term for the meaning given.

Suffix	Meaning of Medical Term	Medical Term
-graphy	process of recording using sound waves	1. _____
-graphy	process of recording a vein	2. _____
-graphy	process of recording the ventricles	3. _____
-graphy	process of recording the aorta	4. _____
-graphy	process of recording a blood vessel	5. _____

Surgical Interventions and Therapeutic Procedures

Term	Pronunciation	Meaning
Related to the Cardiovascular System		
angioplasty	an'jē-ō-plas-tē	surgical repair of a vessel
aortocoronary bypass (ACB)	ā-ōr'tō-kōr'ō-nar-ē bī'pas	attachment of a grafted vessel to the aorta to go around a damaged coronary artery
aneurysmectomy	an'yūr-iz-mek'tŏ-mē	excision of an aneurysm
atherectomy	ath'er-ek'tŏ-mē	surgical removal of fatty plaque from a vessel surgically or using catheterization
cardiac pacemaker	kahr'dē-ak pās'mā-kĕr	surgically placed mechanical device connected to stimulating leads (electrodes) on or within the heart, programmed to help maintain normal heart rate and rhythm (Fig. 7-21)
cardioversion	kahr'dē-ō-vĕr'zhŭn	use of defibrillation or drugs to restore the heart's normal rhythm
coronary artery bypass graft (CABG)	kōr'ŏ-nār-ē ahr'tĕr-ē bī'pās graft	surgical procedure in which a damaged section of a coronary artery is replaced or bypassed with a graft vessel (Fig. 7-22)

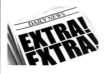

THE EVOLUTION OF CORONARY ARTERY BYPASS SURGERY Advances in technology have led to the development of several types of coronary artery bypass surgery. Traditionally, this procedure involved opening the chest via a large incision through the middle of the sternum; a heart-lung machine circulated the blood while the heart was stopped. A newer type of bypass surgery, called "off-pump," uses special agents to stabilize the heart while the surgery takes place. In addition, surgeons now perform minimally invasive bypass surgery, which uses small incisions in the side of the chest and special instruments for the operation.

(continued)

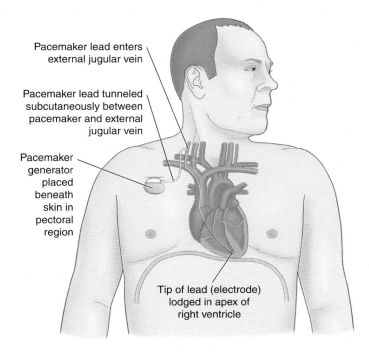

Pacemaker lead enters external jugular vein

Pacemaker lead tunneled subcutaneously between pacemaker and external jugular vein

Pacemaker generator placed beneath skin in pectoral region

Tip of lead (electrode) lodged in apex of right ventricle

Figure 7-21   Insertion of a pacemaker.

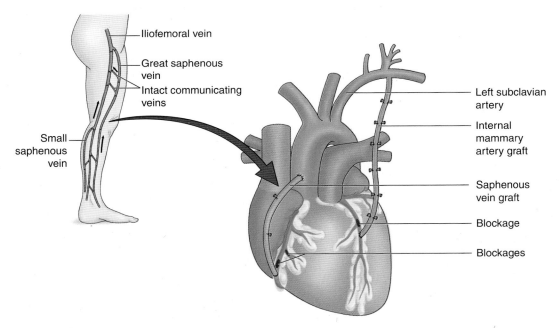

Iliofemoral vein

Great saphenous vein

Intact communicating veins

Small saphenous vein

Left subclavian artery

Internal mammary artery graft

Saphenous vein graft

Blockage

Blockages

Figure 7-22   Coronary artery bypass graft (CABG).

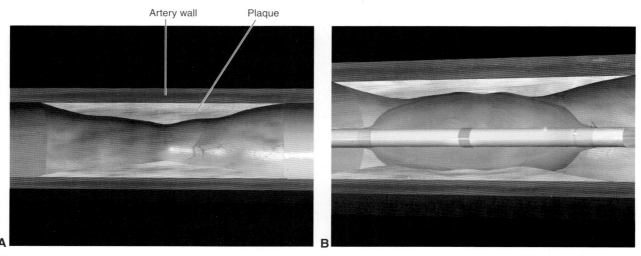

Figure 7-23   Coronary angioplasty (PTCA). **A.** Plaque buildup in an artery. **B.** Balloon inserted and inflated, thus enlarging the lumen.

Surgical Interventions and Therapeutic Procedures *(continued)*

Term	Pronunciation	Meaning
defibrillation	dē-fib′ri-lā′shŭn	use of an electric shock to stop fibrillation or cardiac arrest
embolectomy	em′bō-lek′tŏ-mē	surgical removal of an embolus or blood clot, usually with a catheter
endarterectomy	end′ahr-tĕr-ek′tŏ-mē	surgical removal of atheromatous deposits, usually in a coronary or carotid artery
pericardiocentesis	per′i-kahr′dē-ō-sen-tē′sis	surgical puncture to aspirate fluid from the pericardium
percutaneous transluminal coronary angioplasty (PTCA)	pĕr′kyū-tā′nē-ŭs trans-lū′mĕn-ăl kōr′ŏ-nār-ē an′jē-ō-plas-tē	advancement of a cardiac catheter with a balloon attachment that can be inflated at the site of stenosis, thereby enlarging the lumen (Fig. 7-23)
phlebectomy	fle-bek′tŏ-mē	excision of a vein
stent	stent	intravascular insertion of a hollow mesh tube designed to keep a vessel open or patent (Fig. 7-24)

(continued)

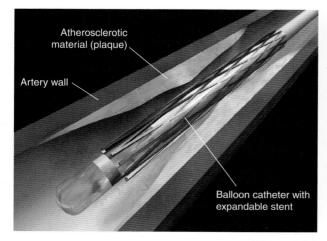

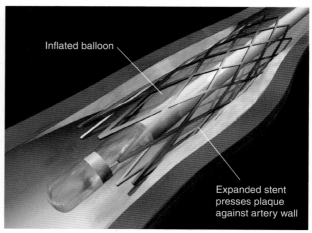

Figure 7-24   Arterial stent.

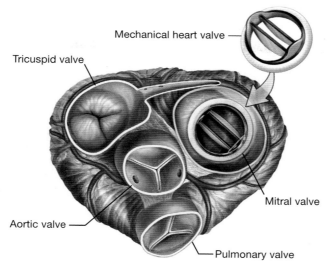

Figure 7-25 Mitral valve prosthesis.

Surgical Interventions and Therapeutic Procedures *(continued)*

Term	Pronunciation	Meaning
valve replacement	valv rĕ-plās'mĕnt	surgical replacement of a valve with a biologic or mechanical device (Fig. 7-25)
valvotomy	val-vot'ŏ-mē	incision into a valve
valvuloplasty	val'vyū-lō-plas-tē	surgical repair of a valve
Related to the Lymphatic System		
adenectomy	ad'ĕ-nek'tŏ-mē	excision of a gland
lymphadenectomy	lim-fad'ĕ-nek'tŏ-mē	excision of a lymph node
lymphadenotomy	lim-fad'ĕ-not'ŏ-mē	incision into a lymph node

■ Exercises: Surgical Interventions and Therapeutic Procedures

SIMPLE
RECALL

Exercise 23

Write the correct medical term for the meaning given.

1. excision of a gland _____

2. inflation of a balloon catheter in a coronary artery _____

3. surgical removal of an embolus or blood clot _____

4. surgical repair of a valve _____

5. surgical removal of fatty plaque _____

6. excision of a lymph node _____

7. incision into a lymph node _____

ADVANCED
RECALL

Exercise 24

Circle the correct term that is appropriate for the meaning of the sentence.

1. Dr. Johansson explained to Mr. Curren that his (*valvuloplasty, valve replacement, atherectomy*) would be with a biologic or mechanical device.

2. A(n) (*angioplasty, cardioversion, valve replacement*) was performed on Mrs. Campbell to correct her irregular and fast heart rate.

3. Mr. Torres had a(n) (*endarterectomy, embolectomy, stent*) to surgically remove the fatty buildup in his carotid artery.

4. After having several syncopal episodes due to bradycardia, Mr. DeHaan was scheduled for implantation of a (*cardiac pacemaker, valve replacement, stent*) to help maintain normal heart rate and rhythm.

5. Dr. LaPenna decided to do a(n) (*ACB, PTCA, CABG*) to open Mr. Thompson's narrowed coronary artery using a catheter with a balloon attachment.

6. A (*pacemaker, PTCA, stent*) was inserted in Ms. Andretti's coronary artery to help keep it open.

7. After documenting the restenosis of his coronary arteries by angiography, Dr. Ayerdi advised Mr. Johnson to have a(n) (*CABG, cardioversion, adenectomy*).

8. Dr. Nowak grafted the saphenous vein to the aorta in a procedure called a(n) (*aortocoronary bypass, endarterectomy, PTCA*).

TERM
CONSTRUCTION

Exercise 25

Using the given suffix, build a medical term for the meaning given.

Suffix	Meaning of Medical Term	Medical Term
-plasty	surgical repair of a blood vessel	1. _____
-ectomy	excision of an aneurysm	2. _____
-centesis	puncture to aspirate fluid from the pericardium	3. _____
-ectomy	excision of a gland	4. _____
-tomy	incision into a valve	5. _____

TERM CONSTRUCTION

Exercise 26

Break the given medical term into its word parts and define each part. Then define the medical term.

For example:

carditis	*word parts:*	cardi/o / -itis
	meanings:	heart / inflammation
	term meaning:	inflammation of the heart

1. valvuloplasty   *word parts:* _____ / _____

meanings: _____ / _____

term meaning: _____

2. angioplasty   *word parts:* _____ / _____

meanings: _____ / _____

term meaning: _____

3. atherectomy   *word parts:* _____ / _____

meanings: _____ / _____

term meaning: _____

4. phlebectomy   *word parts:* _____ / _____

meanings: _____ / _____

term meaning: _____

5. valvotomy   *word parts:* _____ / _____

meanings: _____ / _____

term meaning: _____

Medications and Drug Therapies

Term	Pronunciation	Meaning
anticoagulant	an′tē-kō-ag′yŭ-lănt	drug used to prolong clotting time
antiarrhythmic agent	an′tē-ā-ridh′mik ā′jĕnt	drug used to suppress fast or irregular heart rhythms
hemostatic agent	hē′mō-stat′ik ā′jĕnt	drug that stops the flow of blood within vessels
hypolipidemic agent	hī′pō-lip′id-ē-mĭc a′jĕnt	drug used to lower cholesterol levels
nitroglycerin	nī′trŏ-glĭs′er-in	vasodilator used for angina pectoris
thrombolytic therapy	throm′bō-lit′ik thār′ă-pē	administration of an intravenous drug to dissolve a blood clot
vasoconstrictor	vā′sō-kŏn-strik′tŏr	drug that decreases the size of blood vessels
vasodilator	vā′sō-dī′lā-tŏr	drug that increases the size of blood vessels

■ Exercise: Medications and Drug Therapies

Exercise 27

Write the correct medication or drug therapy term for the meaning given.

1. drug that decreases the size of blood vessels   _____

2. drug that prolongs clotting time   _____

3. administration of an IV drug to dissolve a clot   _____

4. drug that increases the size of blood vessels   _____

5. drug that stops the flow of blood   _____

6. drug that suppresses fast or irregular heart rhythms   _____

7. drug used for angina pectoris   _____

8. drug used to lower cholesterol   _____

Specialties and Specialists

Term	Pronunciation	Meaning
cardiology	kahr′dē-ol′ŏ-jē	medical specialty concerned with diagnosis and treatment of heart disease
cardiologist	kahr′dē-ol′ŏ-jist	physician who specializes in cardiology
cardiac electrophysiology	kahr′dē-ak ĕ-lek′trō-fiz′ē-ol′ŏ-jē	medical speciality concerned with the electrical activities of the heart
cardiac electrophysiologist	kahr′dē-ak ĕ-lek′trō-fiz′ē-ol′ŏ-jist	physician who specializes in cardiac electrophysiology
lymphedema therapy	lim′fĕ-dē′mă thār′ă-pē	medical specialty concerned with the treatment of lymphedema
lymphedema therapist	lim′fĕ-dē′mă thār′ă-pist	one who specializes in lymphedema therapy

■ Exercise: Specialties and Specialists

ADVANCED
RECALL

Exercise 28

Match each medical specialist or specialty with its description.

cardiac electrophysiology   cardiologist   cardiology
lymphedema therapy   lymphedema therapist   cardiac electrophysiologist

1. study of heart disease   _____

2. specialty related to the treatment of lymphedema   _____

3. physician who specializes in heart disease   _____

4. specialty related to the heart's electrical activities _____

5. one who specializes in lymphedema therapy _____

6. physician specialized in the heart's electrical activities _____

Abbreviations

Abbreviation	Meaning
Related to the Cardiovascular System	
ACB	aortocoronary bypass
ACS	acute coronary syndrome
ASHD	arteriosclerotic heart disease
AV	arteriovenous, atrioventricular
BP	blood pressure
CABG	coronary artery bypass graft
CAD	coronary artery disease
CHF	congestive heart failure
DS	Doppler sonography
DVT	deep venous thrombosis
ECG or EKG	electrocardiography
GXT	graded exercise test
HM	Holter monitor
HTN	hypertension
MI	myocardial infarction
MRA	magnetic resonance angiography
MRI	magnetic resonance imaging
MUGA	multiple uptake gated acquisition
PAD	peripheral arterial disease
PTCA	percutaneous transluminal coronary angioplasty
PVC	premature ventricular contraction
RHD	rheumatic heart disease
SPECT	single photon emission computed tomography
TEE	transesophageal echocardiography

■ Exercises: Abbreviations

SIMPLE
RECALL

Exercise 29

Write the meaning for the following abbreviations.

1. CHF _____

2. ACB _____

3. SPECT   _____

4. ASHD   _____

5. DVT   _____

6. PVC   _____

7. BP   _____

8. ACS   _____

9. HTN   _____

10. CABG   _____

Exercise 30

ADVANCED
RECALL

Write the meaning of each abbreviation used in these sentences.

1. Dr. Erickson ordered a **HM** for Mr. Hadley to investigate his complaints of irregular heartbeats.

   _____

2. Mrs. Cuthbert underwent a **PTCA** to enlarge the lumen of her stenotic artery.

   _____

3. The cardiologist ordered an **MRA** of the brain to locate the blocked vessel.

   _____

4. Dr. Anderson's specialty is repair of **AV** defects.

   _____

5. Dr. Macken had difficulty visualizing the heart structures on the echocardiogram, so he ordered a **TEE**, a procedure in which the patient swallows the transducer, to obtain a different perspective.

   _____

6. Angie Smith was diagnosed with **CAD** because of her ischemia.

   _____

7. Mr. Javovich's heart valve was damaged after having **RHD** as a child.

   _____

8. Mr. John's **GXT** was performed using a treadmill.

   _____

9. Dr. Francis diagnosed Ms. Snyder with an **MI** caused by coronary artery occlusion.

_____

10. Mrs. Adkins was diagnosed with **PAD** through the use of Doppler sonography.

_____

Exercise 31

ADVANCED
RECALL

Match each abbreviation with the appropriate description.

DS   MUGA   MRA
MRI   ECG

1. recording of the heart's electrical activity   _____

2. imaging technique using magnetic fields and radiofrequency waves   _____

3. MRI of the heart and blood vessels with an injection of dye   _____

4. technique used to record velocity of blood flow   _____

5. nuclear medicine technique used to assess ventricular function   _____

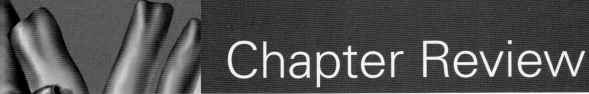

Review of Terms for Anatomy and Physiology

 Exercise 32

VISUAL

Write the correct terms on the blanks for the anatomic structures indicated.

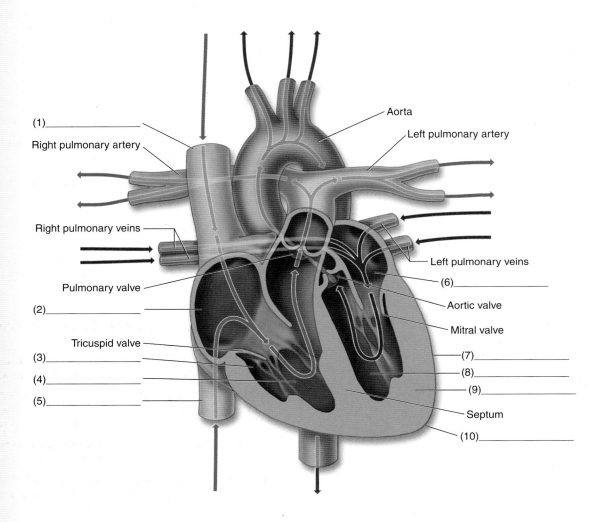

(1)_____

Right pulmonary artery

Aorta

Left pulmonary artery

Right pulmonary veins

Left pulmonary veins

Pulmonary valve

(6)_____

(2)_____

Aortic valve

Tricuspid valve

Mitral valve

(3)_____

(7)_____

(4)_____

(8)_____

(9)_____

(5)_____

Septum

(10)_____

Exercise 33

VISUAL

Write the correct terms on the blanks for the anatomic structures illustrated.

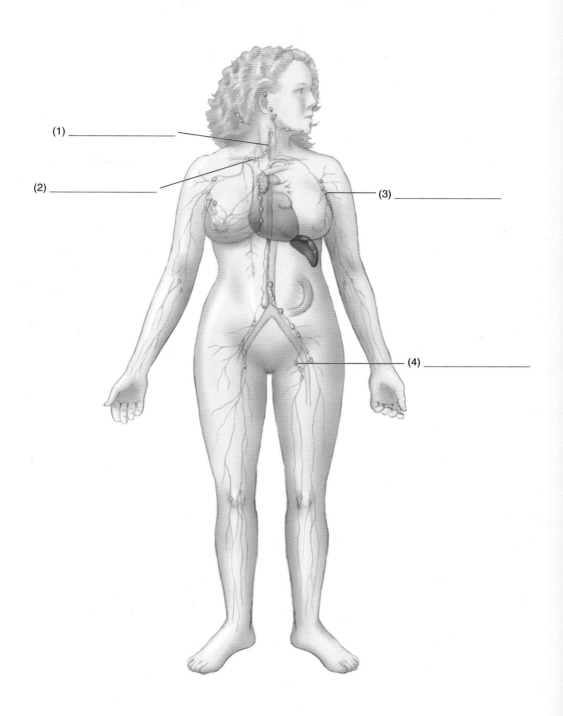

(1) _____

(2) _____

(3) _____

(4) _____

Understanding Term Structure

TERM
CONSTRUCTION

Exercise 34

Break the given medical term into its word parts and define each part. Then define the medical term. (Note: you may need to use word parts from other chapters.)

For example:

carditis	*word parts:*	cardi/o / -itis
	meanings:	heart / inflammation
	term meaning:	inflammation of the heart

1. angiostenosis   *word parts:*   _____ / _____

meanings: _____ / _____

term meaning: _____

2. phlebitis   *word parts:*   _____ / _____

meanings: _____ / _____

term meaning: _____

3. electrocardiography   *word parts:*   _____ / _____ / _____

meanings: _____ / _____ / _____

term meaning: _____

4. atrioventricular   *word parts:*   _____ / _____ / _____

meanings: _____ / _____ / _____

term meaning: _____

5. tachycardia   *word parts:*   _____ / _____ / _____

meanings: _____ / _____ / _____

term meaning: _____

6. interventricular   *word parts:*   _____ / _____ / _____

meanings: _____ / _____ / _____

term meaning: _____

7. thrombosis   *word parts:*   _____ / _____

meanings: _____ / _____

term meaning: _____

8. polyarteritis   *word parts:*   _____ / _____ / _____

                       meanings: _____ / _____ / _____

                       term meaning: _____

9. thrombophlebitis   *word parts:*   _____ / _____ / _____

                       meanings: _____ / _____ / _____

                       term meaning: _____

10. cardiomyopathy   *word parts:*   _____ / _____ / _____

                       meanings: _____ / _____ / _____

                       term meaning: _____

11. arteriosclerosis   *word parts:*   _____ / _____ / _____

                       meanings: _____ / _____ / _____

                       term meaning: _____

12. sphygmic   *word parts:*   _____ / _____

                       meanings: _____ / _____

                       term meaning: _____

13. venography   *word parts:*   _____ / _____

                       meanings: _____ / _____

                       term meaning: _____

14. bradycardia   *word parts:*   _____ / _____ / _____

                       meanings: _____ / _____ / _____

                       term meaning: _____

15. atherosclerosis   *word parts:*   _____ / _____ / _____

                       meanings: _____ / _____ / _____

                       term meaning: _____

16. myocardium   *word parts:*   _____ / _____ / _____

                       meanings: _____ / _____ / _____

                       term meaning: _____

17. valvulotomy   *word parts:*   _____ / _____

                         meanings: _____ / _____

                         term meaning: _____

18. lymphadenopathy *word parts:*   _____ / _____ / _____

                         meanings: _____ / _____ / _____

                         term meaning: _____

19. lymphangiitis   *word parts:*   _____ / _____ / _____

                         meanings: _____ / _____ / _____

                         term meaning: _____

20. thrombolytic   *word parts:*   _____ / _____

                         meanings: _____ / _____

                         term meaning: _____

Comprehension Exercises

Exercise 35

COMPREHENSION **Fill in the blank with the correct term.**

1. The _____ is located between the endocardium and epicardium.

2. The wall that separates the right and left parts of the heart is called the _____.

3. A(n) _____ is one who specializes in the study of the heart.

4. The heart valve between the right ventricle and the pulmonary artery is called the

   _____ valve.

5. The _____ carries oxygenated blood away from the heart.

6. When the ventricles are in the relaxation phase of the heartbeat cycle, it is referred to as

   _____.

7. Dilation of small terminal vessels is a condition called _____.

8. Swollen or twisted veins are referred to as _____.

9. A rhythm of rapid regular contractions of the atria is called atrial _____.

10. A rhythm of rapid irregular contractions of the ventricles is called ventricular

    _____.

11. _____ is the enlargement of the lower extremities due to worms blocking the lymph vessels.

12. Cramping of the legs due to lack of blood flow is called _____.

13. Lack of blood flow is a condition called _____.

14. When the heart muscle is deprived of oxygen or blood flow for a significant amount of time, tissue death may occur. Death of heart muscle is called a(n) _____.

15. Cardiac arrest is complete, sudden cessation of _____ activity.

16. Prolonged immobility during air travel can increase the risk of blood clot formation in the large veins, also called _____.

17. An early contraction of the ventricles is referred to as a(n) _____.

18. Abnormal heart sounds are also referred to as _____.

19. Patent means _____, such as in a patent ductus arteriosus where the fetal circulatory vessels fail to close.

20. C-reactive protein is a blood test used to measure the level of _____ in the body.

Exercise 36

COMPREHENSION

Write a short answer for each question.

1. Which type of drug stops the flow of blood within vessel? _____

2. The pulse is usually felt at which two points on the body? _____

    _____

3. During vascular sonography, where is the catheter placed? _____

    _____

4. What four substances are measured in a lipid panel? _____

    _____

5. What is the difference between hypotension and hypertension? _____

    _____

6. Blood pressure monitoring involves the use of what two instruments? _____

_____

7. The drug nitroglycerin is used to treat what condition? _____

8. What procedure might be used to treat fluid around the pericardium? _____

9. What physical activity does a physician perform during percussion? _____

10. Why might a SPECT scan be performed to diagnose arrhythmias? _____

_____

11. What two types of treatment might be done in cardioversion? _____

12. What is the opposite of tachycardia? _____

13. In what two situations might a defibrillation be performed? _____

_____

14. Which two procedures are done to bypass damaged coronary arteries? _____

_____

15. How does the balloon attachment function in a PTCA? _____

_____

Exercise 37

Circle the letter of the best answer in the following questions.

1. Which of the following would not be used to describe an abnormal heart beat?

A. aneurysm
B. dysrhythmia
C. tachycardia
D. palpitation

2. Using the plural form of the term, the two upper receiving chambers of the heart are called the:

A. aorta
B. atria
C. arterioles
D. atrium

3. Inflammation of the lymph vessels is referred to as:

A. lymphangiitis
B. lymphadenitis

C. lymphedema
D. lymphadenopathy

4. Edema that retains an indentation of a pressed finger is called:

A. dissecting
B. pitting
C. ischemic
D. stenotic

5. Cardiac tamponade is compression of the heart. Which procedure might be used to treat this condition?

A. angioplasty
B. cardioversion
C. myocentesis
D. pericardiocentesis

6. A patient with mitral valve stenosis might have previously had which condition?

   A. rheumatic fever
   B. Raynaud syndrome
   C. murmur
   D. peripheral arterial disease

7. Which of the following is not a diagnostic test designed to record arrhythmias?

   A. lipid profile
   B. graded exercise test
   C. electrocardiogram
   D. Holter monitor

8. ECG electrodes are usually placed at the precordial region or the:

   A. abdomen
   B. anterior left chest
   C. anterior right chest
   D. shoulders

9. CABG stands for:

   A. coronary artery bypass graft
   B. cardiac artery bypass graft
   C. cerebrovascular accident bypass graft
   D. aortocoronary bypass

10. During a PTCA, a catheter is advanced *through a vessel.* Which term pertains to the italicized phrase?

    A. percutaneous
    B. transluminal
    C. coronary
    D. angiogram

11. Which of the following is a hollow mesh tube used to keep a vessel patent?

    A. pacemaker
    B. valvotomy
    C. defibrillation
    D. stent

12. What substance is injected during a cardiac catheterization?

    A. fluid
    B. dye
    C. blood
    D. lymph

13. Which blood test diagnoses an acid-base or pH imbalance?

    A. cardiac enzyme test
    B. C-reactive protein

C. cardiac troponin
D. electrolyte panel

14. Filariae cause elephantiasis by blocking which type of vessels?

    A. arteries
    B. veins
    C. lymph
    D. capillaries

15. A patient who states that she can "feel her heartbeat" is experiencing:

    A. palpitations
    B. tachycardia
    C. bradycardia
    D. percussion

16. Vessels carrying blood to the heart might be tested using which diagnostic procedure?

    A. arteriography
    B. aortography
    C. transesophageal echocardiography
    D. venography

17. Which condition is not a heart rhythm or conduction disorder?

    A bradycardia
    B. tachycardia
    C. phlebitis
    D. dysrhythmia

18. Lack of blood flow to the lower limbs causes:

    A. phlebitis
    B. lymphangitis
    C. intermittent claudication
    D. thrombus

19. Which procedure treats the buildup of plaque or fatty paste inside arterial walls?

    A. pericardiocentesis
    B. atherectomy
    C. valve replacement
    D. aneurysmectomy

20. An ECG produces a recording of the heart's electrical activity in what type of format?

    A. x-ray
    B. three-dimensional image
    C. sonogram
    D. graph

Application and Analysis

APPLICATION

Exercise 38

Read the case reports and circle the letter of your answer choice for the questions that follow.

CASE 7-1

Mr. Terrigo reported to the emergency room with complaints of chest pressure and palpitations. He has a history of a triple CABG done in March 2008 with a history of atrial fibrillation prior to surgery. He was doing well until this morning when he started feeling chest pressure and palpitations. Dr. Francis ordered an ECG that showed evidence of premature ventricular contractions and ST-segment depression. A cardiac catheterization and subsequent PTCA was performed on the stenotic right coronary artery.

1. What of the following best describes a CABG?

    A. noninvasive procedure to open a clogged artery
    B. surgical replacement or bypass of a damaged coronary artery
    C. removal of a clot using catheterization
    D. intravascular insertion of a hollow mesh tube

2. Atrial fibrillation is best described as:

    A. rapid irregular rhythm of the lower heart chambers
    B. rapid regular rhythm of the upper heart chambers
    C. rapid irregular rhythm of the upper heart chambers
    D. rapid regular rhythm of the lower heart chambers

3. Mr. Terrigo's symptoms could best be described as:

    A. acute coronary syndrome
    B. cardiac arrest
    C. intermittent claudication
    D. Raynaud disease

4. Which of the following are waves found on an ECG?

    A. QRS waves
    B. TUV waves
    C. ultrasound waves
    D. Doppler waves

5. Which of the following would typically *not* be true of stenotic coronary arteries?

    A. caused by CAD
    B. caused by a thrombus
    C. caused by atherosclerosis
    D. caused by lymphedema

6. All of the following are true for a PTCA *except*:

    A. attempts to enlarge the vessel lumen
    B. involves a cardiac catheter
    C. involves the use of electric shock
    D. uses a balloon catheter attachment

CASE 7-2

Mr. Peterson had symptoms of fatigue, cough, and a fever over the past few days. Last night he began experiencing chest pain radiating to his back, which was worse lying down and relieved by sitting up. During the precordial exam, Dr. Macken detected by auscultation a "squeaky leather" sound characteristic of a pericardial rub. An ECG and echocardiogram were performed. Mr. Peterson was diagnosed with pericarditis (Fig. 7-26) and placed on antiinflammatory drugs.

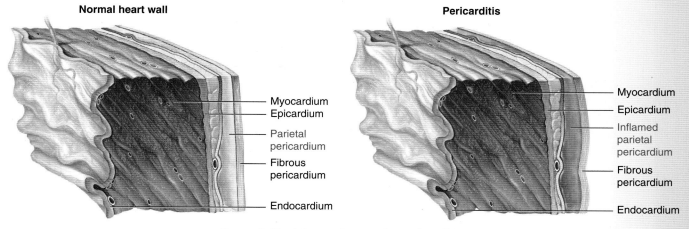

Normal heart wall

- Myocardium
- Epicardium
- Parietal pericardium
- Fibrous pericardium
- Endocardium

Pericarditis

- Myocardium
- Epicardium
- Inflamed parietal pericardium
- Fibrous pericardium
- Endocardium

Figure 7-26   Tissue changes in pericarditis.

7. The pericardium is:

   A. a membrane that protects the heart valves
   B. the heart muscle
   C. inside the heart
   D. the sac surrounding the heart

8. Cardiac tamponade can occur if which condition progresses?

   A. occlusion
   B. chest pain
   C. fatigue
   D. pericarditis

9. Auscultation is an examination by:

   A. microscope
   B. viewing through a scope or tube
   C. palpation
   D. listening

10. The term precordial refers to the:

   A. anterior right chest
   B. anterior left chest
   C. heart
   D. lungs

11. An echocardiogram uses _____ to assess heart structure and function:

   A. radiographic rays
   B. electrical waves
   C. ultrasound waves
   D. nuclear imaging

MEDICAL RECORD ANALYSIS

MEDICAL RECORD 7-1

As a clinical medical assistant working in a cardiac clinic, you work directly with patients, measuring vital signs, assisting with examinations, and performing other procedures as directed by the physician. Last week one of the clinic's patients, Mr. Johnson, was admitted to the hospital for chest pain. He has now been discharged and is returning to the clinic. You are reviewing the history and physical from his hospital admission.

Medical Record

HISTORY AND PHYSICAL

HISTORY

CHIEF COMPLAINT: Chest pain.

HISTORY OF PRESENT ILLNESS: Mr. Johnson presents here today with complaints of chest pressure with pain radiating to left arm and jaw. Onset 4 days ago. These symptoms usually begin when he has been jogging for 1 to 2 miles and get worse when he runs uphill. The pain subsides if he slows down or rests. He has admitted to diaphoresis and shortness of breath during these episodes. He exercises five to seven times per week, usually running or jogging 3–5 miles per day. He is not on any medications at this time other than an over-the-counter daily vitamin.

PAST MEDICAL HISTORY: His family history is positive for heart disease because his father died at the age of 61 from a myocardial infarction.

SOCIAL HISTORY: Nondrinker, nonsmoker.

OCCUPATIONAL HISTORY: Has been working at the executive level for a land development company for 27 years.

REVIEW OF SYSTEMS: On review of systems, his medical history is unremarkable. He denies any cognitive, visual, auditory, musculoskeletal, digestive, or urinary problems.

PHYSICAL EXAM

GENERAL APPEARANCE: On examination this patient is a well-developed, well-nourished 57-year-old man in no acute distress.

VITAL SIGNS: BP 122/78, P 59 reg, R 12, T 98.8 Wt 190# Ht 6'1"

HEENT: Pupils are equal, round, and reactive to light and accommodation.

NECK: The neck is supple. Carotid pulses are strong. No masses or tenderness.

LUNGS: Clear to percussion and auscultation. Breath sounds are easily heard and normal.

HEART: The heart rate and rhythm are regular. Pulse is 59. No murmurs, gallops, or rubs.

EXTREMITIES: No clubbing, cyanosis, or edema.

DIAGNOSTICS: Chest x-ray: suggestive of slight left ventricular enlargement, ECG: positive for ST-segment depression, occasional PVC.

ASSESSMENT

IMPRESSION: Rule out ischemia, rule out cardiovascular disease

PLAN: CBC, chemistry profile, echocardiogram, and GXT today. If positive, schedule cardiac catheterization within a week. Instructions were given to patient to discontinue jogging until further notice. Patient was given a sample of sublingual nitroglycerin and instructed on its use.

Exercise 39

APPLICATION

Write the appropriate medical terms used in this medical record on the blanks after their meanings. Note that not all the terms appear in the chapter, but you should be able to identify these terms based on word parts that are included in this chapter.

1. pertaining to the heart and vessels   _____

2. ultrasound recording of heart structure   _____

3. GXT is an abbreviation for   _____

4. death of heart tissue   _____

5. pertaining to a ventricle   _____

6. abnormal condition characterized by purple or blue discoloration   _____

Bonus Questions

Atherosclerosis is a form of arteriosclerosis. These two medical terms sound similar but have two different meanings. Write in the correct term after each meaning:

7. hardening of the arteries   _____

8. hardening of vessels due to plaque buildup   _____

MEDICAL RECORD 7-2

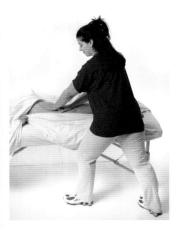

You are a massage therapist seeing Mr. Vanden Berg for the first time for treatment of his lymphedema. He and his wife were missionaries for the past 10 years in Ethiopia, Africa, where he contracted filarial elephantiasis. He has brought his medical record from his last physician visit.

A massage therapist uses touch to assist patients with various conditions.

Medical Record

FOLLOW-UP FOR FILARIAL ELEPHANTIASIS

SUBJECTIVE: Patient returns for follow-up after starting chemotherapy for his condition. He complains of continued edema in both of his lower extremities. This is probably due to lymphangiitis and the interrupted flow of lymph and fluid buildup. He has symptoms of chills, fever, and general malaise, which are all to be expected for this stage of his illness.

OBJECTIVE: Lab results confirm the presence of a bacterial infection from adult filarial worms. His temperature is 100.5°F today. His weight has stayed around 210 lb, which is up 2 lb from last visit. On palpation of lower extremities, there is pitting edema and the right lower leg is erythematic.

ASSESSMENT:
1. Filarial elephantiasis
2. Lymphedema
3. Lymphangiitis
4. Fever
5. General malaise

PLAN:
1. Review appropriate hygiene plan
2. Continue with chemotherapy as prescribed
3. Begin massage therapy as tolerated for lymphedema
4. Follow up in 1 month to monitor signs of lymphadenitis or lymphadenopathy.

Exercise 40

APPLICATION

Read the medical report and circle the letter of your answer choice for the following questions. Note: Although some of the medical terms in these questions do not appear in this chapter, you should understand them from their word parts.

1. What is causing Mr. Vanden Berg's elephantiasis?

   A. red clay soil
   B. filariae
   C. food poisoning
   D. heat

2. What is lymphedema?

   A. infection of a lymph node
   B. inflammation of a lymph node
   C. swelling due to blocked blood vessels
   D. swelling due to blocked lymph vessels and fluid buildup

3. What are filariae?

   A. worms
   B. bacteria
   C. germs
   D. fleas

Bonus Question

6. Although this chapter does not describe this term, what does the word *erythema* mean?

4. What is lymphangiitis?

   A. infection of a lymph vessel
   B. inflammation of a lymph node
   C. inflammation of a lymph vessel
   D. malignant tumor of lymph tissue

5. Which of the following statements about elephantiasis is *not* true?

   A. it occurs most commonly in South America
   B. filariae get into a body via mosquito bites
   C. filariae block lymph vessels
   D. lymphedema and lymphangiitis are common symptoms

Pronunciation and Spelling

Exercise 41

AUDITORY

Review the Chapter 7 terms in the Dictionary/Audio Glossary in the Student Resources and practice pronouncing each term, referring to the pronunciation guide as needed.

Exercise 42

SPELLING

Circle the correct spelling of each term.

1. aneurism   anyerism   aneurysm

2. lymphangeitis   lymphangiitis   lymphanitis

3. valvoplasty   valvuplasty   valvloplasty

4. telangietasia   telengiectasia   telangiectasia

5. Dopplier   Dopler   Doppler

6. sphygmomanometer   sphymonometer   sphymomenometer

7. vasoconstricter   vasoconstrictor   vasoconstitor

8. diastoli   diestole   diastole

9. ascultation   ausultation   auscultation

10. elephantiasis   elephanitis   elephantiosis

11. paroxysmal   paroxismal   paroximal

12. ischimic   iskemic   ischemic

13. dysrhythmia   dysrrythmia   dysrythmia

14. arrhythmia   arrythmia   arythmia

15. claudication   claudacation   claudocation

Media Connection

STUDENT
RESOURCES

Exercise 43

Complete each of the following activities available with the Student Resources. Check off each activity as you complete it, and record your score for the Chapter Quiz in the space provided.

Chapter Exercises

____ Flash Cards   ____ Fill the Gap

____ Concentration   ____ Break It Down

____ Abbreviation Match-Up   ____ True/False Body Building

____ Roboterms   ____ Quiz Show

____ Word Builder   ____ Complete the Case

_____ ⬤ Medical Record Review   _____ 👁 Image Matching

_____ 👁 Look and Label   _____ abc Spelling Bee

_____ **Chapter Quiz**   *Score:* _____%

Additional Resources

_____ 👁 Animation: *Cardiac Cycle*

_____ 👁 Animation: *Hypertension*

_____ 👂 Dictionary/Audio Glossary

_____ Health Professions Careers: Clinical Medical Assistant

_____ Health Professions Careers: Massage Therapist

Blood and Immune System

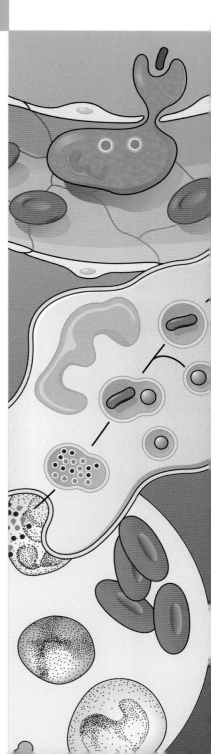

Chapter Outline

Objectives

After completion of this chapter you will be able to:

1. Describe the function and main components of blood and the immune system.

2. Define terms related to the blood, blood cells, blood components, and the immune system.

3. Define combining forms, prefixes, and suffixes related to blood and the immune system.

4. Define common medical terminology related to blood and the immune system, including adjectives and related terms, symptoms and conditions, tests and procedures, surgical interventions and therapeutic procedures, medications and drug therapies, and specialties.

5. Explain abbreviations for terms related to blood and the immune system.

6. Successfully complete all chapter exercises.

7. Explain terms used in case studies and medical records involving blood and the immune system.

8. Successfully complete all pronunciation and spelling exercises, and complete all interactive exercises included with the companion Student Resources.

■ ANATOMY AND PHYSIOLOGY

Functions

- ■ To transport oxygen, carbon dioxide, nutrients, electrolytes, vitamins, hormones, and wastes throughout the body
- ■ To protect the body with circulating white blood cells, antibodies of the immune system, and clotting factors
- ■ To protect the body by naturally and artificially acquired immunity

Structures

- ■ The blood, classified as a connective tissue, is made up of 45% formed elements and 55% liquid or plasma (Fig. 8-1).
- ■ The formed elements are produced in bone marrow and consist of three types of blood cells: erythrocytes, leukocytes, and thrombocytes (Fig. 8-2).
- ■ Erythrocytes, or red blood cells, carry oxygen to body cells.
- ■ Leukocytes, or white blood cells, provide immunity by protecting the body from damaging microorganisms.
- ■ Thrombocytes, or platelets, are instrumental in clotting blood, a process referred to as hemostasis.
- ■ Blood plasma consists of 90% water and 10% components that are transported throughout the body.
- ■ The immune response is a body's reaction to an antigen or a foreign pathogen.

Terms Related to Blood and the Immune System

Term	Pronunciation	Meaning
Whole Blood and Blood Forming Organs		
blood	blŭd	fluid that circulates through the heart, arteries, capillaries, and veins, transporting oxygen and nutritive materials to the tissues
formed elements	fōrmd el'ĕ-mĕnts	blood cells
plasma	plaz'mah	liquid portion of blood that carries formed elements, clotting factors, minerals, and proteins

(continued)

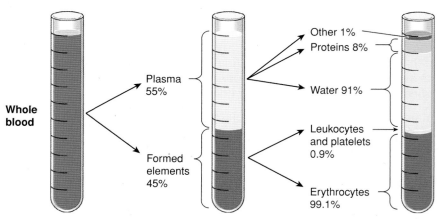

Figure 8-1 Composition of whole blood.

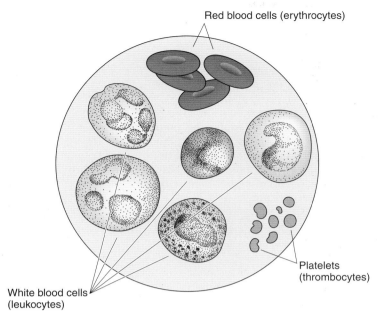

Red blood cells (erythrocytes)

White blood cells
(leukocytes)

Platelets
(thrombocytes)

Figure 8-2   Blood components.

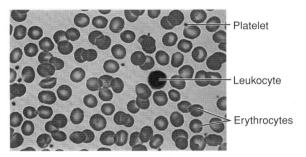

Platelet

Leukocyte

Erythrocytes

Figure 8-3   The three formed elements of blood
as seen under a microscope.

Terms Related to Blood and the Immune System *(continued)*

Term	Pronunciation	Meaning
serum	sēr'ŭm	liquid portion of blood after removal of clotting factors and blood cells
bone marrow	bōn mar'ō	soft tissue within bone, with multiple functions including the production of blood cells
erythropoietin (EPO)	ĕ-rith'rō-poy'ĕ-tin	hormone released by kidneys that stimulates red blood cell production in bone marrow
hematopoiesis	hē'mă-tō-poy-ē'sis	formation of blood cells and other formed elements
spleen	splēn	vascular lymphatic organ responsible for filtering blood, destroying old red blood cells, producing red blood cells before birth, and storing blood
Formed Elements (Fig. 8-3)		
erythrocyte, *syn.* red blood cell (RBC)	ĕ-rith'rō-sīt, red blŭd sel	blood cell that carries oxygen and carbon dioxide (Fig. 8-4)

(continued)

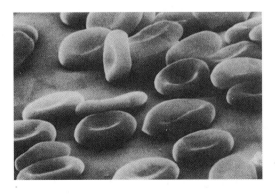

Figure 8-4   Erythrocytes (red blood cells).

Terms Related to Blood and the Immune System *(continued)*

Term	Pronunciation	Meaning
hemoglobin (HGB, Hb, Hgb)	hē′mō-glō′bin	protein in red blood cells that binds to oxygen; gives red blood cells the characteristic color

> **HEMOGLOBIN** The millions of hemoglobin molecules in a red blood cell provide oxygen to the cells of the body. Oxygen molecules bind to the hemoglobin protein and are released in body tissues during the appropriate conditions. The more oxygen carried by the hemoglobin, the brighter red color of blood. Carbon dioxide (CO_2) interferes with the ability of hemoglobin to bind oxygen. Smoking and air pollution can lead to higher-than-normal CO_2 levels and can have an adverse affect on one's health.

Term	Pronunciation	Meaning
iron (Fe)	ī′ŏrn	essential trace element necessary for hemoglobin to transport oxygen on red blood cells
macrocyte	mak′rō-sīt	a large red blood cell
Rh factor	Rh fak′tŏr	protein substance present in the red blood cells of most people (85%) capable of inducing intense antigenic reactions
leukocyte, *syn.* white blood cell (WBC)	lū′kō-sīt, wīt blŭd sel	largest blood cell; protects against pathogens, foreign substances, and cell debris (Fig. 8-5)
granulocyte	gran′yū-lō-sīt	white blood cell with visible granules; the three types of granulocytes are named according to the type of dye each is attracted to
neutrophil	nū′trō-fil	type of granulocyte that fights against bacterial infections; stains a neutral pink
eosinophil	ē′ō-sin′ō-fil	type of granulocyte that functions in allergic reactions and against parasites; stains red
basophil	bā′sō-fil	type of granulocyte that releases histamine in allergic reactions and inflammatory responses; stains a dark blue with a basic dye
agranulocyte	ā-grăn′ŭ-lō-sīt	white blood cell without clearly visible granules

(continued)

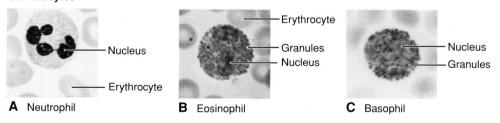

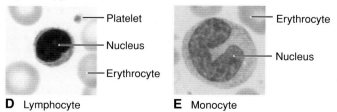

Figure 8-5 Leukocytes (white blood cells).

Terms Related to Blood and the Immune System *(continued)*

Term	Pronunciation	Meaning
lymphocyte	lim′fŏ-sīt	type of agranulocyte that circulates in the lymphatic system and is active in immunity
B lymphocyte, *syn.* B cell	bē lim′fŏ-sīt	white blood cell that, when in contact with a foreign antigen, produces antibodies to inactivate the antigen
T lymphocyte, *syn.* T cell	tē lim′fŏ-sīt	white blood cell that matures in the thymus and specializes in creating an immune response
monocyte	mon′ō-sīt	largest form of white blood cells
macrophage	mak′rō-fāj	enlarged and matured monocytes active in phagocytosis
thrombocyte, *syn.* platelet (PLT)	throm′bō-sīt, plāt′lĕt	cell fragments in the blood that stick together, forming a clot (Fig. 8-6)
Blood Clotting		
clotting factors	kloting fak′tŏrz	any of the various plasma components involved in the clotting process
coagulation	kō-ag′yū-lā′shŭn	clotting; changing from a liquid to a solid state
fibrin	fī′brin	elastic fiber protein needed in clotting and produced by fibrinogen
fibrinogen	fī-brin′ō-jen	plasma protein that is converted into solid threads called fibrin
The Immune System		
antibody (Ab)	an′ti-bod-ē	soldier-like cell that protects the body and inactivates antigens; provides immunity against specific organisms (Fig. 8-7)
antigen (Ag)	an′ti-jen	agent or substance that provokes an immune response
histamine	his′tă-mēn	substance released by damaged cells that increases blood flow to the area, causing an inflammatory process involving heat, redness, swelling, and pain
immunity	i-myū′ni-tē	protection against disease
pathogen	path′ŏ-jĕn	any virus, microorganism, or other substance that causes disease
phagocytosis	fāg-ō-sī-tō′sis	cellular process of eating and destroying substances, usually by the neutrophils and macrophages (Fig. 8-8)

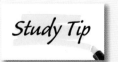 *Study Tip*

Phagocytosis Many of us are familiar with a video arcade game called *Pac-Man*, featuring a round dot that goes around eating things in his way. Phagocytosis is a process in which a particular type of white blood cell performs a similar activity (*phag/o* = eating, *cyt/o* = cell, and *-osis* = process). Leukocytes ingest substances such as other cells, bacteria, foreign particles, and dead tissue. Visualizing a cell as resembling *Pac-Man* may help you to remember the process of phagocytosis.

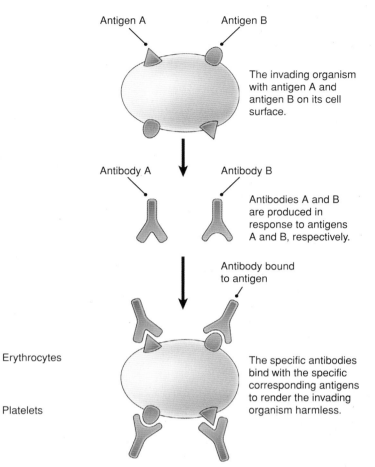

Figure 8-7   Antibodies bind with antigens to provide immunity against specific organisms.

Figure 8-6   Thrombocytes (platelets).

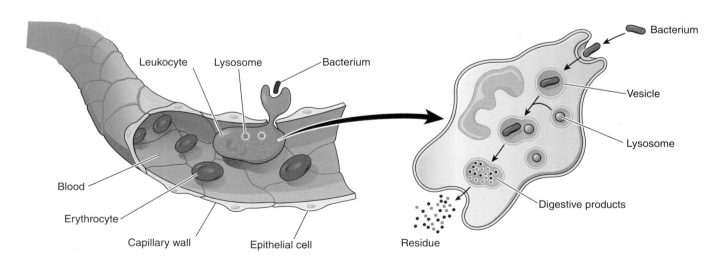

Figure 8-8   Phagocytosis.

■ Exercises: Anatomy and Physiology

SIMPLE
RECALL

Exercise 1

Write the correct anatomic term for the structure described.

1. largest blood cell that protects against pathogens _____

2. cell fragments in blood that form clots _____

3. fluid that circulates through the heart, arteries, capillaries, and veins _____

4. agranulocyte that circulates in the lymphatic system _____

5. liquid portion of blood that carries formed elements _____

6. vascular lymphatic organ _____

7. WBC with visible granules _____

8. WBC lacking visible granules _____

9. largest of the WBCs _____

10. WBC that stains red _____

11. WBC that stains dark blue _____

12. blood cell that carries oxygen and carbon dioxide _____

13. protein in RBCs that binds to oxygen _____

14. soft tissue inside bones _____

15. liquid portion of the blood minus the formed elements _____

SIMPLE
RECALL

Exercise 2

Write the meaning or function of the term given.

1. iron _____

2. antibody _____

3. antigen _____

4. pathogen _____

5. immunity _____

6. erythropoietin _____

7. hematopoiesis _____

8. neutrophil _____

9. clotting factors _____

10. Rh factor _____

Exercise 3

SIMPLE
RECALL

Circle the term that is most appropriate for the meaning of the sentence.

1. The most numerous type of blood cell is the (*leukocyte, erythrocyte, thrombocyte*).

2. (*Stain, Hemoglobin, Granulocytes*) give erythrocytes their red color.

3. The blood cells are also referred to as (*formed elements, histamine, sera*).

4. (*Hemoglobin, Histamine, Fibrin*) is a substance released by damaged cells causing inflammation, redness, and pain.

5. Soldier-like proteins that protect the body are called (*antigens, antibodies, fibrins*).

6. Foreign invaders that can create an immune response are called (*antigens, antibodies, fibrins*).

7. Blood cell production takes place in the (*bone marrow, liver, spleen*).

8. The (*bone marrow, liver, spleen*) is responsible for filtering blood.

9. The kidneys release a hormone called (*erythropoietin, histamine, hematopoiesis*) that stimulates the production of RBCs in bone marrow.

10. The medical term for white blood cell is (*erythrocyte, leukocyte, thrombocyte*).

11. The monocyte active in phagocytosis in tissue is called a (*granulocyte, macrophage, monophage*).

12. The liquid portion of blood (without the clotting factors and blood cells) is called (*serum, plasma, formed elements*).

Exercise 4

ADVANCED
RECALL

Match each term with its meaning.

phagocytosis	leukocyte	antibody
Rh factor	pathogen	fibrin
coagulation	hemoglobin	thrombocyte

Meaning   **Term**

1. may induce intense antigenic reactions _____

2. clotting _____

3. soldier-like protein protecting the body   _____

4. elastic fiber protein used in clotting   _____

5. white blood cell   _____

6. oxygen-binding protein found on RBCs   _____

7. any disease-causing substance   _____

8. platelet   _____

9. cellular process of eating and destroying   _____

ADVANCED
RECALL

Exercise 5

Fill in the blanks with the correct answers.

1. A white blood cell that produces antibodies to inactivate an antigen is called a(n) _____ lymphocyte.

2. A white blood cell that specializes in creating an immune response is called a(n) _____ lymphocyte.

3. The _____ is a lymphatic organ that filters out aging red blood cells.

4. The type of blood cell that carries oxygen and carbon dioxide is a(n) _____.

5. The elastic fiber protein needed in clotting is called _____.

6. A white blood cell with visible granules when stained is referred to as a(n) _____.

7. A large red blood cell is called a(n) _____.

8. _____ is the plasma protein that is converted into solid threads called fibrin.

9. The _____ is an enlarged and mature monocyte active in phagocytosis.

■ WORD PARTS

Note that some word parts that have been introduced earlier in the book may not be repeated here.

Combining Forms

Combining Form	Meaning
chrom/o, chromat/o	color
cyt/o	cell
erythr/o	red
granul/o	granules

(continued)

Combining Forms *(continued)*

Combining Form	Meaning
hem/o, hemat/o	blood
immun/o	immune, safe
leuk/o	white
lymph/o	lymph
neutr/o	neutral
nucle/o	nucleus
path/o	disease
phag/o	eat, swallow
phleb/o	vein
plas/o	formation, growth
thromb/o	blood clot

Prefixes

Prefix	Meaning
auto-	self, same
basi-, baso-	base
macro-	large, long
micro-	small
mono-	one
pro-	before, promoting
poly-	many, much

Suffixes

Suffix	Meaning
-cyte	cell
-emia	blood (condition of)
-sis	condition, process
-gen	origin, production
-lysis	destruction, breakdown, separation
-osis	abnormal condition
-penia	deficiency
-philia	attraction for
-poiesis	production, formation
-rrhage	flowing forth
-y	condition of

■ Exercises: Word Parts

Exercise 6

SIMPLE RECALL

Write the meaning of the combining form(s) given.

1. hem/o, hemat/o _____

2. path/o _____

3. thromb/o _____

4. immun/o _____

5. leuk/o _____

6. erythr/o _____

7. phag/o _____

8. granul/o _____

9. phleb/o _____

10. chrom/o, chromat/o _____

11. neutr/o _____

12. plas/o _____

Exercise 7

SIMPLE RECALL

Write the correct combining form(s) for the meaning given.

1. blood clot _____

2. formation, growth _____

3. lymph _____

4. neutral _____

5. blood _____

6. red _____

7. white _____

8. eat, swallow _____

9. cell _____

10. nucleus _____

SIMPLE
RECALL

Exercise 8

Write the meaning of the prefix or suffix given.

1. auto- _____

2. -rrhage _____

3. mono- _____

4. baso- _____

5. poly- _____

6. -philia _____

7. -penia _____

8. -lysis _____

9. -poiesis _____

10. macro- _____

11. micro- _____

12. -emia _____

13. -gen _____

14. -osis _____

Exercise 9

ADVANCED
RECALL

Considering the meaning of the combining form from which the medical term is made, write the meaning of the medical term. (You have not yet learned many of these terms but can build their meaning from the word parts.)

Combining Form	Meaning	Medical Term	Meaning of Term
phleb/o	vein	phlebology	1. _____
hem/o	blood	hemorrhage	2. _____
thromb/o	blood clot	thrombocyte	3. _____
erythr/o	red	erythrocyte	4. _____
neutr/o	neutral	neutrophil	5. _____

TERM
CONSTRUCTION

Exercise 10

Write the remainder of the term for the meaning given.

Meaning	Medical Term
1. white (blood) cell	leuko _____
2. destruction of a blood clot	_____ lysis
3. abnormal condition of a single nucleus	mono _____ osis
4. deficiency of all blood cells	_____ cytopenia
5. condition of many blood cells	_____ cythemia
6. formation of red (blood cells)	_____ poiesis
7. study of veins	phlebo _____

■ MEDICAL TERMS

Adjectives and Other Related Terms

Term	Pronunciation	Meaning
autoimmunity	aw'tō-i-myū'ni-tē	pertaining to one's immune system attacking its own tissues or cells
cytopathic	sī'tō-path'ik	pertaining to a disease or disorder of a cell or cellular component
hematopoietic	hē'mă-tō-poy-et'ik	pertaining to the formation of blood cells
hemolytic	hē'mō-lit'ik	pertaining to the rupture or destruction of red blood cells
hemorrhagic	hem'ŏr-aj'ik	pertaining to profuse or excessive bleeding
hemostasis	hē'mō-stā'sis	stoppage or arrest of bleeding
hypersensitive	hī'per-sen'si-tiv	condition of excessive response or an exaggerated sensitivity to a stimulus
inflammatory	in-flam'ă-tōr-ē	pertaining to the process of heat, redness, swelling, and pain in response to tissue injury
predisposition	prē'dis-pō-zish'ŭn	condition of being susceptible to disease
proliferative	prō-lif'ěr-ă-tiv	growing and increasing in number of similar cells
rejection	rē-jek'shŭn	immunologic response of incompatibility to a transplanted organ or tissue
systemic	sis-tem'ik	pertaining to the body as a whole
virulent	vir'yū-lĕnt	denotes an extremely toxic pathogen

ANIMATION

To learn more about the inflammatory process and the role that it and phagocytosis play in healing wounds, view the animation Wound Healing *included with the Student Resources.*

■ Exercises: Adjectives and Other Related Terms

Exercise 11

SIMPLE RECALL

Circle the term that is most appropriate for the meaning of the sentence.

1. Hemophilia is a disorder characterized by a tendency to bleed excessively; this may also be called a(n) (*inflammatory, hemorrhagic, proliferative*) disease.

2. Lupus erythematosus is usually referred to as a (*systemic, hypersensitive, hemolytic*) disease because it can affect the body as a whole.

3. (*Autoimmunity, Predisposition, Rejection*) occurs when there is an incompatibility with transplanted tissue.

4. The condition of being susceptible to disease is called (*predisposition, rejection, autoimmunity*).

5. (*Hemorrhagic, Hemolytic, Hemostasis*) means pertaining to the rupture or destruction of red blood cells.

6. The term (*cytopathic, hematopoietic, systemic*) means pertaining to a disease or disorder of a cell or cellular component.

7. When a patient's immune system attacks its own tissues or cells, it is called (*cytopathic, autoimmunity, rejection*).

Exercise 12

ADVANCED RECALL

Match each word with its meaning.

rejection   virulent   hemostasis   hypersensitive
inflammatory   systemic   hematopoietic   proliferative

Meaning   **Term**

1. stopping or arresting bleeding   _____

2. immune response of incompatibility   _____

3. growing and increasing in number of similar cells   _____

4. pertaining to swelling, pain, and redness   _____

5. denoting a very toxic pathogen   _____

6. denoting an exaggerated response to a stimulus   _____

7. pertaining to the formation of blood cells   _____

8. pertaining to the whole body   _____

Symptoms and Medical Conditions

Term	Pronunciation	Meaning
anemia	ă-nē′mē-ă	condition in which the number of red blood cells, hemoglobin, or volume of packed cells is lower than normal
Anemias due to impaired production of red blood cells		
aplastic anemia	ă-plas′tik ă-nē′mē-ă	disorder in which bone marrow does not produce enough red blood cells
iron deficiency anemia	ī′ŏrn dĕ-fish′ĕn-sē ă-nē′mē-ă	disorder in which hemoglobin is unable to transport oxygen due to a lack of iron (Fig. 8-9)
pernicious anemia	pĕr-nish′ŭs ă-nē′mē-ă	disorder in which the number of red blood cells decline with simultaneous enlargement of individual cells (i.e., macrocytes) due to an inability to absorb vitamin B-12; usually in older adults (Fig. 8-10)
Anemias due to the destruction or loss of red blood cells		
hemorrhagic anemia, *syn.* blood loss anemia	hem′ŏr-aj′ik ă-nē′mē-ă, blŭd laws ă-nē′mē-ă	disorder involving lack of red blood cells due to profuse blood loss
thalassemia	thal′ă-sē′mē-ă	disorder caused by a genetic defect resulting in low hemoglobin production
sickle cell anemia	sik′ĕl sel ă-nē′mē-ă	disorder caused by a genetic defect resulting in abnormal hemoglobin causing sickle-shaped red blood cells, which have difficulty moving through small capillary vessels (Fig. 8-11)
autoimmune disease	aw′tō-i-myūn′ di-zēz′	condition in which the immune system attacks normal body tissues
clotting disorder	klot′ing dis-ōr′dĕr	condition characterized by an inability of blood to coagulate
hemophilia	hē′mō-fil′ē-ă	bleeding disorder due to a deficiency of a clotting factor
thrombocytopenia	throm′bō-sī-tō-pē′nē-ă	disorder involving low levels of platelets in blood
idiopathic thrombocytopenic purpura (ITP)	id′ē-ō-path′ik throm′bō-sī-tō-pē′nik pur′pyur-ă	disorder marked by platelet destruction by macrophages resulting in bruising and bleeding from mucous membranes

(continued)

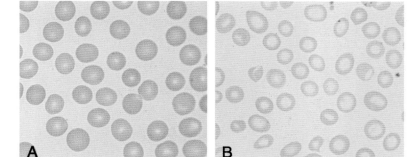

Figure 8-9 A blood smear showing normal erythrocytes (**A**) compared with erythrocytes in a patient with iron deficiency anemia (**B**).

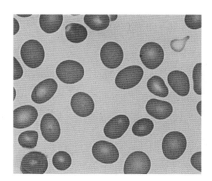

Figure 8-10 Pernicious anemia with few macrocytic red blood cells.

Normal

Red blood cell

Sickle cell anemia

Sickle-shaped red
blood cell

Sickle cell crisis

Obstruction of
blood flow

Sickle-
shaped
cell

A

B

Figure 8-11   Sickle cell anemia. **A.** Sickle cell crisis causes obstruction of blood flow and therefore pain. **B.** The sickle (crescent-shaped) blood cells indicate sickle cell anemia.

Symptoms and Medical Conditions *(continued)*

Term	Pronunciation	Meaning
von Willebrand disease (vWD)	vahn vil'ĕ-brahnt di-zēz'	bleeding disorder characterized by a tendency to bleed primarily from the mucous membranes due to a deficiency of a clotting factor
hemochromatosis	hē'mō-krō-mă-tō'sis	excessive absorption and storage of dietary iron in body tissues causing dysfunction
mononucleosis	mon'ō-nū-klē-ō'sis	increase of mononuclear leukocytes with symptoms of fever, enlarged cervical lymph nodes, and fatigue (Fig. 8-12)

(continued)

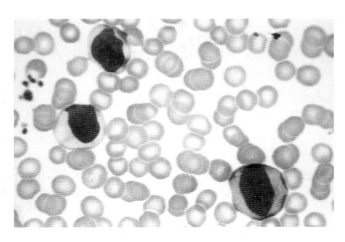

Figure 8-12   Mononucleosis with atypical lymphocytes.

Symptoms and Medical Conditions *(continued)*

Term	Pronunciation	Meaning
pancytopenia	pan'sĭ-tō-pē'nē-ă	deficiency in all types of blood cells
polycythemia	pol'ē-sī-thē'mē-ă	increase of red blood cells
rheumatoid arthritis (RA)	rū'mă-toyd ahr-thrī'tis	autoimmune disease causing progressive destructive changes and inflammation in multiple joints, especially in the hands and feet
septicemia	sep'ti-sē'mē-ă	spread of microorganisms or toxins through circulating blood
Sjögren syndrome	shōr'gren sin'drōm	chronic autoimmune disease in which a person's white blood cells attack their moisture-producing glands
systemic lupus erythematosus (SLE)	sis-tem'ik lū'pŭs ĕr-ith'ĕ-mă-tō'sŭs	inflammatory, autoimmune, connective tissue disease that can affect all organ systems
thrombosis	throm-bō'sis	abnormal presence of clotting within a blood vessel

■ Exercises: Symptoms and Medical Conditions

Exercise 13

SIMPLE RECALL

Select the best term to complete the meaning given.

1. hemophilia = tendency to (*bleed, clot*)

2. hemorrhagic anemia = low red blood cell count due to (*bleeding, clotting*)

3. thrombocytopenia = difficulty with clotting due to low (*RBCs, WBCs, platelets*)

4. iron deficiency anemia = inability of hemoglobin to (*produce, transport*) oxygen

5. hemochromatosis = excessive absorption of (*calcium, iron*)

6. aplastic anemia = inability of bone marrow to (*produce, transport*) red blood cells

7. pernicious anemia = (*destruction, increase*) of red blood cells due to inability to absorb vitamin B-12

8. von Willebrand disease = (*clotting, autoimmune*) disorder

9. polycythemia = (*decrease, increase*) of red blood cells

10. thalassemia = (*high, low*) hemoglobin production

Exercise 14

SIMPLE RECALL

Circle the term that is most appropriate for the meaning of the sentence.

1. Idiopathic thrombocytopenic purpura is a disease due to a destruction of (*leukocytes, platelets, electrolytes*).

2. In (*aplastic, pernicious, virulent*) anemia, there is a decrease in the number of erythrocytes with an increase in size.

3. The disease that affects moisture-producing glands is (*septicemia, SLE, Sjögren syndrome*).

4. Mononucleosis has the symptom of enlarged (*lymph nodes, erythrocytes, thrombocytes*).

5. The condition that causes abnormally shaped red blood cells is called (*aplastic anemia, sickle cell anemia, pernicious anemia*).

6. A condition in which the immune system attacks normal body tissues is called (*thrombocytopenia, sickle cell anemia, autoimmune disease*).

7. A clotting disorder is characterized by an inability of blood to (*form, coagulate, dissolve*).

8. An increase in red blood cells is called (*thrombosis, polycythemia, mononucleosis*).

9. Septicemia is the spread of toxins through circulating (*plasma, serum, blood*).

10. Systemic lupus erythematosus is a(n) (*autoimmune, inherited, cytopathic*) connective tissue disease.

11. Rheumatoid arthritis affects a patient's (*bones, organs, joints*).

Exercise 15

ADVANCED
RECALL

Considering the meaning of the combining form from which the medical term is made, write the meaning of the medical term. (You have not yet learned many of these terms but can build their meaning from the word parts.)

Combining Form	Meaning	Medical Term	Meaning of Term
cyt/o	cell	pancytopenia	1. _____
nucle/o	nucleus	mononucleosis	2. _____
plas/o	formation, growth	aplastic	3. _____
hem/o	blood	hemophilia	4. _____
arthr/o	joint	arthritis	5. _____

Exercise 16

TERM
CONSTRUCTION

Build a medical term from the appropriate combining form(s) and suffix, given their meanings.

Combining Form(s)	Suffix	Term
1. blood; color	abnormal condition	_____
2. blood	attraction for	_____

3. blood clot; cell   deficiency   _____

4. blood clot   abnormal condition   _____

5. blood   flowing forth   _____

Tests and Procedures

Term	Pronunciation	Meaning
Laboratory Tests Related to Hematology		
albumin	al-bū'min	measurement of this protein level; used to diagnose liver or kidney problems, inflammation, malnutrition, or dehydration
bilirubin	bil'i-rū'bin	screen for liver disorders or anemia
blood smear	blŭd smēr	evaluation of the appearance and number of blood cells and the different types of white blood cells (Fig. 8-13)
complete blood count (CBC), *syn.* hemogram	kŏm-plēt' blŭd kownt, hē'mō-gram	automated count of all blood cells (Fig. 8-14)
erythrocyte sedimentation rate (ESR)	ĕ-rith'rŏ-sīt sed'i-mĕn-tā'shŭn rāt	time measurement of red blood cells settling in a test tube over 1 hour; used to diagnose inflammation and anemias
hematocrit (HCT, Hct)	hē-mat'ō-krit	volume of blood occupied by red blood cells; used to diagnose various disorders including anemia (Fig. 8-15)
hemoglobin (HGB, Hgb, Hb) test	hē'mō-glō'bin	test for the red blood cell protein responsible for binding oxygen; used to diagnose various disorders including anemia

(continued)

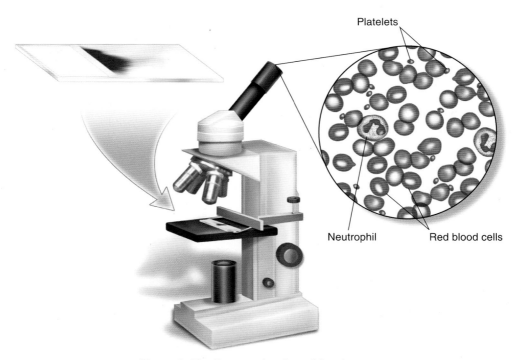

Figure 8-13 Preparation for a blood smear.

Complete Blood Count (CBC) with differential

Test	Result	Units	Reference Interval
White Blood Count	1.5 L	x 10^3/mm^3	5.0-10.0
Red Blood Count	3.50 L	x 106/mm^3	4.1-5.3
Hemoglobin	10.8 L	g/dL	12.0-18.0
Hematocrit	31.1 L	%	37.0-52.0
Platelets	302	x 10^3/mm^3	150-400
Polys (neutrophils)	23 L	%	45-76
Lymphs	68 H	%	17-44
Monocytes	7	%	3-10
Eos	2	%	0-4
Basos	0.6	%	0.2
Polys (absolute)	.34 L	x 10^3/mm^3	1.8-7.8
Lymphs (absolute)	1.0	x 10^3/mm^3	0.7-4.5
Monocytes (absolute)	0.1	x 10^3/mm^3	0.1-1.0
Eos (absolute)	0.1	x 10^3/mm^3	0.0-0.4
Basos (absolute)	0.0	x 10^3/mm^3	0.0-0.2

Figure 8-14 Complete blood count (CBC) report.

Tests and Procedures (continued)

Term	Pronunciation	Meaning
platelet count (PLT)	plăt'lĕt kownt	number of platelets present; used to diagnose bleeding disorders or bone marrow disease
red blood cell count (RBC)	red blŭd sel kownt	number of erythrocytes present; used to diagnose various disorders including anemia

(continued)

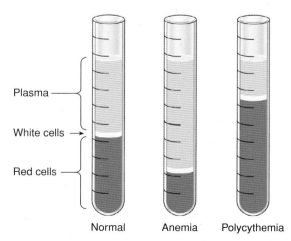

Plasma

White cells →

Red cells

Normal   Anemia   Polycythemia   **Figure 8-15** Hematocrit.

Tests and Procedures *(continued)*

Term	Pronunciation	Meaning
white blood cell count (WBC)	wīt blŭd sel kownt	number of leukocytes present; used to diagnose various disorders, including infections and diseases, and for monitoring treatment
cross-matching	kraws mach'ing	blood typing test for compatibility between donor and recipient blood
culture and sensitivity (C&S)	kŭl'chŭr sen'si-tiv'i-tē	growing of an organism from a specimen from the body to determine its susceptibility to particular medications
prothrombin time (PT)	prō-throm'bin tīm	measurement of time for blood to clot
WBC differential count, *syn.* differential count	dif'ĕr-en'shăl kownt	evaluation of the total percentage of leukocytes
Laboratory Tests for Antibodies		
antinuclear antibody (ANA) test	an'tē-nū'klē-ăr an'ti-bod-ē test	assessment for autoimmune disorders such as systemic lupus erythematosus, rheumatoid arthritis, and others
Epstein-Barr virus (EBV) antibody test	ep'stīn bahr vī'rŭs an'ti-bod-ē test	diagnostic test for mononucleosis and evaluation of Epstein-Barr virus
mononucleosis spot test	mon'ō-nū-klē-ō'sis spot test	assessment for mononucleosis
rheumatoid factor test	rū'mă-toyd fak'tŏr test	test for rheumatoid arthritis and Sjögren syndrome

■ Exercises: Tests and Procedures

Exercise 17

SIMPLE
RECALL

Circle the term that is most appropriate for the meaning of the sentence.

1. The rheumatoid factor test is used to help diagnosis rheumatoid arthritis and (*Epstein-Barr virus, Sjögren syndrome, anemia*).

2. The diagnostic test for mononucleosis and evaluation for Epstein-Barr virus is called the (*EBV antibody test, PLT count, ANA test*).

3. It is important for a blood donor and recipient to have had (*cross-matching, culture and sensitivity, prothrombin time*) tests done to assess compatibility.

4. A test designed to measure the clotting time of blood is a (*bilirubin, prothrombin time, blood smear*).

5. (*HCT, HGB, ESR*) is a test that measures the red blood cell protein responsible for carrying oxygen.

6. In the complete blood count, an increase in the erythrocyte sedimentation rate may signal (*hemophilia, inflammation, erythrocytes*) and/or anemia.

7. To evaluate the total percentage of leukocytes, a (*WBC differential count, white blood cell count, platelet count*) might be ordered.

8. A (*hemoglobin, complete blood count, hematocrit*) measures the percentage of red blood cells in a volume of blood.

9. A culture and sensitivity identifies a (*blood cell, donor, pathogen*) and tests its susceptibility to (*blood transfusion, antibiotic, gene therapy*) treatment.

10. To rule out an autoimmune disease, a physician may order a(n) (*ANA, ESR, BUN*).

ADVANCED
RECALL

Exercise 18

Match each laboratory test with its description.

| platelet count | albumin | white blood cell count | blood smear |
| red blood cell count | hemogram | bilirubin | |

Description   **Term**

1. evaluation of blood cells and different WBCs   _____

2. number of erythrocytes   _____

3. another name for complete blood count   _____

4. diagnosis of bleeding disorders   _____

5. measurement of protein level   _____

6. screen for liver disorders or anemia   _____

7. number of leukocytes   _____

Surgical Interventions and Therapeutic Procedures

Term	Pronunciation	Meaning
apheresis	ă-fĕr-ē'sis	removal and replacement of a patient's own blood or donor blood after specific components have been removed (Fig. 8-16)
blood transfusion (BT)	blŭd trans-fyū'zhŭn	transfer of blood between compatible donor and recipient
autologous blood	aw-tol'ŏ-gŭs blud	blood donated for future use by same patient; usually presurgical
homologous blood	hŏ-mol'ŏ-gŭs blŭd	blood donated from same species for use by a compatible recipient
blood component therapy	blŭd kŏm-pō'nĕnt thār'ă-pē	transfusion of specific blood components such as packed red blood cells, plasma, or platelets

(continued)

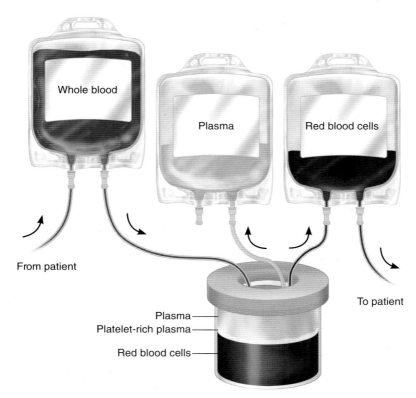

Figure 8-16 Apheresis.

Surgical Interventions and Therapeutic Procedures
(continued)

Term	Pronunciation	Meaning
bone marrow aspiration (BMA)	bōn mar′ō as-pir-ā′shŭn	removal of a small amount of fluid and cells from inside the bone with a needle and syringe (Fig. 8-17)
bone marrow transplant (BMT)	bōn mar′ō trans′plant	transfer of bone marrow from one person to another
immunization, *syn.* vaccination	im′myū-nī-zā′shŭn, vak′si-nā′shŭn	administration of a weakened or killed pathogen, or a protein of a pathogen, to cause the immune system to create antibodies for future protection (Fig. 8-18)
immunosuppression	im′yū-nō-sŭ-presh′ŭn	use of chemotherapy or immunosuppressant drugs to interfere with immune responses; usually prescribed for autoimmune disorders
phlebotomy, *syn.* venipuncture, venotomy	fle-bot′ŏ-mē, ven′i-pŭngk′shŭr, vē-not′ŏ-mē	incision into a vein to inject a solution or withdraw blood (Fig. 8-19)
plasmapheresis	plaz′mă-fĕr-ē′sis	removal and replacement of a patient's own blood after plasma has been removed and replaced with a plasma substitute
splenectomy	splē-nek′tŏ-mē	surgical removal of the spleen

STUDENT RESOURCES

View the video Venipuncture *on the Student Resources for a demonstration of a phlebotomist using a syringe to withdraw blood from a patient.*

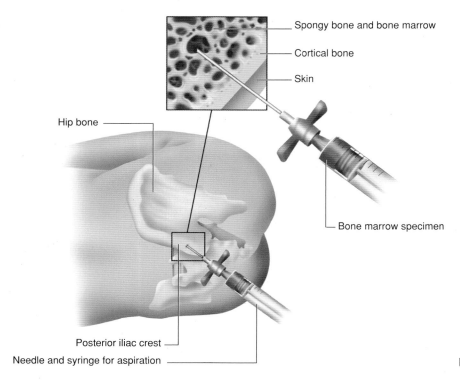

Spongy bone and bone marrow

Cortical bone

Skin

Hip bone

Bone marrow specimen

Posterior iliac crest

Needle and syringe for aspiration

Figure 8-17   Bone marrow aspiration.

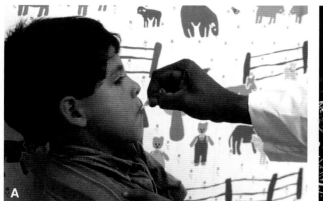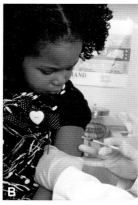

Figure 8-18   Forms of immunization. **A.** Oral administration of an immunization. **B.** Immunization by injection.

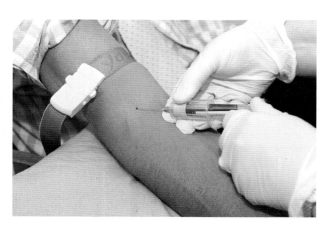

Figure 8-19   Phlebotomy to withdraw blood.

■ Exercises: Surgical Interventions and Therapeutic Procedures

SIMPLE
RECALL

Exercise 19

Write the correct medical term or procedure for the meaning given.

1. removal of plasma from the blood _____

2. bone marrow transfer from one person to another _____

3. removal of the spleen _____

4. transfer of blood between donor and recipient _____

5. transfusion of blood components _____

6. blood donated by same person for future use _____

7. blood donated by another person _____

8. removal and replacement of patient's own blood
   after removal of specific substances _____

ADVANCED
RECALL

Exercise 20

Circle the term that is most appropriate for the meaning of the sentence.

1. Mr. DeHaan was on the surgical schedule for a (*splenectomy, hepatectomy, bone marrow aspiration*), a removal of the immune system organ responsible for removing old blood cells.

2. Mrs. Chon wanted to be protected from pathogens while she traveled abroad, so her physician ordered a series of (*immunosuppressants, immunizations, anticoagulants*).

3. The medical assistant is responsible for drawing blood from patients. This procedure is called (*phlebotomy, venectomy, splenectomy*).

4. The medical technologist who works in the clinical lab occasionally performs cross-matching tests for (*blood transfusions, bone marrow aspirations, vaccinations*).

5. The physician removed a small amount of fluid and cells from inside the bone with a needle and syringe; this procedure is called a bone marrow (*transplant, aspiration, biopsy*).

6. The child had several (*vaccines, vaccinations, transfusions*) to prevent future illnesses.

7. Dr. Adams prescribed (*immunization, immunosuppression, blood transfusion*) therapy to help treat the patient's autoimmune disease.

Medications and Drug Therapies

Term	Pronunciation	Meaning
antibiotic	an'tē-bī-ot'ik	drug that acts against susceptible microorganisms
anticoagulant	an'tē-kō-ag'yŭ-lănt	drug used to prolong blood clotting time
antihistamine	an'tē-his'tă-mēn	drug used to stop the effects of histamine
hemostatic agent, *syn.* procoagulant	hē'mō-stat'ik ā'jĕnt, prō-kō-ag'yŭ-lant	drug that stops the flow of blood within vessels
immune serum	i-myūn' sēr'ŭm	serum prepared from an individual with specific disease antibodies
immunosuppressant	im'yū-nō-sŭ-pres'ănt	drug used to suppress or reduce immune responses in organ transplant recipients or those with severe autoimmune diseases

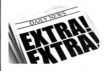

IMMUNOSUPPRESSANT DRUGS When a patient receives an organ transplant, the body treats the transplanted organ as if it were an invader or pathogen and attempts to fight it off. To protect the "new" organ from the recipient's own immune system, the patient is prescribed immunosuppressant drugs. These drugs suppress the person's immune system response, which in turn makes them susceptible to other diseases. It is important that patients receiving immunosuppressants see their physician regularly to screen for untoward side effects that may lead to hypertension and kidney or liver issues.

thrombolytic agent	throm'bō-lit'ik ā'jĕnt	drug that dissolves a blood clot
vaccine	vak-sēn'	preparation composed of a weakened or killed pathogen

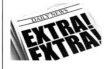

VACCINES AND COWS The Latin word *vaccinus* means relating to a cow. During the mid-1700s, it was known around the English countryside that milkmaids previously infected with the mild cowpox disease would not catch the more deadly smallpox disease. During the devastating smallpox outbreak in 18th-century Europe, Dr. Edward Jenner developed the first vaccination by injecting pus and lymph from a cowpox-infected cow into healthy people. This practice was widely successful and has contributed to the concept of vaccines today.

■ Exercise: Medications and Drug Therapies

Exercise 21

SIMPLE RECALL

Write the correct medication or drug therapy term for the meaning given.

1. drug that prolongs clotting time _____

2. preparation that contains a weakened or killed pathogen _____

3. drug that acts against microorganisms _____

4. serum from an individual with specific antibodies _____

5. drug that stops the flow of blood _____

6. drug used to suppress or reduce immune response _____

7. drug that stops the effects of histamine _____

8. drug to dissolve a blood clot _____

Specialties and Specialists

Term	Pronunciation	Meaning
allergology	al'er-gol'o-jē	medical specialty concerned with diagnosis and treatment of allergy and sensitivity
allergist	al'er-jist	physician who specializes in allergology
hematology	hē'mă-tol'o-jē	medical specialty concerned with diagnosis and treatment of disorders of the blood and blood-forming organs
hematologist	hē'mă-tol'o-jist	physician who specializes in hematology
immunology	im'yū-nol'o-jē	medical specialty concerned with immunity, allergy, and induced sensitivity
immunologist	im'yū-nol'o-jist	one who practices immunology
rheumatology	rū'mă-tol'o-jē	medical specialty concerned with diagnosis and treatment of rheumatic conditions and autoimmune diseases
rheumatologist	rū'mă-tol'o-jist	a physician who specializes in rheumatology

■ Exercise: Specialties and Specialties

ADVANCED
RECALL

Exercise 22

Match each medical specialty and specialist with its description.

hematology	rheumatologist	allergology	immunology
hematologist	immunologist	rheumatology	allergist

Meaning   **Term**

1. medical specialty concerned with allergy and sensitivity _____

2. physician who specializes in rheumatic conditions _____

3. physician who specializes in disorders of the blood _____

4. medical specialty concerned with disorders of blood and blood-forming organs _____

5. medical specialty concerning with immunity, allergy, and induced sensitivity _____

6. physician who specializes in treatment of allergy   _____

7. physician who specializes in immunity and allergy   _____

8. medical specialty concerned with rheumatic conditions and autoimmune diseases   _____

Abbreviations

Abbreviation	Meaning
Ab	antibody
Ag	antigen
ANA	antinuclear antibody test
BMA	bone marrow aspiration
BMT	bone marrow transplant
BT	blood transfusion
CBC	complete blood count
C&S	culture and sensitivity
EBV	Epstein-Barr virus
EPO	erythropoietin
ESR	erythrocyte sedimentation rate
Fe	iron
HCT, Hct, ht	hematocrit
HGB, Hb, Hgb	hemoglobin
ITP	idiopathic thrombocytopenic purpura
PLT	platelet or platelet count
PT	prothrombin time
RA	rheumatoid arthritis
RBC	red blood cell; red blood cell count
SLE	systemic lupus erythematosus
vWD	von Willebrand disease
WBC	white blood cell; white blood cell count

■ Exercises: Abbreviations

ADVANCED
RECALL

Exercise 23

Write the meaning of each abbreviation used in these sentences.

1. Mr. Matthews must have a **PT** done once a month because he has **vWD**, a blood clotting disorder.

   _____

2. It was necessary to perform a **BMA** on the donor before scheduling the **BMT**.

   _____

3. Today, Ms. Tisha will be responsible for performing all **CBC** tests in the clinical lab.

_____

4. An **ESR** test is used to diagnose inflammation.

_____

5. Routinely, an **Hgb** and an **Hct** are performed together.

_____

6. Two types of blood cells are **RBCs** and **WBCs.**

_____

7. A patient with **ITP** will likely need several **BT**s in their lifetime.

_____

8. An **Ab** is a cell that protects the body and inactivates **Ag**s, providing immunity against specific organisms.

_____

9. A **C&S** is performed to identify a pathogen and determine antibiotic treatment.

_____

Exercise 24

ADVANCED
RECALL

Match each abbreviation with the appropriate description.

PLT	SLE	Fe	RA
EPO	ESR	ANA	EBV

Description   **Abbreviation**

1. needed for oxygen transport by hemoglobin   _____

2. platelet count   _____

3. time measurement of RBCs settling in a test tube   _____

4. hormone that stimulates RBC production   _____

5. test for autoimmune diseases   _____

6. test for mononucleosis   _____

7. autoimmune connective tissue disease   _____

8. autoimmune disease causing inflammation
   in multiple joints   _____

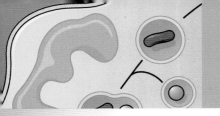
Review of Terms for Anatomy and Physiology

VISUAL

Exercise 25

Write the correct terms on the blanks for the blood cells indicated.

Granulocytes

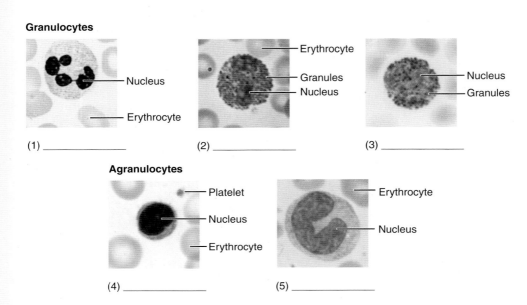

Nucleus

Erythrocyte

(1) _____

Erythrocyte

Granules

Nucleus

(2) _____

Nucleus

Granules

(3) _____

Agranulocytes

Platelet

Nucleus

Erythrocyte

(4) _____

Erythrocyte

Nucleus

(5) _____

Understanding Term Structure

TERM
CONSTRUCTION

Exercise 26

Break the given medical term into its word parts and define each part. Then define the medical term. (Note: you may need to use word parts from other chapters.)

For example:

granulocyte	*word parts:*	granul/o / -cyte
	meanings:	granules / cell
	term meaning:	cell with (visible) granules

1. hemostasis   *word parts:*   _____ / _____

               meanings: _____ / _____

               term meaning: _____

2. erythrocyte

word parts: _____ / _____

meanings: _____ / _____

term meaning: _____

3. hematopoiesis

word parts: _____ / _____

meanings: _____ / _____

term meaning: _____

4. thrombocytopenia

word parts: _____ / _____ / _____

meanings: _____ / _____ / _____

term meaning: _____

5. pathogen

word parts: _____ / _____

meanings: _____ / _____

term meaning: _____

6. cytopathic

word parts: _____ / _____ / _____

meanings: _____ / _____ / _____

term meaning: _____

7. aplastic

word parts: _____ / _____ / _____

meanings: _____ / _____ / _____

term meaning: _____

8. chromatic

word parts: _____ / _____

meanings: _____ / _____

term meaning: _____

9. anemia

word parts: _____ / _____

meanings: _____ / _____

term meaning: _____

10. hemochromatosis

word parts: _____ / _____ / _____

meanings: _____ / _____ / _____

term meaning: _____

11. hemophilia   *word parts:*   _____ / _____

                          meanings: _____ / _____

                          term meaning: _____

12. granulocyte   *word parts:*   _____ / _____

                          meanings: _____ / _____

                          term meaning: _____

13. lymphocytic   *word parts:*   _____ / _____ / _____

                          meanings: _____ / _____ / _____

                          term meaning: _____

14. hemorrhage   *word parts:*   _____ / _____

                          meanings: _____ / _____

                          term meaning: _____

15. mononucleosis   *word parts:*   _____ / _____ / _____

                          meanings: _____ / _____ / _____

                          term meaning: _____

Comprehension Exercises

COMPREHENSION

Exercise 27

Fill in the blank with the correct term.

1. Soldier-like cells that protect the body and inactivate antigens and also provide immunity against specific organisms are called _____ .

2. _____ are agents or substances that induce an immune response.

3. A(n) _____ is the administration of a weakened pathogen for future protection.

4. _____ anemia results from blood loss.

5. _____ is the medical term for low number of blood platelets.

6. _____ is an immune system response causing heat, redness, pain, and swelling.

7. ESR stands for _____ _____ _____ .

8. A differential count usually evaluates _____ blood cells.

Exercise 28

COMPREHENSION   **Write a short answer for each question.**

1. Why would immunosuppressants be given to organ transplant recipients? _____
   _____

2. List the three types of blood cells involved in pancytopenia. _____

   _____

3. What type of drug would not be given to a patient with von Willebrand disease? _____

   _____

4. What red blood cell test might indicate inflammation? _____

5. What is the difference between an antigen and an antibody? _____

   _____

6. In what process is fibrin needed? _____

7. In idiopathic thrombocytopenic purpura, which of the three types of basic formed element is

   attacking the body? _____

8. A positive mononucleosis spot test would indicate the increased presence of which type of

   blood cell? _____

9. What type of transplant might be necessary to treat aplastic anemia? _____

   _____

10. What type of blood transfusion does not require cross-matching? _____

    _____

11. How do immunosuppressant drugs aid in the treatment of rheumatoid arthritis? _____

    _____

12. What is the difference between a vaccine and a vaccination? _____

    _____

13. Why is the term "systemic" included in the term systemic lupus erythematosus? _____

    _____

14. Which blood test looks for a pathogen and possible treatment? _____

    _____

15. Where does most hematopoiesis occur? _____

    _____

Exercise 29

COMPREHENSION   **Circle the letter of the best answer in the following questions.**

1. *Plas/o* is a combining form that means:

   A. chemistry
   B. immune
   C. immature
   D. formation

2. The best definition for the word pathogen is:

   A. a treatment
   B. a lab test
   C. virulent disease
   D. disease-producing agent

3. An erythrocyte is also known as a:

   A. granule
   B. red blood cell
   C. hemoglobin cell
   D. membrane

4. Thrombocytopenia is a condition of:

   A. too many leukocytes
   B. too few leukocytes
   C. too many platelets
   D. too few platelets

5. The procedure for drawing blood from a vein is:

   A. plasmapheresis
   B. phlebotomy
   C. phagocytosis
   D. blood transfusion

6. The word *cell* can be represented by the combining form *cyt/o*, or with the word part *-cyte*, which is a:

   A. combining vowel
   B. combining form
   C. suffix
   D. prefix

7. The monocyte active in phagocytosis in tissue is called a(n):

   A. macrophage
   B. eosinophil
   C. neutrophil
   D. macrocyte

8. Hemoglobin transports oxygen in which type of blood cell?

   A. erythrocyte
   B. leukocyte
   C. thrombocyte
   D. eosinophil

9. The action of a hemostatic agent is to:

   A. prolong bleeding time
   B. prevent clotting
   C. promote clotting
   D. produce blood cells

10. Cells with granules that are stainable with a basic dye are called:

    A. basophils
    B. eosinophils
    C. thrombocytes
    D. neutrophils

11. An immunologist studies:

    A. immunity
    B. allergy
    C. induced sensitivity
    D. all of the above

12. EPO is an abbreviation for a protein that stimulates production of:

    A. thrombocytes
    B. lymphocytes
    C. leukocytes
    D. erythrocytes

Application and Analysis

CASE REPORTS

Exercise 30

APPLICATION   **Read the case reports and circle the letter of your answer choice for the following questions about each case.**

CASE 8-1

Mrs. Ryan is 46 years old and perimenopausal. Dr. Milban, her gynecologist, ordered a CBC after she complained about excessive fatigue for the past 3 months. The results showed a low RBC count of 3.67 [normal 4.00–5.00] and a low Hgb of 10.2 [normal 12.0–16.0]. Mrs. Ryan explained she was currently having more frequent and heavier menstrual periods than normal. Dr. Milban suspected Mrs. Ryan was anemic due to blood loss. He instructed her to take an iron supplement and see her internist for a complete workup.

1. What is the medical term for anemia due to blood loss?

   A. hemolytic anemia
   B. hemorrhagic anemia
   C. hemoglobinuria
   D. hemoglobinemia

2. Which of the following statements does *not* apply to erythrocytes?

   A. they transport oxygen
   B. they transport carbon dioxide
   C. they are disc-shaped with a depression on both sides
   D. their main purpose is immunity

3. Which of the following is *not* an indication of anemia?

   A. low RBC
   B. low Hgb

   C. low clotting factor
   D. low volume of packed cells

4. Which of the following test would not be performed as part of a CBC lab test?

   A. EBV
   B. HGB
   C. ESR
   D. WBC

5. Which of the following is not an abbreviation for hemoglobin?

   A. HGB
   B. Hb
   C. Hgb
   D. Hg

CASE 8-2

Mr. Morozoff has a bleeding disorder that has affected his life since birth. His blood does not clot properly due to a deficiency in clotting factors (Fig. 8-20). The disease is genetically inherited and primarily affects males. As a child, he had to be careful to avoid injuries because even a small bruise could escalate into a life-threatening situation. He has regular lab tests to monitor his blood clotting time.

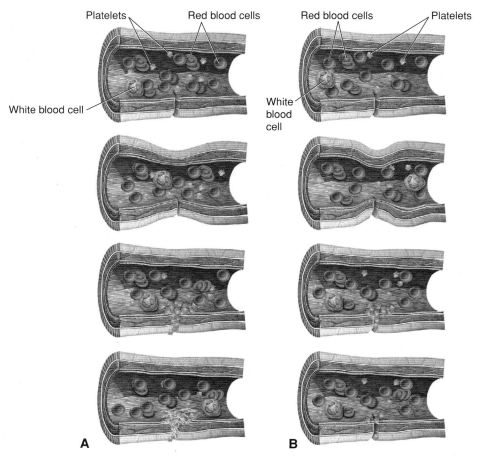

Platelets   Red blood cells   Red blood cells   Platelets

White blood cell   White blood cell

A   **B**

Figure 8-20   A. Normal clotting. **B.** Improper clotting due to deficiency in clotting factors.

6. Based on the information in Case 8-2, what disease do you think Mr. Morozoff has?

   A. hemophilia
   B. hepatitis
   C. hemochromatosis
   D. septicemia

7. What is the medical term for clotting?

   A. coagulopathy
   B. hemostasis
   C. coagulation
   D. fibrinogen

8. What lab test would be used to diagnose a clotting disorder?

   A. C&S
   B. PT
   C. ANA
   D. HCT

9. Which drug used to stop the flow of blood within vessels may be prescribed for Mr. Morozoff's condition?

   A. thrombolytic agent
   B. vaccine
   C. hemostatic agent
   D. anticoagulant

10. Which procedure may be performed to transfer blood from a donor to a recipient in a life-threatening situation?

   A. bone marrow transplant
   B. blood transfusion
   C. immunosuppression
   D. splenectomy

MEDICAL RECORD ANALYSIS

MEDICAL RECORD 8-1

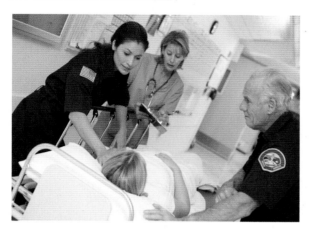

Emergency medical technicians are trained and certified to provide emergency medical services to the ill and injured.

Ms. Stinson sustained a snake bite while hiking in the desert. You are an emergency medical technician who transported her to the hospital and provided care en route. The documentation of her care at the hospital follows.

Medical Record

DISCHARGE SUMMARY

Patient: Carly Stinson   Age: 24 y.o. female   Date: August 24, 20–

FINAL DIAGNOSES:
1. Snake bite
2. Hemolysis
3. Thrombocytopenia
4. Nausea
5. Epistaxis
6. Hematuria
7. Tachycardia
8. Neurotoxicity
9. Hypotension

HOSPITAL COURSE: Patient reported to the emergency room within 3 hours of a presumed rattlesnake bite. She had been hiking in the desert when she was struck on the back of her right lower leg. She saw a large snake, over 6 feet long, with a diamond patterned skin. Her past medical history is unremarkable for chronic illnesses. No known allergies (NKA). Medications are limited to birth control pills. She complained of anxiety, nausea, and tingling of her right lower extremity.

There were two visible entry wounds, with marked edema, ecchymosis, petechiae, and some early blisters. She complained of significant pain in the bite region. Her vital signs were consistent for hypotension at 98/60 and with a tachycardic pulse at 136 BPM. Hemolytic effects from the snakebite venom started with epistaxis and slight hematuria.

TREATMENT:	Administration of 20 vials of antivenin
	Tetanus prophylaxis
	Prophylactic antibiotic ordered because a snake's dirty mouth can cause a bacterial infection
	Admitted to Intensive Care Unit
	Cardiac monitoring with IV
	Coagulation profile ordered q4–12h prn to monitor signs of hemolytic anemia, thrombocytopenia, or fibrinolysis

DISCHARGE INSTRUCTIONS: Patient was discharged after 2 days with symptoms subsiding. Will recheck patient at 1 week and 4 weeks postinjury.

DISCHARGE MEDICATIONS: Patient to complete the 10-day course of antibiotics.

APPLICATION

Exercise 31

Write the appropriate medical terms used in this medical record on the blanks after their meanings. Note that not all the terms appear in the chapter, but you should be able to identify these terms based on word parts that are included in this chapter.

1. pertaining to the rupture or destruction of (red) blood (cells) _____

2. disorder involving low levels of platelets in blood _____

3. abbreviation for no known allergies _____

4. the abbreviation prn means: _____

Bonus Question

5. Break the medical term **<u>antibiotic</u>** into its word parts and define each part. Then define the medical term. (Hint: Refer to *Appendix A: Glossary of Combining Forms, Prefixes, and Suffixes* to recall the meaning of word parts learned earlier in the text.)

   word parts: _____ / _____ / _____

   meanings: _____ / _____ / _____

   term meaning: _____

MEDICAL RECORD 8-2

Following is a clinic note in SOAP (subjective, objective, assessment, plan) format for a 42-year-old patient who was seen 4 weeks ago in an initial consultation by a rheumatologist. As an occupational therapist, you are reviewing her record before meeting with her to identify ways in which she can successfully perform her activities of daily living (ADLs) while managing her disease.

Medical Record

SOAP FOLLOW-UP FOR AUTOIMMUNE DISEASE

S: 42-year-old Debra Conner returns to the clinic for a 1-month follow-up visit. She is married with two children and has a full-time career as a college instructor. She continues to complain of musculoskeletal aches, fatigue, and insomnia, which she admits has contributed to her stress level. She sometimes has trouble with activities of daily living because of her pain. She has had one episode of a urinary tract infection that was treated with a 10-day course of penicillin. She also takes an over-the-counter antiinflammatory drug to reduce her symptoms of muscle aches, which does provide some relief. She denies depressive episodes at this time.

O: Wt: 147   BP: 122/86   HR: 74   T: 98.8   R: 18
Laboratory Results: Positive ANA, ELISA method. Elevated rheumatoid factor, ESR, and complement levels. Negative EBV. CBC: WNL. Chemistry Profile: WNL

A: With the correlation of symptoms and laboratory data, my impressions are as follows:
1. Fibromyalgia
2. Sleep disorder
3. Fatigue
4. Systemic lupus erythematosus

P: Plan to decrease the inflammatory process with the following medications:
prednisone 10 mg daily
mycophenolate mofetil 500 mg b.i.d.

Patient may continue to take over-the-counter ibuprofen, on a prn basis, but not to exceed 1,600 mg/day. Patient instructed on stress reduction and was given written information on living with an autoimmune disease. Have ordered consultation with occupational therapy. Recommended she attend a SLE support group meeting.

Return to clinic in 3 months.

T. Gentry, M.D.
Rheumatology Associates

Exercise 32

APPLICATION   **Read the medical report and circle the letter of your answer choice for the following questions. Note: Although some of the medical terms in these questions do not appear in this chapter, you should understand them from their word parts.**

1. What is the name of Mrs. Conner's autoimmune disease?

   A. fibromyalgia
   B. systemic lupus erythematosus
   C. rheumatoid arthritis
   D. fatigue

2. What does the abbreviation ANA stand for?

   A. antinuclear antigen
   B. antiinflammatory antigen
   C. antinuclear antibody
   D. autonomic nervous system

3. This patient is taking over-the-counter ibuprofen for:

   A. chemotherapy
   B. immunosuppression
   C. NSAID
   D. inflammation

4. An elevated ESR level may indicate:

    A. inflammation
    B. infection
    C. immune disease
    D. clotting disorder

5. What type of medical specialist should Mrs. Conner continue to see to monitor this disease on a regular basis?

    A. rheumatologist
    B. microbiologist
    C. internist
    D. allergologist

Exercise 33

APPLICATION

Write out the complete medical terms from the abbreviations or acronyms used in the medical record above.

1. SLE   _____

2. ESR   _____

3. WBC   _____

4. EBV test   _____

5. ANA test   _____

Bonus Question

6. SLE is an organ-threatening disease in which the kidneys can be a target, resulting in lupus nephritis. Therefore, many physicians will order routine urinalyses for SLE patients. Blood in the urine is an abnormal condition that needs immediate attention. Write in the correct medical term for this condition: _____

Pronunciation and Spelling

Exercise 34

AUDITORY

Review the Chapter 8 terms in the Dictionary/Audio Glossary in the Student Resources and practice pronouncing each term, referring to the pronunciation guide as needed.

Exercise 35

SPELLING

Circle the correct spelling of each term.

1. erythocyte   erythrecyte   erythrocyte

2. granulocyte   granularcyte   granulacyte

3. luekocyte   leukocyte   leukocite

4. neutrophil   nuetrophil   nuetrophyl

5. eaosinphil	eaosinphil	eosinophil
6. agranulicyte	agranulocyte	agranulcyte
7. erhythropoietin	erythropoietin	erythropoetin
8. phagocitosis	phagocytosus	phagocytosis
9. hemoglobin	hemeglobin	hemoglobulin
10. hemorrhagic	hemorhagic	hemmorrhagic
11. virulent	virolent	virulant
12. proliferation	proliforation	preliferation
13. imunosuppressant	immunosuppressant	immunesupressant
14. thallessemia	thalassemia	thalissemia
15. trombocytopinia	thrombocytopenia	thombocytopenia

Media Connection

STUDENT
RESOURCES

Exercise 36

Complete each of the following activities available with the Student Resources. Check off each activity as you complete it.

Chapter Exercises

____ Flash Cards   ____ True/False Body Building

____ Concentration   ____ Quiz Show

____ Abbreviation Match-Up   ____ Complete the Case

____ Roboterms   ____ Medical Record Review

____ Word Builder   ____ Look and Label

____ Fill the Gap   ____ Image Matching

____ Break It Down   ____ Spelling Bee

____ **Chapter Quiz**   *Score:* _____%

Additional Resources

____ Animation: Wound Healing

____ Video: Venipuncture

____ Dictionary/Audio Glossary

____ Health Professions Careers: Emergency Medicine Technician

____ Health Professions Careers: Occupational Therapist

Respiratory System 9

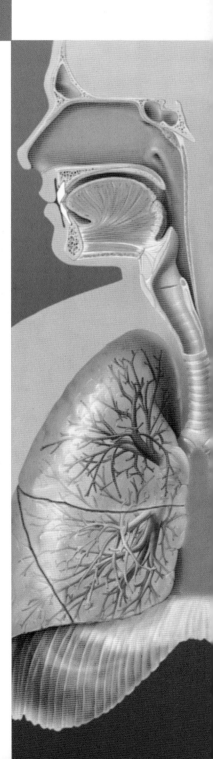

Chapter Outline

Objectives

After completion of this chapter you will be able to:

1. Describe the location of the structures of the respiratory system.

2. Define terms related to the upper and lower respiratory tracts and to respiration.

3. Define combining forms, prefixes, and suffixes related to the respiratory system.

4. Define common medical terminology related to the respiratory system, including adjectives and related terms, symptoms and conditions, tests and procedures, surgical interventions and therapeutic procedures, medications and drug therapies, and specialties.

5. Explain abbreviations for terms related to the respiratory system.

6. Successfully complete all chapter exercises.

7. Explain terms used in case studies and medical records involving the respiratory system.

8. Successfully complete all pronunciation and spelling exercises, and complete all interactive exercises included with the companion Student Resources.

■ ANATOMY AND PHYSIOLOGY

Functions

- ■ To supply oxygen to body cells and tissues
- ■ To eliminate carbon dioxide from the body
- ■ To provide airflow between the upper and lower respiratory tracts through the larynx and vocal cords, making human vocal sounds possible

Organs and Structures

- ■ The respiratory system consists of an upper respiratory tract and a lower respiratory tract.
- ■ The upper and lower respiratory tracts work together to supply oxygen to the lungs and to eliminate carbon dioxide from the lungs (Fig. 9-1).

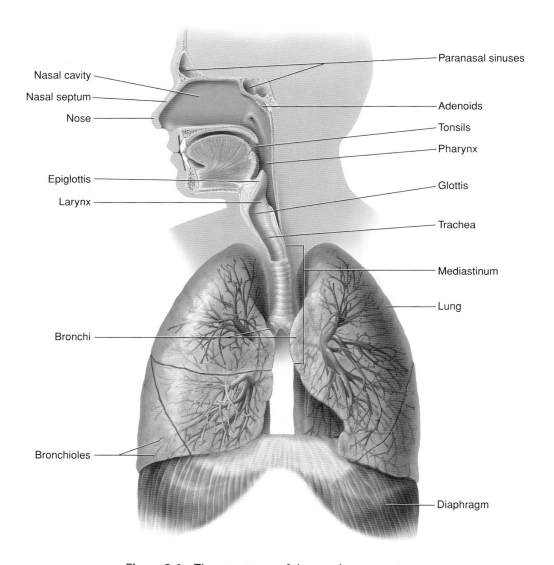

Figure 9-1 The structures of the respiratory system.

Terms Related to the Respiratory System

Term	Pronunciation	Meaning
The Upper Respiratory Tract (Fig. 9-2)		
nose	nōz	anatomic structure positioned above the hard palette that provides an air passageway, which acts as a filter to moisten and warm inhaled air
cilia	sil'ē-ă	fine hairlike projections on the mucous membranes inside the nose
nasal septum	nā'zăl sep'tŭm	dividing wall between the right and left nasal cavities
paranasal sinuses	par'ă-nā'zăl sīnŭ-ez'	paired air-filled cavities in the bones of the face that are connected to the nasal cavity
pharynx, *syn.* throat	far'ingks, thrōt	space behind the mouth that serves as a passage for food from the mouth to the esophagus and for air from the nose and mouth to the larynx
adenoids	ad'ĕ-noydz	two lymphatic structures located on the posterior wall of the nasopharynx that enlarge during childhood and shrink during puberty
tonsils, *syn.* palatine tonsils	ton'silz, pal'ă-tīn ton'şilz	two structures of lymphoid tissue located on either side of the throat
The Lower Respiratory Tract (Fig. 9-3)		
larynx	lar'ingks	air passageway located between the pharynx and the trachea that holds the vocal cords
epiglottis	ep'i-glot'is	flap of cartilage that covers the upper region of the larynx during swallowing to prevent food or other matter from entering the lungs
glottis, *syn.* vocal cords	glot'is, vō'kăl kōrdz	vocal structure of the larynx

(continued)

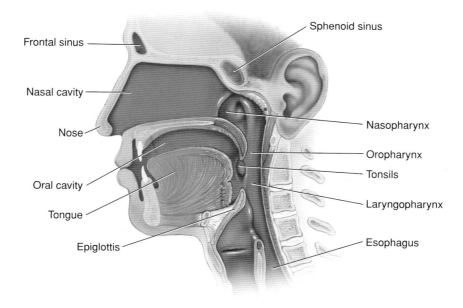

Figure 9-2   The structures of the upper respiratory tract.

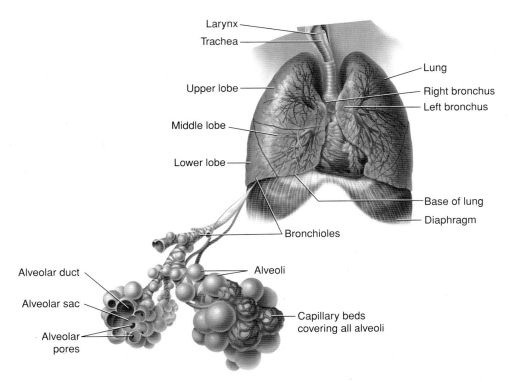

Figure 9-3   The structures of the lower respiratory tract.

Terms Related to the Respiratory System *(continued)*

Term	Pronunciation	Meaning
trachea, *syn.* windpipe	tră′kē-ă, wind′pīp	air passage extending from the larynx into the thorax
bronchi	brong′kī	the two subdivisions of the trachea serving to convey air to and from the lungs
carina, *syn.* tracheal bifurcation	kă-rī′nă, trā′kē-ăl bĭ′fŭr-kă′shŭn	cartilaginous ridge that divides into, and is continuous with, the two main or principal bronchi
alveoli	al-vē′ō-lī	saclike cavities located off the bronchioles where gas is exchanged between the lungs and blood
bronchioles	brong′kē-ōlz	finer subdivisions of the bronchi located in the lungs
lungs	lŭngz	pair of spongy organs of respiration in which blood is aerated
lobes	lōbz	subdivisions of the lungs: three on the right (upper, middle and lower) and two on the left (upper and lower)
pleura	plūr′ă	membrane surrounding the lungs and lining the walls of the pleural cavities
parietal layer	pă-rī′ĕ-tăl lā′ĕr	outer layer of the pleura that attaches to the chest wall

(continued)

ANIMATION

Learn more about the structures and functions of the respiratory system by viewing the animation *The Respiratory System* included with the Student Resources.

Terms Related to the Respiratory System *(continued)*

Term	Pronunciation	Meaning
pleural cavity	plūr'ăl kav'i-tē	space between the layers of the pleura
visceral layer	vis'ĕr-ăl lā'ĕr	inner layer of the pleura that attaches to the lungs
thorax, *syn.* chest	thō'raks, chest	anatomic region formed by the sternum, the thoracic vertebrae, and the ribs, extending from the neck to the diaphragm
diaphragm	dī'ă-fram	muscular partition between the abdominal and thoracic cavities; the contraction and relaxation of the diaphragm causes inspiration and expiration

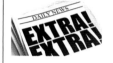 **THE DIAPHRAGM** The diaphragm assists in breathing. When air is taken into the lungs (inspiration), the diaphragm contracts, or is pushed down. As the muscle relaxes, it forces air back out of the lungs (expiration). People who experience a "stitch" while exercising are actually experiencing a spasm of the diaphragm. Physicians agree that the way to prevent a stitch is to breathe deeply when exercising. This puts less stress on the diaphragm.

mediastinum	me'dē-as-tī'nŭm	area of the thoracic cavity between the lungs that contains the heart, aorta, esophagus, trachea, and thymus

Respiration		
airway	ār'wā	any part of the respiratory tract through which air passes during breathing
eupnea	yūp-nē'ă	normal breathing
expiration, *syn.* exhalation	eks'pi-rā'shŭn, eks'hă-lā'shŭn	the process of breathing out (Fig. 9-4)
external respiration, *syn.* breathing	eks-tĕr'năl res'pi-rā'shŭn, brēdh'ing	the process of inspiration and expiration
inspiration, *syn.* inhalation	in-spi-rā'shŭn, in'hă-lā'shŭn	the process of breathing in (Fig. 9-4)
internal respiration	in-ter'năl res'pi-rā'shŭn	the exchange of gases between the blood in the capillaries and the cells of the body
patent	pā'tĕnt	open or exposed (as in the airway)
respiration	res'pi-rā'shŭn	the process involving the exchange of oxygen and carbon dioxide between the environment and body cells

(continued)

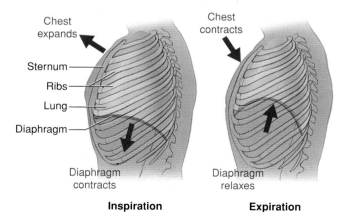

Figure 9-4   The external process of breathing.

Terms Related to the Respiratory System *(continued)*

Term	Pronunciation	Meaning
sputum	spyū'tŭm	expectorated matter, especially mucus or mucopurulent matter expectorated in diseases of the air passages
ventilation	ven-ti-lā'shŭn	the distribution of gas into and out of the lungs

ANIMATION

To see a visual representation of the ventilation process, view the animation *Pulmonary Ventilation* in the electronic Student Resources.

■ Exercises: Anatomy and Physiology

SIMPLE
RECALL

Exercise 1

Write the correct anatomic term for the definition given.

1. subdivisions of the left and right lungs _____

2. the process of breathing out _____

3. prevents food or other materials from entering the lungs during swallowing _____

4. normal breathing _____

5. air passageway located between the pharynx and the trachea _____

6. space behind the mouth where food and air pass _____

7. process of breathing in _____

8. muscular partition between the thoracic and abdominal cavities _____

9. structure above the hard palette that filters air _____

10. process of breathing in and out _____

11. dividing wall between the nasal cavities _____

12. the two subdivisions of the trachea _____

13. space where gas is exchanged between the lungs and blood _____

14. inner layer of pleura that attaches to the lungs _____

15. expectorated matter _____

SIMPLE
RECALL

Exercise 2

Circle the term that is most appropriate for the meaning of the sentence.

1. The major structures of the upper respiratory system are the (*nose and pharynx, pharynx and lungs, larynx and diaphragm*).

2. The (*paranasal sinuses, cilia*) are fine hairlike projections on the mucous membranes inside the (*cilia, nose*).

3. When the (*sputum, airway, ventilation*) is blocked, air cannot pass through the respiratory tract.

4. Human speech is made possible when air enters the (*pharynx, larynx, pleura*).

5. The (*laryngopharynx, epiglottis, palate*) prevents food from entering the lower respiratory tract.

6. The (*bronchus, trachea, pharynx*) is the air passage extending from the larynx into the thorax.

7. The bronchi further divide into finer subdivisions in the lungs called (*bronchioles, alveoli, cilia*).

8. The (*mediastinum, diaphragm, thorax*) separates the thoracic cavity from the abdominal cavity.

9. The air-filled cavities in the bones of the face are called (*alveoli, adenoids, paranasal sinuses*).

10. The (*carina, alveoli, diaphragm*) divides into and is continuous with the bronchi.

11. The outer layer of the pleura that attaches to the chest wall is called the (*visceral layer, pleural cavity, parietal layer*).

12. The (*mediastinum, pleural cavity, thorax*) is the space between the layers of the pleura.

13. The process involving the exchange of oxygen and carbon dioxide between the environment and body cells is called (*ventilation, expiration, respiration*).

ADVANCED
RECALL

Exercise 3

Match each medical term with its meaning.

| glottis | patent | pleura | mediastinum |
| lungs | thorax | adenoids | internal respiration |

Meaning   **Term**

1. the exchange of gases between the blood in the capillaries   _____
   and the cells of the body

2. structure also known as the vocal cords   _____

3. lymphatic structures located on the wall of the nasopharynx   _____

4. part of the thoracic cavity between the lungs   _____

5. structure consisting of spongy organs of respiration in which   _____
   blood is aerated

6. the membrane surrounding the lungs _____

7. open or exposed (as in the airway) _____

8. region of the body formed by the sternum, thoracic vertebrae, and ribs _____

■ WORDS PARTS

Note that some word parts that have been introduced earlier in the book may not be repeated here.

Combining Forms

Combining Form	Meaning
adenoid/o	adenoids
alveol/o	alveolus
aspir/o	to breathe in or suck in
atel/o	incomplete
ausculat/o	listening
bronchi/o, bronch/o	bronchus
capn/o, capn/i	carbon dioxide
cost/o	rib
diaphragmat/o, phren/o	diaphragm
epiglott/o	epiglottis
laryng/o	larynx
lob/o	lobe
mediastin/o	mediastinum
muc/o	mucus
nas/o, rhin/o	nose
ox/o, ox/a	oxygen
pector/o	chest
pharyng/o	pharynx
phon/o	sound, voice
pleur/o	pleura
pneum/o, pneumat/o, pneumon/o	lung, air
pulmon/o	lung
sept/o	septum
sinus/o	sinus
spir/o	breathe
thorac/o	thorax, chest
tonsill/o	tonsil
trache/o	trachea

Prefixes

Prefix	Meaning
a-, an-	without, not
dys-	painful, difficult, abnormal
em-	in
eu-	good, normal
hypo-	below, deficient
in-	not
pan-	all, entire
per-	through
tachy-	rapid, fast

Suffixes

Suffix	Meaning
-algia	pain
-al, -ar, -ary, -ic	pertaining to
-cele	herniation, protrusion
-centesis	puncture to aspirate
-ectasis	dilation, stretching
-ectomy	excision, surgical removal
-emia	blood (condition of)
-graphy	process of recording
-itis	inflammation
-metry	measurement of
-phonia	condition of the voice
-plasty	surgical repair, reconstruction
-plegia	paralysis
-pnea	breathing
-rrhagia	flowing forth
-rrhea	flow, discharge
-scopy	process of examining, examination
-spasm	involuntary movement
-stomy	surgical opening
-tomy	incision

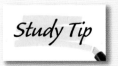

Study Tip

tonsil and tonsill/o: The word tonsil just has one "l" but the combining form for tonsil contains two "ls". Any word built from this combining form will have two "ls."

■ Exercises: Word Parts

Exercise 4

Write the meaning of the combining form given.

1. capn/o _____

2. trache/o _____

3. epiglott/o _____

4. thorac/o _____

5. aspir/o _____

6. sept/o _____

7. pleur/o _____

8. mediastin/o _____

9. bronchi/o _____

10. muc/o _____

11. tonsill/o _____

12. ausculat/o _____

13. pneumat/o _____

14. pulmon/o _____

15. atel/o _____

Exercise 5

Write the correct combining form(s) for the meaning given.

1. chest _____

2. tonsils _____

3. sound, voice _____

4. thorax, chest _____

5. pharynx _____

6. larynx _____

7. pleura _____

8. breathe _____

9. lobe _____

10. bronchus _____

11. sinus _____

12. nose _____

13. diaphragm _____

14. oxygen _____

15. carbon dioxide _____

SIMPLE
RECALL

Exercise 6

Write the meaning of the suffix or prefix given.

1. per- _____

2. hypo- _____

3. em- _____

4. -pnea _____

5. tachy- _____

6. -rrhagia _____

7. pan- _____

8. -spasm _____

9. -plegia _____

10. -cele _____

11. -ectomy _____

12. -emia _____

13. -scopy _____

14. a-, an- _____

15. -graphy _____

Exercise 7

SIMPLE RECALL

Write the correct suffix or prefix for the meaning given.

1. measurement of _____

2. pertaining to _____

3. flow, discharge _____

4. condition of the voice _____

5. blood (condition of) _____

6. puncture to aspirate _____

7. dilation, stretching _____

8. painful, difficult, abnormal _____

9. surgical opening _____

10. through _____

11. good, normal _____

12. surgical repair _____

13. inflammation _____

14. protrusion _____

15. incision _____

Exercise 8

ADVANCED RECALL

Considering the meaning of the combining form from which the medical term is made, write the meaning of the medical term. (You have not yet learned many of these terms but can build their meaning from the word parts.)

Combining Form	Meaning	Medical Term	Meaning of Term
adenoid/o	adenoids	adenoidectomy	1. _____
alveol/o	alveolus	alveolitis	2. _____
bronch/o	bronchus	bronchoscope	3. _____
diaphragmat/o	diaphragm	diaphragmatocele	4. _____
epiglott/o	epiglottis	epiglottitis	5. _____
laryng/o	larynx	laryngoscope	6. _____

lob/o	lobe	lobar	7. _____
nas/o	nose	nasal	8. _____
pharyng/o	pharynx	pharyngospasm	9. _____
pleur/o	pleura	pleuritis	10. _____

TERM
CONSTRUCTION

Exercise 9

Using the given combining form and a word part learned previously, build a medical term for the meaning given.

Combining Form	Meaning of Medical Term	Medical Term
pneum/o	inflammation of the lung	1. _____
sept/o	surgical repair of the septum	2. _____
trache/o	incision of the trachea	3. _____
thorac/o	surgical opening into the chest	4. _____
tonsill/o	inflammation of the tonsils	5. _____
sinus/o	inflammation of sinus	6. _____
laryng/o	inflammation of larynx	7. _____
lob/o	pertaining to the lobes (of the lungs)	8. _____
alveol/o	pertaining to the alveolus	9. _____
pharyng/o	inflammation of pharynx	10. _____

■ MEDICAL TERMS

Adjectives and Other Related Terms

Term	Pronunciation	Meaning
alveolar	al-vē′ŏ-lăr	pertaining to the alveoli
anoxic	an-ok′sik	pertaining to the absence of oxygen
apneic	ap′nē-ik	pertaining to or suffering from apnea
bronchial	brong′kē-ăl	pertaining to the bronchus
diaphragmatic	dī′ă-frag-mat′ik	pertaining to the diaphragm
endotracheal	en′dō-trā′kē-ăl	pertaining to within the trachea

(continued)

Adjectives and Other Related Terms *(continued)*

Term	Pronunciation	Meaning
hypoxic	hī-pok'sik	pertaining to a low level of oxygen
intercostal	in'tĕr-kos'tăl	pertaining to the area between the ribs
laryngeal	lă-rin'jē-ăl	pertaining to the larynx
lobar	lō'bahr	pertaining to any lobe of the lungs
mediastinal	mē'dē-as-tī'năl	pertaining to the mediastinum
mucous	myū'kŭs	pertaining to mucus or a mucous membrane
nasal	nā'zăl	pertaining to the nose
pectoral	pek'tō-răl	pertaining to the chest
pharyngeal	făr-in'jē-ăl	pertaining to the pharynx
phrenic	fren'ik	pertaining to the diaphragm
pleural	plūr'ăl	pertaining to the pleura
pleuritic	plū-rit'ik	pertaining to pleurisy
pulmonary	pul'mŏ-nār-ē	pertaining to the lungs
respiratory	res'pi-ră-tōr'ē	pertaining to respiration
thoracic	thō-ras'ik	pertaining to the thorax (chest)
tonsillar	ton-sil'lăr	pertaining to the tonsil
tracheal	trā'kē-ăl	pertaining to the trachea

■ Exercises: Adjectives and Other Related Terms

Exercise 10

SIMPLE
RECALL

Write the meaning of the term given.

1. apneic   _____

2. tracheal   _____

3. phrenic   _____

4. hypoxic   _____

5. pleuritic   _____

6. respiratory   _____

7. tonsillar   _____

8. endotracheal   _____

9. mediastinal _____

10. mucous _____

ADVANCED
RECALL

Exercise 11

Match each medical term with its meaning.

alveolar	thoracic	pharyngeal	bronchial	intercostal
diaphragmatic	anoxic	pleural	pectoral	lobar

Meaning   **Term**

1. pertaining to the thorax   _____

2. pertaining to the bronchus   _____

3. pertaining to the pleura   _____

4. pertaining to the alveoli   _____

5. pertaining to the diaphragm   _____

6. pertaining to any lobe   _____

7. pertaining to the absence of oxygen _____

8. pertaining to the pharynx   _____

9. pertaining to the area between the ribs _____

10. pertaining to the chest   _____

ADVANCED
RECALL

Exercise 12

Circle the term that is most appropriate for the meaning of the sentence.

1. Mr. Mullins was treated in the emergency department for a (*pleuritic, pulmonary*) infection within the lower right (*lobar, thoracic*) portion of his lung.

2. Ms. Lane was diagnosed with a fractured rib based on her report of pain and the results of the x-ray of the (*thoracic, pharyngeal, nasal*) cavity.

3. When the physician asked Gabriel where he felt pain, the child pointed at his throat. The physician noted that the reported pain was in the (*pharyngeal, laryngeal, pectoral*) area.

4. Mr. Bolling's left lung biopsy involved surgery within the (*laryngeal, tracheal, mediastinal*) cavity.

5. Diagnosing Ms. Hatfield's respiratory condition required an examination of each of the (*lobar, thoracic, pleural*) areas within the lung.

Exercise 13

TERM CONSTRUCTION

Write the combining form used in the medical term, followed by the meaning of the combining form.

Term	Combining Form	Meaning of Combining Form
1. lobar	_____	_____
2. phrenic	_____	_____
3. pleural	_____	_____
4. nasal	_____	_____
5. pulmonary	_____	_____

Symptoms and Medical Conditions

Term	Pronunciation	Meaning
acute respiratory distress syndrome (ARDS)	ă-kyūt' res'pi-ră-tōr'ē dis-tres' sin'drōm	respiratory failure that can occur with underlying illnesses or injury
aphonia	ă-fō'nē-ă	loss of the voice as a result of disease or injury to the larynx
apnea	ap'nē-ă	absence of breathing
asthma	az'mă	chronic severe breathing disorder characterized by attacks of wheezing due to inflammation and narrowing of the airways (Fig. 9-5)
atelectasis	at-ĕ-lek'tă-sis	decrease or loss of air in the lung, causing loss of lung volume and possible lung collapse

(continued)

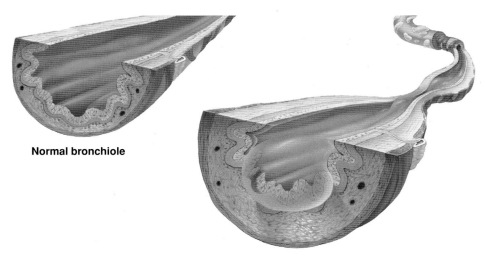

Normal bronchiole

Asthmatic bronchiole

Figure 9-5 Asthma as characterized by obstructed airway.

Symptoms and Medical Conditions *(continued)*

Term	Pronunciation	Meaning
bronchiectasis	brong′kē-ek′tă-sis	an irreversible widening of portions of the bronchi resulting from damage to the airway wall
bronchitis	brong-kī′tis	inflammation of the bronchi
bronchiolitis obliterans with organizing pneumonia (BOOP)	brong′kē-ō-lī′tis ob-lit′ĕr-ă′nz with ŏr′gă-ni-zing nū-mō′nē-ă	obstructive lung condition characterized by granulation tissue plugs in the bronchioles that extend into the alveoli
chronic obstructive pulmonary disease (COPD)	kron′ik ob-strŭk′tiv pul′mō-nār′ē di-zēz′	general term used for those disorders with permanent or temporary narrowing of small bronchi, in which forced expiratory flow is slowed
Cheyne-Stokes respiration	chān-stōks res′pi-rā′shŭn	respiratory pattern that involves alternating periods of apnea and deep, rapid breathing
croup	krūp	acute obstruction of the upper airway in infants and children characterized by a barking cough with difficult and noisy respiration
diaphragmatocele	dī′ă-frag-mat′ō-sēl	hernia of the diaphragm
dysphonia	dis-fō′nē-ă	vocal difficulty
dyspnea	disp-nē′ă	difficulty breathing
emphysema	em′fi-sē′mă	lung condition that involves the permanent destruction of very fine airways and alveoli, thus decreasing respiratory function (Fig. 9-6)
empyema	em′pī-ē′mă	localized collection of pus in the thoracic cavity resulting from an infection in the lungs

(continued)

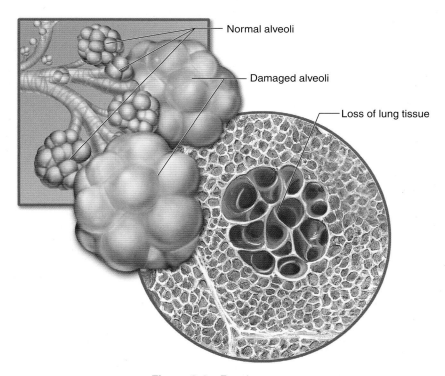

Figure 9-6   Emphysema.

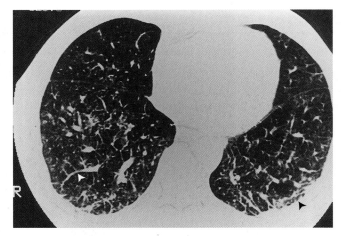

Figure 9-7 Cross-section computed tomography of the chest revealing markings in the lungs consistent with interstitial lung disease (*arrows*).

Symptoms and Medical Conditions *(continued)*

Term	Pronunciation	Meaning
epistaxis	ep'i-stak'sis	bleeding from the nose
hemothorax	hē'mō-thōr'aks	blood located in the pleural cavity
hypoxemia	hī'pok-sē'mē-ă	decreased level of oxygen in the blood
hypoxia	hī-pok'sē-ă	decreased levels of oxygen in the tissues
influenza, *syn.* flu	in-flū-en'ză, flū	an acute contagious respiratory illness caused by influenza viruses
interstitial lung disease (ILD), *syn.* pulmonary fibrosis	in'tĕr-stish'ăl lŭng di-zēz, pul'mŏ-nār-ē fī-brō'sis	a group of chronic lung disorders affecting the tissue between the air sacs of the lungs causing irreversible inflammation and fibrosis, or scarring (Fig. 9-7)
laryngitis	lar'in-jī'tis	inflammation of the larynx
laryngospasm	lă-ring'gō-spazm	involuntary movement of the larynx
nasopharyngitis	nā-so-fă-rin-jī'tis	inflammation of the nasal cavity and pharynx
orthopnea	ōr'thop-nē'ă	discomfort in breathing that is brought on or aggravated by lying flat
pansinusitis	pan-sī-nŭ-sī'tis	inflammation of all sinuses
pertussis, *syn.* whooping cough	per-tŭs'is, hūp'ing kawf	an acute infectious inflammation of the larynx, trachea, and bronchi caused by the bacterium *Bordetella pertussis*
pharyngitis	fă-rin-jī'tis	inflammation of the pharynx
pleural effusion	plūr'ăl e-fyū'zhŭn	collection of fluid or blood in the pleural space around the lung
pleuritis	plū-rī'tis	inflammation of the pleura
pneumonia	nū-mō'nē-ă	bacterial infection and inflammation within the lobes of the lungs (Fig. 9-8)
bacterial pneumonia	bak-tēr'ē-ăl nū-mō'nē-ă	pneumonia caused by a bacterial infection
bronchopneumonia	brong'ko-nū-mō'nē-ă	infection of the smaller bronchial tubes of the lungs

(continued)

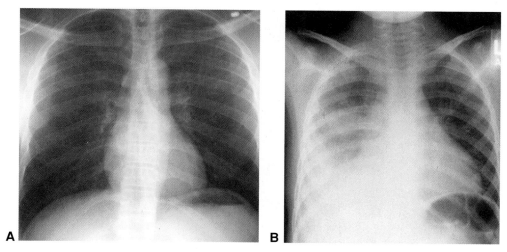

Figure 9-8 **A.** Radiograph of a normal lung. **B.** Radiograph of the lungs of a child with bacterial pneumonia. The white area of the right lung signifies pneumonia.

Symptoms and Medical Conditions *(continued)*

Term	Pronunciation	Meaning
lobar pneumonia	lō'bar nū-mō'nē-ă	infection of the alveoli caused by fluid and pus filling an entire lobe of the lung
pneumococcal pneumonia	nū'mō-kok'ăl nū-mō'nē-ă	form of pneumonia caused by the bacterial species *Streptococcus pneumoniae*
pneumonitis	nū'mō-nī'tis	inflammation of the lungs
pneumothorax	nū'mō-thōr'aks	the presence of air or gas in the pleural cavity (Fig. 9-9)
pulmonary edema	pul'mō-nār'ē e-dē'mă	buildup of fluid in the lungs
pulmonary embolism	pul'mō-nār'ē em'bō-lizm	obstruction of the pulmonary circulation by a blood clot (Fig. 9-10)
rales, *syn.* crackles	rahlz, krak'ĕlz	crackling or bubbling lung noises heard on inspiration that indicate fluid in the alveoli or fibrosis
reactive airway disease (RAD)	rē-ak'ti-v ār'wā di-zēz'	respiratory condition characterized by wheezing, shortness of breath, and coughing after exposure to an irritant

(continued)

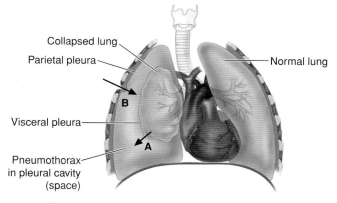

Collapsed lung
Parietal pleura
Normal lung
B
Visceral pleura
Pneumothorax in pleural cavity (space)
A

Figure 9-9 Pneumothorax can be caused by lung disease **(A)** or a perforation in the chest wall **(B)**.

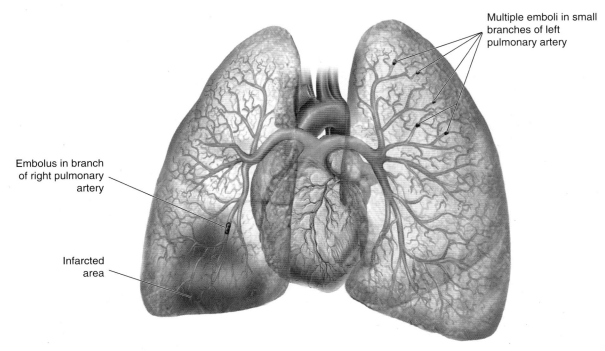

Multiple emboli in small
branches of left
pulmonary artery

Embolus in branch
of right pulmonary
artery

Infarcted
area

Figure 9-10   Pulmonary embolism.

Symptoms and Medical Conditions *(continued)*

Term	Pronunciation	Meaning
respiratory failure (RF)	res'pi-ră-tōr'ē făl'yūr	condition in which the level of oxygen in the blood becomes dangerously low and/or the level of carbon dioxide becomes dangerously high
rhinitis	rī-nī'tis	inflammation of the mucous membranes within the nasal cavity
rhonchi	rong'kī	abnormal whistling, humming, or snoring sounds heard during inspiration or expiration
rubs	rŭbz	friction sounds in the lungs caused by inflammation of the pleura
sinusitis	sī'nŭ-sī'tis	inflammation of the sinus
stridor	strī'dōr	a whistling sound heard on inspiration that indicates partial obstruction of the trachea or larynx
tachypnea	tak-ip-nē'ă	abnormally fast rate of respiration
tonsillitis	ton'si-lī'tis	inflammation of one or both tonsils
tracheitis	trā-kē-ī'tis	inflammation of the trachea
tracheorrhagia	trā'kē-ō-rā'jē-ă	bleeding from the lining of the trachea
tuberculosis (TB)	tū-ber'kyū-lō'sis	infection caused by *Mycobacterium tuberculosis*, a bacterium that attacks the lungs and is spread through the air from one person to another (Fig. 9-11)
upper respiratory infection (URI)	ŭp'r res'pi-ră-tōr'ē in-fek'shŭn	acute infection involving the nose, sinus, larynx, or pharynx; commonly called a cold
wheeze	wēz	an airy, whistling type sound made on inspiration and expiration

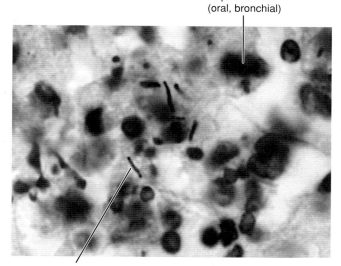

Sputum cells
(oral, bronchial)

Mycobacterium tuberculosis

Figure 9-11 *Mycobacterium tuberculosis,* the bacterium
that causes tuberculosis, as viewed under a microscope.

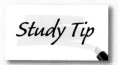

Study Tip

Pulmonary Embolism: A pulmonary embolism is a traveling clot (thrombus) from an
injured or inflamed blood vessel in the body, or a clot that has formed and broken
loose from the right side of the heart. The clot travels into the pulmonary artery,
where it lodges in the vessel.

■ Exercises: Symptoms and Medical Conditions

SIMPLE
RECALL

Exercise 14

Write the correct medical term for the meaning given.

1. decreased level of oxygen in the blood _____

2. inflammation of the tonsils _____

3. an acute infection involving the nose, sinus, larynx,
   or pharynx _____

4. chronic enlargement of the bronchi _____

5. inflammation within the bronchi of the lung _____

6. buildup of fluid in the space around the lungs _____

7. inflammation of the mucous membranes in
   the nasal cavity _____

8. bleeding from the lining of the trachea _____

9. bleeding from the nose _____

10. infection of the alveoli caused by fluid and pus filling an entire lobe of the lung

_____

11. inflammation of the pharynx

_____

12. inflammation of all sinuses

_____

13. decrease or loss of air in the lung

_____

14. inflammation of the lungs

_____

15. abnormal whistling, humming, or snoring sounds

_____

16. difficulty breathing

_____

17. friction sounds caused by inflammation of the pleura

_____

18. airy, whistling type of sound made while breathing

_____

19. group of disorders involving narrowing of small bronchi

_____

Exercise 15

ADVANCED
RECALL

Match each medical term with its meaning.

pertussis	bronchopneumonia	adult respiratory distress syndrome	hemothorax
pansinusitis	influenza	pulmonary embolism	pulmonary edema
empyema	tuberculosis	pleuritis	

Meaning   **Term**

1. buildup of fluid in the lung

_____

2. an infection of the smaller bronchial tubes of the lungs

_____

3. acute highly contagious viral infection, also known as flu

_____

4. blood located in the pleural cavity

_____

5. a localized collection of pus in the thoracic cavity

_____

6. an acute infectious inflammation of the larynx, trachea, and bronchi caused by the bacterium _Bordetella pertussis_

_____

7. inflammation of all sinuses

_____

8. respiratory failure that can occur with underlying illnesses or injury

_____

9. inflammation of the pleura

_____

10. an infection caused by _Mycobacterium tuberculosis_

_____

11. an obstruction of the pulmonary circulation by a blood clot

_____

ADVANCED
RECALL

Exercise 16

Circle the term that is most appropriate for the meaning of the sentence.

1. When Timmy Smith presented with a barking cough and difficult and noisy respirations, his physician diagnosed (*asthma, croup, dysphonia*).

2. Mr. Hannah was seen in follow-up for (*asthma, emphysema, empyema*), a chronic severe breathing disorder that includes attacks of wheezing.

3. Dr. Thomas informed Mr. Jenkins that severe (*stridor, hypoxia, pulmonary embolism*) can occur in respiratory failure.

4. Mrs. Lin was diagnosed with (*bacterial pneumonia, lobar pneumonia, pneumococcal pneumonia*) when the lab discovered *Streptococcus pneumonia* in her sputum.

5. On auscultation of the child's chest, Dr. Daughtry heard these two types of breath sounds: rhonchi and (*rales, rhinitis, dyspnea*).

6. Dr. Bazel explained to the patient that (*bacterial pneumonia, interstitial lung disease, chronic obstructive pulmonary disease*) is a group of chronic lung disorders affecting the tissue between the air sacs of the lungs.

7. After his x-ray report showed an obstruction of pulmonary circulation due to a blood clot, the patient was told that he had a (*pneumothorax, pulmonary embolism, pneumonitis*).

8. Mrs. Green had (*chronic obstructive pulmonary disease, interstitial lung disease, bronchiolitis obliterans with organizing pneumonia*), a condition in which her bronchioles were filled with granulated tissue plugs.

9. The physician diagnosed Ms. Thatcher with (*emphysema, empyema, dyspnea*) after testing showed permanent destruction of very fine airways and alveoli.

10. Mr. McGrath was diagnosed with (*respiratory failure, reactive airway disease, rales*) after he inhaled a toxic substance and began wheezing, coughing, and experiencing shortness of breath.

11. Jon Burns suffered from alternating periods of apnea and deep, rapid breathing known as (*respiratory failure, dyspnea, Cheyne-Stokes respiration*).

TERM
CONSTRUCTION

Exercise 17

Break the given medical term into its word parts and define each part. Then define the medical term.

For example:

bronchoplasty	*word parts:*	bronch/o / -plasty
	meanings:	bronchus / surgical repair, reconstruction
	term meaning:	surgical repair of the bronchus

1. pneumonia   *word parts:*   _____ / _____

   meanings: _____ / _____

   term meaning: _____

2. aphonia   *word parts:* _____ / _____

                    meanings: _____ / _____

                    term meaning: _____

3. bronchiectasis   *word parts:* _____ / _____

                    meanings: _____ / _____

                    term meaning: _____

4. bronchopneumonia   *word parts:* _____ / _____ / _____

                    meanings: _____ / _____ / _____

                    term meaning: _____

5. laryngospasm   *word parts:* _____ / _____

                    meanings: _____ / _____

                    term meaning: _____

6. pleuritis   *word parts:* _____ / _____

                    meanings: _____ / _____

                    term meaning: _____

7. apnea   *word parts:* _____ / _____

                    meanings: _____ / _____

                    term meaning: _____

8. laryngitis   *word parts:* _____ / _____

                    meanings: _____ / _____

                    term meaning: _____

9. pneumonitis   *word parts:* _____ / _____

                    meanings: _____ / _____

                    term meaning: _____

10. sinusitis   *word parts:* _____ / _____

                    meanings: _____ / _____

                    term meaning: _____

11. tracheitis   *word parts:* _____ / _____

                       meanings: _____ / _____

                       term meaning: _____

12. diaphragmatocele   *word parts:* _____ / _____

                       meanings: _____ / _____

                       term meaning: _____

13. nasopharyngitis   *word parts:* _____ / _____ / _____

                       meanings: _____ / _____ / _____

                       term meaning: _____

14. dysphonia   *word parts:* _____ / _____

                       meanings: _____ / _____

                       term meaning: _____

15. pharyngitis   *word parts:* _____ / _____

                       meanings: _____ / _____

                       term meaning: _____

Tests and Procedures

Term	Pronunciation	Meaning
Laboratory Tests		
acid-fast bacilli (AFB) smear	as′id-fast bă-sil′ī smĕr	clinical test performed on sputum to determine the presence of acid-fast bacilli, the bacteria that cause tuberculosis
arterial blood gases (ABGs)	ahr-tĕr′ē-ăl blŭd gas′ĕz	test performed on arterial blood to determine levels of oxygen, carbon dioxide, and other gases present
purified protein derivative (PPD) skin test	pyū′ri-fied prō′tēn dĕ-riv′ă-tiv skin test	skin test used to determine whether the patient has developed an immune response to the bacteria that cause tuberculosis
Diagnostic Procedures		
Imaging Studies		
chest radiograph (CXR)	chest rā′dē-ō-graf	radiographic image of chest used to evaluate the lungs and the heart
computed tomography (CT) scan	kŏm-pyū′tĕd tŏ-mog′ră-fē skan	x-ray technique producing computer-generated cross-sectional images
magnetic resonance imaging (MRI)	mag-net′ik rez′ŏ-năns im′ăj-ing	imaging technique that uses magnetic fields and radiofrequency waves to visualize anatomic structures; often used to diagnose lung disorders

(continued)

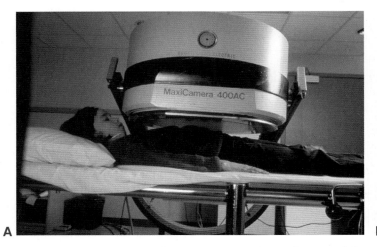

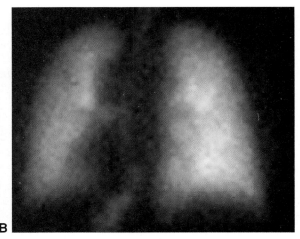

A   **B**

Figure 9-12   Ventilation-perfusion scanning. **A.** Nuclear medicine scanner. **B.** Ventilation-perfusion scan showing posterior view of the lungs.

Tests and Procedures *(continued)*

Term	Pronunciation	Meaning
radiography	rā'dē-og'ră-fē	examination of any part of the body for diagnostic purposes by means of x-rays with the record of the findings exposed onto photographic film
ventilation-perfusion (V/Q) scan	ven'ti-lā'shŭn-pĕr-fyū' zhŭn skan	test used to assess distribution of blood flow and ventilation through both lungs (Fig. 9-12)
Other Diagnostic Procedures		
auscultation	aws'kŭl-tā'shŭn	physical examination method of listening to body sounds with a stethoscope (Fig. 9-13)
bronchoalveolar lavage (BAL)	brong'kō-al-vē'ō-lăr lă-vahzh'	procedure performed during bronchoscopy to collect cells of the alveoli; saline solution is instilled into distal bronchi and then that solution is withdrawn along with the alveolar cells
bronchoscopy	brong-kos'kŏ-pē	endoscopic examination of the larynx and airways (Fig. 9-14)
laryngoscopy	lar'ing-gos'kŏ-pē	endoscopic examination of the larynx

(continued)

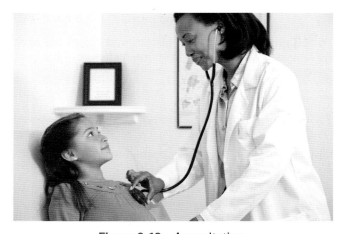

Figure 9-13   Auscultation.

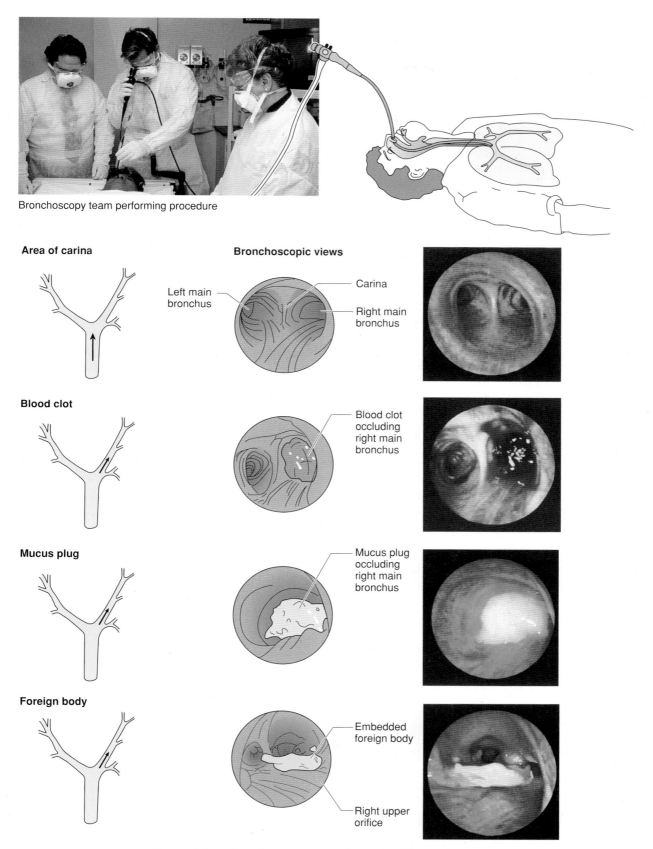

Figure 9-14   Bronchoscopy done through a fiberoptic scope.

Tests and Procedures *(continued)*

Term	Pronunciation	Meaning
nasopharyngoscopy	nā′zō-far-in-gos′kŏ-pē	endoscopic examination of the nasal passages and the pharynx
peak flow monitoring	pēk flō mon′i-tŏr′ing	test that measures the rate of air flow, or how fast air is able to pass through the airways
percussion	pĕr-kŭsh′ŭn	physical examination method of tapping over the body to elicit vibrations and sounds to estimate the size, border, or fluid content of a cavity, such as the chest
pharyngoscopy	far′ing-gos′kŏ-pē	endoscopic examination of the pharynx
polysomnography	pol′ē-som-nog′ră-fē	monitoring and recording normal and abnormal activity during sleep, including neural and respiratory functions
pulmonary function tests (PFTs)	pul′mŏ-nār-ē fŭngk′shŭn tests	group of tests performed to measure breathing; used to determine respiratory function or abnormalities; useful in distinguishing chronic obstructive pulmonary diseases from asthma
pulse oximetry	pŭls ok-sim′ĕ-trē	measurement of oxygen saturation in the blood (Fig. 9-15)

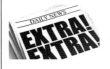 **PULSE OXIMETRY MEASUREMENTS** Pulse oximetry is measured via a probe placed on either the finger or the ear of the patient. If placed on the patient's finger, it is important to note that a patient should not have fingernail polish on the digit used for monitoring. Readings between 95% and 100% are acceptable ranges for pulse oximetry. When measurements are documented, it is noted if the reading was obtained on room air or on supplemental oxygen. If a patient is receiving oxygen, then the amount of oxygen the patient is receiving is also documented.

Term	Pronunciation	Meaning
rhinoscopy	rī-nos′kŏ-pē	endoscopic examination of the nasal cavity
spirometry	spī-rom′ĕ-trē	procedure for measuring air flow and volume of air inspired and expired by the lungs using a device called a spirometer
thoracoscopy	thōr-ă-kos′kŏ-pē	endoscopic examination of the thorax done through a small opening in the chest wall
video-assisted thorascopic surgery (VATS)	vid′ē-o ă-sis′ted thō′ra-skop′ik sŭr′jĕr-ē	thoracic surgery performed using endoscopic cameras, optical systems, and display screens, as well as specially designed surgical instruments, which enables surgeons to view the inside of the chest cavity and remove tissue to test for disease (Fig. 9-16)

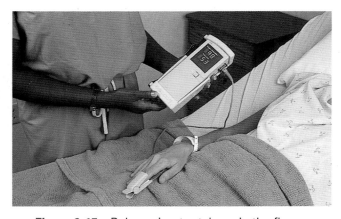

Figure 9-15 Pulse oximetry taken via the finger.

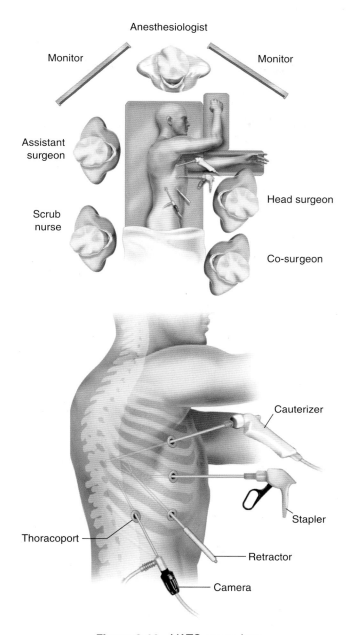

Figure 9-16   VATS procedure.

For a visual and audio tour of some of the sounds heard on auscultation, view the animation *Change in Breathing Sounds* on the electronic Student Resources.

■ Exercises: Tests and Procedures

Exercise 18

SIMPLE
RECALL

Circle the term that is most appropriate for the meaning of the sentence.

1. (*Computed tomography, Thoracoscopy, Bronchoscopy*) is an x-ray technique producing computer-generated cross-sectional images.

2. An x-ray procedure used to evaluate the lungs and the heart is called a(n) (*arthrogram, chest radiograph, bronchoscopy*).

3. (*Magnetic resonance imaging, Computed tomography, V/Q scan*) is a test used to assess distribution of blood flow and ventilation through both lungs.

4. The skin test used to determine immune response to the bacteria that cause tuberculosis is called (*AFB smear, PPD test, ABGs*).

5. (*Thoracoscopy, Computed tomography, Bronchoalveolar lavage*) is performed during bronchoscopy to collect cells of the alveoli.

6. The imaging technique that uses magnetic fields and radiofrequency waves is called (*magnetic resonance imaging, computed tomography, chest radiography*).

7. (*CT, VATS, MRI*) allows surgeons to view the inside of the chest cavity and remove tissue for testing.

8. A procedure for measuring air flow and volume of air inspired and expired by the lungs is called (*spirometry, radiography, pulse oximetry*).

Exercise 19

ADVANCED
RECALL

Complete each sentence by writing in the correct medical term.

1. The measurement of oxygen saturation in the blood is called _____.

2. A test performed on arterial blood to determine levels of oxygen, carbon dioxide, and other gases present is called _____.

3. A method of physical examination that uses a tapping motion over the body to elicit vibrations and sounds to estimate the size, border, or fluid content of a cavity is called

   _____.

4. The test performed on sputum to determine the presence of acid-fast bacilli, the bacteria that causes tuberculosis, is called _____.

5. Examination of any part of the body for diagnostic purposes by means of x-rays with the record of the findings exposed onto photographic film is called _____.

6. An endoscopic examination of the larynx is called a(n) _____.

7. A group of tests used to determine respiratory function or abnormalities that is useful in distinguishing chronic obstructive pulmonary diseases from asthma is called _____.

8. The monitoring and recording of normal and abnormal activity during sleep, including neural and respiratory function, is called _____.

9. A physical examination method of listening to the sounds of the respiratory system with the aid of a stethoscope is called _____.

10. A test that measures the rate of air flow, or how fast air is able to pass through the airways, is called _____.

Exercise 20

TERM CONSTRUCTION

Using the given combining form, build a medical term for the meaning given.

Combining Form	Meaning of Medical Term	Medical Term
thorac/o	endoscopic examination of the thorax	1._____
rhin/o	endoscopic examination of the nasal cavity	2._____
pharyng/o	endoscopic examination of the pharynx	3._____
bronch/o	endoscopic examination of the larynx and airways	4._____
laryng/o	endoscopic examination of the larynx	5._____

Surgical Interventions and Therapeutic Procedures

Term	Pronunciation	Meaning
adenoidectomy	ad'ĕ-noyd-ek'tŏ-mē	excision of the adenoids
aspiration	as'pi-rā'shŭn	removal of accumulated fluid by suction
bronchoplasty	brong'kō-plas-tē	surgical repair of the bronchus
cardiopulmonary resuscitation (CPR)	kar'dē-ō-pŭl'mo-nār-ē rē-sŭs'i-tā'shŭn	medical procedure to ventilate the lungs and artificially circulate the blood if a patient has stopped breathing and the heart has stopped
continuous positive airway pressure (CPAP) therapy	kon-tin'yū-us poz'i-tiv ār'wā presh'ŭr thăr'ă-pē	breathing apparatus that pumps constant pressurized air through the nasal passages via a mask to keep the airway open (Fig. 9-17)
endotracheal intubation	en'dō-trā'kē-ăl in'tū-bā'shŭn	medical procedure in which a tube is inserted between the vocal cords in the larynx and into the trachea to establish an airway for breathing purposes, either manually or mechanically (Fig. 9-18)
hyperbaric medicine	hī'pĕr-băr'ik med'i-sin	medicinal use of high barometric pressure, usually in specially constructed chambers, to increase oxygen content of blood and tissues

(continued)

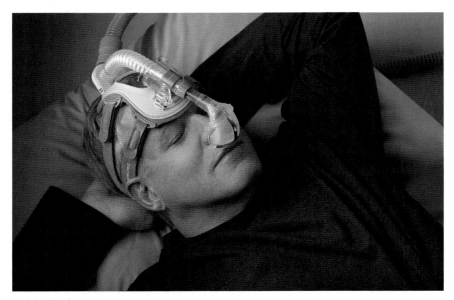

Figure 9-17 Continuous positive airway pressure (CPAP) therapy.

Surgical Interventions and Therapeutic Procedures *(continued)*

Term	Pronunciation	Meaning
incentive spirometry	in-sen'tiv spī-rom'ĕ-trē	medical procedure to encourage patients to breathe deeply by using a portable plastic device called a spirometer that gives visual feedback as the patient inhales forcefully (Fig. 9-19)
laryngectomy	lar'in-jek'tŏ-mē	excision of the larynx
laryngotracheotomy	lă-ring'gō-trākē-otŏ-mē	incision of the larynx and trachea
lobectomy	lō-bek'tŏ-mē	excision of a lobe (of the lung)
mechanical ventilation	mĕ-kan'i-kăl ven-ti-lā'shŭn	use of an automatic mechanical device to perform all or part of the work of breathing (Fig. 9-20)

(continued)

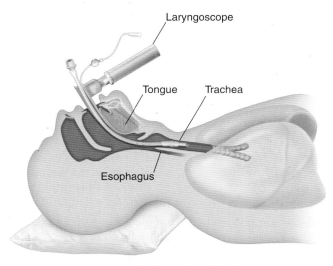

Laryngoscope

Tongue   Trachea

Esophagus

Figure 9-18 Endotracheal intubation.

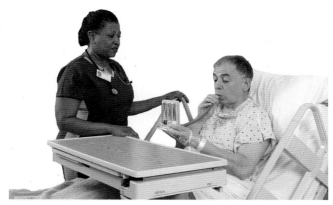

Figure 9-19   Incentive spirometry.

Surgical Interventions and Therapeutic Procedures *(continued)*

Term	Pronunciation	Meaning
pneumonectomy	nū′mō-nek′tŏ-mē	excision of the lung
rhinoplasty	rī′nō-plas-tē	surgical repair of the nose
septoplasty	sep′tō-plas-tē	surgical repair of the (nasal) septum
sinusotomy	sī′nŭ-sot′ŏ-mē	incision of the sinus
thoracentesis	thōr′ă-kō-sen-tē′sis	surgical puncture to aspirate fluid from the chest cavity
thoracotomy	thōr′ă-kot′ŏ-mē	incision of the chest cavity
tonsillectomy	ton′si-lek′tŏ-mē	surgical removal of one or both tonsils
tracheoplasty	trā′kē-ō-plas-tē	surgical repair of the trachea
tracheostomy	trā′kē-os′tŏ-mē	creation of an artificial opening in the trachea (Fig. 9-21)
tracheotomy	trā′kē-ot′ŏ-mē	incision of the trachea (Fig. 9-21)

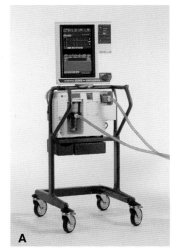
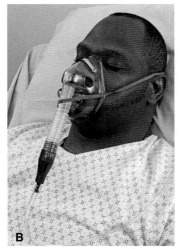

A   **B**

Figure 9-20   A. Mechanical ventilation system. **B.** Patient on mechanical ventilation via mask attached to system.

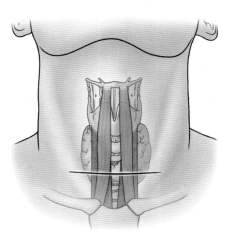

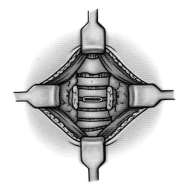

Incision in trachea
after retracting
infrahyoid muscles
and
incising isthmus
of thyroid gland

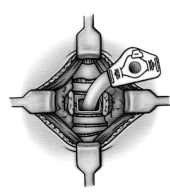

Tracheostomy tube
inserted in tracheal opening

Skin incision for tracheostomy

Figure 9-21   Tracheotomy and tracheostomy.

■ Exercises: Surgical Interventions and Therapeutic Procedures

SIMPLE
RECALL

Exercise 21

Write the correct medical term for the meaning given.

1. incision of the chest cavity _____

2. excision of the adenoids _____

3. surgical repair of the trachea _____

4. use of high barometric pressure to increase oxygen
   content of blood and tissues _____

5. use of an automatic mechanical device to perform all or part
   of the work of breathing _____

6. removal of accumulated fluid by suction _____

7. breathing apparatus that pumps air through the nasal
   passages to keep the airway open _____

8. incision of the trachea _____

9. incision of the larynx and trachea _____

10. insertion of a tube between the vocal cords and into the
    trachea to establish an airway for breathing _____

11. surgical repair of the bronchus _____

12. creation of an artificial opening in the trachea _____

13. excision of the lung _____

14. medical procedure to encourage patients to breathe deeply _____

Exercise 22

ADVANCED
RECALL

Circle the term that is most appropriate for the meaning of the sentence.

1. Mr. Martinez required a (*tracheostomy, tracheoplasty, tracheotomy*) to create an opening to ensure normal breathing processes could occur.

2. Mr. Browder had long had a very sore throat and inflamed left tonsil but was, nonetheless, reluctant to undergo (*adenoidectomy, tonsillectomy, laryngectomy*) to remove it.

3. The boxer's nose was injured during the ninth round of the match, which required (*rhinoplasty, tracheoplasty, bronchoplasty*) surgery to fix his nasal injury.

4. Following surgical removal of a tumor in the right lung, Mr. Hunnicutt required extensive (*thoracentesis, thoracoscopy, thoracotomy*) to remove the buildup of fluid in the thoracic cavity.

5. The patient's heart stopped, causing the medical team to begin (*BOOP, CPAP, CPR*) immediately.

Exercise 23

TERM
CONSTRUCTION

Using the given suffix, build a medical term for the meaning given.

Suffix	Meaning of Medical Term	Medical Term
-plasty	surgical repair of the nasal septum	1. _____
-ectomy	excision of the larynx	2. _____
-centesis	surgical puncture of the chest cavity	3. _____
-scopy	process of examining the bronchus	4. _____
-tomy	surgical opening of the thorax	5. _____

Exercise 24

TERM
CONSTRUCTION

Break the given medical term into its word parts and define each part. Then define the medical term.

For example:
pleuritis

word parts:	pleur/o / -itis
meanings:	pleura / inflammation
term meaning:	inflammation of the pleura

1. laryngoscope

word parts: _____ / _____

meanings: _____ / _____

term meaning: _____

2. rhinoplasty   *word parts:*   _____ / _____

                          meanings: _____ / _____

                          term meaning: _____

3. laryngostomy   *word parts:*   _____ / _____

                          meanings: _____ / _____

                          term meaning: _____

4. pneumonectomy   *word parts:*   _____ / _____

                          meanings: _____ / _____

                          term meaning: _____

5. sinusotomy   *word parts:*   _____ / _____

                          meanings: _____ / _____

                          term meaning: _____

6. bronchoplasty   *word parts:*   _____ / _____

                          meanings: _____ / _____

                          term meaning: _____

7. thoracentesis   *word parts:*   _____ / _____

                          meanings: _____ / _____

                          term meaning: _____

8. tracheotomy   *word parts:*   _____ / _____

                          meanings: _____ / _____

                          term meaning: _____

9. adenoidectomy   *word parts:*   _____ / _____

                          meanings: _____ / _____

                          term meaning: _____

10. tracheostomy   *word parts:*   _____ / _____

                          meanings: _____ / _____

                          term meaning: _____

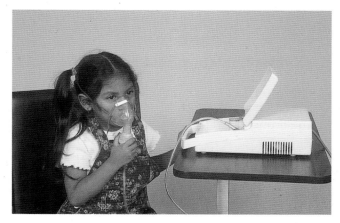

Figure 9-22   Child using a portable nebulizer.

Medications and Drug Therapies

Term	Pronunciation	Meaning
antibiotic	an'tē-bī-ot'ik	drug that acts against susceptible microorganisms
antihistamine	an'tē-his'tă-mēn	drug used to stop the effects of histamine in the respiratory tract
antitubercular	an'tē-tū-ber'kyū-lăr	drug contained in a vaccine used to lower the risk of getting tuberculosis in people who may be exposed to the disease
antitussive	an'tē-tŭs'iv	drug that suppresses the cough center in the brain to stop repeated or productive coughing
bronchodilator	brong'kō-dī-lā'ter	drug that dilates the bronchial wall, allowing air to pass through and relieving breathing difficulties
corticosteroid	kōr'ti-kō-stĕr'oyd	drug that reduces bronchial inflammation and airway obstruction and thereby improves lung function
decongestant	dē'kon-jes'tant	drug that relieves congestion by shrinking swollen nasal tissues and blood vessels
expectorant	ek-spek'tō-rănt	drug that helps bring up mucus and other material from the lungs, bronchi, and trachea and helps to lubricate the irritated respiratory tract
nebulizer, *syn.* atomizer	neb'yū-līz'ĕr, at'ŏm-ī-zĕr	device for administering a drug by spraying a fine mist into the nose (Fig. 9-22)

■ Exercise: Medications and Drug Therapies

SIMPLE RECALL

Exercise 25

Write the correct medication or drug therapy term for the meaning given.

1. device for administering a medication by spraying a fine mist   _____
   into the nose

2. drug that helps bring up mucus and other material from   _____
   the lungs, bronchi, and trachea

3. drug that reduces bronchial inflammation and airway obstruction

_____

4. drug that suppresses the cough center in the brain

_____

5. drug used to stop the effects of histamine

_____

6. drug that dilates the bronchial wall

_____

7. drug that that acts against susceptible microorganisms

_____

8. drug that relieves congestion by shrinking swollen nasal tissues and blood vessels

_____

9. drug contained in a vaccine used to lower the risk of getting tuberculosis

_____

Specialties and Specialists

Term	Pronunciation	Meaning
otorhinolaryngology	ō′tō-rī′nō-lar-in-gol′ŏ-jē	medical specialty concerned with diagnosis and treatment of diseases of the ear, nose, and throat
otorhinolaryngologist	ō′tō-rī′nō-lar-in-gol′ŏ-jist	physician who specializes in otorhinolaryngology
pulmonology	pul′mō-nol′ŏ-jē	medical specialty concerned with diseases of the lungs and the respiratory tract
pulmonologist	pul′mō-nol′ŏ-jist	physician who specializes in pulmonology

■ Exercise: Specialties and Specialists

Exercise 26

ADVANCED
RECALL

Match each medical specialist or specialty with its description.

otorhinolaryngology   pulmonology
otorhinolaryngologist   pulmonologist

Description   **Term**

1. physician who specializes in otorhinolaryngology

_____

2. physician who specializes in pulmonology

_____

3. medical specialty concerned with diseases of the ear, nose, and throat

_____

4. medical specialty concerned with diseases of the lungs and the respiratory tract

_____

Abbreviations

Abbreviation	Meaning
ABG	arterial blood gas
AFB	acid-fast bacilli
ARDS	acute respiratory distress syndrome
BAL	bronchoalveolar lavage
BOOP	bronchiolitis obliterans with organizing pneumonia
COPD	chronic obstructive pulmonary disease
CPAP	continuous positive airway pressure
CPR	cardiopulmonary resuscitation
CT	computed tomography (scan)
CXR	chest x-ray
ILD	interstitial lung disease
MRI	magnetic resonance imaging
PFTs	pulmonary function tests
PPD	purified protein derivative
RAD	reactive airway disease
RF	respiratory failure
TB	tuberculosis
URI	upper respiratory infection
V/Q	ventilation-perfusion (scan)
VATS	video-assisted thorascopic surgery

■ Exercises: Abbreviations

SIMPLE
RECALL

Exercise 27

Write the meaning of each abbreviation.

1. RAD   _____

2. CT   _____

3. URI   _____

4. V/Q   _____

5. TB   _____

6. CPR   _____

7. MRI   _____

8. PPD   _____

9. VATS _____

10. ABG _____

11. CPAP _____

12. BAL _____

Exercise 28

SIMPLE RECALL

Write the meaning of each abbreviation used in these sentences.

1. After completing the examination, Dr. Gaskill diagnosed Mr. Stewart with **COPD** complicated with **ILD**.

   _____   _____

2. A college student underwent **PFTs** when members of her family developed symptoms related to **RF.**

   _____   _____

3. The physician concluded the patient suffered from **ARDS** and was admitted to the hospital for treatment.

   _____

4. The physician ordered an **AFB** test to help determine if the patient had tuberculosis or **BOOP**.

   _____   _____

5. The patient's **CXR** showed a small nodule in the left upper lobe.

   _____

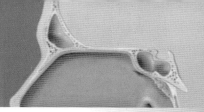

Review of Terms for Anatomy and Physiology

Exercise 29

VISUAL

Write the correct terms on the blanks for the anatomic structures indicated.

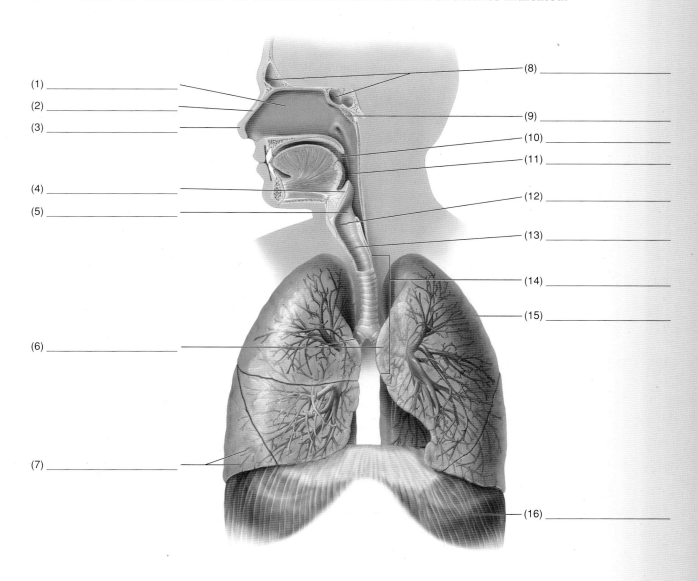

(1) _____

(2) _____

(3) _____

(4) _____

(5) _____

(6) _____

(7) _____

(8) _____

(9) _____

(10) _____

(11) _____

(12) _____

(13) _____

(14) _____

(15) _____

(16) _____

Exercise 30

VISUAL

Write the correct terms on the blanks for the anatomic structures indicated.

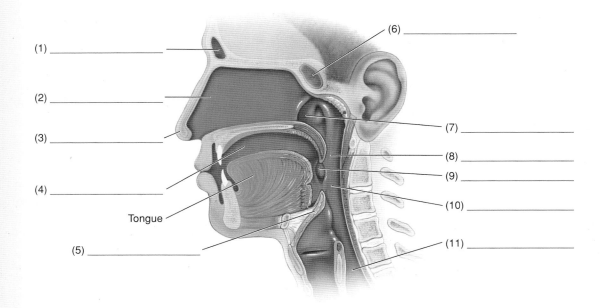

(1) _____

(2) _____

(3) _____

(4) _____

Tongue

(5) _____

(6) _____

(7) _____

(8) _____

(9) _____

(10) _____

(11) _____

Understanding Term Structure

Exercise 31

TERM CONSTRUCTION

Break the given medical term into its word parts and define each part. Then define the medical term. (Note: you may need to use word parts from other chapters.)

For example:

laryngospasm	*word parts:*	laryng/o / -spasm
	meanings:	larynx / involuntary movement
	term meaning:	involuntary movement of the larynx

1. laryngeal   *word parts:*   _____ / _____

    meanings: _____ / _____

    term meaning: _____

2. rhinorrhea   *word parts:*   _____ / _____

    meanings: _____ / _____

    term meaning: _____

3. pulmonary   *word parts:* _____ / _____

   meanings: _____ / _____

   term meaning: _____

4. phrenospasm   *word parts:* _____ / _____

   meanings: _____ / _____

   term meaning: _____

5. thoracotomy   *word parts:* _____ / _____

   meanings: _____ / _____

   term meaning: _____

6. tachypnea   *word parts:* _____ / _____

   meanings: _____ / _____

   term meaning: _____

7. thoracic   *word parts:* _____ / _____

   meanings: _____ / _____

   term meaning: _____

8. bronchospasm   *word parts:* _____ / _____

   meanings: _____ / _____

   term meaning: _____

9. pulmonology   *word parts:* _____ / _____

   meanings: _____ / _____

   term meaning: _____

10. bronchoscopy   *word parts:* _____ / _____

   meanings: _____ / _____

   term meaning: _____

Comprehension Exercises

COMPREHENSION

Exercise 32

Fill in the blank with the correct term.

1. The layer of the pleura that is closest to the lung is known as the _____.

2. The smallest divisions of the bronchial tree are the _____.

3. The _____ acts as a lid over the entrance to the esophagus.

4. Abnormally fast breathing is termed _____.

5. _____ is a term used to describe blood located in the chest.

6. During a(n) _____ attack, a person has attacks of wheezing due to obstruction of the airways from excessive amounts of secretions.

7. A sudden involuntary movement of the larynx is a(n) _____.

8. The _____ tract is comprised of the nose and pharynx.

9. _____ is a sound indicating obstruction of the airway.

10. Inflammation of the _____ is commonly known as a sore throat.

Exercise 33

COMPREHENSION

Write a short answer for each question.

1. What body structures make up the lower respiratory tract? _____

_____

2. Name the structure that allows humans to form sounds. _____

3. Describe the thoracic region. _____

_____

4. How many lobes are present within each lung? _____

5. What is the term for a procedure that requires the creation of an artificial opening in the trachea? _____

6. What is another name for interstitial lung disease? _____

7. Why would a thoracentesis be performed? _____

_____

8. How does a CPAP work? _____

_____

9. What does a spirometer measure? _____

10. What is another name for the trachea? _____

Exercise 34

COMPREHENSION   **Circle the letter of the best answer in the following questions.**

1. The term that most specifically applies to inflammation of the structure between the pharynx and trachea is:

A. epiglottitis
B. laryngitis
C. pharyngitis
D. pleuritis

2. Which procedure would be performed when a patient's heart and breathing stop?

A. CPR
B. VATS
C. CXR
D. CPAP

3. What is the condition that causes a progressive loss of lung function?

A. asthma
B. diphtheria
C. pneumonia
D. emphysema

4. Which term describes the condition commonly known as whooping cough?

A. pyothorax
B. pertussis
C. pleuritis
D. pneumonitis

5. Which of the following tests sputum for tuberculosis?

A. arterial blood gases
B. peak flow monitoring
C. purified protein derivative test
D. acid-fast bacilli smear

6. Every year, a highly contagious viral infection causes many adults and children to seek medical treatment for a disease, commonly known as the flu. The medical term for this infection is:

A. emphysema
B. influenza
C. croup
D. asthma

7. What is the name of the test used to examine the nasal passages and the pharynx to diagnose structural abnormalities?

A. auscultation
B. nasopharyngoscopy
C. laryngopharyngoscopy
D. laryngoscopy

8. A group of tests performed to measure breathing are referred to as:

A. PPD
B. PFTs
C. PEFR
D. PF

9. Even if you had never heard of this condition, you might assume that sinusitis refers to:

A. surgical repair of the sinus
B. incision of the sinus
C. inflammation of the sinus
D. excision of the sinus

10. Which combining form refers to the structure that takes in air?

A. sinus/o
B. sept/o
C. adenoid/o
D. rhin/o

Application and Analysis

CASE REPORTS

APPLICATION

Exercise 35

Read the case reports and circle the letter of your answer choice for the questions that follow each case.

CASE 9-1

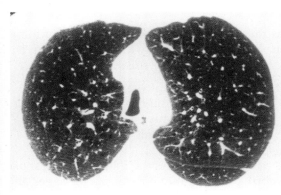

Figure 9-23 CT scan of the chest of a patient diagnosed with COPD.

After working 25 years in the coal-mining industry, Mr. Orbin Davis, age 65, is undergoing a series of pulmonary function tests to investigate issues related to his progressive loss of lung function and inability to breathe normally. During the procedures, an instrument was used to measure Mr. Davis's breathing rate by estimating the amount of air exhaled after normal inspiration. Ms. Whalen, a nurse practitioner, also performed a test that measured the amount of air exhaled after a maximal inspiration. This group of tests will assist in ascertaining whether Mr. Davis suffers from COPD or from asthma. Depending on the test results, a CT scan may also be ordered to confirm COPD (Fig. 9-23).

1. The term for an instrument used to measure breathing is:

   A. spirometry
   B. spirometer
   C. percussion
   D. capnometer

2. The abbreviation COPD stands for:

   A. chronic obstructive pneumonia dyspnea
   B. chronic olfactory pharyngitis disease
   C. caustic other pneumonic disease
   D. chronic obstructive pulmonary disease

3. What group of tests will assist in ascertaining whether the patient has COPD or asthma?

   A. PFTs
   B. RRs

   C. AFBs
   D. ABGs

4. A symptom related to asthma is:

   A. a progressive loss of lung function
   B. lack of expansion of a lung
   C. wheezing
   D. severe headaches

5. Mr. Davis' pulmonary function test revealed an abnormal amount of fluid inside various lobes within the lungs. This condition is known as:

   A. pleurodesis
   B. pleural effusion
   C. pulmonary edema
   D. pneumothorax

CASE 9-2

Ms. Beverly Bonner, age 58, requested an office appointment. Ms. Bonner stated she suffered from a sore throat, fever, chills, and depression. Dr. Wallace physically examined her, took a chest x-ray, measured her breathing, and established the amount of fluid in her lungs with the use of a stethoscope and vibration within her pleural cavity. After reviewing the results of the tests and exam, Dr. Wallace diagnosed Ms. Bonner with pneumococcal pneumonia.

6. What bacterial species is the cause of pneumococcal pneumonia?

   A. *Pneumococcus aureus*
   B. *Streptococcus pneumoniae*
   C. *Mycopneumonia streptococcus*
   D. *Pneumococcus pneumoniae*

7. The throat is the common name for which structure?

   A. pharynx
   B. larynx
   C. nasopharynx
   D. glottis

8. An instrument that measures breathing is called a(n):

   A. oximeter
   B. peak flow meter
   C. spirometer
   D. tidal volume meter

9. What is the name of the physical exam involving listening inside the pleural cavity that relies on the use of a stethoscope?

   A. percussion
   B. auscultation
   C. polysomnography
   D. spirometry

10. What is the name of the physical examination of the pleural cavity that relies on the use of tapping over the body to elicit vibrations and sounds?

   A. percussion
   B. auscultation
   C. polysomnography
   D. spirometry

MEDICAL RECORD ANALYSIS

MEDICAL RECORD 9-1

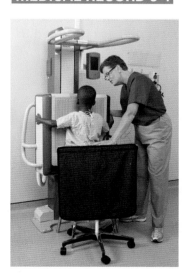

Travis Reynolds is a patient who is returning to the office with his mother after a routine tuberculosis skin test was performed a couple of days ago. As the radiologic technologist, you are reviewing the record in preparation for performing his chest x-ray.

A radiologic technician prepares patients for and performs radiologic examinations.

Medical Record

POSITIVE TUBERCULIN SKIN TEST

SUBJECTIVE: This is a 4-year-old African American boy patient of our clinic who came here today for tuberculosis test reading. The patient had a TB test placed previously and today, 48 hours later, shows a positive reaction. TB test was present in the left forearm, and there is an area of erythema and induration corresponding to about 20 mm. This was measured by the nurse and verified for me.

Mom denies child being exposed to anyone with tuberculosis. He had been tested a couple of times during the past year, but mom had never come in for the reading. She said there was no reaction to it on either occasion except this one time. She also says that he is only around the family and the kids in school. She is not aware of anyone being diagnosed with tuberculosis and child has been completely fine, alert, active, and feeding well with no problems.

OBJECTIVE: Temperature 98.8, blood pressure 80/60, weight 32 pounds, heart rate 80. General: Alert, active, well nourished. Neck: Supple, no lymphadenopathy. Heart: Regular rate and rhythm, no heart murmurs. Lungs: Clear to auscultation bilaterally. No rhonchi, rales, crackles, or wheezing.

ASSESSMENT AND PLAN: Patient is a 4-year-old boy with positive tuberculin skin test result, recent converter. I ordered chest x-rays to rule out active tuberculosis. The patient very likely has latent TB and mom was told that her son would be a good candidate for INH prophylaxis. The patient is to return to clinic in the next couple of weeks. Mom voiced understanding and agrees to follow up accordingly.

Exercise 36

APPLICATION

Write the appropriate medical terms used in this medical record on the blanks after their definitions. Note that not all the terms appear in the chapter, but you should be able to identify these terms based on word parts that are included in this chapter.

1. redness   _____

2. infection by a bacterium that attacks
the lungs   _____

3. abnormal whisting, humming, or snoring
sounds during breathing   _____

4. listening with aid of a stethoscope   _____

5. an airy, whistling type sound   _____

6. pertaining to both sides   _____

Bonus Question

7. Why were chest x-rays ordered?   _____

MEDICAL RECORD 9-2

You are a respiratory therapist working at a VA hospital and will be treating Mr. Samuel Burnett, who suffers from chronic obstructive pulmonary disease. Prior to his appointment, you are reviewing the medical record from his recent hospitalization.

Medical Record

BRONCHITIS WITH COPD

DIAGNOSES:

1. (1)_____.
2. Chronic obstructive pulmonary disease.
3. Coronary artery disease.

PROCEDURES: Chest x-ray that had the following result: The patient had increased markings in left lower lung, possibly early left lower lobe pneumonia versus chronic fibrosis, minimal hyperinflation with flattened diaphragms, decreased lung markings both upper lungs and increased AP diameter. Chest compatible with emphysema. Moderate diffuse osteoporosis. Wedging one midthoracic vertebral body.

HISTORY AND HOSPITAL COURSE: The patient was admitted with a chief complaint of cough with white (2)_____ with shortness of breath and (3)_____ on exertion, worse for 3 days.

This is an 83-year-old male with COPD and diagnosed with a non-ST-elevation MI 1-1/2 months ago. Patient underwent cardiac catheterization at that time and was discharged on Plavix. The patient reports ongoing dyspnea on exertion and shortness of breath since then. Most recently, the patient complained of very severe cough with white sputum. The patient denies chest pain. He does have nocturia and paroxysmal nocturnal dyspnea, subjective hot and cold flashes, but denies night sweats or weight loss.

I believe the patient has severe COPD but the patient does not want to have PFTs done because he does not want to pay the expense since he can get them done for free at the VA. The patient also does not want to have a CT to make sure he does not have a (4)_____, although my previous assessment of probability for a PE was low. The patient also refuses to be transferred to the VA where he can receive these studies for free. The patient decided he would rather be discharged.

The patient was treated for bronchitis with doxycycline with improvement in his symptoms. He was discharged to home in stable condition. He will be discharged on Atrovent MDI 2 puffs every 6 hours and doxycycline 100 mg by mouth 2 times per day for 10 days. The patient was told to go to the VA to set up home physical therapy and (5)_____ rehab. No activity restrictions but he should walk with assistance. He should continue to be active. He will call the VA to set up home physical therapy and pulmonary rehabilitation.

Exercise 37

APPLICATION

Fill in the blanks in the medical record above with the correct medical terms. The definitions of the missing terms are listed below.

1. inflammation of the bronchi

2. expectorated matter

3. difficulty breathing

4. blockage of the pulmonary artery by a blood clot

5. pertaining to the lungs

Bonus Question

6. Which type of physician specialist would most likely have treated this patient?

Pronunciation and Spelling

Exercise 38

AUDITORY

Review the Chapter 9 terms in the Dictionary/Audio Glossary in the Student Resources and practice pronouncing each term, referring to the pronunciation guide as needed.

Exercise 39

SPELLING

Check the spelling of each term. If it is correct, check off the correct box. If incorrect, write the correct spelling on the line.

1. alveolor ☐ _____

2. pulomonary ☐ _____

3. bronchiolitis ☐ _____

4. diaphram ☐ _____

5. pneumopluritis ☐ _____

6. pleuraglia ☐ _____

7. rhinorrhea ☐ _____

8. bronchography ☐ _____

9. tonsilar ☐ _____

10. dispena ☐ _____

Media Connection

STUDENT
RESOURCES

Exercise 40

**Complete each of the following activities available with the Student Resources.
Check off each activity as you complete it.**

Chapter Exercises

_____ Flash Cards   _____ True/False Body Building

_____ Concentration   _____ Quiz Show

_____ Abbreviation Match-Up   _____ Complete the Case

_____ Roboterms   _____ Medical Record Review

_____ Word Builder   _____ Look and Label

_____ Fill the Gap   _____ Image Matching

_____ Break It Down   _____ Spelling Bee

_____ **Chapter Quiz**   _Score:_ _____%

Additional Resources

_____ Animation: _The Respiratory System_

_____ Animation: _Pulmonary Ventilation_

_____ Animation: _Change in Breathing Sounds_

_____ Dictionary/Audio Glossary

_____ Health Professions Careers: Radiologic Technician

_____ Health Professions Careers: Respiratory Therapist

Male Reproductive System

10

Chapter Outline

Objectives

After completion of this chapter you will be able to:

1. Describe the location of main structures in the male reproductive system.

2. Define terms related to the male reproductive system.

3. Define combining forms, prefixes, and suffixes related to the male reproductive system.

4. Define common medical terminology related to the male reproductive system, including adjectives and related terms, symptoms and conditions, tests and procedures, surgical interventions and therapeutic procedures, medications and drug therapies, and specialties.

5. Explain abbreviations for terms related to the male reproductive system.

6. Successfully complete all chapter exercises.

7. Explain terms used in case studies and medical records involving the male reproductive system.

8. Successfully complete all pronunciation and spelling exercises, and complete all interactive exercises included with the companion Student Resources.

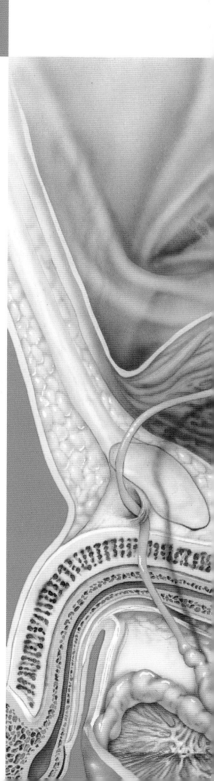

■ ANATOMY AND PHYSIOLOGY

Functions

- ■ To produce testosterone, which is the male hormone
- ■ To produce and store spermatozoa, the male reproductive cells
- ■ To produce, transport, and release semen

Organs and Structures

- ■ The prostate gland, bulbourethral glands, and the seminal vesicles produce fluids that aid in the movement of spermatozoa.
- ■ The primary male reproductive organs are the two testes (or testicles), which produce spermatozoa and testosterone.
- ■ The epididymis and the vas deferens transport spermatozoa and semen.
- ■ The sac containing the testes and the epididymis is called the scrotum.
- ■ The penis is the external organ of urination and sexual intercourse.
- ■ Testosterone is the male sex hormone.
- ■ Spermatozoa are the male reproductive (sex) cells.
- ■ Semen is the fluid produced by the glands in the male reproductive system.

Terms Related to the Male Reproductive System (Fig. 10-1)

Term	Pronunciation	Meaning
bulbourethral glands	bŭl'bō-yū-rē'thrăl glandz	the two glands below the prostate that secrete a sticky fluid that becomes a component of semen
epididymis	ep'i-did'i-mis	long duct coiled on top of each testis that transports and stores mature spermatozoa
penis	pē'nis	external male organ used in urination and sexual intercourse
glans penis	glanz pē'nis	bulbous tip at the end of the penis
prepuce, *syn.* foreskin	prē'pyŭs	layer of skin that covers the glans penis in uncircumcised males
prostate gland	pros'tāt gland	gland that surrounds the top of the urethra (immediately below the bladder) that secretes a fluid that becomes part of semen
scrotum	skrō'tŭm	sac that is suspended on either side of and behind the penis that encloses the testes and epididymis
semen	sē'mĕn	viscous fluid containing spermatozoa and secretions of the testes and seminal glands, prostate, and bulbourethral glands
seminal vesicles	sem'i-năl ves'i-kălz	two glands behind the urinary bladder that produce seminal fluid, which becomes a component of semen
seminiferous tubules	sem'i-nif'ĕr-ŭs tū'byūlz	coiled tubes in the testes in which spermatozoa are formed
sperm, *syn.* spermatozoon	spĕrm, spĕr'mă-tō-zō'on	male reproductive (sex) cell produced by the testes that can fertilize an ovum in a female to produce offspring
testis, *syn.* testicle	tes'tis, tes'ti-kĕl	male reproductive gland (found in pairs) located in the scrotum that produces spermatozoa and testosterone

(continued)

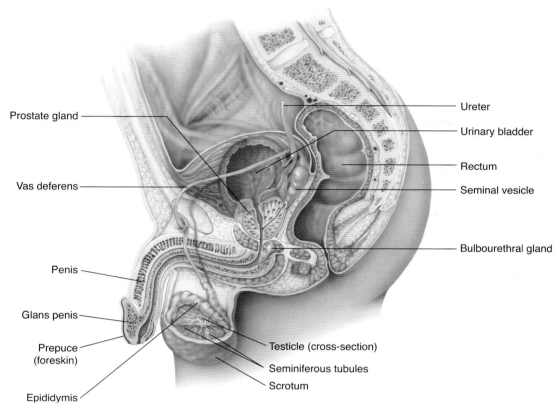

Prostate gland

Vas deferens

Penis

Glans penis

Prepuce
(foreskin)

Epididymis

Ureter

Urinary bladder

Rectum

Seminal vesicle

Bulbourethral gland

Testicle (cross-section)

Seminiferous tubules

Scrotum

Figure 10-1   The male reproductive system.

Terms Related to the Male Reproductive System *(continued)*

Term	Pronunciation	Meaning
testosterone	tes-tos'tĕ-rōn	male hormone produced by the testes
vas deferens	vas def'ĕr-enz	ducts that carry spermatozoa from the epididymis to the urethra

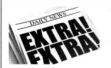

MALE URETHRA   The male urethra has two separate functions. It carries urine from the bladder during urination. It also transports semen from the vas deferens during ejaculation. A muscle contracts during sexual intercourse to prevent the escape of urine during ejaculation.

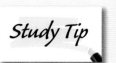

Prostate vs. Prostrate: Be careful when writing or saying the word *prostate* (one *r*). It is frequently mistaken for *prostrate* (two *r*'s). *Prostate* refers to the gland, whereas *prostrate* means completely overcome or lying in a face-down position.

■ Exercises: Anatomy and Physiology

SIMPLE
RECALL

Exercise 1

Write the correct anatomic structure for the definition given.

1. layer of skin covering the glans penis   _____

2. sac that contains the testes and epididymis   _____

3. glands behind the bladder that produce fluid   _____

4. male sex cell   _____

5. ducts carrying spermatozoa from the epididymis to the urethra   _____

6. glands below the prostate that secrete a sticky fluid   _____

7. external male organ of urination and intercourse   _____

8. coiled tubes in the testes where spermatozoa are formed   _____

ADVANCED
RECALL

Exercise 2

Match each medical term with its meaning.

epididymis	semen	testis
testosterone	glans penis	prostate gland

Definition   **Term**

1. male hormone produced by the testes   _____

2. bulbous tip of the penis   _____

3. coiled duct on top of testes that transports spermatozoa   _____

4. fluid containing spermatozoa and fluids from glands   _____

5. gland that surrounds the top of the urethra   _____

6. male reproductive gland that produces spermatozoa and testosterone   _____

■ WORD PARTS

Note that some word parts that have been introduced earlier in the book may not be repeated here.

Combining Forms

Combining Form	Meaning
andr/o	male
balan/o	glans penis
epididym/o	epididymis
orch/o, orchi/o, orchid/o, test/o, testicul/o	testis, testicle
prostat/o	prostate
sperm/o, spermat/o	sperm, spermatozoon
vas/o	duct, vessel, vas deferens*
vesicul/o	fluid-filled sac (seminal vesicle)*

*In this chapter, the combining form *vas/o* will refer specifically to the vas deferens and the combining form *vesicul/o* will refer to the seminal vesicle.

Prefixes

Prefix	Meaning
an-	without, not
crypt-	hidden

Suffixes

Suffix	Meaning
-cele	herniation, protrusion
-genesis	originating, producing
-ism	condition of
-lith	stone, calculus
-lysis	destruction, breakdown, separation
-pathy	disease
-pexy	surgical fixation
-plasty	surgical repair, reconstruction
-rrhea	flow, discharge
-stomy	surgical opening
-tomy	incision

■ Exercises: Word Parts

SIMPLE
RECALL

Exercise 3

Write the meaning for the combining form given.

1. prostat/o _____

2. sperm/o _____

3. andr/o   _____

4. vesicul/o   _____

5. orchid/o   _____

6. balan/o   _____

7. epididym/o   _____

8. spermat/o   _____

9. vas/o   _____

10. test/o   _____

Exercise 4

SIMPLE
RECALL

Write the correct prefix or suffix for the meaning given.

1. hidden   _____

2. destruction, breakdown   _____

3. condition of   _____

4. herniation   _____

5. incision   _____

6. without   _____

7. surgical fixation   _____

8. surgical repair   _____

9. surgical opening   _____

Exercise 5

ADVANCED
RECALL

Match each combining form with its meaning.

orchi/o   balan/o   prostat/o
vas/o   vesicul/o

Meaning   **Term**

1. male reproductive gland that produces spermatozoa
and testosterone   _____

2. bulbous tip of the penis   _____

3. fluid-filled sac (seminal vesicle)   _____

4. a duct or a vessel   _____

5. gland that surrounds the top of the urethra   _____

TERM CONSTRUCTION

Exercise 6

Build a medical term for each definition, using one of the listed combining forms and one of the listed suffixes.

Combining forms	Suffixes
orchi/o	-genesis
andr/o	-rrhea
vas/o	-ectomy
spermat/o	-lith
balan/o	-pathy
prostat/o	-itis
vesicul/o	-pexy

1. excision of the vas deferens _____

2. disease found only in males _____

3. stone in the prostate _____

4. inflammation of a seminal vesicle _____

5. formation of spermatozoa _____

6. discharge from the glans penis _____

7. surgical fixation of a testicle _____

■ MEDICAL TERMS

Adjectives and Other Related Terms

Term	Pronunciation	Meaning
balanic	ba-lan'ik	pertaining to the glans penis
coitus	kō'i-tŭs	sexual intercourse
condom	kŏn'dom	sheath for the penis worn during intercourse for prevention of conception or infection
ejaculation	ē-jak'yū-lā'shŭn	expulsion of semen from the male urethra
epididymal	ep'i-did'i-măl	pertaining to the epididymis
prostatic	pros-tat'ik	pertaining to the prostate
puberty	pyū'bĕr-tē	period of development when secondary sex characteristics develop and the ability to reproduce begins
spermatic	spĕr-mat'ik	pertaining to sperm
spermicide	spĕr'mi-sīd	agent that kills spermatozoa
testicular	tes-tik'yū-lăr	pertaining to a testicle

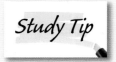

Study Tip

Prostatic vs. Prosthetic: Avoid confusing these sound-alike terms. Prostatic means relating to the prostate. A prosthetic is a fabricated substitute for a damaged or missing part of the body.

■ Exercises: Adjectives and Other Related Terms

SIMPLE
RECALL

Exercise 7

Write the correct medical term for the definition given.

1. pertaining to the prostate   _____

2. pertaining to a testicle   _____

3. sheath for the penis worn during intercourse   _____

4. expulsion of semen from a male urethra   _____

5. pertaining to the epididymis   _____

6. pertaining to sperm   _____

7. pertaining to the glans penis   _____

ADVANCED
RECALL

Exercise 8

Circle the term that is most appropriate for the meaning of the sentence.

1. Mrs. Perez's preferred form of birth control is a(n) (*coitus, spermicide, ejaculation*).

2. Dr. Smyth suspected that Mr. Lee had a problem with his testes, so he performed a (*prostatic, balanic, testicular*) examination.

3. The patient reported fluid coming from his penis; this is known as a(n) (*balanic, testicular, epididymal*) discharge.

4. Dr. Jovan explained that the patient's prostate had increased in size, a condition also referred to as (*testicular, prostatic, spermatic*) enlargement.

5. Because of his developmental changes, 13-year-old Jimmy Petit was thought to be going through (*ejaculation, puberty, spermatic*).

6. Mr. Cuomo was diagnosed with a(n) (*epididymal, balanic, spermatic*) infection, which is located in the coiled duct on top of the testes.

7. The physician asked Mr. Ackerman if he knew the correct way to use a (*coitus, puberty, condom*).

Exercise 9

TERM CONSTRUCTION

Write the combining form used in the medical term, followed by the meaning of the combining form.

Term	Combining Form	Combining Form Definition
1. testicular	_____	_____
2. prostatic	_____	_____
3. balanic	_____	_____
4. epididymal	_____	_____
5. spermicide	_____	_____

Symptoms and Medical Conditions

Term	Pronunciation	Meaning
andropathy	an-drop′ă-thē	disease found only in males
anorchism	an-ōr′kizm	condition of being without a testis or testes
aspermia	ă-spĕr′mē-ă	absence of sperm; inability to produce sperm
balanitis	bal′ă-nī′tis	inflammation of the glans penis
balanorrhea	bal′ă-nō-rē′ă	abnormal discharge from the glans penis
benign prostatic hyperplasia (BPH), *syn.* benign prostatic hypertrophy (BPH)	bē-nīn′ pros-tat′ik hī-pĕr-plā′zhē-ă, hī-pĕr′trō-fē	enlargement of the prostate gland (Fig. 10-2)
cryptorchidism	krip-tōr′ki-dizm	condition of hidden testis (or testes); failure of the testes to descend into the scrotum before birth (Fig. 10-3)

(continued)

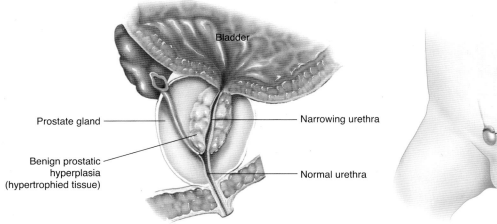

Figure 10-2 Benign prostatic hyperplasia.

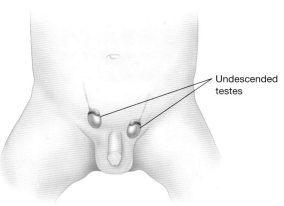

Figure 10-3 Cryptorchidism.

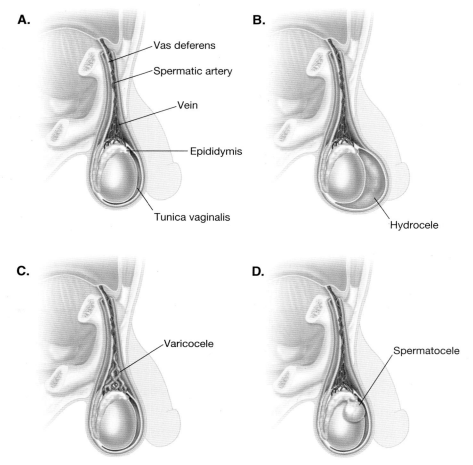

Figure 10-4 Abnormalities of the scrotum. **A.** Normal scrotum. **B.** Hydrocele. **C.** Varicocele. **D.** Spermatocele.

Symptoms and Medical Conditions *(continued)*

Term	Pronunciation	Meaning
epididymitis	ep′i-did-i-mī′tis	inflammation of the epididymis
erectile dysfunction (ED)	ē-rek′tĭl dis-fŭngk′shŭn	inability of a male to attain or maintain an erection
hydrocele	hī′drō-sēl	accumulation of fluid in the scrotum (Fig. 10-4B)
oligospermia	ol′i-gō-spĕr′mē-ă	scanty production of sperm
orchitis, *syn.* orchiditis, testitis	ōr-kī′tis, ōr′ki-dī′tis, tes-tī′tis	inflammation of a testis or testicle
Peyronie disease	pā-rō-nē′ di-zēz′	development of abnormal scar tissue, or plaques, in tissues inside the penis, causing bending of an erect penis
phimosis	fī-mō′sis	narrowing of the opening of the prepuce that prevents it from being drawn back over the glans penis (Fig. 10-5)

(continued)

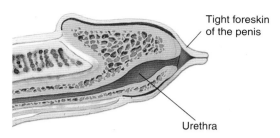

Figure 10-5 Phimosis.

Tight foreskin of the penis

Urethra

Symptoms and Medical Conditions *(continued)*

Term	Pronunciation	Meaning
priapism	prī′ă-pizm	abnormal persistent erection of the penis
prostatitis	pros′tă-tī′tis	inflammation of the prostate
prostatolith	pros-tat′ō-lith	stone or calculus in the prostate
prostatorrhea	pros′tă-tō-rē′ă	discharge from the prostate
spermatocele	spĕr′mă-tō-sēl′	cyst in the epididymis containing spermatozoa (Fig. 10-4D)
testicular torsion	tes-tik′yū-lăr tōr′shŭn	twisting of the spermatic cord, causing a decrease in blood flow to the penis
varicocele	var′i-kō-sēl′	enlargement of veins in the spermatic cord (Fig. 10-4C)
Sexually Transmitted Diseases (STDs)		
acquired immunodeficiency syndrome (AIDS)	ă-kwīrd′ im′yū-nō-dē-fish′ĕn-sē sin′drōm	disease of the immune system caused by infection with human immunodeficiency virus (HIV)
chlamydia	klă-mid′ē-ă	bacterial sexually transmitted disease that can occur with no symptoms (sometimes referred to as the silent sexually transmitted disease) until it progresses to where it damages organs; the most common STD in the United States
condyloma	kon′di-lō′mă	a wartlike lesion on the genitals
genital herpes	jen′i-tăl hĕr′pēz	inflammatory sexually transmitted disease caused by the herpes simplex virus; symptoms include blisters or ulcerative lesions on the genitals
gonorrhea	gon′ŏ-rē′ă	contagious, inflammatory, sexually transmitted disease affecting mucous membranes of the genitals and urinary system
human immunodeficiency virus (HIV)	hyū′măn im′yū-nō-dē-fish′ĕn-sē vī′rŭs	a virus that weakens the body's immune system and can cause AIDS
human papillomavirus (HPV)	hyū′măn pap′i-lō′mă-vī′rŭs	viral sexually transmitted disease that causes genital warts and other symptoms (Fig. 10-6)
sexually transmitted disease (STD) *syn.* venereal disease (VD)	sek′shū-ă-lē tranz-mit′ĕd di-zēz′, vĕ-nēr′ē-ăl di-zēz′	a communicable disease spread from one person to another primarily through sexual contact
syphilis	sif′i-lis	bacterial sexually transmitted disease that causes sores called chancres; can spread to other parts of the body (Fig. 10-7)

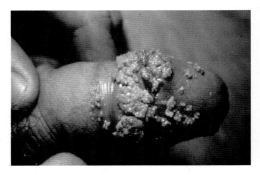

Figure 10-6 Genital warts caused by human papillomavirus.

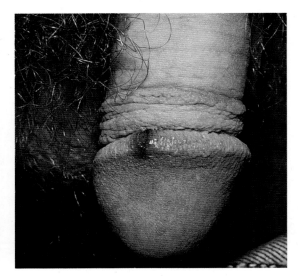

Figure 10-7 Syphilitic chancre.

■ Exercises: Symptoms and Medical Conditions

Exercise 10

Write the meaning of the term given.

1. prostatitis _____

2. priapism _____

3. aspermia _____

4. balanorrhea _____

5. epididymitis _____

6. phimosis _____

7. condyloma _____

Exercise 11

Circle the term that is most appropriate for the meaning of the sentence.

1. The bacterial sexually transmitted disease that can occur with no symptoms until it reaches a serious stage is called (*syphilis, chlamydia, gonorrhea*).

2. (*Gonorrhea, Human papillomavirus, Genital herpes*) is a sexually transmitted disease that causes blisters or ulcerative lesions on the genitals.

3. When veins in the spermatic cord enlarge, it is called a (*phimosis, varicocele, prostatolith*).

4. (*Gonorrhea, Condyloma, Genital herpes*) is a sexually transmitted disease that affects the mucous membranes of the genitals and urinary system.

5. A disease of the immune system caused by infection with HIV is called (*human papillomavirus, syphilis, acquired immunodeficiency syndrome*).

6. A patient with an accumulation of fluid in the scrotum has a (*spermatocele, condyloma, hydrocele*).

7. (*Erectile dysfunction, Benign prostatic hypertrophy, Priapism*) is a condition in which the prostate is enlarged.

8. When a patient cannot attain or maintain an erection, he has a condition called (*chlamydia, phimosis, erectile dysfunction*).

ADVANCED
RECALL

Exercise 12

Complete each sentence by writing in the correct medical term.

1. A sexually transmitted disease that causes genital warts is _____.

2. Enlargement of the prostate gland is called _____.

3. The virus that weakens the body's immune system and causes AIDS is known as

   _____.

4. Any disease transmitted through sexual contact is known as a(n)

   _____.

5. An epididymal cyst containing spermatozoa is a(n) _____.

6. A condition where there is twisting of the spermatic cord is a(n) _____.

7. A sexually transmitted disease that causes chancres is _____.

8. Development of abnormal scar tissue, or plaques, in tissues inside the penis is called

   _____.

TERM
CONSTRUCTION

Exercise 13

Build the correct medical term for the meaning given. Write the term in the blank indicating the word parts (P, prefix; CF, combining form; S, suffix).

1. cyst in the epididymis containing spermatozoa   _____ / _____

                                                            CF   S

2. inflammation of the prostate   _____ / _____

                                                            CF   S

3. abnormal discharge from the glans penis   _____ / _____
                                                                   CF   S

4. absence of sperm   _____ / _____ / _____
                                                          P   CF   S

5. inflammation of a testis   _____ / _____
                                                                   CF   S

6. inflammation of the glans penis   _____ / _____
                                                                   CF   S

7. condition of hidden testes   _____ / _____ / _____
                                                          P   CF   S

8. inflammation of the epididymis   _____ / _____
                                                                   CF   S

TERM
CONSTRUCTION

Exercise 14

Break the given medical term into its word parts and define each part. Then define the medical term.

For example:
orchitis   *word parts:*   orchi/o / -itis
                meanings: testicle / inflammation of
                term meaning: inflammation of the testicles

1. andropathy   *word parts:*   _____ / _____

                     meanings: _____ / _____

                     term meaning: _____

2. prostatolith *word parts:*   _____ / _____

                     meanings: _____ / _____

                     term meaning: _____

3. balanitis   *word parts:*   _____ / _____

                     meanings: _____ / _____

                     term meaning: _____

4. oligospermia *word parts:*   _____ / _____ / _____

                     meanings: _____ / _____ / _____

                     term meaning: _____

5. anorchism   *word parts:*   _____ / _____ / _____

                              meanings: _____ / _____ / _____

                              term meaning: _____

6. prostatorrhea   *word parts:*   _____ / _____

                              meanings: _____ / _____

                              term meaning: _____

7. cryptorchidism   *word parts:*   _____ / _____ / _____

                              meanings: _____ / _____ / _____

                              term meaning: _____

Tests and Procedures

Term	Pronunciation	Meaning
Laboratory Test		
prostate-specific antigen (PSA) test	pros′tāt-spĕ-sif′ik an′ti-jen	blood test that measures the amount of prostate-specific antigen in the blood to screen for benign prostatic hyperplasia (BPH) or prostate cancer
Diagnostic Procedures		
digital rectal examination (DRE)	dij′i-tăl rek′tăl eg-zam′i-nā′shŭn	assessment done by inserting a finger into the male rectum to determine the size and shape of the prostate through the rectal wall (Fig. 10-8)
transrectal ultrasound (TRUS)	trans-rek′tăl ŭl′tră-sownd	ultrasound imaging of the prostate done through the rectum

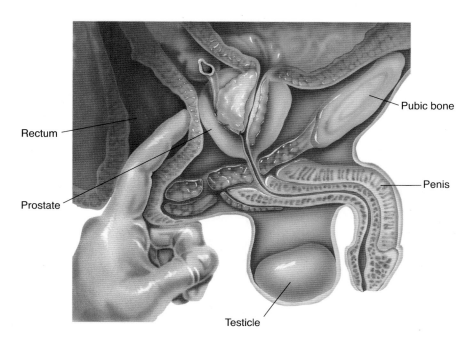

Rectum

Prostate

Testicle

Pubic bone

Penis

Figure 10-8 Digital rectal examination.

■ Exercise: Tests and Procedures

ADVANCED RECALL

Exercise 15

Match each medical term with its meaning.

digital rectal examination   prostatic-specific antigen   transrectal ultrasound

Definition   **Term**

1. ultrasound imaging of the prostate through the rectum   _____

2. examination of the prostate by inserting a
   finger into the rectum   _____

3. blood test that screens for BPH or prostate cancer   _____

Surgical Interventions and Therapeutic Procedures

Term	Pronunciation	Meaning
balanoplasty	bal'ăn-ō-plas'tē	surgical repair or reconstruction of the glans penis
circumcision	ser'kŭm-sizh'ŭn	excision of the prepuce (foreskin) from the penis (Fig. 10-9)
epididymectomy	ep'i-did-i-mek'tŏ-mē	excision of an epididymis
orchidectomy, *syn.* orchiectomy	ōr'ki-dek'tŏ-mē, ōr'kē-ek'tŏ-mē	excision of a testis
orchidopexy, *syn.* orchiopexy	ōr-kid'ō-peks'ē, ōr'kē-ō-peks'ē	surgical fixation of a testis; used to bring an undescended testicle into the scrotum
orchidotomy, *syn.* orchiotomy	ōr'kid-ot'ŏ-mē, ōr'kē-ot'ŏ-mē	incision into a testis
orchioplasty	ōr'kē-ō-plas'tē	surgical repair or reconstruction of a testis

(continued)

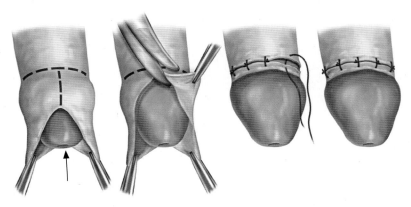

Figure 10-9 Circumcision.

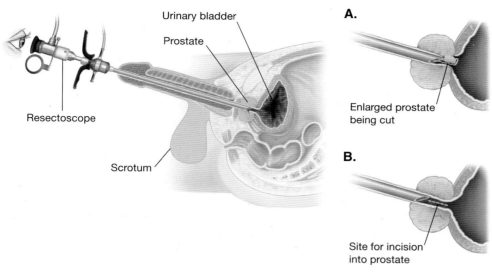

Figure 10-10   Transurethral resection of the prostate (TURP).

Surgical Interventions and Therapeutic Procedures *(continued)*

Term	Pronunciation	Meaning
penile implant	pē′nīl im′plant	surgical procedure to place a penile prosthesis for patients with erectile dysfunction
prostatectomy	pros′tă-tek′tŏ-mē	excision of the prostate
prostatolithotomy	pros′tă-tō-li-thot′ŏ-mē	incision to remove a stone from the prostate
transurethral incision of the prostate (TUIP)	trans′yū-rē′thrăl in-sizh′ŭn of the pros′tāt	surgical procedure that widens the urethra by making small incisions in the bladder and the prostate gland to facilitate urination
transurethral resection of the prostate (TURP)	trans′yū-rē′thrăl rē-sek′shŭn of the pros′tāt	removal of prostatic tissue through the urethra using a resectoscope; used for treatment of benign prostatic hyperplasia (Fig. 10-10)
vasectomy	va-sek′tŏ-mē	excision of a segment of the vas deferens to cause male sterility (Fig. 10-11)

(continued)

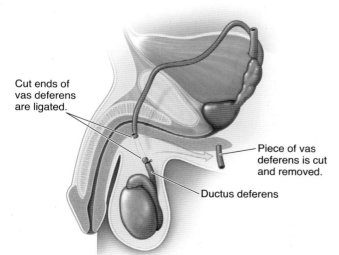

Figure 10-11   In a vasectomy, a piece of the vas deferens is cut and removed.

Surgical Interventions and Therapeutic Procedures *(continued)*

Term	Pronunciation	Meaning
vasovasostomy	vā'sō-vă-sos'tŏ-mē	creation of a new opening using an incision between two pieces of vas deferens to reverse the effects of a vasectomy
vesiculectomy	vĕ-sik'yū-lek'tŏ-mē	excision of a seminal vesicle

■ Exercises: Surgical Interventions and Therapeutic Procedures

Exercise 16

SIMPLE RECALL

Write the meaning of the term given.

1. vasovasostomy   _____

2. circumcision   _____

3. orchiectomy   _____

4. prostatolithotomy   _____

5. transurethral resection of the prostate   _____

6. penile implant   _____

Exercise 17

ADVANCED RECALL

Match each medical term with its meaning.

prostatolithotomy   orchioplasty   epididymectomy
vasectomy   prostatectomy   orchiectomy

Definition   **Term**

1. surgical repair of a testicle   _____

2. excision of an epididymis   _____

3. incision to remove a stone from the prostate   _____

4. excision of a testicle   _____

5. male sterilization procedure   _____

6. excision of the prostate   _____

TERM
CONSTRUCTION

Exercise 18

Write the remainder of the term for the meaning given.

1. excision of the epididymis   _____ectomy

2. surgical repair or reconstruction of a testis   orchio_____

3. excision of a seminal vesicle   vesicul_____

4. incision into a testis   orchido_____

5. excision of the vas deferens   _____ectomy

TERM
CONSTRUCTION

Exercise 19

Break the given medical term into its word parts and define each part. Then define the medical term.

For example:
   orchitis   *word parts:*   orchi/o / -itis
                  meanings: testicle / inflammation of
                  term meaning: inflammation of the testicles

1. orchiotomy   *word parts:*   _____ / _____

                  meanings: _____ / _____

                  term meaning: _____

2. balanoplasty   *word parts:*   _____ / _____

                  meanings: _____ / _____

                  term meaning: _____

3. prostatectomy   *word parts:*   _____ / _____

                  meanings: _____ / _____

                  term meaning: _____

4. orchiopexy   *word parts:*   _____ / _____

                  meanings: _____ / _____

                  term meaning: _____

5. vasectomy   *word parts:*   _____ / _____

                  meanings: _____ / _____

                  term meaning: _____

Medications and Drug Therapies

Term	Pronunciation	Meaning
antiretroviral	an'tē-ret'rō-vī'răl	drug used for the treatment of infection by a retrovirus, primarily human immunodeficiency virus (HIV)
antiviral	an'tē-vī'răl	drug used specifically for treating viral infections
impotence agent	im'pŏ-tĕns ā'jĕnt	drug used to treat erectile dysfunction
vasodilator	vā'sō-dī'lā-tŏr	drug used to open blood vessels; may be used to treat benign prostatic hypertrophy and erectile dysfunction

■ Exercise: Medications and Drug Therapies

Exercise 20

SIMPLE
RECALL

Write the correct medication or drug therapy term for the definition given.

1. drug used to treat erectile dysfunction   _____

2. drug used to treat infection caused by a retrovirus   _____

3. drug used to open blood vessels   _____

4. drug used specifically to treat viral infections   _____

Specialties and Specialists

Term	Pronunciation	Meaning
urology	yūr-ol'ŏ-jē	medical specialty focusing on the study and treatment of conditions of the urinary system and male reproductive system
urologist	yūr-ol'ŏ-jist	physician who specializes in urology

■ Exercise: Specialties and Specialists

Exercise 21

SIMPLE
RECALL

Write the correct medical term for the definition given.

1. specialty concerned with conditions of the urinary system   _____

2. physician who specializes in urology   _____

Abbreviations

Abbreviation	Meaning
AIDS	acquired immunodeficiency syndrome
BPH	benign prostatic hyperplasia; benign prostatic hypertrophy
DRE	digital rectal examination
ED	erectile dysfunction
HIV	human immunodeficiency virus
HPV	human papillomavirus
PSA	prostate-specific antigen
STD	sexually transmitted disease
TRUS	transrectal ultrasound
TUIP	transurethral incision of the prostate
TURP	transurethral resection of the prostate
VD	venereal disease

■ Exercises: Abbreviations

SIMPLE
RECALL

Exercise 22

Write the meaning of each abbreviation.

1. BPH _____

2. TUIP _____

3. ED _____

4. HIV _____

5. PSA _____

6. VD _____

7. TRUS _____

ADVANCED
RECALL

Exercise 23

Write the meaning of each abbreviation used in these sentences.

1. The patient had an enlarged prostate, so the physician scheduled him for a **TURP**.

2. The physician counseled the patient about the risks of getting an **STD**.

_____

3. At the patient's annual physical, the physician performed a **DRE**.

_____

4. The patient's genital warts were caused by an **HPV** infection.

_____

5. The human immunodeficiency virus caused the patient to develop **AIDS**.

_____

6. The patient's oliguria was determined to be caused by **BPH**.

_____

Review of Terms for Anatomy and Physiology

VISUAL

Exercise 24

Write the correct terms on the blanks for the anatomic structures indicated.

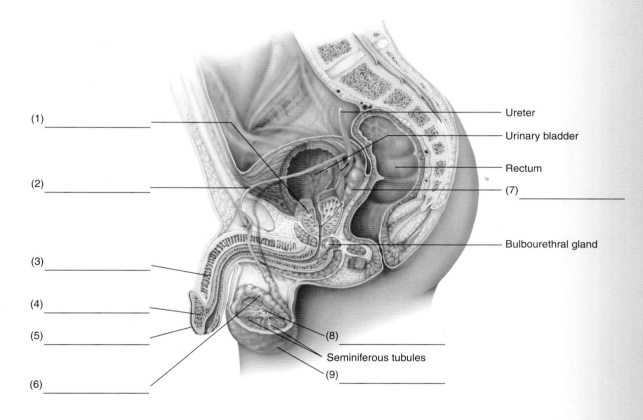

(1) _____

(2) _____

(3) _____

(4) _____

(5) _____

(6) _____

Ureter

Urinary bladder

Rectum

(7) _____

Bulbourethral gland

(8) _____

Seminiferous tubules

(9) _____

Understanding Term Structure

TERM CONSTRUCTION

Exercise 25

Write the combining form used in the medical term, followed by the meaning of the combining form.

Term	Combining Form	Combining Form Definition
1. testicular	_____	_____
2. prostatitis	_____	_____

3. balanorrhea _____ _____

4. anorchism _____ _____

5. epididymectomy _____ _____

6. spermatic _____ _____

7. vesiculectomy _____ _____

8. andropathy _____ _____

Exercise 26

TERM
CONSTRUCTION

For each term, first write the meaning of the term. Then write the meaning of the word parts in that term.

1. vasectomy _____

vas/o _____

-ectomy _____

2. prostatorrhea _____

prostat/o _____

-rrhea _____

3. balanitis _____

balan/o _____

-itis _____

4. epididymal _____

epididym/o _____

-al _____

5. orchidopexy _____

orchid/o _____

-pexy _____

6. prostatolith _____

prostat/o _____

-lith _____

7. orchioplasty _____

orchid/o _____

-plasty _____

8. vesiculectomy _____

vesicul/o _____

-ectomy _____

Comprehension Exercises

Exercise 27

COMPREHENSION **Write a short answer for each question.**

1. How is gonorrhea transmitted? _____

2. Why would a patient undergo a vasovasostomy? _____

_____

3. What is the name of the hormone produced by the testes? _____

4. In addition to sperm, what other substances constitute semen? _____

_____

5. What is a cyst in the epididymis that contains sperm called? _____

6. Genital warts are a symptom of what sexually transmitted disease? _____

7. What structure is assessed during a digital rectal examination? _____

8. What layer of skin is left intact on an uncircumcised male penis? _____

9. Which medical condition involves the testes and occurs before birth? _____

10. Males who no longer want to produce offspring often have which procedure? _____

_____

11. Where does abnormal scar tissue form in a patient with Peyronie disease? _____

_____

Exercise 28

COMPREHENSION **Circle the letter of the best answer in the following questions.**

1. Which procedure involves the removal of prostatic tissue with a resectoscope?

    A. vasovasostomy
    B. transurethral resection of the prostate
    C. orchiectomy
    D. circumcision

2. An examination of the prostate might reveal which condition?

    A. phimosis
    B. condyloma
    C. varicocele
    D. benign prostatic hyperplasia

3. Reproduction is not possible until a male goes through what period of development?

    A. prepuce
    B. puberty
    C. balanorrhea
    D. epididymis

4. Which test is performed to screen for BPH?

    A. transrectal ultrasound
    B. transurethral resection of the prostate
    C. prostate-specific antigen test
    D. balanoplasty

5. Another term for sexual intercourse is:

    A. coitus
    B. prepuce
    C. priapism
    D. puberty

6. When there is an abnormal persistent erection of the penis, the condition is called:

    A. benign prostatic hypertrophy
    B. erectile dysfunction
    C. priapism
    D. syphilis

7. Which of the following conditions is an STD?

    A. condyloma
    B. hydrocele
    C. varicocele
    D. anorchism

8. What is the name of the male sex cell needed to fertilize an ovum?

    A. testosterone
    B. bulbourethral glands
    C. glans penis
    D. spermatozoon

9. A patient with chancres would likely be diagnosed with which condition?

    A. AIDS
    B. gonorrhea
    C. syphilis
    D. chlamydia

10. Twisting of the spermatic cord is known as:

    A. anorchism
    B. testicular torsion
    C. testicular cancer
    D. spermatocele

11. The procedure that involves an ultrasound of the prostate done through the rectum is called a:

    A. digital rectal examination
    B. prostatolithotomy
    C. circumcision
    D. transrectal ultrasound

12. A sheath for the penis worn during intercourse to prevent conception or infection is a:

    A. condyloma
    B. semen
    C. condom
    D. coitus

13. A patient wanting to reverse his vasectomy needs to undergo a(n):

    A. orchioplasty
    B. vasovasostomy
    C. transurethral resection of the prostate
    D. vesiculectomy

14. When semen is expelled from the male urethra, it is called:

    A. ejaculation
    B. orchiotomy
    C. erectile dysfunction
    D. priapism

15. The sexually transmitted disease that can occur with no symptoms until it becomes severe is:

    A. chlamydia
    B. syphilis
    C. gonorrhea
    D. human papillomavirus

16. An agent that is used to prevent pregnancy by killing the male sex cell is called:

    A. prostate-specific antigen
    B. testosterone
    C. ejaculation
    D. spermicide

17. Which condition might be resolved as a result of circumcision?

    A. varicocele
    B. phimosis
    C. priapism
    D. testicular torsion

18. The male hormone produced by the testes is:

    A. semen
    B. testosterone
    C. prostatorrhea
    D. balanorrhea

Application and Analysis

CASE REPORTS

APPLICATION

Exercise 29

Read the case reports and circle the letter of your answer choice for the following questions.

CASE 10-1

Mr. Kendall was seen in the office because of a lump he discovered in his testes when he performed a testicular self-examination. He was concerned about the possibility of having testicular cancer. He denied having any balanorrhea. Examination revealed a circumcised male with an enlargement in the scrotum consistent with a varicocele.

1. The term that means abnormal discharge from the glans penis is:

    A. semen
    B. testosterone
    C. prostatorrhea
    D. balanorrhea

2. The term that means enlargement of veins in the spermatic cord is:

    A. spermatocele
    B. varicocele
    C. hydrocele
    D. cystocele

3. The term that refers to the sac that contains the testes is:

    A. testicular
    B. varicocele
    C. scrotum
    D. circumcised

CASE 10-2

Mr. Glower was seen in the office today for consideration of a vasovasostomy. He underwent a vasectomy 5 years ago. He had a past history of an STD. Findings of genital examination today were significant for a single condylomatous lesion on the penis as well as for phimosis. After discussion of the risks and benefits of surgery, he has decided to go ahead with it. The procedure has been scheduled for next week.

4. The term that involves creating a new opening between two severed pieces of vas deferens is:

    A. vasectomy
    B. vasovasostomy
    C. phimosis
    D. balanoplasty

5. The condyloma on the patient's penis could be described as a(n):

    A. blister or ulcerative lesion
    B. enlargement of the veins

    C. agent that kills sperm
    D. wartlike lesion

6. The term *phimosis* means there is a(n):

    A. narrowing of the glans penis
    B. enlargement of the penis
    C. enlargement of the veins in the spermatic cord
    D. accumulation of fluid in the scrotum

MEDICAL RECORD ANALYSIS

MEDICAL RECORD 10-1

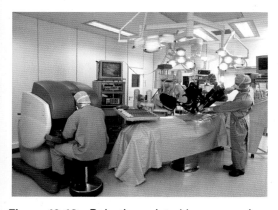

Tim Mullins, the patient in the History and Physical report that follows, was previously diagnosed with prostate cancer and is being admitted to County General Hospital for a prostatectomy. As a diagnostic medical sonographer, you performed the transrectal ultrasound that helped to confirm the presence of this patient's tumor.

Figure 10-12 Robotic-assisted laparoscopic prostatectomy.

Medical Record

HISTORY AND PHYSICAL

HPI: The patient was seen in the office 1 month ago for symptoms of dysuria, oliguria, and nocturia, which had been worsening over the preceding 3 weeks. He was concerned about possible recurrence of BPH.

PMH: Past medical history was remarkable for benign prostatic hyperplasia, which was treated medically 3 years ago with good results. He also reported having a hydrocele approximately 5 years ago and an orchiopexy as a child for cryptorchidism. He also has hypertension, which is under good control with medication and diet.

PE: Physical examination revealed no tenderness to palpation of the pubic area. A digital rectal exam was performed and revealed enlargement of the prostate gland. The gland was notably firm and nodular. Examination was otherwise unremarkable.

Laboratory and radiologic testing was ordered. A PSA was highly elevated at 25 ng/mL. A prostatic acid phosphatase test revealed elevated enzyme levels. Transrectal ultrasound was also performed and confirmed the presence of a tumor. Using ultrasound guidance, a needle biopsy of the prostate was also performed and revealed the presence of malignant cells.

Dx: Diagnosis was prostate cancer.

PLAN: Patient is admitted at this time for a robotic-assisted laparoscopic prostatectomy for minimally invasive removal of his tumor.

APPLICATION

Exercise 30

Write the appropriate medical terms used in this medical record on the blanks after their definitions. Note that not all the terms appear in the chapter, but you should be able to identify these terms based on word parts that are included in this chapter.

1. exam by feeling the prostate through the rectal wall _____

2. painful urination _____

3. accumulation of fluid in the scrotum _____

4. surgical fixation of a testis _____

5. imaging of the prostate done through the rectum _____

APPLICATION

Exercise 31

Read the medical report and circle the letter of your answer choice for the following questions.

1. The medical record indicates that the patient's PSA level was highly elevated. The abbreviation PSA stands for:

   A. prostatic acid phosphatase

   B. prostate-specific alkaline

   C. prostate symptom analysis

   D. prostate-specific antigen

2. Which of the patient's symptoms indicates he is urinating frequently at night?

   A. oliguria
   B. nocturia
   C. dysuria
   D. hematuria

3. As a child, the patient underwent surgery to correct:

   A. an undescended testicle
   B. enlargement of veins in the spermatic cord
   C. condition of being without a testis or testes
   D. abnormal persistent erection of the penis

4. The patient is admitted for a prostatectomy, or:

   A. excision of a segment of the vas deferens
   B. incision into a testis
   C. surgical fixation of a testis
   D. removal of the prostate

5. The abbreviation for enlargement of the prostate gland is:

   A. DRE
   B. PSA
   C. UTI
   D. BPH

Bonus Question

6. In what two procedures was ultrasound imaging used? _____

_____

MEDICAL RECORD 10-2

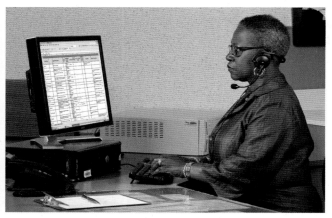

A medical transcriptionist transcribes the physician's dictated report.

Mr. Roberts was recently seen by his physician, who dictated his findings on completion of the exam. You, as a medical transcriptionist, transcribed the physician's dictated report to become a permanent part of the patient's medical record. The final transcribed record is as follows:

Medical Record

PROGRESS NOTE

SUBJECTIVE: The patient presents today with complaints of burning during urination, orchialgia, and balanorrhea for the past week. He denies having any condylomata, chancres, or other sores in the genital area or elsewhere on his body. He had one episode of syphilis many years ago, which was successfully treated with antibiotics. He admits to having unprotected coitus in the past few weeks. Contraceptive method is spermicide. The patient denies any previous history of STDs.

OBJECTIVE: Examination is within normal limits with the exception of scant yellow discharge from the glans penis, urethritis, and testicular edema. A culture was taken from the discharge and Gram stain was performed revealing gonorrhea bacterium. A urine sample was obtained and will be sent to the lab for STD screening to rule out concurrent chlamydial infection.

ASSESSMENT: Gonorrhea. Rule out chlamydia.

PLAN: Rocephin 1 g injection as administered for treatment of gonorrhea. Should the lab testing prove positive for chlamydia, oral antibiotics will be prescribed. The patient was also counseled regarding the transmission of STDs and safe sex measures, including the use of condoms. He was advised to notify his sexual partners about his diagnosis so they can be tested too. He was further advised to return should his symptoms return or not resolve following antibiotic therapy.

APPLICATION

Exercise 32

Write the appropriate medical terms used in this medical record on the blanks after their definitions. Note that not all these terms appear in the chapter, but you should be able to identify these terms based on word parts that are included in this chapter.

1. testicular pain   _____

2. discharge from the glans penis   _____

3. agent that kills sperm   _____

4. genital warts   _____

5. inflammation of the urethra   _____

APPLICATION

Exercise 33

Read the medical report and circle the letter of your answer choice for the following questions.

1. The STD that affects the mucous membranes of the genitals and urinary system is:

   A. genital herpes
   B. chlamydia
   C. syphilis
   D. gonorrhea

2. The term for a sore caused by syphilis is:

   A. chancre
   B. genital herpes
   C. condyloma
   D. chlamydia

3. The term for the silent STD is:

    A. human papillomavirus
    B. chlamydia
    C. syphilis
    D. genital herpes

4. _____ is the medical term for sexual intercourse.

    A. prepuce
    B. edema

    C. coitus
    D. priapism

5. _____ is the STD that causes chancres and can spread to other parts of the body.

    A. gonorrhea
    B. syphilis
    C. genital herpes
    D. chlamydia

Bonus Question

6. Using your medical dictionary, look up the word edema and write the definition here:

_____

Pronunciation and Spelling

AUDITORY

Exercise 34

Review the Chapter 10 terms in the Dictionary/Audio Glossary in the Student Resources and practice pronouncing each term, referring to the pronunciation guide as needed.

SPELLING

Exercise 35

Circle the correct spelling of each term.

1. skrotum	scrotum	scrotim
2. spermatazoon	spermatozoun	spermatozoon
3. semin	semun	semen
4. prostate	prostrate	prostat
5. coytus	coitis	coitus
6. epididimis	epididymus	epididymis
7. balanorrhea	balanorhea	balanorrhia
8. aspermea	aspermia	aspirmea
9. fimosis	phimosis	phemosis
10. hidrocele	hydrocele	hydroseal

11. prostatitis	prostratitis	prostatittis
12. vericocele	varicoseal	varicocele
13. chlamydia	clamydia	chlamidia
14. condiloma	condyloma	condylloma
15. sifilus	syphillis	syphilis

Media Connection

STUDENT
RESOURCES

Exercise 38

Complete each of the following activities available with the Student Resources. Check off each activity as you complete it, and record your score for the Chapter Quiz in the space provided.

Chapter Exercises

____ Flash Cards

____ Concentration

____ Abbreviation Match-Up

____ Roboterms

____ Word Builder

____ Fill the Gap

____ Break It Down

____ **Chapter Quiz**

____ True/False Body Building

____ Quiz Show

____ Complete the Case

____ Medical Record Review

____ Look and Label

____ Image Matching

____ Spelling Bee

Score: _____%

Additional Resources

____ Dictionary/Audio Glossary

____ Health Professions Careers: Diagnostic Medical Sonographer

____ Health Professions Careers: Medical Transcriptionist

Female Reproductive System, Obstetrics, and Neonatology

11

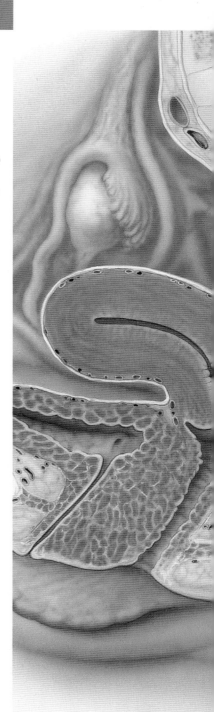

Chapter Outline

Objectives

After completion of this chapter you will be able to:

1. Describe the location of primary structures in the female reproductive system.

2. Describe terms related to the process of the menstrual cycle and obstetrics.

3. Define combing forms, prefixes, and suffixes related to the female reproductive system, obstetrics, and neonatology.

4. Define common medical terminology related to the female reproductive system, obstetrics, and neonatology, including adjectives and related terms, symptoms and conditions, tests and procedures, surgical interventions and therapeutic procedures, medications and drug therapies, and specialties.

5. Explain abbreviations for terms related to the female reproductive system, obstetrics, and neonatology.

6. Successfully complete all chapter exercises.

7. Explain terms used in case studies and medical records involving the female reproductive system and obstetrics.

8. Successfully complete all pronunciation and spelling exercises, and complete all interactive exercises included with the companion Student Resources.

■ ANATOMY AND PHYSIOLOGY

Functions

- To produce the female sex hormones
- To propagate life by producing and sustaining ova
- To transport ova to a site where they may be fertilized by spermatozoa
- To support and nurture a developing fetus in a favorable environment until birth
- To provide an infant's first source of nutrition and protective antibodies after birth through breast milk

Organs and Structures

- The external genital organs enable spermatozoa to enter the body, protect the internal genital organs from infectious organisms, and provide sexual pleasure.
- The internal genital organs are the structures involved in human reproduction and together form a pathway called the genital tract.
- The breasts are functionally a part of the female reproductive system because they contain the milk-producing organs that nourish an infant.

Terms Related to the Female Reproductive System
(Figs. 11-1 and 11-2)

Term	Pronunciation	Meaning
breasts	brests	female organs of milk secretion (Fig. 11-3)
areola	ă-rē'ō-lă	pigmented area around the breast nipple
lactiferous ducts	lak-tif'ĕr-ŭs dŭkts	channels that carry breast milk to the nipple
lactiferous lobules	lak-tif'ĕr-ŭs lob'yūlz	glands in the breast that make breast milk
mammary glands	măm'ă-rē glandz	modified sweat glands located in the breasts that prepare for milk production in anticipation of the birth of a fetus
mammary papilla	măm'ă-rē pă-pil'ă	breast nipple
genitalia	jen'i-tā'lē-ă	external and internal organs of reproduction
mons pubis	monz pyū'bis	rounded mound of fatty tissue that covers the pubic bone
ovaries	ō'vă-rēz	pair of oval reproductive glands attached to the uterus, which produce hormones and release ova (Fig. 11-4)
corpus luteum	kōr'pŭs lū'tē-ŭm	temporary endocrine gland formed in the ovary that secretes progesterone during the second half of the menstrual cycle
vesicular ovarian follicles, *syn.* graafian follicles	vĕ-sik'yū-lăr ō-var'ē-ăn fol'i-kĕlz, grah'fē-ăn fol'i-kĕlz	fluid-filled sacs in the ovaries, each containing an immature ovum (Fig. 11-5)
oocyte	ō'ō-sīt	an immature ovum contained in a follicle
ovum, *pl.* ova	ō'vŭm, ō'vă	an egg cell (Fig. 11-5)

(continued)

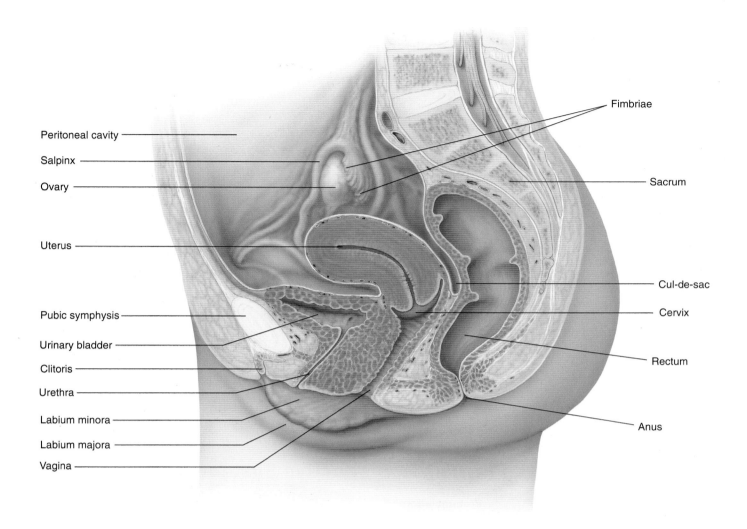

Peritoneal cavity

Salpinx

Ovary

Uterus

Pubic symphysis

Urinary bladder

Clitoris

Urethra

Labium minora

Labium majora

Vagina

Fimbriae

Sacrum

Cul-de-sac

Cervix

Rectum

Anus

Figure 11-1   The female reproductive system.

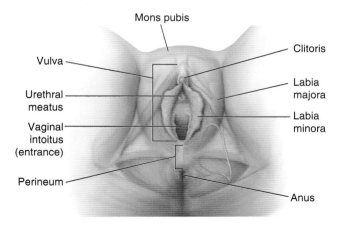

Mons pubis

Vulva

Urethral meatus

Vaginal intoitus (entrance)

Perineum

Clitoris

Labia majora

Labia minora

Anus

Figure 11-2   External female genitalia.

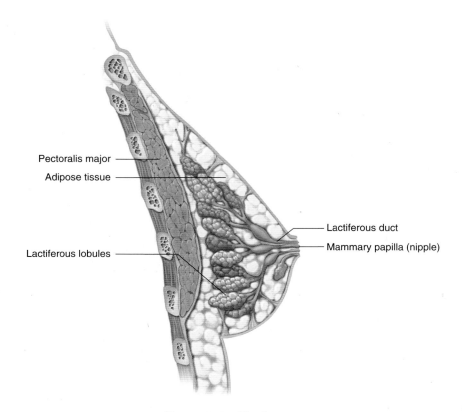

Figure 11-3 The breast.

Terms Related to the Female Reproductive System *(continued)*

Term	Pronunciation	Meaning
perineum	per'i-nē'ŭm	surface area between the thighs extending from the coccyx to the pubis that includes the anus posteriorly and the external genitalia anteriorly
salpinges, *syn.* fallopian tubes	sal-pin'jēz, fă-lō'pē-ăn tūbz	tubular structures that carry the ovum from the ovary to the uterus (Fig. 11-4)
fimbriae	fim'brē-ē	finger-like extensions of the salpinx that drape over the ovary

(continued)

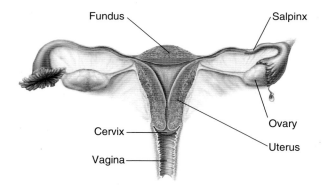

Figure 11-4 Ovaries and salpinges.

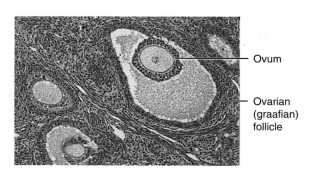

Figure 11-5 Microscopic view of the ovary.

Terms Related to the Female Reproductive System *(continued)*

Term	Pronunciation	Meaning
uterus, *syn.* womb	yū'těr-ŭs, wŭm	pear-shaped organ located in the middle of the pelvis that supports a growing fetus and is the site of menses (Fig. 11-6)
adnexa	ad-nek'să	appendages or adjunct parts; the adnexa of the uterus consist of the salpinges, ovaries, and the ligaments that hold them together
endometrium	en'dō-mē'trē-ŭm	inner lining of the uterus
myometrium	mī'ō-mē'trē-ŭm	thick, muscular middle layer of the uterus
perimetrium	per'i-mē'trē-ŭm	outer layer of the uterus that covers the body of the uterus and part of the cervix
cervix	sěr'viks	tubular, lower portion of the uterus that opens into the vagina
cervical os	sěr'vi-kăl os	opening of the cervical canal
fundus	fŭn'dŭs	dome-shaped top portion of the uterus that lies above the entrance of the salpinges
vagina, *syn.* birth canal	vă-jī'nă, bĭrth kă-nal'	muscular tube projecting inside a female that connects the uterus to the outside of the body

(continued)

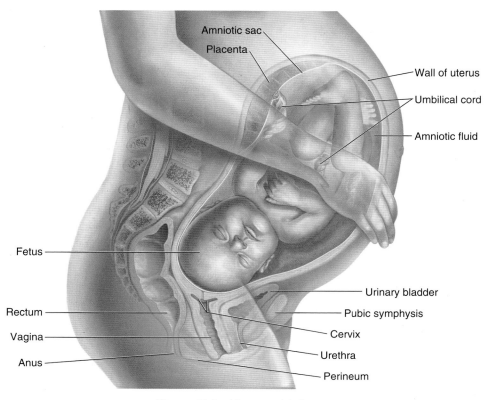

Figure 11-6 Uterus with fetus.

Terms Related to the Female Reproductive System (continued)

Term	Pronunciation	Meaning
greater vestibular glands, *syn.* Bartholin glands	grā'tĕr ves-tib'yū-lăr glandz, bahr'tō-lin glandz	glands that keep the vaginal mucosa moist and provide a lubricant for the vagina during sexual intercourse
introitus	in-trō'i-tŭs	opening of the vagina
vulva	vŭl'vă	the female external genital organs
clitoris	klit'ŏr-is	small (less than 2 cm) mass of erectile tissue in females that responds to sexual stimulation
labia	lā'bē-ă	two sets of skin folds that serve to cover the female external genital organs and tissues
labia majora	lā'bē-ă mă-jōr'ă	part of the labia that covers and protects the female external genital organs
labia minora	lā'bē-ă mi-nō'ră	inner folds of the labia that surround the openings to the vagina and urethra

Terms Related to Obstetrics

Term	Pronunciation	Meaning
amnion	am'nē-on	inner layer of membrane surrounding the fetus and containing the amniotic fluid
amniotic fluid	am'nē-ot'ik flū'id	fluid that encases the fetus and provides a cushion for the fetus as the mother moves
chorion	kōr'ē-on	outermost membrane surrounding the fetus
conception, *syn.* fertilization	kŏn-sep'shŭn, fĕr'til-ī-zā'shŭn	instant at which the spermatozoa and egg unite
effacement	ē-fās'mĕnt	thinning of the cervix in preparation for delivery
embryo	em'brē-ō	fertilized ovum from the time of implantation in the uterus until about the eighth week of gestation (Fig. 11-7)
fetus	fē'tŭs	developing embryo from the eighth week of gestation until delivery (Fig. 11-7)
gamete	gam'ēt	an organism's reproductive cell, such as sperm or egg cells
human chorionic gonadotropin (hCG)	hyū'măn kōr'ē-on'ik gō-nad'ō-trō'pin	hormone secreted by the fertilized ovum soon after conception
lactation	lak-tā'shŭn	production of breast milk by the mammary glands after childbirth
lochia	lō'kē-ă	discharges from the vagina of mucus, blood, and tissue debris following childbirth
ovulation	ov'yū-lā'shŭn	process of discharging one ovum from an ovary
placenta	plă-sen'tă	temporary organ implanted in the uterus through which the fetus receives nutrients and oxygen from the mother's blood and passes waste

(continued)

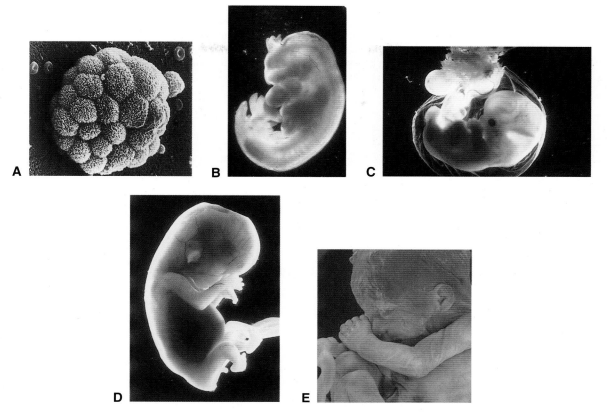

Figure 11-7   Human embryos and early fetus. **A.** Implantation in uterus 7 to 8 days after conception. **B.** Embryo at 32 days. **C.** Embryo at 37 days. **D.** Embryo at 41 days. **E.** Fetus between 12 and 15 weeks.

Terms Related to Obstetrics *(continued)*

Term	Pronunciation	Meaning
pregnancy, *syn.* gestation	preg'năn-sē, jes-tā'shŭn	state of a female after conception and until delivery
prolactin	prō-lak'tin	lactation-stimulating hormone
umbilical cord	ŭm-bil'i-kăl kōrd	cord composed of blood vessels and connective tissue that is connected to the fetus from the placenta

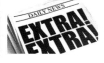 **STEM CELLS**   The umbilical cord is one of several sites where stem cells can be harvested. Stem cells are self-renewing—that is, they reproduce through cell division—and can produce many different types of specialized cells, such as blood cells, heart muscle tissue, or pancreatic cells. These cells are retrieved from the blood in the umbilical cord.

zygote	zī'gōt	cell resulting from the union of a sperm and oocyte

ANIMATION

View the animation *Ovulation and Fertilization* included with the Student Resources for an illustration of the process of ovulation.

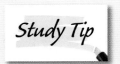

Study Tip   **Endometrium and Perimetrium:** When memorizing these parts of the uterus, let the prefixes guide you. Remember that *endo-* means *in, within*, thus endometrium is the inner lining of the uterus. *Peri-* means *around, surrounding,* so perimetrium is the outer layer that covers (surrounds) the body of the uterus.

■ Exercises: Anatomy and Physiology

SIMPLE
RECALL

Exercise 1

Write the correct anatomic structure for the definition given.

1. temporary organ implanted in the uterus   _____

2. channels that carry breast milk to the nipple   _____

3. inner lining of the uterus   _____

4. female organs of milk secretion   _____

5. organs of reproduction   _____

6. an egg cell   _____

7. membrane that surrounds the fetus   _____

8. cord that connects the placenta to the fetus   _____

9. breast nipple   _____

10. dome-shaped top portion of the uterus   _____

11. pigmented area around the nipple   _____

12. temporary endocrine gland   _____

13. sacs containing an immature ovum   _____

14. glands that keep vaginal mucosa moist   _____

15. cell resulting from union of sperm and oocyte   _____

Exercise 2

SIMPLE
RECALL

Write the meaning of the term given.

1. perimetrium   _____

2. amniotic fluid   _____

3. cervix _____

4. human chorionic gonadotropin _____

5. oocyte _____

6. chorion _____

7. salpinges _____

8. pregnancy _____

9. lactiferous lobules _____

10. prolactin _____

11. uterus _____

12. labia majora _____

13. embryo _____

Exercise 3

ADVANCED
RECALL

Circle the term that is most appropriate for the meaning of the sentence.

1. The (*corpus luteum, clitoris, mammary gland*) secretes progesterone.

2. The (*labia, ovaries, adnexa*) cover the female external genital organs.

3. (*Oocytes, Fimbriae, Lobules*) are like fingers that extend over the ovaries.

4. The fatty tissue that covers the pubic bone is called the (*mons pubis, perineum, vulva*).

5. An ovum is discharged from the ovary in a process called (*pregnancy, ripening, ovulation*).

6. Another name for the vaginal opening is the (*uterus, introitus, vulva*).

7. The (*labia minora, labia majora, mons pubis*) surround the opening of the vagina.

8. One purpose of the (*salpinges, uterus, ovaries*) is to release eggs.

9. Another name for the (*uterus, cervix, vagina*) is the "birth canal."

10. A(n) (*fetus, zygote, ovum*) is an early embryo.

Exercise 4

ADVANCED RECALL

Match each medical term with its meaning.

lactiferous lobules	gamete	ovaries	effacement
vulva	vagina	fetus	cervical os
lochia	lactation		

1. area containing the external genital organs _____

2. embryo from week eight until delivery _____

3. opening of the cervical canal _____

4. the production of breast milk _____

5. thinning of the cervix for delivery _____

6. an organism's reproductive cell _____

7. vaginal discharges following childbirth _____

8. the birth canal _____

9. glands in the breasts that make milk _____

10. they produce hormones and release eggs _____

Exercise 5

ADVANCED RECALL

Complete each sentence by writing in the correct medical term.

1. The inner lining of the uterus is called the _____.

2. The _____ is a structure that responds to sexual stimulation.

3. The _____ are the two sets of skin folds that cover the external genital organs and tissues.

4. The surface area between the thighs from the coccyx to the mons pubis is called the

    _____.

5. The _____ prepare for milk production for a newborn.

6. The organs of reproduction are generally referred to as _____.

7. A general term for appendages or adjunct parts is _____.

8. The _____ is the thick, muscular middle layer of the uterus.

■ WORD PARTS

Note that some word parts that have been introduced earlier in the book may not be repeated here.

Combining Forms

Combining Form	Meaning
Related to the Female Reproductive System	
cervic/o	neck, cervix (neck of uterus)
gyn/o, gynec/o	woman
hyster/o, metr/o, metri/o, uter/o	uterus
men/o, menstru/o	menstruation
my/o	muscle (uterus)
ovari/o, oophor/o	ovary
pelv/i	pelvis, pelvic cavity
perine/o	perineum
salping/o	salpinx, fallopian tube
vagin/o, colp/o	vagina
vulv/o, episi/o	vulva
Related to Obstetrics and Neonatology	
amni/o, amnion/o	amnion
cephal/o	head
chori/o	chorion
embry/o, embryon/o	embryo, immature form
fet/o	fetus
fund/o	fundus
galact/o, lact/o	milk
gestat/o	from conception to birth
gravid/o	pregnancy
hydr/o	water, fluid
mamm/o, mast/o	breast, mammary gland
nat/o	birth
olig/o	scanty, few
omphal/o	umbilicus, navel
pub/o	pubis
toc/o	labor, birth

Prefixes

Prefix	Meaning
ante-, pre-	before
dys-	painful, difficult, abnormal

(continued)

Prefixes *(continued)*

Prefix	Meaning
ecto-	outer, outside
endo-	in, within
micro-	small
multi-	many
neo-	new
nulli-	none
poly-	many, much
post-	after, behind
supra-	above

Suffixes

Suffix	Meaning
-arche	beginning
-asthenia	weakness
-cele	herniation, protrusion
-centesis	puncture to aspirate
-ia, -ism	condition of
-metry	measurement of
-partum	childbirth, labor
-pexy	surgical fixation
-plasia	formation, growth
-plasty	surgical repair, reconstruction
-rrhage, -rrhagia	flowing forth
-rrhaphy	suture
-rrhea	flow, discharge
-scopy	process of examining, examination
-tomy	incision

■ Exercises: Word Parts

SIMPLE
RECALL

Exercise 6

Write the meaning of the combining form given.

1. fund/o _____

2. pelv/i _____

3. cervic/o _____

4. mast/o _____

5. gestat/o   _____

6. pub/o   _____

7. salping/o   _____

8. colp/o   _____

9. gravid/o   _____

10. olig/o   _____

11. uter/o   _____

12. galact/o   _____

13. nat/o   _____

14. chori/o   _____

15. perine/o   _____

SIMPLE
RECALL

Exercise 7

Write the correct combining form or forms for the meaning given.

1. vagina   _____

2. woman   _____

3. muscle (uterus)   _____

4. salpinx   _____

5. breast, mammary gland   _____

6. head   _____

7. pregnancy   _____

8. perineum   _____

9. water, fluid   _____

10. labor, birth   _____

11. menstruation   _____

12. cervix   _____

13. milk   _____

14. vulva   _____

15. pubis   _____

Exercise 8

SIMPLE RECALL

Write the meaning of the prefix or suffix given.

1. supra- _____

2. -plasty _____

3. -tomy _____

4. nulli- _____

5. -cele _____

6. -metry _____

7. -rrhea _____

8. -ia _____

9. neo- _____

10. -arche _____

11. -rrhaphy _____

12. -centesis _____

13. ante- _____

14. endo- _____

15. -partum _____

Exercise 9

ADVANCED RECALL

Considering the meaning of the combining form from which the medical term is made, write the meaning of the medical term. (You have not yet learned many of these terms but can build their meaning from the word parts.)

Combining Form	Meaning	Medical Term	Meaning of Term
metr/o	uterus	metrorrhagia	1. _____
gynec/o	woman	gynecology	2. _____
hyster/o	uterus	hysterectomy	3. _____
mamm/o	breast	mammogram	4. _____
episi/o	vulva	episiotomy	5. _____
colp/o	vagina	colporrhaphy	6. _____

oophor/o	ovary	oophorectomy	7. _____
cervic/o	cervix	cervicitis	8. _____
vagin/o	vagina	vaginoplasty	9. _____
salping/o	salpinx	salpingectomy	10. _____

TERM
CONSTRUCTION

Exercise 10

Using the given combining form and word part from the earlier tables, build a medical term for the meaning given.

Combining Form	Meaning of Medical Term	Medical Term
gynec/o	one who specializes in the study of women	1. _____
hyster/o	process of examining the uterus	2. _____
colp/o	suturing of the vagina	3. _____
omphal/o	herniation of the umbilical cord	4. _____
vagin/o	inflammation of the vagina	5. _____
mamm/o	process of recording the breast	6. _____
amni/o	incision of the amnion (to induce labor)	7. _____
fet/o	pertaining to a fetus	8. _____
embry/o	study of an embryo	9. _____
mast/o	excision or surgical removal of a breast	10. _____

■ MEDICAL TERMS

Adjectives and Other Related Terms

Term	Pronunciation	Meaning
abdominopelvic	ab-dom′i-nō-pel′vik	pertaining to the abdomen and pelvis
chorionic	kōr′ē-on′ik	pertaining to the chorion
congenital	kŏn-jen′i-tăl	existing at birth
cystic	sis′tik	pertaining to or containing cysts
date of birth (DOB)	dāt bĭrth	the day of birth of a patient
embryonic	em′brē-on′ik	pertaining to an embryo
endometrial	en′dō-mē′trē-ăl	pertaining to or composed of endometrium

(continued)

Adjectives and Other Related Terms *(continued)*

Term	Pronunciation	Meaning
estimated date of confinement (EDC), *syn.* estimated date of delivery (EDD)	es′ti-mā′ted dāt kŏn-fīn′mĕnt, es′ti-mā′ted dāt dē-liv′ĕr-ē	the date at which an infant is expected to be born, calculated from the date of the mother's last menstrual period

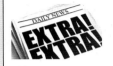 **CALCULATING THE EDC** A pregnant woman's "due date" is usually determined by the 280-day rule, which is based on a regular 28-day menstrual cycle. Assuming that the patient has regular periods every 28 days, the estimated date of confinement is calculated by counting 40 weeks, or 280 days, from the first day of her last cycle. If the patient's cycles are not right on target, then the resulting date is only a very good estimate of the actual due date.

Term	Pronunciation	Meaning
fetal	fē′tăl	pertaining to a fetus
gestational	jes-tā′shŭn-ăl	pertaining to pregnancy
gravida	grav′i-dă	a pregnant woman
in vitro	in vē′trō	in an artificial environment
intrauterine	in′tră-yū′tĕr-in	within the uterus
last menstrual period (LMP)	last men′strū-ăl pĕr′ē-ŏd	the date indicating the first day of a patient's last menstrual period
meconium	mē-kō′nē-ŭm	greenish-black first stool of a newborn
menarche	men′ahr′kē	a girl's first menstrual period
menstruation, *syn.* menses	men′strū-ā′shŭn, men′sēz	cyclic shedding of endometrial lining and discharge of bloody fluid from the uterus; occurs approximately every 28 days
neonatal	nē′ō-nā′tăl	pertaining to the period immediately succeeding birth and continuing through the first 28 days of life
neonate, *syn.* newborn	nē′ō-nāt, nū′bōrn	a newborn infant
nulligravida	nŭl-i-grav′i-dă	a woman who has never conceived a child
nullipara	nŭ-lip′ă-ră	a woman who has never given birth to a child
ovarian	ō-var′ē-ăn	pertaining to an ovary
para	par′ă	a woman who has given birth
pelvic	pel′vik	pertaining to the pelvis
perineal	per′i-nē′ăl	pertaining to the perineum
postpartum	pōst-pahr′tŭm	the period of time after birth
prenatal	prē-nā′tăl	the period of time preceding birth
primigravida	prī′mi-grav′i-dă	a woman who has had one pregnancy
suprapubic	sū′pră-pyū′bik	above the pubic bone
transabdominal	tranz′ab-dom′ĭ-năl	across or through the abdomen
transvaginal	trans-vaj′i-năl	across or through the vagina
stillbirth	stil′bĭrth	the birth of an infant who has died before delivery
uterine	yū′tĕr-in	pertaining to the uterus

■ Exercises: Adjectives and Other Related Terms

SIMPLE
RECALL

Exercise 11

1. The area above the pubic bone is referred to as the (*transvaginal, intrauterine, suprapubic*) area.

2. Birth control products implanted in the uterus are typically called (*ovarian, intrauterine, perineal*) devices.

3. The word that describes a female's first menstrual period is (*nulligravida, menarche, meconium*).

4. A patient's due date is also called the (*last menstrual period, date of birth, estimated date of confinement*).

5. The birth of an infant who has died before delivery is called a (*stillbirth, gravida, neonate*).

6. The word that describes a woman who has given birth is (*gravida, para, congenital*).

7. The period of time preceding birth is known as the (*postnatal, perinatal, prenatal*) period.

8. A newborn's first stool is called (*menstruation, meconium, menarche*).

9. The term (*nulligravida, gravida, primigravida*) refers to a woman who has had one pregnancy.

ADVANCED
RECALL

Exercise 12

Match each medical term with its meaning.

congenital	cystic	chorionic	gravida
nullipara	transabdominal	neonate	gestational

Definition   **Term**

1. relating to the chorion   _____

2. woman who has never given birth   _____

3. across or through the abdomen   _____

4. a newborn infant   _____

5. existing at birth   _____

6. containing cysts   _____

7. relating to pregnancy   _____

8. a pregnant woman   _____

Exercise 13

ADVANCED
RECALL

Circle the correct term that is appropriate for the meaning of the sentence.

1. After having failed at conception several times, Mr. and Mrs. Timmeney decided to undergo fertilization in an artificial environment, also known as (*in vitro, congenital, transvaginal*) fertilization.

2. The physician diagnosed a(n) (*ovarian, chorionic, suprapubic*) cyst, which is a very painful cyst on an ovary.

3. On pelvic examination, Mrs. Veras displayed no (*uterine, nulligravida, in vitro*) tenderness.

4. Ms. Smith will return 6 weeks after the delivery of her child for (*postpartum, prenatal, perineal*) care.

5. Our practice provides (*neonatal, gestational, congenital*) care for the infant for the first 28 days of life.

6. Mrs. Wu came in complaining of a rash involving the surface area between her thighs, also known as the (*perineal, peritoneal, endometrial*) area.

7. An adolescent girl typically begins her (*neonatal, para, menses*), or cyclic shedding of the endometrial lining, around the age of 12.

8. Ms. Patton was born on September 20, 1978; that day is called her (*estimated date of confinement, due date, date of birth*).

9. Mrs. Lau indicated that her menses had started on July 12; this date was noted in her medical record as her (*estimated date of confinement, date of birth, last menstrual period*).

10. Mrs. Johnson has not been able to conceive; her medical record would note that she is (*gravida, nullipara, nulligravida*).

Exercise 14

TERM
CONSTRUCTION

Write the combining form(s) used in the medical term, followed by the meaning of the combining form(s).

Term	Combining Form(s)	Combining Form Definition(s)
1. fetal	_____	_____
2. transvaginal	_____	_____
3. pelvic	_____	_____
4. endometrial	_____	_____
5. abdominopelvic	_____	_____
6. embryonic	_____	_____
7. transabdominal	_____	_____
8. ovarian	_____	_____

Symptoms and Medical Conditions

Term	Pronunciation	Meaning
Related to the Female Reproductive System		
adenomyosis	ad′ĕ-nō-mī-ō′sis	the presence of endometrial tissue growing through the myometrium
amenorrhea	ā-men-ŏr-ē′ă	absence of menstrual bleeding
atrophic vaginitis	ā-trō′fik vaj′i-nī′tis	inflammation of the vagina due to the thinning and shrinking of the tissues, as well as decreased lubrication
bacterial vaginosis	bak-tēr′ē-ăl vaj′i-nō′sis	infection of the vagina caused by the disruption of the normal balance of bacteria, in which "good" bacteria is replaced by "harmful" bacteria
cervical dysplasia	sĕr′vi-kăl dis-plā′zē-ă	development of abnormal cells in the lining of the cervix
cervicitis	sĕr′vi-sī′tis	inflammation of the cervix (Fig. 11-8)
dysmenorrhea	dis-men′ŏr-ē′ă	difficult or painful menstruation
dyspareunia	dis′păr-ū′nē-ă	condition of experiencing pain during sexual intercourse
endometriosis	en′dō-mē-trē-ō′sis	the presence of endometrial tissue somewhere other than in the lining of the uterus (Fig. 11-9)
endometritis	en′dō-mē-trī′tis	inflammation of the endometrium
mastitis	mas-tī′tis	inflammation of the breast(s)
mastodynia	mas′tō-din′ē-ă	pain in the breast(s)
menopause	men′ō-pawz	permanent cessation of menses
menorrhagia	men′ō-rā′jē-ă	irregular or excessive bleeding during menstruation
metrorrhagia	mē′trō-rā′jē-ă	irregular bleeding from the uterus between menstrual periods
myoma, *syn.* uterine fibroid, fibromyoma	mī-ō′mă, yū′tĕr-in fī′broyd, fī′brō-mī-ō′mă	benign growth that develops from the smooth muscular tissue of the uterus (Fig. 11-10)
pelvic inflammatory disease (PID)	pel′vik in-flam′ă-tōr-ē di-zēz′	inflammation of the female pelvic organs (ovaries, salpinges, and uterus) caused by infection by any of several microorganisms, such as gonococci and chlamydia

(continued)

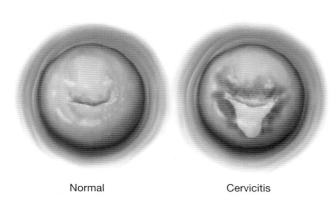

Normal   Cervicitis

Figure 11-8 Inflammation and discharge are symptoms of cervicitis.

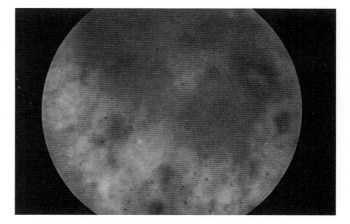

Figure 11-9 Cervical endometriosis appears as blue-black spots on the walls of the endocervical canal.

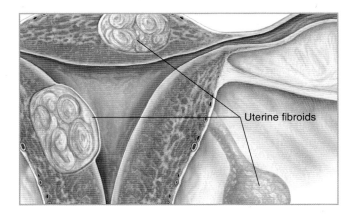

Figure 11-10 Myomas.

Symptoms and Medical Conditions *(continued)*

Term	Pronunciation	Meaning
polycystic ovary syndrome	pol′ē-sis′tik ō′văr-ē sin′drōm	hormone secretion disorder in women, characterized by irregular menstrual periods, excess hair growth, obesity, and numerous other symptoms (Fig. 11-11)
salpingitis	sal′pin-jī′tis	inflammation of the salpinx
sexually transmitted disease (STD)*	sek′shū-ă-lē tranz-mit′ĕd di-zēz′	a communicable disease spread from one person to another primarily through sexual contact
uterine prolapse	yū′tĕr-in prō′laps	protrusion of the uterus into or through the vagina
vulvodynia	vŭl′vō-din′ē-ă	chronic vulvar discomfort with complaints of burning and superficial irritation
Related to Obstetrics		
abortion (AB), *syn.* spontaneous abortion (SAB)	ă-bōr′shŭn, spon-tā′nē-ŭs ă-bōr′shŭn	expulsion of an embryo or fetus from the uterus before viability
incomplete abortion	in′kŏm-plēt′ ă-bōr′shŭn	abortion without expulsion of all of the products of conception
abruptio placentae	ăb-rŭp′shē-ō plă-sen′tē	premature detachment of a normally situated placenta

*See Chapter 10: Male Reproductive System for coverage of specific sexually transmitted diseases.

(continued)

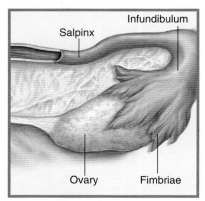

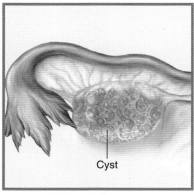

Normal ovary   **Polycystic ovary**

Figure 11-11 Polycystic ovary syndrome.

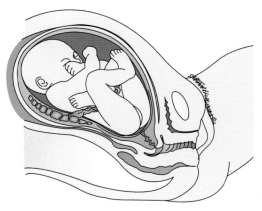

Figure 11-12 Breech pregnancy.

Symptoms and Medical Conditions *(continued)*

Term	Pronunciation	Meaning
Braxton Hicks contractions, *syn.* false labor	braks′tŏn-hiks kŏn-trak′shŭns, fawls lā′bŏr	painless uterine contractions that happen throughout pregnancy
breech pregnancy	brēch preg′năn-sē	pregnancy in which the buttocks of the baby present at the bottom of the uterus, while the head remains in the upper part of the uterus (Fig. 11-12)
dystocia	dis-tō′sē-ă	difficult childbirth
eclampsia	ek-lamp′sē-ă	seizures or coma in a patient with pregnancy-induced hypertension
ectopic pregnancy	ek-top′ik preg′năn-sē	a pregnancy that occurs when the egg implants itself outside the uterus
gestational diabetes	jes-tā′shŭn-ăl dī-ă-bē′tēz	diabetes that develops or first occurs during pregnancy
infertility	in′fĕr-til′i-tē	inability of a couple to conceive, regardless of the cause
nuchal cord	nū′kăl kōrd	loop(s) of umbilical cord around the neck of the fetus, posing risk of intrauterine hypoxia, fetal distress, or death (Fig. 11-13)
oligohydramnios	ol′i-gō-hī-dram′nē-os	presence of an insufficient amount of amniotic fluid
placenta previa	plă-sen′tă prē′vē-ă	condition in which the placenta is implanted in the lower segment of the uterus instead of the upper part (Fig. 11-14)
postpartum depression	pōst-pahr′tŭm dĕ-presh′ŭn	form of clinical depression that occurs soon after giving birth
preeclampsia	prē′ē-klamp′sē-ă	development of hypertension with proteinuria, edema, or both, due to pregnancy

(continued)

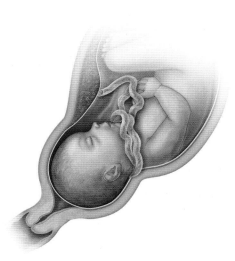

Figure 11-13 Nuchal cord (umbilical cord wrapped around the neck of the fetus).

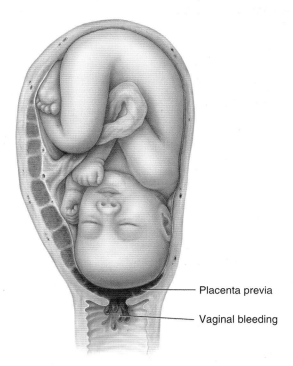
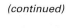

Placenta previa

Vaginal bleeding

Figure 11-14 Placenta previa.

Symptoms and Medical Conditions *(continued)*

Term	Pronunciation	Meaning
prolapsed cord	prō-lapst kōrd	slipping of the umbilical cord into the vagina before delivery
rupture of membranes	rŭp'chŭr membrānz	spontaneous rupture of the amniotic sac with release of fluid preceding childbirth
toxoplasmosis	tok'sō-plaz-mō'sis	infection caused by protozoan parasites transmitted to humans from the droppings of infected cats; if contracted by a pregnant woman, can affect the fetus in many ways, including profound physical abnormalities
Related to Neonatology		
atresia	ă-trē'zē-ă'	congenital absence of a normal opening, such as the esophagus or anus
atrial septal defect (ASD)	ā'trē-ăl sep'tăl dē'fekt	failure of an opening or foramen to close between the atria after birth
cleft lip	kleft lip	congenital facial defect of the lip (Fig. 11-15)
cleft palate	kleft pal'ăt	congenital fissure in the median line of the palate, often associated with cleft lip (Fig. 11-15)
Down syndrome	down sin'drōm	congenital, chromosomal condition characterized by mental retardation, retarded growth, and various other physical abnormalities (Fig. 11-16)
gastroschisis	gas-tros'ki-sis	congenital defect in the anterior abdominal wall, usually accompanied by protrusion of the intestines

(continued)

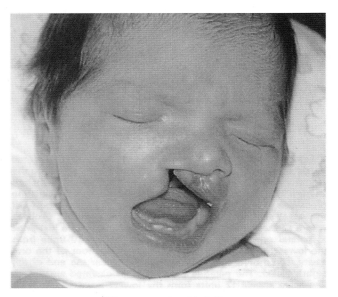

Figure 11-15   Cleft lip.

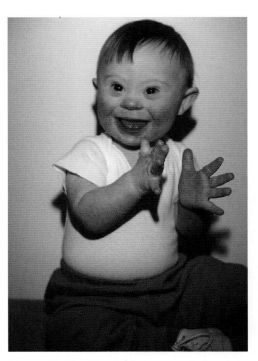

Figure 11-16   Physical characteristics due to Down syndrome.

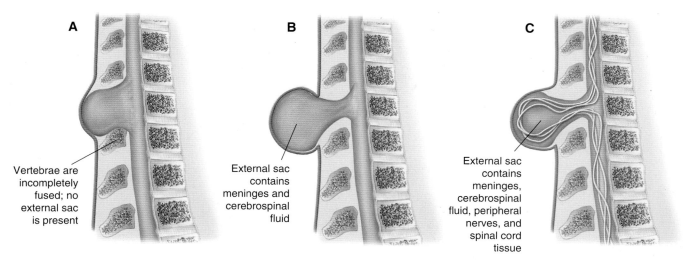

A

Vertebrae are incompletely fused; no external sac is present

B

External sac contains meninges and cerebrospinal fluid

C

External sac contains meninges, cerebrospinal fluid, peripheral nerves, and spinal cord tissue

Figure 11-17 Types of spina bifida. **A.** Spina bifida occulta. **B.** Meningocele. **C.** Myelomeningocele.

Symptoms and Medical Conditions *(continued)*

Term	Pronunciation	Meaning
jaundice of newborn	jawn′dis nū′bōrn	inability of an infant's liver to metabolize bilirubin; usually disappears within 48 to 72 hours after birth
microcephaly	mī′krō-sef′ă-lē	congenital condition characterized by an abnormally small head; usually associated with mental retardation
omphalocele	om-fal′ŏ-sēl	congenital herniation at the umbilical cord
patent ductus arteriosus (PDA)	pā′tent dŭk′tŭs ahr-tē-rē-ō′sus	failure of a fetal circulatory vessel to close after birth
spina bifida	spī′nă bif′i-dă	congenital condition in which the vertebral column does not close properly; usually is accompanied by protrusion of the spinal cord and or meninges (Fig. 11-17)
tetralogy of Fallot	te-tral′ŏ-jē fahl-ō′	set of four congenital heart defects: ventricular septal defect, pulmonic valve stenosis, malposition of the aorta, and right ventricular hypertrophy
Turner syndrome	tŭr′nĕr sin′drōm	congenital abnormality of the X chromosome that alters the development of females
ventricular septal defect (VSD)	ven-trik′yū-lăr sep′tăl dē-fekt′	failure of an opening or foramen to close between the ventricles after birth

■ Exercises: Symptoms and Medical Conditions

Exercise 15

SIMPLE RECALL

Write the correct medical term for the definition given.

1. communicable disease spread through sexual contact _____

2. an insufficient amount of amniotic fluid _____

3. congenital defect in the abdominal wall _____

4. abnormal cells in the lining of the cervix _____

5. congenital abnormality of the X chromosome _____

6. a pregnancy that develops outside the uterus _____

7. cessation of menses _____

8. failure of the foramen of the atria to close after birth _____

9. congenital facial defect of the lip _____

10. loops of umbilical cord around the neck of the fetus _____

11. expulsion of an embryo or fetus before viability _____

12. an infection caused by parasites transmitted by cats _____

13. loss of fluid from the amniotic sac preceding childbirth _____

14. failure of a fetal circulatory vessel to close after birth _____

15. premature detachment of the placenta _____

16. syndrome involving four congenital heart defects _____

17. disruption of the normal balance of bacteria in the vagina _____

18 inflammation of the female pelvic organs _____

19. congenital absence of a normal opening _____

20. pregnancy in which the buttocks of the baby present first _____

ADVANCED
RECALL

Exercise 16

Circle the term that is most appropriate for the meaning of the sentence.

1. Mrs. Murphy experienced irregular bleeding from the uterus between menstrual periods, which is referred to as (*menorrhagia, metrorrhagia, vulvodynia*).

2. After hearing the patient's symptoms of painful intercourse, the physician diagnosed her with (*bacterial vaginosis, oophoritis, dyspareunia*).

3. The couple was suffering from (*endometriosis, eclampsia, infertility*) because they could not conceive a child.

4. Dr. Jones noticed excess hair growth in Ms. Allen, which is a characteristic of a hormonal disorder known as (*salpingitis, menopause, polycystic ovary syndrome*).

5. The baby suffered from a(n) (*atrial septal defect, tetralogy of Fallot, ventricular septal defect*) characterized by the failure of the foramen to close between the ventricles after birth.

6. My sister suffered from (*Braxton Hicks, eclampsia, syphilis*) contractions, or false labor, during all three of her pregnancies.

7. Mrs. Tobias was diagnosed with (*preeclampsia, erythroblastosis fetalis, gestational diabetes*), which is a type of diabetes that develops during pregnancy.

8. The patient's preeclampsia developed into (*ectopic pregnancy, abruption placentae, eclampsia*), which caused her to have a seizure.

9. Some women suffer from (*postpartum depression, oligohydramnios, nuchal cord*) after the birth of their babies.

10. The physician explained to Mrs. Lane that her (*atrophic vaginitis, bacterial vaginosis, dyspareunia*) was due to thinning and shrinking of vaginal tissues.

11. The baby was diagnosed with (*spina bifida, cleft palate, microcephaly*), a congenital condition in which the spinal cord does not close properly.

12. The woman developed a protrusion of the uterus through the vagina, which is known as (*vaginitis, uterine prolapse, pelvic inflammatory disease*).

13. The infant had difficulty feeding because of a (*cleft chin, cleft palate, cleft mouth*), a congenital fissure that is often associated with a cleft lip.

14. The pregnancy was complicated by (*menopause, infertility, placenta previa*).

15. Mrs. Brown experienced a slipping of the umbilical cord into the vagina before delivery, which is called (*premature cord, prolapsed cord, presenting cord*).

16. Mr. Marfin's daughter was born with Down syndrome, a (*contracted, contraindicated, congenital*) chromosomal condition.

17. The baby suffered from (*Down syndrome, Turner syndrome, jaundice of newborn*), which cleared within 48 hours of birth.

18. Ms. Lloyd experienced a(n) (*spontaneous abortion, rupture of membranes, incomplete abortion*) when all the products of conception were not expelled.

19. The patient was diagnosed with (*endometriosis, endometritis, adenomyosis*) after endometrial tissue was found growing in the muscular lining of her uterus.

TERM
CONSTRUCTION

Exercise 17

Break the given medical term into its word parts and define each part. Then define the medical term. (Note: This exercise uses some suffixes learned previously.)

For example:

urethritis	*word parts:*	urethr/o / -itis
	meanings:	urethra / inflammation
	term meaning:	inflammation of the urethra

1. amenorrhea   *word parts:*   _____ / _____ / _____

   meanings: _____ / _____ / _____

   term meaning: _____

2. salpingitis   *word parts:* _____ / _____

                        meanings: _____ / _____

                        term meaning: _____

3. mastitis   *word parts:* _____ / _____

                        meanings: _____ / _____

                        term meaning: _____

4. endometriosis   *word parts:* _____ / _____ / _____

                        meanings: _____ / _____ / _____

                        term meaning: _____

5. vulvodynia   *word parts:* _____ / _____

                        meanings: _____ / _____

                        term meaning: _____

6. microcephaly   *word parts:* _____ / _____ / _____

                        meanings: _____ / _____ / _____

                        term meaning: _____

7. myoma   *word parts:* _____ / _____

                        meanings: _____ / _____

                        term meaning: _____

8. omphalocele   *word parts:* _____ / _____

                        meanings: _____ / _____

                        term meaning: _____

9. mastodynia   *word parts:* _____ / _____

                        meanings: _____ / _____

                        term meaning: _____

10. dysmenorrhea   *word parts:* _____ / _____ / _____

                        meanings: _____ / _____ / _____

                        term meaning: _____

Tests and Procedures

Term	Pronunciation	Meaning
Laboratory Tests Related to the Female Reproductive System and Obstetrics		
group B streptococcus	grūp B strep'tō-kok'ŭs	test for bacterium that, if transmitted from the mother, can cause life-threatening infections in newborns
Papanicolaou (Pap) test	pa-pă-ni'kō-lō (pap) test	microscopic examination of cells collected from the vagina and cervix to detect abnormal changes (e.g., cancer)
pregnancy test	preg'năn-sē test	blood test to determine the presence of the hormone human chorionic gonadotropin (hCG) secreted by the fertilized ovum
quad marker screen	kwahd mahrk'ĕr skrēn	blood test to determine the risk of having a baby with a birth defect
TORCH panel	tōrch pan'ĕl	group of tests to screen for antibodies to four organisms (toxoplasmosis, rubella, cytomegalovirus infection, and herpes simplex) that can be transmitted from mother to fetus and cause congenital infections (Fig. 11-18)
Diagnostic Procedures Related to the Female Reproductive System, Obstetrics, and Neonatology		
amniocentesis	am'nē-ō-sen-tē'sis	transabdominal aspiration of fluid from the amniotic sac to test for certain problems in the fetus (Fig. 11-19)
Apgar score	ap'gahr skōr	numeric result of a test conducted on an infant immediately after delivery to evaluate a newborn's physical condition quickly

APGAR SCORE Part of a pediatrician's examination of an infant immediately after birth includes assigning an Apgar score. Developed in 1952 by anesthesiologist Virginia Apgar, the test is designed to evaluate quickly a newborn's physical condition after delivery and to determine any immediate need for extra medical or emergency care. The score evaluates pulse, breathing, color, tone, and reflex irritability, which are rated 0, 1, or 2 at 1 and 5 minutes after birth. Each set of ratings is totaled, and both totals are reported.

chorionic villus sampling (CVS)	kōr'ē-on'ik vil'ŭs samp'ling	removal of a small piece of placenta tissue from the uterus during early pregnancy to test for fetal abnormalities

(continued)

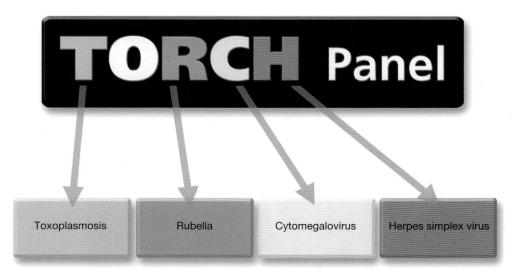

Figure 11-18 TORCH panel.

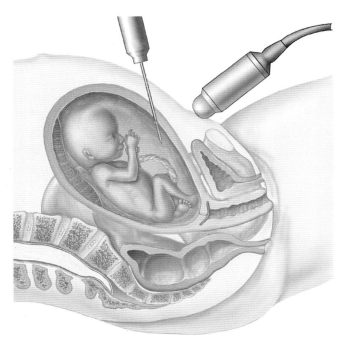

Figure 11-19   Amniocentesis.

Tests and Procedures *(continued)*

Term	Pronunciation	Meaning
colposcope	kol'pō-skōp	a thin lighted endoscope inserted into the vagina to allow for direct visualization of the vagina and cervix
colposcopy	kol-pos'kŏ-pē	visual examination of the tissues of the cervix and vagina (Fig. 11-20)
fetal ultrasound, *syn.* obstetric ultrasound	fē'tăl ŭl'tră-sownd, ob-stet'rik ŭl'tră-sownd	ultrasound done during pregnancy that uses reflected sound waves to produce a picture of a fetus, the placenta that nourishes it, and the amniotic fluid that surrounds it

(continued)

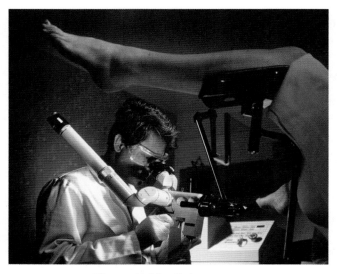

Figure 11-20   Colposcopy.

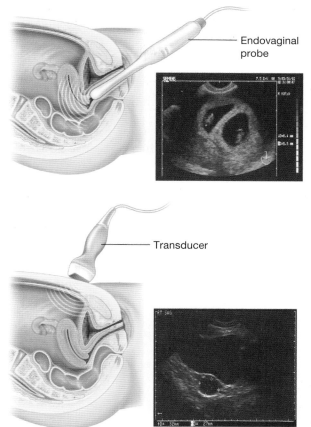

Figure 11-21   Ultrasound: transvaginal and pelvic.

Tests and Procedures *(continued)*

Term	Pronunciation	Meaning
fetoscope	fē'tō-skōp	special type of stethoscope used for listening to a fetus in the womb, usually used after about 18 weeks' gestation
hysterosalpingography (HSG)	his'tĕr-ō-sal-ping-gog'ră-fē	x-ray examination of the uterus and salpinges after injection of contrast dye
mammography	mă-mog'ră-fē	x-ray examination of the breasts; used to detect breast tumors
pelvic ultrasound	pel'vik ŭl'tră-sownd	ultrasound of the pelvic area (Fig. 11-21)
transvaginal ultrasound	trans-vaj'i-năl ŭl'tră-sownd	ultrasound using a transducer inserted into the vagina to view the internal female reproductive organs (Fig. 11-21)

■ Exercises: Tests and Procedures

SIMPLE
RECALL

Exercise 18

Circle the term that is most appropriate for the meaning of the sentence.

1. The physician listened to the fetus in the womb by using a (*hysteroscope, stethoscope, fetoscope*).

2. An ultrasound using a transducer inserted into the vagina to view the internal female reproductive organs is called a (*fetal ultrasound, transvaginal ultrasound, pelvic ultrasound*).

3. An x-ray examination of the uterus and salpinges is called a (*colposcopy, pelvimetry, hysterosalpingography*).

4. The (*pelvimetry, CVS, Apgar*) is a numeric score that indicates an infant's condition immediately after birth.

5. A test for bacterium that, if transmitted from the mother, can cause life-threatening infections in newborns is called a (*TORCH panel, group B streptococcus, pregnancy test*).

6. A (*quad marker screen, chorionic villus sampling, pelvic ultrasound*) is a blood test to determine the risk of carrying a baby with a birth defect.

7. The (*pregnancy test, quad marker screen, Papanicolaou test*) is the microscopic examination of cells collected from the vagina and cervix to detect abnormal changes.

ADVANCED
RECALL

Exercise 19

Complete each sentence by writing in the correct medical term.

1. An ultrasound of the pelvic area that can be used to reproduce images of a fetus is called _____.

2. A visual examination of the cervix and vagina is called a(n) _____.

3. A blood test to determine the presence of the hormone human chorionic gonadotrophin secreted by the fertilized ovum is called a(n) _____.

4. An x-ray examination of the breasts used to detect breast tumors is called _____.

5. A procedure whereby a sample of placental tissue is removed from the uterus to detect fetal abnormalities is called _____.

6. Transabdominal aspiration of fluid from the amniotic sac to test for certain problems in the fetus is called a(n) _____.

7. A group of tests for antibodies to four organisms that cause congenital infections transmitted from mother to fetus is called a(n) _____.

TERM
CONSTRUCTION

Exercise 20

Considering the meaning of the combining form(s) from which the medical term is made, write the meaning of the medical term.

Combining Form(s)	Meaning(s)	Medical Term	Meaning of Term
amni/o	amnion	amniocentesis	1. _____
colp/o	vagina	colposcope	2. _____

hyster/o, salping/o	uterus, salpinges	hysterosalpingography	3. _____
mamm/o	breast	mammography	4. _____
fet/o	fetus	fetoscope	5. _____
colp/o	vagina	colposcopy	6. _____

Surgical Interventions and Therapeutic Procedures

Term	Pronunciation	Meaning
Related to the Female Reproductive System		
colporrhaphy, *syn.* anterior/posterior repair	kol-pōr′ă-fē, an-tēr′ē-ŏr-pos-tēr′ē-ŏr rē-pār′	surgical procedure that repairs a defect in the wall of the vagina
cryosurgery	krī′ō-sŭr′jĕr-ē	in gynecology, a procedure that uses liquid nitrogen to freeze a section of the cervix to destroy abnormal or precancerous cervical cells
dilation and curettage (D&C)	dī-lā′shŭn kūr′ĕ-tahzh′	surgical procedure in which the cervix is dilated and the endometrial lining of the uterus is scraped with a curette (Fig. 11-22)
hysterectomy	his′tĕr-ek′tŏ-mē	surgical excision of the uterus (Fig. 11-23)
total abdominal hysterectomy (TAH)	tō′tăl ab-dom′i-năl his′tĕr-ek′tŏ-mē	surgical excision of the uterus and cervix (with or without removal of the ovaries or salpinges) through an incision in the abdomen
vaginal hysterectomy	vaj′i-năl his′tĕr-ek′tŏ-mē	surgical excision of the uterus and cervix through an incision deep inside the vagina
loop electrosurgical excision procedure (LEEP)	lūp ĕ-lek′trō-sĭr′jik-ăl ek-sizh′ŭn prŏ-sē′jŭr	gynecologic procedure that uses a thin, low-voltage electrified wire loop to cut out abnormal tissue in the cervix
mammoplasty	mam′ō-plas-tē	surgical repair of the breast
mastopexy	mas′tō-pek-sē	fixation procedure that raises and firms the breasts by removing excess skin and tightening the surrounding tissue to reshape the breast
myomectomy	mī′ō-mek′tŏ-mē	surgical removal of myomas

(continued)

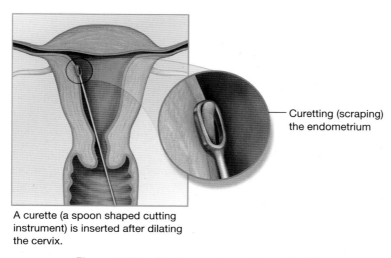

A curette (a spoon shaped cutting instrument) is inserted after dilating the cervix.

Curetting (scraping) the endometrium

Figure 11-22 Dilation and curettage (D&C).

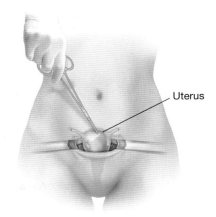

Abdominal hysterectomy

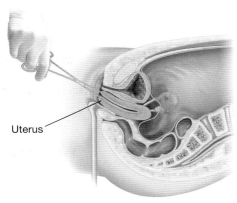

Vaginal hysterectomy

Figure 11-23 Hysterectomy: abdominal and vaginal.

Surgical Interventions and Therapeutic Procedures *(continued)*

Term	Pronunciation	Meaning
oophorectomy	ō'of-ōr-ek'tŏ-mē	surgical excision of an ovary
pessary	pes'ă-rē	appliance of varied form, introduced into the vagina to support the uterus or to correct any displacement
salpingectomy	sal'pin-jek'tŏ-mē	surgical excision of a salpinx
salpingo-oophorectomy	sal-ping'gō-ō-of'ŏr-ek'tŏ-mē	surgical excision of a salpinx and an ovary
uterotomy, *syn.* hysterotomy	yū'tĕr-ot'ŏ-mē, his'tĕr-ot'ŏ-mē	incision of the uterus
vulvectomy	vŭl-vek'tŏ-mē	surgical removal of all or part of the vulva
Related to Obstetrics		
amniotomy, *syn.* artificial rupture of membranes	am'nē-ot'ŏ-mē, ahr'ti-fish'ăl rup'shŭr mem'brānz	artificial tearing of the amniotic sac to induce or expedite labor

(continued)

Surgical Interventions and Therapeutic Procedures *(continued)*

Term	Pronunciation	Meaning
cerclage	ser-klazh′	placement of a nonabsorbable suture around an incompetent cervical opening
cesarean section	se-zăr′ē-ăn sek′shŭn	surgical incision made through the abdominal wall and the uterus to extract the fetus
episiotomy	e-piz′ē-ot′ŏ-mē	surgical incision through the perineum to enlarge the vagina and assist childbirth
induction of labor	in-duk′shŭn lā′bŏr	attempt to start the childbirth process artificially by administering a drug to start labor or by puncturing the amniotic sac
in vitro fertilization (IVF)	in vē′trō fĕr′til-ĭ-zā′shŭn	process whereby ova are placed in a medium to which spermatozoa are added for fertilization, which produces a zygote; the zygote is then introduced into the uterus with the objective of full-term development
therapeutic abortion (TAB)	thăr-ă-pyū′tik ă-bōr′shŭn	abortion performed for medical reasons (such as when the mother's life is threatened by the pregnancy)
tubal ligation	tū′băl lī-gā′shŭn	sterilization procedure for women in which the salpinges are tied in two places and the tubes in between the ligations are removed

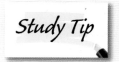

Study Tip

Salpingo-oophorectomy The spelling of salpingo-oophorectomy (surgical excision of the ovary and salpinx) includes a hyphen because of the presence of three like vowels in a row. Always include the hyphen whether the term is handwritten or typed.

◼ Exercises: Surgical Interventions and Therapeutic Procedures

SIMPLE
RECALL

Exercise 21

Write the correct medical term for the definition given.

1. procedure whereby the cervix is dilated and the uterus is scraped _____

2. surgical removal of myomas _____

3. appliance introduced into the vagina to support the uterus _____

4. surgical excision of the uterus and cervix through the abdomen _____

5. placement of a nonabsorbable suture around an incompetent cervical opening _____

6. surgical excision of the uterus and cervix through a vaginal incision _____

7. inducing childbirth artificially with drugs or by puncturing the amniotic sac _____

8. process whereby ova and spermatozoa are placed in a medium to produce a zygote _____

9. procedure using an electrified wire loop to cut out abnormal tissue in the cervix _____

10. artificial rupture of the amniotic sac to induce or expedite labor _____

ADVANCED
RECALL

Exercise 22

Circle the term that is most appropriate for the meaning of the sentence.

1. After having four children, Ms. Thompson decided on a (*vulvectomy, episiotomy, tubal ligation*) as a permanent contraceptive measure.

2. Dr. Adams used (*LEEP, cryosurgery, colporrhaphy*) to freeze abnormal cells from the patient's cervix.

3. Mrs. Kumar's surgeon performed a bilateral (*salpingo-oophorectomy, oophorectomy, salpingectomy*), a procedure whereby both the ovaries and salpinges are removed.

4. Mrs. Grace underwent a (*vulvectomy, lumpectomy, salpingectomy*) to remove a diseased portion of her salpinx.

5. After her car accident, Mrs. Nabors had a (*therapeutic abortion, missed abortion, spontaneous abortion*) to save her life.

6. As a vaginal birth was not possible, Mrs. Nguyen delivered the child by means of (*cesarean section, hysterectomy, myomectomy*).

TERM
CONSTRUCTION

Exercise 23

Using the given suffix, build a medical term for the meaning given.

Suffix	Meaning of Medical Term	Medical Term
-plasty	surgical repair of the breast	1. _____
-tomy	incision into the amniotic sac	2. _____
-pexy	surgical fixation of the breast	3. _____
-plasty	surgical repair of the uterus	4. _____
-tomy	surgical incision of the vulva to assist in childbirth	5. _____

TERM CONSTRUCTION

Exercise 24

Break the given medical term into its word parts and define each part. Then define the medical term.

For example:

mastitis	*word parts:*	mast/o / -itis
	meanings:	breast / inflammation
	term meaning:	inflammation of the breast

1. salpingo-oophorectomy   *word parts:* _____ / _____ / _____

   meanings: _____ / _____ / _____

   term meaning: _____

2. colporrhaphy   *word parts:* _____ / _____

   meanings: _____ / _____

   term meaning: _____

3. uterotomy   *word parts:* _____ / _____

   meanings: _____ / _____

   term meaning: _____

4. mammoplasty   *word parts:* _____ / _____

   meanings: _____ / _____

   term meaning: _____

5. hysterectomy   *word parts:* _____ / _____

   meanings: _____ / _____

   term meaning: _____

6. episiotomy   *word parts:* _____ / _____

   meanings: _____ / _____

   term meaning: _____

7. salpingectomy   *word parts:* _____ / _____

   meanings: _____ / _____

   term meaning: _____

8. oophorectomy   *word parts:* _____ / _____

                           meanings: _____ / _____

                           term meaning: _____

9. mastopexy   *word parts:* _____ / _____

                           meanings: _____ / _____

                           term meaning: _____

10. vulvectomy   *word parts:* _____ / _____

                           meanings: _____ / _____

                           term meaning: _____

Medications and Drug Therapies

Term	Pronunciation	Meaning
Related to the Female Reproductive System		
contraceptive	kon'tră-sep'tiv	agent that prevents conception
hormone replacement therapy (HRT)	hōr'mōn rĕ-plăs'mĕnt thăr'ă-pē	administration of hormones (e.g., estrogen, progesterone) to women after menopause or oophorectomy
Related to Obstetrics		
abortifacient	ă-bōr'ti-fā'shĕnt	agent that produces abortion
ovulation induction	ov'yū-lā'shŭn in-dŭk'shŭn	use of hormone therapy to stimulate the development of mature eggs
oxytocin	ok'sē-tō'sin	hormone that causes contractions and promotes milk release during lactation; also used to induce or stimulate labor
tocolytic agent	tō'kō-lit'ik ā'jĕnt	agent used to arrest uterine contractions, often used in an attempt to arrest premature labor contractions

■ Exercise: Medications and Drug Therapies

SIMPLE
RECALL

Exercise 25

Write the correct medication or drug therapy term for the definition given.

1. a hormone that causes uterine contractions and promotes milk   _____

2. agent that produces abortion   _____

3. agent that prevents conception   _____

4. hormone therapy to stimulate the development of mature eggs _____

5. agent used to arrest uterine contractions _____

6. administration of hormones to women after menopause _____

Specialties and Specialists

Term	Pronunciation	Meaning
gynecology (GYN)	gī′nĕ-kol′ŏ-jē	medical specialty concerned with diseases of the female genital tract, as well as endocrinology and reproductive physiology of the female
gynecologist (GYN)	gī′nĕ-kol′ŏ-jist	physician who specializes in gynecology
midwifery	mid-wif′ĕ-rē	practice of providing holistic health care to the childbearing woman and newborn
midwife	mid′wīf	health professional who practices midwifery
neonatal intensive care unit (NICU)	nē′ō-nā′tăl in-ten′siv kār yū′nit	hospital department designed for care of critically ill premature and full-term infants
neonatology	nē′ō-nā-tol′ŏ-jē	medical subspecialty of pediatrics concerned with the medical needs of newborn babies through the 28th day of life
neonatologist	nē′ō-nā-tol′ŏ-jist	pediatrician specializing in neonatology
obstetrics (OB)	ob-stet′riks	medical specialty concerned with childbirth and care of the mother
obstetrician (OB)	ob-stĕ-trish′ŭn	physician who specializes in obstetrics
pediatrics	pē-dē-at′riks	medical specialty concerned with the study and treatment of children in health and disease during development from birth through adolescence
pediatrician	pē′dē-ă-trish′ăn	physician who specializes in pediatrics
reproductive endocrinology	rē′prō-dŭk′tiv en′dō-kri-nol′ŏ-jē	medical subspecialty within gynecology and obstetrics that addresses hormonal functioning as it pertains to reproduction as well as the issue of infertility
reproductive endocrinologist	rē′prō-dŭk′tiv en′dō-kri-nol′ŏ-jist	physician who practices reproductive endocrinology

■ Exercise: Specialties and Specialists

ADVANCED
RECALL

Exercise 26

Match each medical specialty or specialist with its description.

gynecology   neonatology   obstetrics   reproductive endocrinology
midwifery   pediatrics   gynecologist   neonatal intensive care unit
pediatrician   midwife   obstetrician   neonatologist
reproductive endocrinologist

Description   **Term**

1. provider of holistic healthcare to the childbearing woman _____

2. hospital unit caring for critically ill infants _____

3. addresses hormonal functioning as it relates to pregnancy and infertility   _____

4. medical subspecialty that focuses on care and treatment of newborns up to 28 days   _____

5. branch of medicine dealing with childbirth and care of the mother   _____

6. the study and treatment of children from birth through adolescence   _____

7. pediatrician who specializes in caring and treating newborns up to 28 days   _____

8. practice that focuses on providing holistic health care to the childbearing woman and newborn   _____

9. physician who specializes in hormonal functioning as it relates to pregnancy and infertility   _____

10. the study and treatment of diseases of the female genital tract   _____

11. physician who specializes in childbirth and care of the mother   _____

12. physician who studies and treats children from birth through adolescence   _____

13. physician who specializes in diseases of the female genital tract   _____

Abbreviations

Abbreviation	Meaning
AB	abortion
CVS	chorionic villus sampling
D&C	dilation and curettage
DOB	date of birth
EDC	estimated date of confinement
EDD	estimated date of delivery
GYN	gynecology; gynecologist
hCG	human chorionic gonadotropin
HRT	hormone replacement therapy
HSG	hysterosalpingogram
IVF	in vitro fertilization
LEEP	loop electrosurgical excision procedure
LMP	last menstrual period

(continued)

Abbreviations *(continued)*

Abbreviation	Meaning
NICU	neonatal intensive care unit
OB	obstetrics; obstetrician
PID	pelvic inflammatory disease
SAB	spontaneous abortion
STD	sexually transmitted disease
TAB	therapeutic abortion
TAH	total abdominal hysterectomy

■ Exercises: Abbreviations

Exercise 27

SIMPLE
RECALL

Write the meaning of each abbreviation.

1. TAH _____

2. SAB _____

3. AB _____

4. PID _____

5. STD _____

Exercise 28

ADVANCED
RECALL

Write the meaning of each abbreviation used in these sentences.

1. The infant was born 6 weeks prematurely and was sent to the **NICU** for further care.

   _____

2. Ms. McNeal saw her **OB** regularly until the birth of her baby last year.

   _____

3. Mrs. Hajdu's gynecologist started her on **HRT** to help minimize the symptoms of menopause.

   _____

4. A **TAH** is a common type of surgery performed on women who require removal of the uterus and cervix.

   _____

5. A **TAB** may be performed when the mother's life is threatened by the pregnancy.

_____

6. Given the date of conception, the obstetrician placed Ms. Ellys's **EDD** at December 25th.

_____

7. Part of Mrs. Winn's gynecologic record includes the date of her **LMP**, which was sometime in March.

_____

8. Ms. Hernandez underwent **IVF** because she could not conceive a child normally.

_____

9. The patient underwent a **D&C** following her therapeutic abortion to remove any remaining products of conception.

_____

10. Theresa underwent a **LEEP** to remove abnormal tissue in her cervix.

_____

Exercise 29

ADVANCED RECALL

Match each abbreviation with the appropriate description.

| GYN | DOB | CVS |
| hCG | D&C | HSG |

1. removal of endocervical tissue using a curette _____

2. examination of placental tissue _____

3. x-ray examination of the uterus and salpinges _____

4. one who practices gynecology _____

5. date of birth of a patient _____

6. hormone produced in pregnancy _____

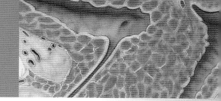

Chapter Review

Review of Terms for Anatomy and Physiology

VISUAL

Exercise 30

Write the correct terms on the blanks for the anatomic structures indicated.

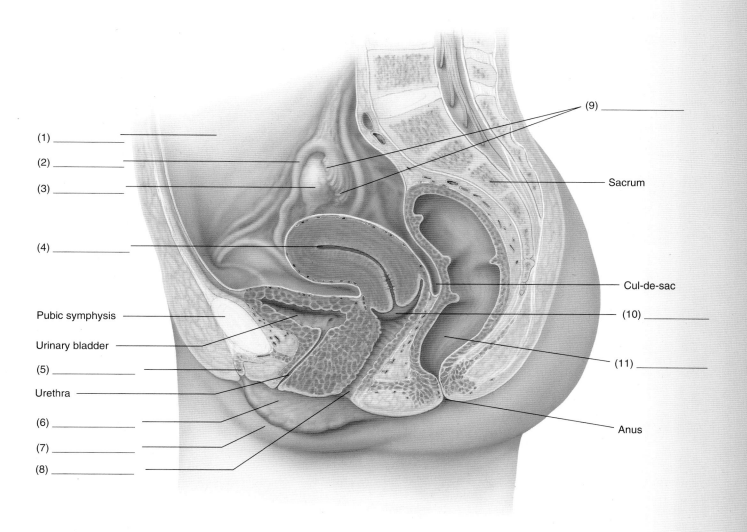

(1) _____

(2) _____

(3) _____

(4) _____

Pubic symphysis _____

Urinary bladder _____

(5) _____

Urethra _____

(6) _____

(7) _____

(8) _____

(9) _____

Sacrum _____

Cul-de-sac _____

(10) _____

(11) _____

Anus _____

Understanding Term Structure

TERM CONSTRUCTION

Exercise 31

Break the given medical term into its word parts and define each part. Then define the medical term. (Note: You may need to use word parts from other chapters.)

For example:

mastitis	*word parts:*	mast/o / -itis
	meanings:	breast / inflammation
	term meaning:	inflammation of the breast

1. hysterosalpingography

word parts: _____ / _____ / _____

meanings: _____ / _____ / _____

term meaning: _____

2. episiotomy

word parts: _____ / _____

meanings: _____ / _____

term meaning: _____

3. colporrhaphy

word parts: _____ / _____ / _____

meanings: _____ / _____ / _____

term meaning: _____

4. endocervical

word parts: _____ / _____

meanings: _____ / _____

term meaning: _____

5. pelvimetry

word parts: _____ / _____

meanings: _____ / _____

term meaning: _____

6. oophorectomy

word parts: _____ / _____

meanings: _____ / _____

term meaning: _____

7. mammography

word parts: _____ / _____ / _____

meanings: _____ / _____ / _____

term meaning: _____

8. metrorrhagia   *word parts:*   _____ / _____ / _____

                              meanings: _____ / _____ / _____

                              term meaning: _____

9. oligomenorrhea   *word parts:*   _____ / _____

                              meanings: _____ / _____

                              term meaning: _____

10. mammoplasty   *word parts:*   _____ / _____

                              meanings: _____ / _____

                              term meaning: _____

11. salpingectomy   *word parts:*   _____ / _____

                              meanings: _____ / _____

                              term meaning: _____

12. colposcopy   *word parts:*   _____ / _____ / _____

                              meanings: _____ / _____ / _____

                              term meaning: _____

13. vaginitis   *word parts:*   _____ / _____

                              meanings: _____ / _____

                              term meaning: _____

14. cervicitis   *word parts:*   _____ / _____

                              meanings: _____ / _____

                              term meaning: _____

Comprehension Exercises

Exercise 32

COMPREHENSION **Fill in the blank with the correct term.**

1. A(n) _____ pregnancy occurs when a fertilized ovum implants itself outside the uterus.

2. The term _____ means no pregnancies.

3. _____ is the inability of a couple to achieve fertilization.

4. _____ is a method of conception that takes place outside of the uterus.

5. _____ is a method to extract the fetus other than through the birth canal.

6. A(n) _____ poses the risk of intrauterine hypoxia, fetal distress, and death.

Exercise 33

COMPREHENSION   **Write a short answer for each question.**

1. In what surgical procedure is the adnexa of the uterus removed?_____

   _____

2. What is the name given to a developing infant between the zygote and fetus stages?_____

   _____

3. What structure enables an ovum to travel from the ovary to the uterus?_____

   _____

4. How do the meanings of the terms *nulligravida, primigravida,* and *gravida* differ?_____

   _____

5. Name the three layers making up the wall of the uterus. _____

   _____

6. What is the difference between gynecology and obstetrics?_____

   _____

7. Where can endometriosis occur?_____

   _____

8. What is the difference between rupture of membranes and an amniotomy?_____

   _____

9. For what reason would a physician perform amniocentesis?_____

   _____

Exercise 34

COMPREHENSION   **Circle the letter of the best answer in the following questions.**

1. Which of the following structures might be involved if a woman has PID?

    A. ovaries
    B. uterus
    C. salpinges
    D. all of the above

2. The cervix is a part of which structure?

    A. uterus
    B. vagina
    C. it is a separate structure
    D. none of the above

3. The structures that store eggs and produce hormones are the:

    A. salpinges
    B. ovaries
    C. labia
    D. fimbriae

4. A girl's first onset of menses is referred to as:

    A. menarche
    B. primimenses
    C. monomenses
    D. menstruation

5. A _____ can be performed either transvaginally or through the abdomen.

    A. mastectomy
    B. laparotomy
    C. hysterectomy
    D. myomectomy

6. The estimated date of confinement is calculated from the patient's:

    A. EDC
    B. LMP
    C. DOB
    D. EDD

7. Which test is done to examine tissues inside the uterus?

    A. Apgar score
    B. chorionic villus sampling
    C. quad marker screen
    D. pregnancy test

8. The term that indicates a patient's obstetric history in which there have been no deliveries of viable offspring is:

    A. gravida
    B. nulligravida
    C. primigravida
    D. nullipara

Application and Analysis

CASE REPORTS

Exercise 35

APPLICATION   **Read the case reports and circle the letter of your answer choice for the questions that follow about each case.**

CASE 11-1

Mrs. Andresson, who had been seen in the emergency room for vaginal bleeding last week, came into the medical office for follow-up. She had a positive pregnancy test result more than 11 weeks ago and had recently begun passing several clots. A specimen was sent for testing. It was explained to her that this was a spontaneous abortion because her hCG levels have declined and the specimen showed products of conception. She was provided emotional support and given instructions to take a multivitamin as needed.

1. What is hCG?

   A. a hormone produced in the pancreas
   B. a growth hormone
   C. a hormone produced in pregnancy that is made by the developing embryo soon after conception
   D. a hormone that causes pregnancy

2. What was the patient's diagnosis?

   A. a therapeutic abortion
   B. a spontaneous abortion
   C. a missed abortion
   D. a D&C

3. Declining levels of hCG probably indicate:

   A. a spontaneous abortion
   B. a growing baby

   C. a conflict in blood types between mother and baby
   D. a twin gestation

4. What was the initial symptom that brought the patient to the emergency room?

   A. headaches
   B. declining hCG levels
   C. vaginal bleeding
   D. a positive pregnancy test

5. The specimen showed products of conception that also indicated a:

   A. spontaneous abortion
   B. rupture of membranes
   C. congenital defect
   D. placenta previa

CASE 11-2

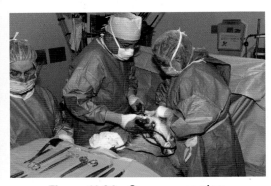

Ms. Jamesly is seen in the office for follow-up. She was admitted to the hospital last week to deliver her baby. On examination, the baby was found to be in a breech presentation. Ms. Jamesly was taken to the operating room where a cesarean section was performed. She also had a tubal ligation. Her incision appears normal and she says that her breast milk is coming in. She states that baby is being treated for jaundice but is feeding well.

Figure 11-24   Cesarean section.

6. In a breech presentation, the infant's buttocks:

   A. appear last
   B. appear first
   C. do not appear at all
   D. none of the above

7. What is the medical term for production of breast milk?

   A. lactation
   B. lochia
   C. prolactin
   D. milk production

8. A cesarean section involves removing the fetus via an incision in the abdominal wall and the:

   A. perineum
   B. vagina

   C. uterus
   D. peritoneum

9. A tubal ligation is a _____ procedure for women.

   A. sterilization
   B. uterine
   C. conception
   D. in vitro fertilization

10. Jaundice is the inability of the infant's liver to metabolize:

   A. prolactin
   B. fat
   C. breast milk
   D. bilirubin

MEDICAL RECORD ANALYSIS

MEDICAL RECORD 11-1

Ms. Brown is a patient who is being observed for suspicious-looking lesions on a Pap test with subsequent evaluation of those lesions, as detailed in the medical record that follows. She is now returning for a followup Pap test. You are the cytotechnologist who will be analyzing the specimen from the test.

Medical Record

CLINIC NOTE

SUBJECTIVE: This patient is a 36-year-old gravida 3, para 3-0-0-3 with a history of conization in September 20xx, which showed precancerous cells and a negative endocervical curettage. Patient, prior to that, had had a colposcopy revealing precancerous cells in August 20xx. The patient has had followup after her colposcopy with a Pap test.

Later the patient had another Pap test that was negative and a colposcopy performed that was negative. No lesions or metastases were seen at that time and no biopsies were taken, as such. The Pap test, again, returned as normal. Today the patient comes back for a Pap test. She has no changes in her interval history. She denies any sexually transmitted diseases.

OBJECTIVE: On examination, the external genitalia appeared to be within normal limits and without any obvious lesions. The speculum was inserted into the vaginal canal, and the vaginal mucosa appeared to be pink and healthy. The cervix was visualized and noted to be free of lesions, although at the 9 o'clock position, a suture was seen. A Pap test was performed. There was some stenosis of the cervical os. The patient tolerated the procedure well.

ASSESSMENT AND PLAN: The test results and plan for follow-up will be mailed to patient when available.

Exercise 36

APPLICATION   **Write the appropriate medical terms used in this medical record on the blanks after their definitions. Note that not all the terms appear in the chapter, but you should be able to identify these terms based on word parts that are included in this chapter.**

1. communicable disease spread through sexual contact   _____

2. scraping within the cervix with a curette   _____

3. process of examining the vagina and cervix   _____

4. narrowing of a structure   _____

Bonus Questions

5. What is meant by the phrase *gravida 3*?   _____

6. What is the full term for Pap test?   _____

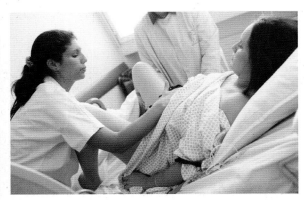

Nurse midwife assisting a patient in labor.

As a nurse midwife, you have cared for the patient in the following medical record throughout her pregnancy and delivery. You are now documenting the delivery through this medical record.

Medical Record

DELIVERY NOTE

PROCEDURES:
1. Controlled vaginal delivery.
2. Repair of episiotomy.

PROCEDURE IN DETAIL: The patient is a primigravida 27-year-old white female who received

(1) _____ care throughout her pregnancy. She has remained normotensive throughout her pregnancy, and dipsticks remained negative. Maternal blood type is O negative, so RhoGAM was administered postdelivery.

The patient arrived in active labor with a good mechanism at 0430 hours. She was 80% effaced with the

(2) _____ dilated to 4 cm. The fetus was noted to be in a vertex presentation at a -2 station. She progressed rapidly in labor, and by 1045 hours, she was 100% effaced and dilated to 5 cm. An epidural was started by anesthesia at the patient's request. The fetus remained in the vertex presentation and had normal fetal monitoring strips throughout labor, with a heart rate ranging from 120 to 152.

At 1205 hours, the patient was moved to delivery. The epidural was continued. The patient's vagina and perineum were prepped, and drapes were applied after the patient was placed in Allen stirrups

in the lithotomy position. It was felt necessary to do a midline (3) _____. The infant's head was delivered, and the nose and oropharynx were suctioned with a bulb. The shoulders were gently rotated, and the infant was delivered and placed on the mother's abdomen. The infant cried spontaneously and vigorously. The mouth and nose were once again suctioned. The cord was clamped and cut. Cord blood was obtained from a three-vessel cord. The infant was handed off the

field to the (4) _____ in attendance. The infant's blood type will be determined, and the infant will be closely monitored for any signs of Rh incompatibility, but none was apparent at birth.

The patient delivered a viable male infant weighing 7 pounds 9 ounces with an (5)_____

_____ of 8 at 1 minute and 10 at 5 minutes. RhoGAM will be administered. The midline episiotomy was repaired without complications. The infant was sent to the newborn nursery, and the mother will be closely observed prior to returning to her room for recovery.

Exercise 37

APPLICATION   **Fill in the blanks in the medical record above with the correct medical terms. The definitions of the missing terms are listed below.**

1. period of time preceding birth

2. tubular, lower portion of the uterus

3. surgical incision of the perineum to assist childbirth

4. pediatrician specializing in neonatology

5. numeric result of a test to evaluate a newborn's physical condition quickly

Bonus Question

6. Why was an episiotomy performed? _____

_____

Pronunciation and Spelling

Exercise 38

AUDITORY   **Review the Chapter 11 terms in the Dictionary/Audio Glossary in the Student Resources and practice pronouncing each term, referring to the pronunciation guide as needed.**

Exercise 39

SPELLING   **Circle the correct spelling of each term.**

1. histerectomy	hysterectomy	hystirectomy
2. suprepublic	suprapubic	suprepubic
3. servicitis	cervicitis	cervisitis
4. cistic	cystik	cystic
5. laperotomy	laparotomy	laprotome
6. mastectomy	mestectomy	mastectome
7. endometrial	indometrial	endometreal
8. oveulation	ovulation	ovvulation
9. parimetrium	perimetrum	perimetrium

10. mamography   mammographe   mammography

11. plecenta   placenta   plasenta

12. cleitoris   clitoris   clytoris

13. areola   ariola   areolla

14. colposcopy   culposcopy   colposcopey

15. zygote   zygoote   zygotte

Media Connection

STUDENT
RESOURCES

Exercise 40

Complete each of the following activities available with the Student Resources. Check off each activity as you complete it, and record your score for the Chapter Quiz in the space provided.

Chapter Exercises

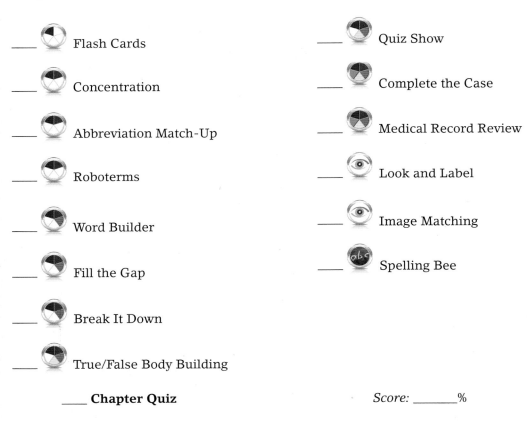

____ Flash Cards

____ Concentration

____ Abbreviation Match-Up

____ Roboterms

____ Word Builder

____ Fill the Gap

____ Break It Down

____ True/False Body Building

____ Quiz Show

____ Complete the Case

____ Medical Record Review

____ Look and Label

____ Image Matching

____ Spelling Bee

____ **Chapter Quiz**   *Score:* _____%

Additional Resources

____ 👁 Animation: *Ovulation and Fertilization*

____ 👂 Dictionary/Audio Glossary

____ Health Professions Careers: Cytotechnologist

____ Health Professions Careers: Nurse-Midwife

Nervous System and Mental Health

12

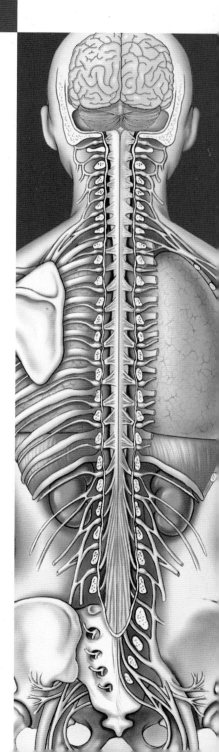

Chapter Outline

Objectives

After completion of this chapter you will be able to:

1. Describe the location of the main structures in the nervous system.

2. Define terms related to the central and peripheral nervous systems.

3. Define combining forms, prefixes, and suffixes related to the nervous system and mental health.

4. Define common medical terminology related to the nervous system and mental health, including adjectives and related terms, symptoms and conditions, diagnostic procedures, surgical interventions and therapeutic procedures, medications and drug therapies, and specialties.

5. Explain abbreviations for terms related to the nervous system and mental health.

6. Successfully complete all chapter exercises.

7. Explain terms used in medical records and case studies involving the nervous system and mental health.

8. Successfully complete all pronunciation and spelling exercises, and complete all interactive exercises included with the companion Student Resources.

■ ANATOMY AND PHYSIOLOGY

Functions

■ To carry impulses between the brain, neck, head, and spinal nerves
■ To release chemicals called neurotransmitters
■ To control voluntary and involuntary body functions

Organs and Structures

■ The nervous system may be divided into two parts: the central nervous system and the peripheral nervous system (Fig. 12-1).

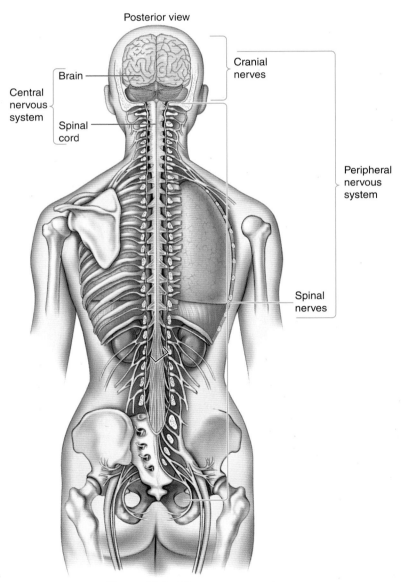

Posterior view

Brain

Cranial nerves

Central nervous system

Spinal cord

Peripheral nervous system

Spinal nerves

Figure 12-1 The nervous system.

■ The central nervous system consists of the brain and the spinal cord.

■ The brain consists of four parts: the cerebrum, the diencephalon, the brainstem, and the cerebellum.

■ The spinal cord begins at the medulla oblongata in the brainstem and tapers to end at the first and second lumbar vertebrae.

■ The terminal ends of the spinal nerves culminate in a structure called the cauda equina.

■ The peripheral nervous system consists of all of the other nerves throughout the body.

■ Each nerve ends with two roots; the dorsal (posterior) root carries sensory impulses to the spinal cord, and the ventral (anterior) root carries motor impulses away from the cord to muscles or glands.

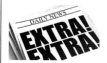

CAUDA EQUINA The name cauda equina is Latin for "horse's tail." This name was given because the spinal nerves end at various levels and branch off from the end of the spinal cord, giving it the appearance of a horse's tail.

Terms Related to the Nervous System

Term	Pronunciation	Meaning
Terms Related to the Central Nervous System		
central nervous system (CNS)	sen′trăl nĕr′vŭs sis′tĕm	the brain and the spinal cord
brain	brān	part of the central nervous system contained within the cranium (Fig. 12-2)
brainstem	brān′stem	connects the brain to the spinal cord; assists in breathing, heart rhythm, vision, and consciousness
pons	ponz	part of the brainstem that connects different regions of the brain
medulla oblongata	mĕ-dŭl′ă ob-long-gah′tă	part of the brainstem that connects the brain and the spinal cord; controls respiration and heartbeat
midbrain, *syn.* mesencephalon	mid′brān, mes′en-sef′ă-lon	part of the brainstem that connects the brainstem to the cerebellum; controls sensory processes
cerebellum, *syn.* hindbrain	ser-ĕ-bel′ŭm, hīnd′brān	posterior portion of the brain that coordinates the voluntary muscles and maintains balance and muscle tone
cerebrum	ser′ĕ-brŭm	largest and uppermost portion of the brain; divided into right and left halves (called cerebral hemispheres) and subdivided into lobes
cerebral cortex	ser′ĕ-brăl kŏr′teks	outer layer of the cerebrum; controls higher mental functions
frontal lobe	frŏn′tăl lōb	front portion of the cerebrum that controls voluntary muscle movement and is involved in emotions
gyrus	jī′rŭs	raised convolution on the surface of the cerebrum
occipital lobe	ok-sip′i-tăl lōb	back portion of the cerebrum that controls vision
parietal lobe	pă-rī′ĕ-tăl lōb	middle-top portion of the cerebrum involved in perception of touch, temperature, and pain

(continued)

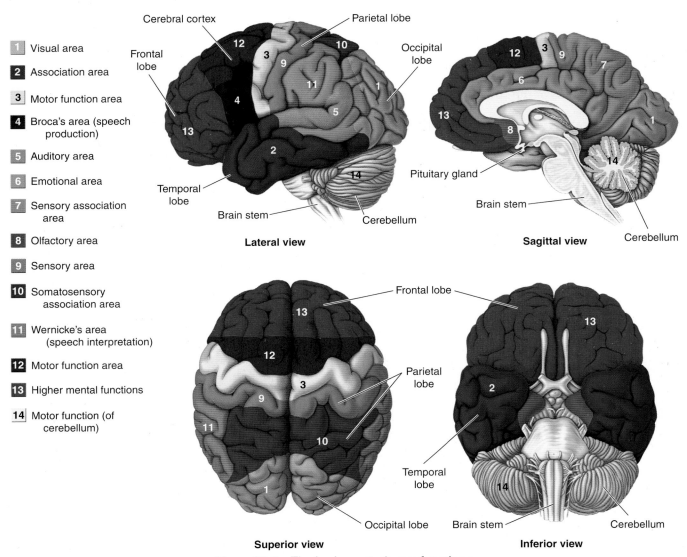

1 Visual area

2 Association area

3 Motor function area

4 Broca's area (speech production)

5 Auditory area

6 Emotional area

7 Sensory association area

8 Olfactory area

9 Sensory area

10 Somatosensory association area

11 Wernicke's area (speech interpretation)

12 Motor function area

13 Higher mental functions

14 Motor function (of cerebellum)

Figure 12-2   The brain controls our functions.

Terms Related to the Nervous System *(continued)*

Term	Pronunciation	Meaning
sulcus	sŭl′kŭs	groove or fissure on the surface of the brain
temporal lobe	tem′pŏr-ăl lōb	portion of the cerebrum below the frontal lobe; controls senses of hearing and smell as well as memory, emotion, speech, and behavior
diencephalon, *syn.* hypophysis	dī′en-sef′ă-lon, hī-pŏf′-i-sis	area deep within the brain that contains the thalamus, hypothalamus, and pituitary gland; responsible for directing sensory information to the cortex
cerebrospinal fluid (CSF)	ser′ĕ-brō-spī′năl flū′id	colorless fluid that circulates in and around the brain and spinal cord; acts as a protector and transports nutrients

(continued)

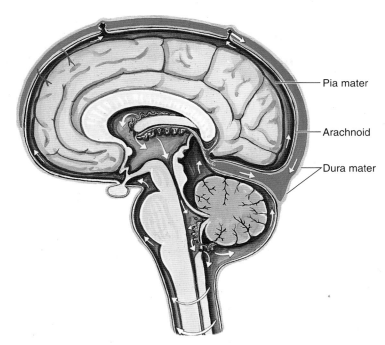

Pia mater

Arachnoid

Dura mater

Figure 12-3 The meninges protect the brain and spinal cord. Arrows indicate the flow of cerebrospinal fluid.

Terms Related to the Nervous System *(continued)*

Term	Pronunciation	Meaning
meninges	mĕ-nin'jēz	membranous covering of the brain and spinal cord (Fig. 12-3)
arachnoid	ă-rak'noyd	delicate fibrous membrane forming the middle layer of the meninges
dura mater	dūr'ă mā'tĕr	strong fibrous outermost layer of the meninges
pia mater	pī'ă mā'tĕr	thin inner layer of the meninges that attaches directly to the brain and spinal cord
spinal cord	spī'năl kōrd	portion of the central nervous system contained in the spinal or vertebral canal; responsible for nerve conduction to and from the brain and body
ventricle	ven'tri-kĕl	one of four interconnected cavities within the brain that secrete cerebrospinal fluid
Terms Related to the Peripheral Nervous System		
peripheral nervous system	pĕr-if'ĕr-ăl nĕr'vŭs sis'tĕm	part of the nervous system external to the brain and spinal cord that consists of all other nerves throughout the body
nerve	nĕrv	whitish cordlike structure that transmits stimuli from the central nervous system to another area of the body or from the body to the central nervous system
ganglion	gang'glē-ŏn	group of nerve cell bodies located along the pathway of a nerve

(continued)

Terms Related to the Nervous System *(continued)*

Term	Pronunciation	Meaning
neuroglia, *syn.* glia	nŭr-og'lē-ă, glī'ă	cells that support and protect nervous tissue

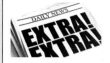 **GLIAL CELLS** Glial cells provide support and protection for neurons, or nerve cells, the other main type of cell in the nervous system. They were identified as the "glue" of the nervous system. The Greek word for glue is *glio*.

Term	Pronunciation	Meaning
neuron	nŭr'on	nerve cells; cells that make up the basic structure of the nervous system and conduct impulses
cranial nerves	krā'nē-ăl něrvz	the 12 pairs of nerves that emerge from the cranium
spinal nerves	spī'năl něrvz	the 31 pairs of nerves that emerge from the spine

■ Exercises: Anatomy and Physiology

SIMPLE
RECALL

Exercise 1

Write the correct anatomic structure for the meaning given.

1. part of the brainstem that connects different regions of the brain

   _____

2. back portion of the cerebrum that controls vision

   _____

3. largest and uppermost portion of the brain

   _____

4. the brain and spinal cord, collectively

   _____

5. portion of the brain that coordinates voluntary muscles

   _____

6. cavity within the brain that secretes cerebrospinal fluid

   _____

7. portion of the cerebrum below the frontal lobe that controls the senses of hearing and smell

   _____

8. middle-top portion of the cerebrum involved in perception of touch, temperature, and pain

   _____

9. front portion of the cerebrum that controls voluntary muscle movement and is involved in emotions

   _____

10. connects the brain to the spinal cord

   _____

Exercise 2

SIMPLE RECALL

Write the meaning of the term given.

1. spinal cord _____

2. cerebral cortex _____

3. nerve _____

4. sulcus _____

5. pia mater _____

6. peripheral nervous system _____

7. midbrain _____

8. cranial nerves _____

9. brain _____

10. meninges _____

Exercise 3

ADVANCED RECALL

Match each medical term with its meaning.

gyrus   arachnoid   ganglion
dura mater   neuron   diencephalon
spinal nerves   cerebrospinal fluid   neuroglia

Meaning   **Term**

1. group of nerve cell bodies along the pathway of a nerve _____

2. 31 pairs of nerves emerging from the spine _____

3. cells that conduct impulses _____

4. the middle layer of the meninges _____

5. colorless fluid in and around the brain and spinal cord _____

6. convolution on the surface of the cerebrum _____

7. cells that support and protect nervous tissue _____

8. fibrous outermost layer of the meninges _____

9. area deep within the brain responsible for directing sensory information to the cortex _____

■ WORD PARTS

Note that some word parts that have been introduced earlier in the book may not be repeated here.

Combining Forms

Combining Form	Meaning
Related to the Nervous System	
cerebell/o	cerebellum (little brain)
cerebr/o	brain, cerebrum
cortic/o	cortex (as in cerebral cortex)
crani/o	cranium, skull
dur/o	hard, dura mater
encephal/o	entire brain
esthesi/o	sensation, perception
gangli/o, ganglion/o	ganglion
gli/o	glue, neuroglia
mening/o, meningi/o	meninges
myel/o	bone marrow, spinal cord
narc/o	stupor, numbness, sleep
neur/o	nerve
phas/o	speech
poli/o	gray
radicul/o	nerve root
somn/o, somn/i	sleep
spin/o	spine
spondyl/o, vertebr/o	vertebra
thalam/o	thalamus
ventricul/o	ventricle
Related to Mental Health	
anxi/o	fear, worry
hallucin/o	to wander in one's mind
hypn/o	sleep, hypnosis
ment/o, psych/o, phren/o	mind, mental
schiz/o	split
soci/o	social, society
thym/i, thym/o	mind, soul, emotion

Prefixes

Prefix	Meaning
Related to the Nervous System	
epi-	on, following
hemi-	half
hyper-	above, excessive
hypo-	below, deficient
para-	beside
poly-	many, much
quadri-	four
Related to Mental Health	
bi-	two, twice
de-	away from, cessation, without
eu-	good, normal

Suffixes

Suffix	Meaning
Related to the Nervous System	
-al, -ar	pertaining to
-gram	record, recording
-ia	condition of
-ictal, -lepsy	seizure
-logist	one who specializes in
-paresis	partial or incomplete paralysis
-phrenia	the mind
-plegia	paralysis
-tomy	incision
Related to Mental Health	
-iatrist	one who specializes in
-mania	excited state, obsession
-philia, -phile	attraction for
-phobia	abnormal fear, aversion to, sensitivity to

■ Exercises: Word Parts

Exercise 4

SIMPLE
RECALL

Write the meaning for the combining form given.

   1. encephal/o _____

   2. gli/o _____

   3. cerebr/o _____

   4. neur/o _____

   5. dur/o _____

   6. meningi/o _____

   7. cerebell/o _____

   8. radicul/o _____

   9. somn/i _____

  10. ment/o _____

  11. gangli/o _____

  12. thalam/o _____

  13. crani/o _____

  14. esthesi/o _____

  15. phas/o _____

  16. spondyl/o _____

  17. myel/o _____

  18. spin/o _____

  19. psych/o _____

  20. poli/o _____

Exercise 5

SIMPLE
RECALL

Write the correct combining form for the meaning given.

   1. glue _____

   2. ventricle _____

   3. entire brain _____

   4. fear, worry _____

   5. spinal cord _____

   6. cerebellum _____

7. cortex   _____

8. ganglion   _____

9. thalamus   _____

10. split   _____

11. spine   _____

12. mind, soul, emotions   _____

13. cerebrum   _____

14. mind   _____

15. vertebra   _____

16. sensation, perception   _____

17. dura mater, hard   _____

18. to wander in one's mind _____

19. stupor, numbness, sleep _____

Exercise 6

SIMPLE RECALL

Write the meaning of the prefix or the suffix given.

1. -iatrist   _____

2. hemi-   _____

3. -philia, -phile   _____

4. -mania   _____

5. -phobia   _____

6. poly-   _____

7. quadri-   _____

8. -ia   _____

9. -tomy   _____

10. hyper-   _____

11. -paresis   _____

12. hypo-   _____

13. -plegia   _____

14. epi-   _____

15. -ictal   _____

ADVANCED
RECALL

Exercise 7

Considering the meaning of the combining form(s) from which the medical term is made, write the meaning of the medical term.

Combining Form	Meaning	Medical Term	Meaning of Term
encephal/o	entire brain	encephalitis	1. _____
crani/o	cerebrum, skull	craniotomy	2. _____
myel/o	spinal cord	myelogram	3. _____
gli/o	glue, neuroglia	glial	4. _____
phas/o	speech	dysphasia	5. _____
spin/o	spine	spinal	6. _____
cerebell/o	cerebellum	cerebellar	7. _____
psych/o	mind	psychologist	8. _____
schiz/o; phren/o	split; mind	schizophrenia	9. _____
esthesi/o	sensation	anesthesia	10. _____
radicul/o	nerve root	radiculopathy	11. _____
neur/o	nerve	polyneuropathy	12. _____

TERM
CONSTRUCTION

Exercise 8

Using the given combining form and a word part from the earlier tables, build a medical term for the meaning given.

Combining Form	Meaning of Medical Term	Medical Term
myel/o	inflammation of the spinal cord	1. _____
crani/o	incision into the skull	2. _____
neur/o	disease of the nerves	3. _____
gli/o	tumor of the glial cells	4. _____
crani/o	pertaining to the skull	5. _____

esthesi/o	condition of painful sensation	6. _____
meningi/o	inflammation of the membranes of the spinal cord	7. _____
dur/o	pertaining to below the dura mater	8. _____
meningi/o	tumor of the membranes of the spinal cord	9. _____
encephal/o	disease of the brain	10. _____

■ MEDICAL TERMS

Adjectives and Other Related Terms

Term	Pronunciation	Meaning
bipolar	bī-pō′lăr	having two ends or extremes
cerebral	ser′ĕ-brăl	pertaining to the cerebrum
cerebellar	ser-ĕ-bel′ăr	pertaining to the cerebellum
cranial	krā′nē-ăl	pertaining to the cranium or skull
dural	dūr′ăl	pertaining to the dura mater
epidural	ep′i-dūr′ăl	pertaining to on or outside the dura mater
glial	glī′ăl	pertaining to the glia
ictal	ik′tăl	pertaining to or caused by a stroke or seizure
ischemic	is-kē′mik	pertaining to a lack of blood flow
meningeal	men′in-jē′ăl	pertaining to the meninges
mental	men′tăl	pertaining to the mind
neural	nūr′ăl	pertaining to the nerves or any structure consisting of nerves
postictal	pōst-ik′tăl	pertaining to following a seizure
radicular	ră-dik′yū-lăr	pertaining to a root (nerve)
subdural	sŭb-dūr′ăl	pertaining to below the dura mater

■ Exercises: Adjectives and Other Related Terms

SIMPLE
RECALL

Exercise 9

Write the meaning of the term given.

1. meningeal _____

2. cranial _____

3. epidural   _____

4. cerebral   _____

5. ischemic   _____

6. radicular   _____

7. mental   _____

Exercise 10

ADVANCED
RECALL

Match each medical term with its meaning.

neural	cerebellar	bipolar
postictal	subdural	ischemic
ictal	glial	dural

Meaning   **Term**

1. having two ends or extremes   _____

2. pertaining to the dura mater   _____

3. pertaining to the nerves or any
structure consisting of nerves   _____

4. pertaining to the glia   _____

5. pertaining to or caused by a stroke
or seizure   _____

6. pertaining to following a seizure   _____

7. pertaining to the cerebellum   _____

8. pertaining to a lack of blood flow   _____

9. pertaining to below the dura mater   _____

Exercise 11

**Write the combining form used in the medical term, followed by the meaning
of the combining form.**

Term	Combining Form	Combining Form Meaning
1. cerebral	_____	_____
2. radicular	_____	_____

3. mental   _____   _____

4. epidural   _____   _____

5. spinal   _____   _____

6. cerebellar   _____   _____

Symptoms and Medical Conditions

Term	Pronunciation	Meaning
Related to the Nervous System		
Alzheimer disease	awlts′hī-mĕr di-zĕz′	a degenerative progressive brain disease that results in impairment of language function, inability to calculate, and deterioration of judgment
amnesia	am-nē′zē-ă	loss of long-term memory
amyotrophic lateral sclerosis (ALS), *syn.* Lou Gehrig disease	ă-mī′ō-trō′fik lat′ĕr-ăl skler-ō′sis, lū ger′ig di-zĕz′	condition marked by a progressive deterioration of motor nerve cells; leads to muscle weakness and eventually paralysis and death (Fig. 12-4)

(continued)

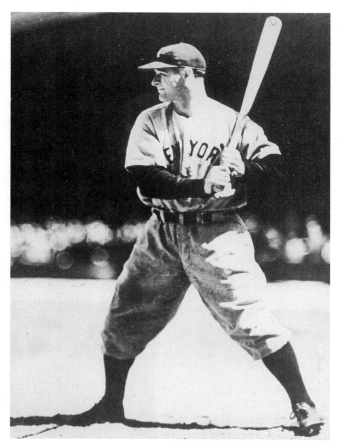

Figure 12-4 ALS is also called Lou Gehrig disease after Gehrig, a major league baseball player who was diagnosed with the disease in 1939.

Symptoms and Medical Conditions *(continued)*

Term	Pronunciation	Meaning
aphasia	ă-fā′zē-ă	impaired comprehension or formulation of speech, reading, or writing caused by damage to the brain
ataxia	ă-tak′sē-ă	lack of muscle coordination; may involve the limbs, head, or trunk
Bell palsy	bel pawl′zē	paralysis of facial muscles, often on one side of the face, caused by a dysfunction of a cranial nerve

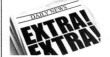 **BELL PALSY** Bell palsy is believed to be an inflammation of the facial nerve. The diagnosis is made by ruling out infections by Lyme disease, herpes infection, or even a stroke.

Term	Pronunciation	Meaning
cerebral aneurysm	ser′ĕ-brăl an′yūr-izm	widening of a blood vessel in the brain, usually due to a weakness in the wall of the artery
cerebral embolism	ser′ĕ-brăl em′bŏ-lizm	obstruction or occlusion of a vessel in the brain by an embolus (Fig. 12-5)
cerebral palsy (CP)	ser′ĕ-brăl pawl′zē	defect of motor power and coordination related to damage to the brain that occurred prenatally, perinatally, or in the first 3 years of life
cerebral thrombosis	ser′ĕ-brăl throm-bō′sis	clot within a blood vessel of the brain (Fig. 12-5)
cerebrovascular accident (CVA), *syn.* stroke	ser′ĕ-brō-vas′kyū-lăr ak′si-dĕnt, strōk	damage to the brain caused by an interruption of blood supply to a region of the brain (Fig. 12-6)

(continued)

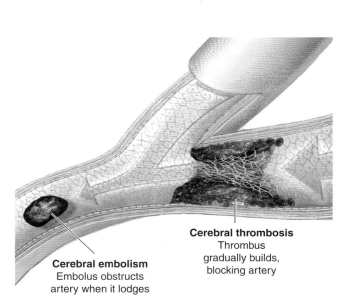

Figure 12-5 Cerebral embolism and cerebral thrombosis.

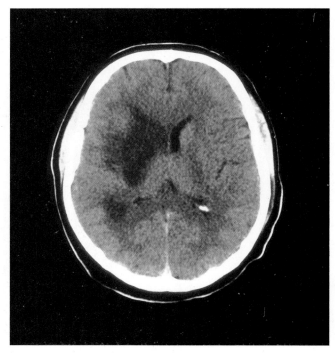

Figure 12-6 Computed tomography scan of the brain. The darker shaded area of this scan indicates damage from a cerebrovascular accident.

Symptoms and Medical Conditions *(continued)*

Term	Pronunciation	Meaning
coma	kō'mă	a state of profound unconsciousness
concussion	kŏn-kŭsh'ŭn	injury to the brain resulting from a blow or violent shaking
disorientation	dis-ōr'ē-ĕn-tā'shŭn	loss of sense of familiarity with one's surroundings (time, place, and self)

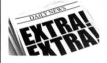 **"ORIENTED ×3"** When trying to determine if a person is aware of their surroundings, usually after an accident or a temporary loss of consciousness, medical personnel will typically ask the victim if they know their name, if they know where they are, and if they know the day, week, month, or year. This is known as *orientation times 3*. It is charted as A&O ×3 which means "alert and oriented ×3."

Term	Pronunciation	Meaning
encephalitis	en-sef'ă-lī'tis	inflammation of the entire brain
epilepsy	ep'i-lep'sē	disorder of the central nervous system that is usually characterized by seizure activity and some alteration of consciousness
herpes zoster, *syn.* shingles	hĕr'pēz zos'tĕr, shing'gĕlz	painful viral infection that affects the peripheral nerves and causes an eruption of blisters that follows the course of the affected nerves; closely related to varicella
incoherence	in'kō-hēr'ens	confusion; denoting unconnected speech or thoughts
lethargy	leth'ăr-jē	a feeling of sluggishness or stupor
hemiparesis	hem'ē-pă-rē'sis	partial or incomplete paralysis affecting one side of the body (Fig. 12-7)

(continued)

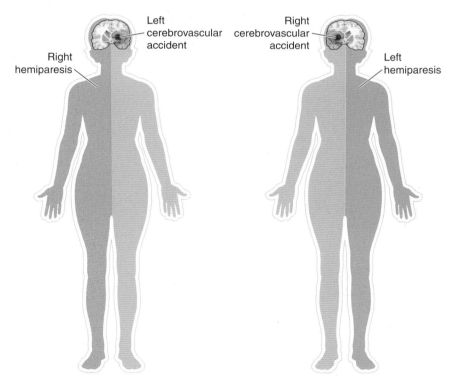

Figure 12-7 Right and left hemiparesis caused by CVA.

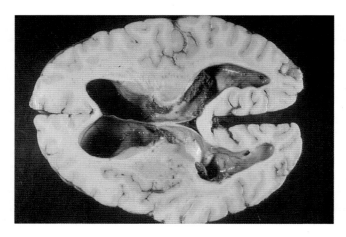

Figure 12-8   Cerebral ventricles have become enlarged from hydrocephalus.

Symptoms and Medical Conditions *(continued)*

Term	Pronunciation	Meaning
hydrocephalus	hī′drō-sef′ă-lŭs	a condition involving increased cerebrospinal fluid; leads to enlargement of the cerebral ventricles and an increase in intracranial pressure; may cause cranial enlargement (Fig. 12-8)
meningitis	men′in-jī′tis	inflammation of the meninges
meningomyelocele	mĕ-ning′gō-mī′ĕ-lō-sēl	protrusion of the meninges and spinal cord through a defect in the vertebra (Fig. 12-9)

(continued)

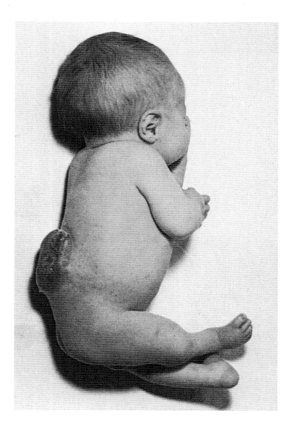

Figure 12-9   Meningomyelocele.

Symptoms and Medical Conditions *(continued)*

Term	Pronunciation	Meaning
migraine	mī′grān	recurrent syndrome characterized by unilateral head pain, vertigo, nausea, and sensitivity to light
multiple sclerosis (MS)	mŭl′ti-pĕl skler-ō′sis	common disorder of the central nervous system that causes sclerotic patches (plaques) in the brain and spinal cord; symptoms may include visual loss, weakness, paresthesias, bladder abnormalities, and mood alterations
narcolepsy, *syn.* excessive sleep disorder	nahr′kō-lep-sē, eks-es′iv slēp dis-ōr′dĕr	neurologic condition consisting of recurring episodes of sleep during the day and often disrupted nocturnal sleep
neuralgia	nūr-al′jē-ă	pain in a nerve
neuritis	nūr-ī′tis	inflammation of a nerve
neuropathy	nūr-op′ă-thē	disease of the nerves
paraplegia	par′ă-plē′jē-ă	paralysis of the legs and lower part of the body
paresthesia	par-es-thē′zē-ă	an abnormal sensation, such as numbness, tingling, or "pins and needles"
parkinsonism, *syn.* Parkinson disease	pahr′kin-sŏn-izm, pahr′kin-sŏn di-zēz′	degenerative disorder of the central nervous system that often impairs the sufferer's motor skills and speech; most notably characterized by tremors of the limbs
poliomyelitis	pō′lē-ō-mī-ĕ-lī′tis	inflammation of the gray matter of the spinal cord
polyneuritis	pol′ē-nūr-ī′tis	inflammation of a number of peripheral nerves
radiculitis	ră-dik′yū-lī′tis	inflammation of the nerve roots
radiculopathy	ră-dik′yū-lop′ă-thē	disease of the nerve roots
seizure	sē′zhŭr	violent spasm or series of jerky movements of the face, trunk, or limbs
sleep apnea	slēp ap′nē-ă	disorder marked by interruptions of breathing during sleep
stupor	stū′pŏr	state of impaired consciousness in which the person shows a marked reduction in reactivity to environmental stimuli
subdural hematoma	sŭb-dūr′ăl hē′mă-tō′mă	a collection of blood below the dura mater resulting from a broken blood vessel, usually due to trauma (Fig. 12-10)
syncope, *syn.* syncopal episode	sing′kŏ-pē, sing′kŏ-păl ep′i-sōd	fainting, or an episode of fainting, usually due to lack of blood supply to the cerebrum
Tourette syndrome	tūr-et′ sin′drōm	tic disorder characterized by intermittent motor and vocal manifestations that begins in childhood
transient ischemic attack (TIA)	tran′sē-ĕnt is-kē′mik ă-tak′	sudden, brief, and temporary cerebral dysfunction usually caused by interruption of blood flow to the brain
Related to Mental Health		
anxiety	ang-zī′ĕ-tē	feeling of fear, worry, uneasiness, or dread
attention deficit hyperactivity disorder (ADHD)	ă-ten′shŭn def′i-sit hī′pĕr-ak-tiv′i-tē dis-ōr′dĕr	condition that begins in childhood and is characterized by short attention span, rapid boredom, impulsive behavior, and hyperactivity
agoraphobia	ag′ŏr-ă-fō′bē-ă	type of mental disorder with an irrational fear of leaving home and going out into the open; usually associated with panic attacks

(continued)

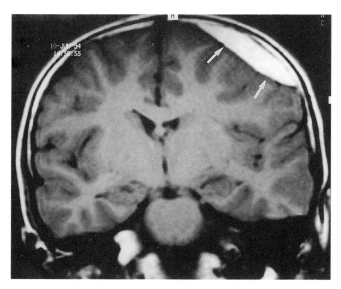

Figure 12-10 Coronal magnetic resonance image showing a subdural hematoma (*arrows*).

Symptoms and Medical Conditions *(continued)*

Term	Pronunciation	Meaning
autism	aw'tizm	disorder of unknown cause consisting of self-absorption, withdrawal of social contacts, repetitive movements and other mannerisms; severity varies from mild (functional) to severe (catatonic)
bipolar disorder	bī-pō'lăr dis-ōr'děr	disorder characterized by the occurrence of alternating periods of euphoria (mania) and depression (Fig. 12-11)
catatonia	kat'ă-tō'nē-ă	a phase of schizophrenia in which the patient is unresponsive, sometimes remaining in a fixed position without moving or talking

(continued)

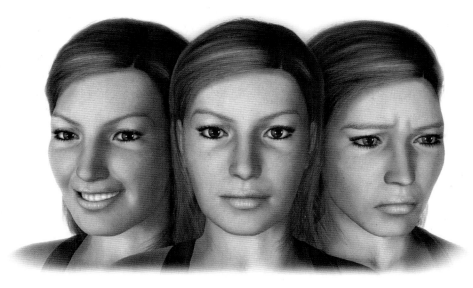

Figure 12-11 Bipolar disorder.

Symptoms and Medical Conditions (continued)

Term	Pronunciation	Meaning
claustrophobia	klaw'strŏ-fō'bē-ă	fear of being shut in or enclosed
compulsion	kŏm-pŭl'shŭn	uncontrollable impulses to perform an act, often repetitively, to relieve anxiety; if the compulsive act is prevented, the anxiety becomes fully manifested
delirium	dĕ-lir'ē-ŭm	an altered state with confusion, distractibility, hallucinations, and overactivity caused by medication or a metabolic disorder
delusion	dĕ-lū'zhŭn	a false belief or decision that is strongly held and remains unchanged regardless of any outside factors
dementia	dĕ-men'shē-ă	usually progressive loss of cognitive and intellectual functions, without impairment of perception or consciousness; most commonly associated with structural brain disease
depression	dĕ-presh'ŭn	mental state characterized by profound feelings of sadness, emptiness, hopelessness, and lack of interest or pleasure in activities (Fig. 12-12)
euphoria	yū-fōr'ē-ă	an exaggerated feeling of well-being
hallucination	hă-lū'si-nā'shŭn	false perception unrelated to reality or external stimuli; can be visual, auditory, or related to the other senses
mania	mā'nē-ă	emotional disorder characterized by euphoria or irritability as well as rapid speech, decreased need for sleep, distractibility, and poor judgment; usually occurs in bipolar disorder
neurosis	nūr-ō'sis	psychological or behavioral disorder characterized by excessive anxiety

(continued)

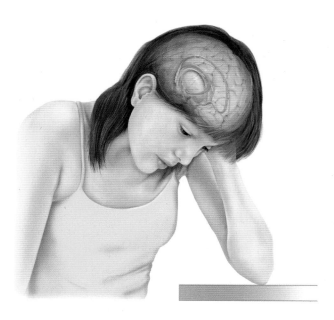

Figure 12-12 Depression.

Symptoms and Medical Conditions *(continued)*

Term	Pronunciation	Meaning
obsessive-compulsive disorder (OCD)	ob-ses'iv-kŏm-pŭl'siv dis-ōr'dĕr	condition associated with recurrent and intrusive thoughts, images, and repetitive behaviors performed to relieve anxiety
panic disorder	pan'ik dis-ōr'dĕr	form of anxiety disorder marked by episodes of intense fear of social or personal situations
paranoia	par'ă-noy'ă	mental state characterized by jealousy, delusions of persecution, or perceptions of threat or harm
phobia	fō'bē-ă	extreme persistent fear of a specific object or situation
posttraumatic stress disorder (PTSD)	pŏst'traw-mat'ik stres dis-ōr'dĕr	persistent emotional disturbances that follow exposure to life-threatening catastrophic events such as trauma, abuse, natural disasters, and war
psychosis	sī-kō'sis	mental disorder extreme enough to cause gross misperception of reality with delusions and hallucinations
schizophrenia	skits'ō-frē'nē-ă	common type of psychosis, characterized by abnormalities in perception, content of thought, hallucinations and delusions, and withdrawn or bizarre behavior

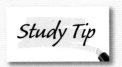

Aphasia vs. Aphagia: Avoid confusing these sound-alike terms. Aphasia means impaired comprehension or formulation of speech, reading, or writing caused by damage to the brain, whereas aphagia means the inability to eat. To prevent mix-ups, use this hint: Aphasia has an "s" (as in speech), and aphagia has a "g" (as in gastrointestinal, which is related to eating).

■ Exercises: Symptoms and Medical Conditions

Exercise 12

SIMPLE RECALL

Write the correct medical term for the meaning given.

1. injury to the brain resulting from a blow or violent shaking   _____

2. state of impaired consciousness in which the person shows a marked reduction in reactivity to environmental stimuli   _____

3. a state of profound unconsciousness   _____

4. degenerative disorder of the central nervous system   _____

5. loss of sense of familiarity with one's surroundings   _____

6. damage to the brain caused by an interruption of blood supply to a region of the brain   _____

7. disorder that causes sclerotic patches (plaques) in the brain and spinal cord   _____

8. widening of a blood vessel in the brain   _____

9. obstruction or occlusion of a vessel in the brain   _____

10. loss of long-term memory   _____

11. progressive deterioration of motor nerve cells   _____

12. paralysis of the legs and lower part of the body   _____

Exercise 13

ADVANCED
RECALL

Complete each sentence by writing in the correct medical term.

1. A person who repeatedly washes household items that are already clean because of an intrusive fear they will get infected with germs is suffering from a condition called

_____.

2. A person who worries or is overly fearful about a situation may be diagnosed as having

_____.

3. Children and even adults who cannot focus on their tasks without being easily distracted and who display impulsive behavior may be diagnosed with _____.

4. A person with _____ experiences persistent emotional disturbances following exposure to life-threatening catastrophic events.

5. Patients suffering from _____ feel persecuted and think that others are out to cause them harm.

6. Persons who strongly hold a false belief that remains unchanged despite outside factors may be diagnosed with _____.

7. Someone with an uncontrollable impulse to gamble at every opportunity may be exhibiting a(n) _____ for the activity.

8. Patients who have profound feelings of sadness, emptiness, hopelessness, and lack of interest or pleasure in activities are often diagnosed with _____.

9. The phase of schizophrenia in which a patient is unresponsive is called _____.

10. Patients with _____ have difficulty leaving their home because of an irrational fear of going out in the open.

11. Children who suffer from _____ withdraw from social contacts and exhibit repetitive movements.

12. A patient who is in an altered state with confusion, distractibility, hallucinations, and overactivity might be suffering from _____.

TERM
CONSTRUCTION

Exercise 14

Break the given medical terms into its word parts and define each part. Then define the medical term. (Note: This exercise uses some word parts learned previously in this text.)

For example:
neuritis   *word parts:*   neur/o   /   -itis
               meanings: nerve   /   inflammation
               term meaning: inflammation of a nerve

1. polyneuritis   *word parts:*   _____ / _____ / _____

                    meanings: _____ / _____ / _____

                    term meaning: _____

2. radiculopathy   *word parts:*   _____ / _____

                    meanings: _____ / _____

                    term meaning: _____

3. aphasia   *word parts:*   _____ / _____ / _____

                    meanings: _____ / _____ / _____

                    term meaning: _____

4. meningomyelocele   *word parts:*   _____ / _____ / _____

                    meanings: _____ / _____ / _____

                    term meaning: _____

5. encephalitis   *word parts:*   _____ / _____

                    meanings: _____ / _____

                    term meaning: _____

6. hemiparesis   *word parts:*   _____ / _____

                    meanings: _____ / _____

                    term meaning: _____

7. neuralgia   *word parts:*   _____ / _____

                    meanings: _____ / _____

                    term meaning: _____

8. schizophrenia   *word parts:* _____ / _____

                   meanings: _____ / _____

                   term meaning: _____

9. subdural   *word parts:* _____ / _____ / _____

                   meanings: _____ / _____ / _____

                   term meaning: _____

10. poliomyelitis   *word parts:* _____ / _____ / _____

                   meanings: _____ / _____ / _____

                   term meaning: _____

Diagnostic Procedures

Term	Pronunciation	Meaning
Babinski sign	bă-bin′skē sīn	toe movement elicited by manipulation in a neurologic test performed on the sole of the foot to indicate injury to the brain or spinal nerves (Fig. 12-13)
cerebral angiography	ser′ĕ-brăl an′jē-og′ră-fē	radiography of blood vessels in the brain after injection of radiopaque contrast material
deep tendon reflex (DTR)	dēp ten′dŏn rē′fleks	evaluation of the response of a muscle to stimuli to provide information on the integrity of the central and peripheral nervous system; generally, decreased reflexes indicate a problem with the *peripheral* nervous system, and lively or exaggerated reflexes indicate a problem with the *central* nervous system

(continued)

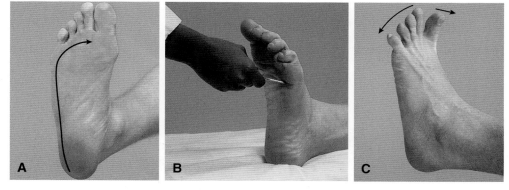

Figure 12-13 **Babinski sign.** The physician uses an instrument to stroke the sole of the patient's foot, beginning at the heel and curving upward, causing toe flexion (negative Babinski sign). (A and B). Toes that fan outward (positive Babinski sign) may indicate injury to the brain or spinal nerves.

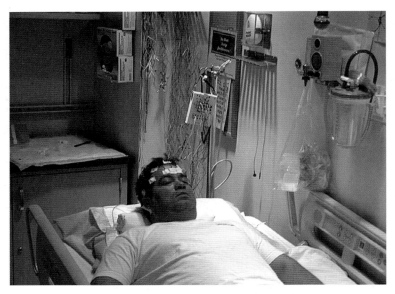

Figure 12-14 Electroencephalography.

Diagnostic Procedures *(continued)*

Term	Pronunciation	Meaning
electroencephalogram (EEG)	ĕ-lek′trō-en-sef′ă-lō-gram	electrical recording of activity of the brain (Fig. 12-14)
evoked potential studies	ē-vōkt′ pŏ-ten′shăl stŭd′ēz	diagnostic tests that use an EEG to record changes in brain waves during various stimuli
Glasgow coma scale	glas′gō kō′mă skāl	a neurologic scale used to assess level of consciousness
lumbar puncture (LP)	lŭm′bahr pungk′shŭr	the process of inserting a needle into the subarachnoid space of the lumbar spine to obtain cerebrospinal fluid for analysis (Fig. 12-15)

(continued)

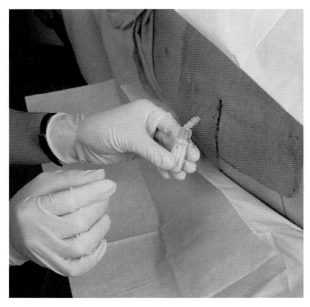

Figure 12-15 Obtaining a sample of cerebrospinal fluid after a lumbar puncture.

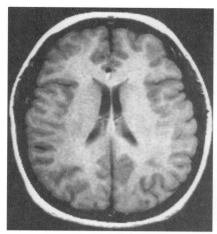 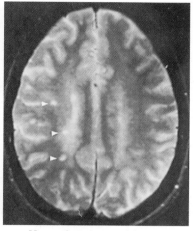

Magnetic resonance image, normal brain, horizontal view

Magnetic resonance image, multiple sclerosis, horizontal view

Figure 12-16 Magnetic resonance imaging of the brain.

Diagnostic Procedures *(continued)*

Term	Pronunciation	Meaning
magnetic resonance imaging (MRI)	mag-net′ik rez′ŏ-năns im′ăj-ing	imaging technique that uses magnetic fields and radio-frequency waves to visualize anatomic structures; often used for diagnosing soft tissue (Fig. 12-16)
myelogram	mī′ĕ-lō-gram	radiographic contrast study of the spinal subarachnoid space and its contents
polysomnography	pol′ē-som-nog′ră-fē	monitoring and recording of normal and abnormal activity during sleep to diagnose sleep disorders
positron emission tomography (PET)	poz′i-tron ĕ-mish′ŭn tŏ-mog′ră-fē	a nuclear medicine procedure that shows blood flow in the brain that can correspond to various brain activity (Fig. 12-17)

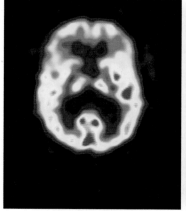 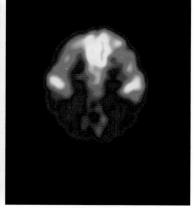

PET scan of healthy brain

PET scan of Alzheimer brain

Figure 12-17 Positron-emission tomography (PET) scans of the brain.

■ Exercises: Diagnostic Procedures

Exercise 15

SIMPLE RECALL

Write the correct medical term for the meaning given.

1. neurologic scale to assess level of consciousness _____

2. group of tests to record changes in brain waves _____

3. result of neurologic test performed on the sole of the foot _____

4. test that shows blood flow in the brain corresponding to brain activity _____

5. radiography of blood vessels in the brain after injection of radiopaque contrast material _____

Exercise 16

ADVANCED RECALL

Complete each sentence by writing the correct medical term.

1. The process of inserting a needle into the low back area to extract a small amount of cerebrospinal fluid for analysis is called a(n) _____.

2. During _____, various aspects of sleep are recorded to diagnose sleep disorders.

3. Before undergoing _____, which generates images by using a magnetic field, patients are thoroughly questioned to determine if they have any metal within their bodies.

4. The test that evaluates how a muscle responds to stimuli is called _____.

5. The procedure in which sensors are applied to a patient's head to produce an electrical recording of brain activity is called a(n) _____.

6. A(n) _____ is a type of contrast study that allows visualization of the spinal subarachnoid space and its contents.

Surgical Interventions and Therapeutic Procedures

Term	Pronunciation	Meaning
craniectomy	krā′nē-ek′tŏ-me	excision of part of the cranium to access the brain (Fig. 12-18)
craniotomy	krā′nē-ot′ŏ-mē	incision into the skull to access the brain (Fig. 12-18)
ganglionectomy	gang′glē-ō-nek′tŏ-mē	excision of a ganglion
laminectomy	lam′i-nek′tŏ-mē	excision of the thin plate of the vertebra to relieve pressure on the spinal cord

(continued)

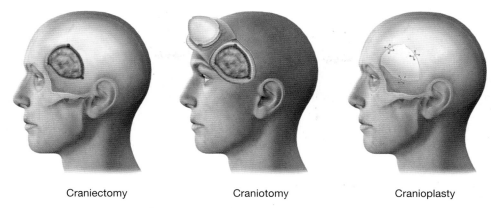

Craniectomy   Craniotomy   Cranioplasty

Figure 12-18   Surgeries of the skull.

Surgical Interventions and Therapeutic Procedures *(continued)*

Term	Pronunciation	Meaning
neurolysis	nūr-ol'i-sis	separation of a nerve from inflammatory adhesions
neuroplasty	nūr'ō-plas-tē	surgical repair of the nerves
psychotherapy	sī'kō-thār'ă-pē	the general term for an interaction in which a trained mental health professional tries to help a patient resolve emotional and mental distress
radicotomy, *syn.* rhizotomy	rad'i-kot'ŏ-mē, rī-zot'ŏ-mē	incision into the spinal nerve roots to relieve pain or spastic paralysis

■ Exercises: Surgical Interventions and Therapeutic Procedures

ADVANCED
RECALL

Exercise 17

Match each medical term with its meaning.

neuroplasty   craniectomy   neurolysis   ganglionectomy
craniotomy   radicotomy   laminectomy   psychotherapy

1. surgical repair of the nerves   _____

2. excision of part of the skull   _____

3. removal of the thin plate of the vertebra   _____

4. incision into the skull   _____

5. incision into the spinal nerve roots   _____

6. separation of a nerve from inflammatory adhesions   _____

7. excision of a ganglion   _____

8. intervention to help a patient deal with emotional distress   _____

Exercise 18

TERM CONSTRUCTION

Build a medical term from an appropriate combining form and suffix, given their meanings.

Use Combining Form for	Use Suffix for	Term
1. nerve	surgical repair	_____
2. ganglion	excision	_____
3. nerve root	incision	_____
4. cranium	excision	_____

Medications and Drug Therapies

Term	Pronunciation	Meaning
analgesic	an'ăl-jē'zik	drug that relieves pain
anesthetic	an'es-thet'ik	compound that provides temporary loss of sensation
antianxiety agent, *syn.* anxiolytic	an'tē-ang-zī'ĕ-tē ă'jĕnt, ang'zē-ō-lit'ik	category of drugs used to treat anxiety without causing excessive sedation
anticonvulsant	an'tē-kŏn-vŭl'sănt	drug that prevents or arrests seizures
antidepressant	an'tē-dĕ-pres'ănt	drug used to treat depression
antiinflammatory	an'tē-in-flam'ă-tōr-ē	drug that reduces inflammation
epidural injection	ep'i-dūr'ăl in-jek'shŭn	subcutaneous or intramuscular injection of an analgesic into the epidural space
hypnotic	hip-not'ik	drug that promotes sleep
neuroleptic	nūr'ō-lep'tik	class of psychotropic drugs used to treat psychosis, particularly schizophrenia
psychotropic	sī'kō-trō'pik	drug used to treat mental illnesses
sedative	sed'ă-tiv	drug that quiets nervous excitement

■ Exercises: Medications and Drug Therapies

Exercise 19

SIMPLE RECALL

Write the correct medication or drug therapy term for the meaning given.

1. a drug that prevents or arrests seizures _____

2. a drug used to treat depression _____

3. a category of drugs used to treat anxiety _____

4. a drug that reduces inflammation   _____

5. a drug that quiets nervous excitement   _____

6. a drug that relieves pain   _____

7. a class of psychotropic drugs   _____

8. subcutaneous injection of an analgesic into the epidural space   _____

Exercise 20

ADVANCED
RECALL

Considering the meaning of the combining form from which the medication or drug therapy is made, write the meaning of the term.

Combining Form	Meaning	Medical Term	Meaning of Term
anxi/o	anxiety	anxiolytic	**1.** _____
psych/o	mind, mental	psychotropic	**2.** _____
esthesi/o	sensation	anesthetic	**3.** _____
hypn/o	sleep, hypnosis	hypnotic	**4.** _____

Specialties and Specialists

Term	Pronunciation	Meaning
electroencephalography (EEG) technician	ĕ-lek′trō-en-sef′ă-log′ră-fē tek-nish′ŭn	a person who is trained to set up and perform electroencephalograms (EEGs) (tests that evaluate the electrical functions of the brain)
neurology	nūr-ol′ŏ-jē	medical specialty concerned with the study and treatment of conditions involving the nervous system
neurologist	nūr-ol′ŏ-jist	physician who specializes in neurology
psychiatry	sī-kī′ă-trē	medical specialty concerned with the diagnosis and treatment of mental disorders as practiced by a licensed medical doctor who may prescribe medications
psychiatrist	sī-kī′ă-trist	physician who specializes in psychiatry
psychology	sī-kol′ŏ-jē	medical specialty concerned with the study and treatment of mental processes, behaviors and abnormal/irregular mood disorders as practiced by a trained professional who is not a medical doctor and is not authorized to prescribe psychotropic medications
psychologist	sī-kol′ŏ-jist	one who specializes in psychology

■ Exercise: Specialties and Specialists

ADVANCED
RECALL

Exercise 21

Match each medical specialty or specialist with its description.

psychologist	psychology	neurology	psychiatry
psychiatrist	neurologist	EEG technician	

1. professional who specializes in psychology _____

2. study and treatment of nervous system _____
   conditions

3. specialty concerned with the diagnosis and _____
   treatment of mental disorders as practiced
   by a licensed medical doctor who may
   prescribe medications

4. physician who specializes in psychiatry _____

5. specially trained person who performs tests _____
   that evaluate the electrical current of the brain

6. medical specialty concerned with the study _____
   and treatment of mental processes, behaviors,
   and abnormal or irregular mood disorders

7. physician who specializes in the nervous _____
   system

Abbreviations

Abbreviation	Meaning
ADHD	attention deficit hyperactivity disorder
ALS	amyotrophic lateral sclerosis
CNS	central nervous system
CP	cerebral palsy
CSF	cerebrospinal fluid
CVA	cerebrovascular accident
DTR	deep tendon reflex
EEG	electroencephalogram
LP	lumbar puncture
MRI	magnetic resonance imaging
MS	multiple sclerosis
OCD	obsessive-compulsive disorder
PET	positron emission tomography
PTSD	posttraumatic stress disorder
TIA	transient ischemic attack

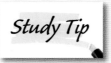

Study Tip

EEG vs. ECG or EKG: Be very careful when using EEG—the abbreviation for electroencephalogram. Do not confuse it with ECG or EKG—the abbreviations for electrocardiogram.

■ Exercises: Abbreviations

ADVANCED
RECALL

Exercise 22

Write the meaning of each abbreviation used in these sentences.

1. The child was diagnosed with **CP** as a result of damage to the brain that occurred prenatally.

   _____

2. Mr. Jackowski was admitted with strokelike symptoms, but testing revealed that he had suffered a **TIA.**

   _____

3. Mrs. Wu had to undergo an **LP** to check for bacteria in her cerebrospinal fluid.

   _____

4. Patients with **MS** may become weak and lethargic, and may have problems with coordination.

   _____

5. **CSF** is normally clear without any evidence of cells or bacteria.

   _____

6. Mrs. Merriman received a written warning at work because she has **OCD** and was constantly in the ladies room washing her hands.

   _____

7. The patient had an **MRI** to assess his injuries after a car accident.

   _____

8. The effects of a **CVA** can be either minimal, with a short recovery period, or debilitating, requiring extensive rehabilitation.

   _____

ADVANCED
RECALL

Exercise 23

Match the abbreviations with the appropriate meaning.

PET	PTSD	ADHD	CNS
EEG	ALS	DTR	CVA

Meaning   **Abbreviation**

1. study that measures brain waves, function and status   _____

2. condition that results in a stroke   _____

3. progressive deterioration of motor nerve cells   _____

4. persistent emotional disturbances that follow   _____
   exposure to life-threatening catastrophic events

5. condition characterized by an inability to sit still, lack   _____
   of focus, and easy distraction

6. procedure that shows blood flow in the brain   _____

7. the brain and the spinal cord system, collectively   _____

8. assessment of reflexes by tapping or stimulating   _____
   at certain points

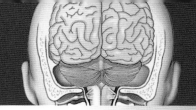

Chapter Review

Review of Terms for Anatomy and Physiology

VISUAL

Exercise 24

Write the correct terms on the blanks for the anatomic structures indicated.

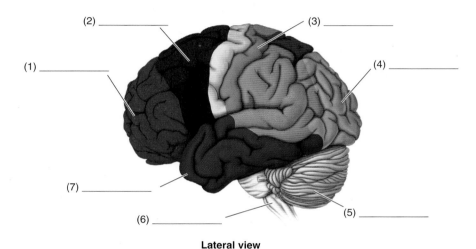

(1) _____
(2) _____
(3) _____
(4) _____
(5) _____
(6) _____
(7) _____

Lateral view

VISUAL

Exercise 25

Write the correct terms on the blanks for the anatomic structures indicated.

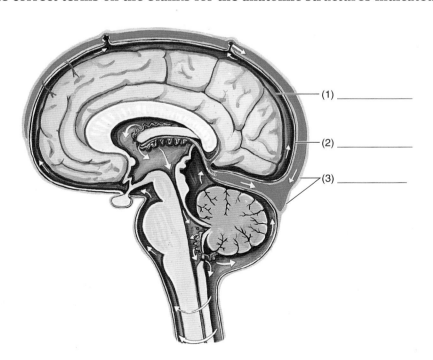

(1) _____
(2) _____
(3) _____

Understanding Term Structure

TERM CONSTRUCTION

Exercise 26

Break the given medical term into its word parts and define each part. Then define the medical term.

For example:

encephalitis	*word parts:*	encephal/o / -itis
	meanings:	entire brain / inflammation
	term meaning:	inflammation of the entire brain

1. meningocyte

word parts: _____ / _____

meanings: _____ / _____

term meaning: _____

2. neuropathy

word parts: _____ / _____

meanings: _____ / _____

term meaning: _____

3. craniocerebral

word parts: _____ / _____ / _____

meanings: _____ / _____ / _____

term meaning: _____

4. quadriparesis

word parts: _____ / _____

meanings: _____ / _____

term meaning: _____

5. radiculomyelopathy

word parts: _____ / _____ / _____

meanings: _____ / _____ / _____

term meaning: _____

6. electroencephalography

word parts: _____ / _____ / _____

meanings: _____ / _____ / _____

term meaning: _____

7. encephaloscopy

word parts: _____ / _____

meanings: _____ / _____

term meaning: _____

8. poliodystrophy   *word parts:*   _____ / _____ / _____

    meanings: _____ / _____ / _____

    term meaning: _____

9. spondylosis   *word parts:*   _____ / _____

    meanings: _____ / _____

    term meaning: _____

10. ganglionectomy   *word parts:*   _____ / _____

    meanings: _____ / _____

    term meaning: _____

Comprehension Exercises

Exercise 27

COMPREHENSION **Fill in the blank with the correct term.**

1. A patient with auditory and visual _____ may be admitted into the psychiatric ward of the hospital.

2. _____ is a feeling of sluggishness or state of impaired consciousness.

3. The inability to walk because of a lack of muscle coordination is called _____.

4. The patient had _____, a condition involving paralysis on one side of the face.

5. The disorder that causes patients to stop breathing for short periods in their sleep is called _____.

6. A degenerative brain disease that results in a patient's inability to assess situations and make appropriate decisions is called _____.

7. Loss of sensation, usually caused by administration of a medication, is called _____.

8. A(n) _____ is a procedure that is done to check brain activity.

9. Herpes zoster, also known as _____, causes blisters on the course of affected nerves.

10. Patients with _____ constantly fear that they are going to be harmed.

11. _____ is caused by brain damage that occurs during the first 3 years of life or prenatally.

12. Inflammation of the membranous covering of the brain and spinal cord is called

_____.

13. _____ is a disease of the nerve roots.

14. A patient experiencing a(n) _____ usually has pain on only one side of the head.

15. A(n) _____ impairs circulation to the brain due to a blood clot.

16. The _____ is the part of the brain that is divided into two hemispheres, a right and left.

17. Prominent rounded elevations that form the cerebral hemispheres are called

_____.

18. The _____ connects the brain to the portion of the central nervous system that is contained in the spinal canal.

19. _____ is the medical term for fainting.

20. A neurologic disorder characterized by temporary loss of consciousness and violent spasms or series of jerky movements of the face, trunk, or limbs is called _____.

Exercise 28

COMPREHENSION **Circle the letter of the best answer in the following questions.**

1. A patient who is having problems formulating thoughts into words is experiencing:

   A. paraplegia
   B. aphagia
   C. ataxia
   D. aphasia

2. A person who exhibits involuntary vocal or motor dysfunctions in a tic-like manner suffers from:

   A. a stroke
   B. Alzheimer disease
   C. Tourette syndrome
   D. dementia

3. A patient visits her physician complaining of a severe headache and nausea. She states that she must lie down in a darkened room. Her likely diagnosis is:

   A. migraine
   B. claustrophobia
   C. myelitis
   D. delusion

4. Patients with diabetes who have long-term manifestations often have pain in the nerves of their feet. This is called:

   A. neurology
   B. neuralgia
   C. stupor
   D. amnesia

5. A child was hit in the head by a foul ball at a baseball game. At the hospital, he was found to have a collection of blood under the skull, just inside the brain. The diagnosis was:

   A. neuritis
   B. a subdural hematoma
   C. a temporal lobe
   D. a frontal lobe

6. A patient suddenly appears to be staring off into space. Her face droops slightly at the mouth, and she does not respond to verbal stimuli. After about 30 minutes, she appears fine and is speaking clearly and coherently. Her face no longer

droops at the mouth. She most likely had a(n):

A. EEG
B. TIA
C. CNS
D. CSF

7. A sleep disturbance in which a person cannot sleep at night but can often fall asleep without notice is called:

A. Alzheimer disease
B. sleep apnea
C. narcolepsy
D. meningitis

8. A patient suddenly has difficulty speaking and her right arm feels stiff and weak. Her face has a right-sided droop and her speech is slurred. She most likely suffered a(n):

A. EEG
B. LP
C. CSF
D. CVA

9. In elderly patients, a progressive loss of thought processes without loss of awareness is called:

A. sleep apnea
B. meningitis
C. dementia
D. neuropathy

10. Symptoms of this disorder mimic a stroke and are thought to be caused by a dysfunction of a nerve. This illness is called:

A. shingles
B. Bell palsy

C. autism
D. anxiety

11. The accumulation of excessive fluid that circulates in and around the brain and spinal cord with resulting increased intracranial pressure is called:

A. encephalitis
B. hydrocephalus
C. hydromeningitis
D. hydrocraniosis

12. A patient who lacks normal clarity of speech and also is confused is said to be suffering from:

A. lethargy
B. incoherence
C. stupor
D. phobia

13. A patient complains of feeling "pins and needles." The medical term for this abnormal sensation is:

A. paralysis
B. hemiplegia
C. paresthesia
D. hydrocephalus

14. A young man suddenly falls to the floor convulsing and appears unconscious. He is thought to be having a(n):

A. migraine
B. autism
C. seizure
D. amnesia

Application and Analysis

Exercise 29

APPLICATION

Read the case reports and circle the letter of your answer choice for the following questions about each case.

CASE 12-1

Mr. Parker, age 78, was found at home on the bathroom floor somewhat confused and disoriented. He does not recall exactly what happened. He remembers going to the bathroom, talks about falling, and then speaks about moving things around that did not belong in the bathroom. When asked about the type of objects being moved, the patient was not able to name anything specific. Some expressive aphasia is noted during our discussion. It was determined he does not have a mental disorder. Neurologically, he is oriented to person (self) but not to time or place.

1. Based on the information provided in the case, what specialist might be called to see this patient?

   A. psychiatrist
   B. neurology
   C. neurologist
   D. psychologist

2. Aphasia is:

   A. the inability to walk
   B. the inability to swallow
   C. the inability to respond or communicate appropriately
   D. the inability to see

3. Disorientation can include the loss of familiarity with:

   A. time
   B. place
   C. person (self)
   D. all of the above

4. This patient might have had an episode of fainting, also called:

   A. syncope
   B. seizures
   C. lethargy
   D. ataxia

CASE 12-2

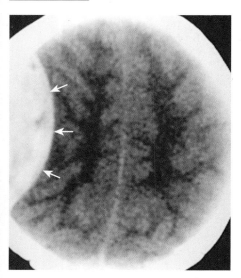

Figure 12-19 Computed tomography (CT) scan revealing epidural hematoma (*arrows*).

A 16-year-old boy was riding his bike when he skidded on a patch of sand. The bike made a sudden turn, and the boy flipped over the handlebars, hitting his head in the street; he suffered lacerations, a concussion, and a hematoma. He was taken to the emergency room where he was found to be disoriented, lethargic, and suffering from amnesia. A CT scan was done, and he was found to have an epidural hematoma (Fig. 12-19). He was immediately brought to the operating room for surgical intervention to open up the skull and evacuate the blood clot.

5. Where is the hematoma located?

   A. beneath the dura
   B. outside of the dura
   C. in the dura
   D. above the dura

6. A procedure to open up the skull and remove the clot was performed. The medical term for "incision into the skull" is:

   A. craniectomy
   B. cranioplasty
   C. craniotomy
   D. craniocele

7. A concussion is an injury to the:

    A. spine
    B. spinal cord
    C. cranial nerves
    D. brain

8. The medical term for the loss of long-term memory is:

    A. ataxia
    B. amnesia
    C. aphasia
    D. stupor

MEDICAL RECORD ANALYSIS

MEDICAL RECORD 12-1

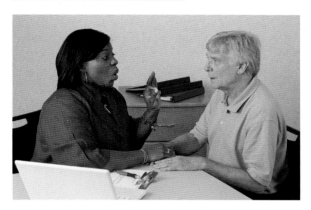

Following is the admission history and physical for a patient who sustained a cerebrovascular accident and is now undergoing rehabilitation. As a speech therapist, you will be working with the physician to develop a speech therapy plan for this patient. You take this opportunity to review the medical record.

Speech therapists work with patients to improve or regain their speech.

Medical Record

CEREBROVASCULAR ACCIDENT REHABILITATION HISTORY AND PHYSICAL

REASON FOR ADMISSION: Cerebrovascular accident (CVA), left hemiparesis, for advanced rehabilitation.

PATIENT GOAL: To be able to return home to live independently.

HISTORY OF PRESENT ILLNESS: This is a 64-year-old male. He developed sudden onset of left-sided weakness in early November. He was on the floor of his home approximately 1 week before being found. He was taken to the local hospital. In the emergency room, he was found to have a high CPK of greater than 5,000, which was felt to be secondary to rhabdomyolysis from lying on the floor. He also had left-sided hemiparesis. CT scan of the head showed advanced periventricular malacia, compatible with deep white matter ischemia. There was a superimposed edema to this infarct in the right basal ganglia. MRI of the head showed small vessel ischemic changes with an acute infarction of the right basal ganglia.

PAST MEDICAL HISTORY: Significant for hypertension.

ALLERGIES: He has no known drug allergies.

SOCIAL HISTORY: He lives at home alone. He has all of his arrangements on the first floor. The patient is right-handed.

HABITS: He admits to smoking cigarettes. He denies drinking alcohol or using illicit drugs.

FAMILY HISTORY: Significant for CVA, diabetes mellitus, and cancer.

REVIEW OF SYSTEMS

GENERAL: He denies weight gain, weight loss, chills, fevers, night sweats. Head, Ears, Eyes, Nose, and Throat: Review is significant for mild dysphasia.

CARDIOVASCULAR: Significant for hypertension.

NEUROLOGIC: As above.

All other systems are negative.

PHYSICAL EXAMINATION

VITAL SIGNS: Temperature 98.8°F, pulse 78, respirations 20, blood pressure 150/98, weight 158 pounds.

EXTREMITIES: His right upper and lower limbs have functional range of motion and strength.

PULMONARY: Chest is clear.

CARDIOVASCULAR: Heart has regular rate and rhythm.

ABDOMEN: Abdomen is soft with normal active bowel sounds. Foley catheter is in place.

NEUROLOGIC: This is a well-developed, thin male in no acute distress. He is alert and oriented ×3. Pupils equal and reactive to light and accommodation. Pays attention bilaterally. Has left central facial weakness. Tongue deviates to the left. He has moderate dysphasia. His swallowing reflex appears intact. He has dense left hemiparesis without appreciable moving of the upper or lower extremity. Sensation remains intact on the left. Babinski sign is positive on the left. He has 1 to 2 beats of clonus at the left ankle.

IMPRESSION
1. Cerebrovascular accident, dense left hemiparesis.
2. Rhabdomyolysis.
3. Hypertension.

PLAN: The patient will be admitted for a comprehensive inpatient rehabilitation program consisting of physical therapy, occupational therapy, speech therapy, recreational therapy, and case management support. Goals will be directed toward patient-and-family goals, to allow the patient to return home hopefully to live independently or else live with support.

Exercise 30

APPLICATION   **Read the medical report and circle the letter of your answer choice for the following questions. Note: Although some of the medical terms do not appear in this chapter, you should understand them from their word parts.**

1. The patient had a CVA or a cerebrovascular accident. What is another name for this medical problem?

   A. stupor
   B. stroke
   C. hallucination
   D. Alzheimer disease

2. The patient is admitted for rehabilitation because he has weakness on only his left side. This is called:

   A. paraplegia
   B. quadriplegia
   C. hemiparesis
   D. paraparesis

3. A Babinski sign is a neurologic test performed on the:

   A. top of the foot
   B. sole of the foot

   C. back of the calf
   D. big toe

4. What two radiologic tests were performed?

   A. echocardiogram and CPK
   B. MRI and CT scan
   C. CPK and CT scan
   D. MRI and echocardiogram

5. The patient has moderate dysphasia. This means that he has:

   A. difficulty swallowing
   B. difficulty walking
   C. difficulty speaking
   D. difficulty breathing

MEDICAL RECORD 12-2

You are a physician working in an acute hospital setting and are completing the discharge summary on an elderly patient. She will be discharged home with her daughter.

Medical Record

ACUTE SEIZURES DISCHARGE SUMMARY

CHIEF COMPLAINT: Mental status changes and expressive aphasia.

HISTORY OF PRESENT ILLNESS: This is an elderly white female who has a history of multiple hospitalizations in the past with the same complaint, who presented to the hospital with expressive (1)_____, mental status changes.

PAST MEDICAL HISTORY: Past medical history significant for the patient having similar episode with seizures, (2)_____, hypertension, CAD, CABG, CHF, atrial fibrillation, hypothyroidism, (3)_____, respiratory arrest, UTI, right carotid endarterectomy, cholecystectomy, hysterectomy, CABG, and peripheral vascular disease.

HOSPITAL COURSE: On admission to the hospital, the patient had expressive aphasia. The whole time she was alert and oriented x1. She could move all four extremities well. She was seen by the neurologist, who recommended that we maintain her Dilantin 100 mg t.i.d. and also recommended increasing the Lamictal to 200 mg b.i.d. She tolerated the increase of the Lamictal with no problems. Her expressive aphasia improved while she was in the hospital. She continued to mentate well, was alert and oriented x1.

Also on admission she was noted to have atrial fibrillation, RVR. She was seen by a cardiologist, who recommended increasing her sotalol and decreasing the metoprolol. Her heart rate came down. She was also continued on Coumadin while she was in the hospital.

She was running a low-grade temperature on admission. UA was positive for UTI, and she was put on Macrobid. She had defervescence of her fever.

The (4)_____ was positive for (5)_____ disorder. Again, we felt that her expressive aphasia and mental status changes were probably secondary to acute seizures. She had no evidence of any tonic-clonic seizures. At this point she is alert and essentially back to baseline.

DISCHARGE DIAGNOSES: Acute seizures, history of cerebrovascular accident, atrial fibrillation, rapid ventricular response, hypertension, coronary artery bypass graft, and urinary tract infection.

DISCHARGE MEDICATIONS: Sotalol 80 mg b.i.d. for atrial fibrillation, Macrobid 100 mg b.i.d. for UTI, metoprolol 50 mg once a day for hypertension, Lamictal 100 mg 2 tablets b.i.d. for seizures, Dilantin 100 mg t.i.d. for seizures She is also to continue her Lasix, Lipitor, Cozaar, Coumadin as before, and Synthroid and Trental.

FOLLOWUP CARE: See the doctor in 1 week. Have a Coumadin check once a week.

APPLICATION

Exercise 31

Fill in the blanks in the medical report with the correct medical terms. The meanings of the missing terms are listed below.

1. impaired comprehension or formulation of speech, reading, or writing caused by damage to the brain

2. damage to the brain caused by an interruption of blood supply to a region of the brain

3. a sudden, brief, and temporary cerebral dysfunction usually caused by interruption of blood flow to the brain

4. an electrical recording of the activity of the brain

5. violent spasm or series of jerky movements of the face, trunk, or limbs

Bonus Questions

6. Which two medications prescribed to the patient on discharge are anticonvulsants?

   _____

7. Using what you have learned about other body systems, what procedure did the patient have

   that removed the plaque from the main artery in her neck? _____

Pronunciation and Spelling

Exercise 32

AUDITORY

Review the Chapter 12 terms in the Dictionary/Audio Glossary in the Student Resources and practice pronouncing each term, referring to the pronunciation guide as needed.

Exercise 33

SPELLING   Circle the correct spelling of each term.

1.	cerebrum	cerebrim	ceribrum
2.	encephalopithy	encepholopathy	encephalopathy
3.	temporil	temporal	temperal
4.	delusiun	delusion	delusian
5.	Alzheirmer	Alazheimer	Alzheimer
6.	schizophrenia	scziophrenia	schzerphrenia
7.	radiculopithy	radicolopathy	radiculopathy
8.	catatonia	catotonia	catitonia
9.	cerebelum	cerebellum	cerabellum
10.	mylopathy	myeleopathy	myelopathy
11.	anasthesia	anestesia	anesthesia
12.	nuropathy	niropathy	neuropathy
13.	paraital	parietal	perietal
14.	hallucination	hallocination	hellucination
15.	siezure	seizure	sizeure

Media Connection

STUDENT
RESOURCES

Exercise 34

Complete each of the following activities available with the Student Resources. Check off each activity as you complete it, and record your score for the Chapter Quiz in the space provided.

Chapter Exercises

_____ Flash Cards

_____ Concentration

_____ Abbreviation Match-Up

_____ Roboterms

_____ Word Builder

_____ Fill the Gap

_____ Break It Down

_____ True/False Body Building

_____ Quiz Show

_____ Complete the Case

_____ Medical Record Review

_____ Image Matching

_____ Spelling Bee

_____ **Chapter Quiz**   _Score:_ _____%

Additional Resources

_____ Dictionary/Audio Glossary

_____ Health Professions Careers: Speech Therapist

_____ Health Professions Careers: Physician

Sensory Systems

Chapter Outline

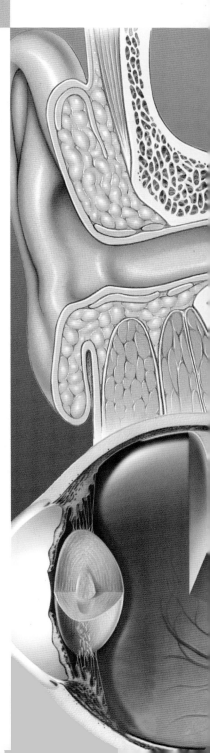

Objectives

After completion of this chapter you will be able to:

1. Identify the organs and structures of the eyes and ears.

2. Define terms related to the eyes and ears.

3. Define combining forms, prefixes, and suffixes related to the eyes and ears.

4. Define common medical terminology related to the eyes and ears, including adjectives and related terms, symptoms and conditions, tests and procedures, surgical interventions and therapeutic procedures, medications and drug therapies, and specialties.

5. Explain abbreviations for terms related to the eyes and ears.

6. Successfully complete all chapter exercises.

7. Explain terms used in case studies and medical records involving the eyes and ears.

8. Successfully complete all pronunciation and spelling exercises and complete all interactive exercises included with the companion Student Resources.

■ ANATOMY AND PHYSIOLOGY OF THE EYE

Function

■ To provide vision in conjunction with the brain to translate light rays into visual images

Organs and Structures

■ Each eye is located in a body socket in the skull called the orbit.
■ The eyes are protected by the movable folds of the eyelids.
■ The eyes are lubricated by fluids produced by the lacrimal glands.

Terms Related to the Eye (Fig. 13-1)

Term	Pronunciation	Meaning
orbit	ōr'bit	bony cavity of the skull that encases the eye
conjunctiva	kon'jŭnk-tī'vă	mucous membrane that lines the eyelids and outer surface of the eyeball
lacrimal glands	lak'ri-măl glandz	glands that secrete tears (Fig. 13-2)
lacrimal ducts	lak'ri-măl dŭktz	channels that carry tears to the eye (Fig. 13-2)
nasolacrimal ducts	nā'zō-lak'ri-măl dŭktz	ducts that carry tears from the lacrimal glands to the nose

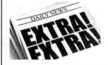 **NASOLACRIMAL DUCTS** Do you know why your nose runs when you cry? The nasolacrimal duct carries tears that are released from the tear glands into your nose.

| tarsal glands, *syn.* meibomian glands | tahr'săl glandz, mī-bō'mē-ăn glandz | oil glands along the edges of the eyelids that lubricate the eye |

(continued)

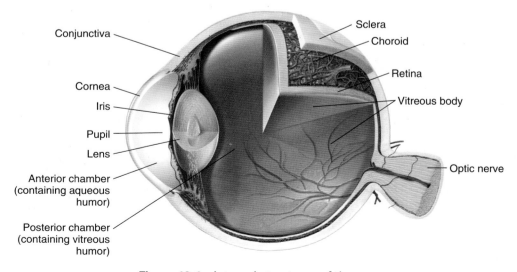

Figure 13-1   Internal structures of the eye.

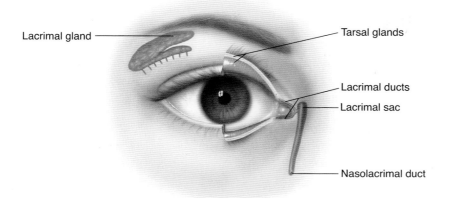

Figure 13-2   Right lacrimal gland and ducts.

Terms Related to the Eye *(continued)*

Term	Pronunciation	Meaning
Outer Layer of the Eye		
sclera	sklē′ră	tough outer layer of the eye (the white of the eye) that extends from the cornea to the optic nerve
cornea	kōr′nē-ă	transparent outer covering of the anterior portion of the eye
aqueous humor	ā′kwē-ŭs hyū′mŏr	watery fluid that fills the anterior chamber of the eye
iris	ī′ris	colored muscular part of the eye located behind the cornea that allows light to pass through
Middle Layer of the Eye		
pupil	pyū′pil	opening in the middle of the iris through which light passes
lens	lenz	transparent structure behind the pupil that bends and focuses light rays
choroid	kor′oyd	middle layer of the eye that contains blood vessels
vitreous humor	vit′rē-ŭs hyū′mŏr	jellylike fluid that fills the posterior chamber of the eye
Inner Layer of the Eye		
retina	ret′i-nă	innermost layer of the eye that contains visual receptors
optic nerve	op′tik nerv	nerve that carries impulses from the retina to the brain to provide the sense of sight
fundus	fŭn′dŭs	posterior portion of the interior of the eyeball, visible through the ophthalmoscope

■ Exercises: Anatomy and Physiology of the Eye

SIMPLE
RECALL

Exercise 1

Write the correct anatomic structure for the definition given.

1. part of the eye that bends and focuses light rays _____

2. jellylike fluid in the posterior chamber of the eye _____

3. layer of the eye that contains blood vessels _____

4. bony cavity of the skull that encases the eye _____

5. colored muscular part of the eye _____

6. mucous membrane that lines the eyelids and eye surface _____

7. opening in the iris through which light passes _____

8. transparent outer covering of the anterior eye _____

9. nerve that carries impulses to the brain to provide sight _____

10. ducts that carry tears from the lacrimal glands to the nose _____

ADVANCED
RECALL

Exercise 2

Complete each sentence by writing in the correct medical term.

1. The _____ is the part of the eye that contains vision receptors.

2. The _____ is the white outer layer of the eye.

3. Tears are carried through the _____ to the eye.

4. The _____ is the layer of the eye that contains blood vessels.

5. Oil that lubricates the eyes is produced by the _____.

6. The _____ is behind the pupil and bends and focuses light rays.

7. The _____ is the mucous membrane that lines the eyelid and eye surface.

8. Tears are secreted by the _____.

9. The opening in the middle of the iris through which light passes is the _____.

10. The _____ is a watery fluid filling the anterior chamber of the eye.

Exercise 3

ADVANCED RECALL

Match each medical term with its meaning.

vitreous humor   retina   iris
lacrimal glands   cornea   aqueous humor
optic nerve   sclera   tarsal glands

Meaning   **Term**

1. oil-producing glands of the eye   _____

2. layer of the eye that contains visual receptors   _____

3. watery fluid in the anterior chamber of the eye   _____

4. nerve that carries vision impulses to the brain   _____

5. transparent outer covering of the anterior portion of the eye   _____

6. jellylike fluid in the posterior chamber of the eye   _____

7. tear-producing glands of the eye   _____

8. colored part of the eye behind the cornea   _____

9. hard white outer layer of the eye   _____

■ WORD PARTS FOR THE EYE

Note that some word parts that have been introduced earlier in the book may not
be repeated here.

Combining Forms

Combining Form	Meaning
blephar/o	eyelid
conjunctiv/o	conjunctiva
corne/o	cornea
cry/o	cold
dacry/o, lacrim/o	tears or tear ducts
dipl/o	double, two
ir/o, irid/o	iris
kerat/o	cornea
ocul/o, ophthalm/o	eye

(continued)

Combining Forms *(continued)*

Combining Form	Meaning
opt/o	vision, eye
phot/o	light
presby/o	related to aging
pupill/o, cor/e, cor/o	pupil
retin/o	retina
scler/o	hard, sclera
ton/o	tension, pressure

Prefixes

Prefix	Meaning
bi-, bin-	two, twice

Suffixes

Suffix	Meaning
-ectasia, -ectasis	dilation, stretching
-lysis	destruction, breakdown, separation
-malacia	softening
-meter	instrument for measuring
-metry	measurement of
-opia, -opsia	vision
-pexy	surgical fixation
-phobia	abnormal fear, aversion to, sensitivity to
-plasty	surgical repair, reconstruction
-plegia	paralysis
-ptosis	prolapse, drooping, sagging
-rrhea	flow, discharge
-scopy	process of examining, examination
-spasm	involuntary movement
-trophia	to turn

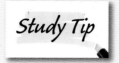

Study Tip

Spelling: The combining form for the eye—*ophthalm/o*—can be tricky to spell. To avoid errors, check that you have an "h" before *and* after the "t."

■ Exercises: Word Parts Related to the Eye

SIMPLE
RECALL

Exercise 4

Write the meaning of the combining form given.

1. ocul/o _____

2. lacrim/o _____

3. ir/o _____

4. cor/o _____

5. dacry/o _____

6. kerat/o _____

7. ophthalm/o _____

8. pupill/o _____

9. corne/o _____

10. blephar/o _____

SIMPLE
RECALL

Exercise 5

Write the correct combining form(s) for the meaning given.

1. conjunctiva _____

2. hard, sclera _____

3. light _____

4. eyelid _____

5. tension, pressure _____

6. related to aging _____

7. double _____

8. vision _____

9. iris _____

10. retina _____

Exercise 6

SIMPLE RECALL

Write the meaning of the prefix or suffix given.

1. -plegia   _____

2. -opia   _____

3. -ptosis   _____

4. bin-   _____

5. -lysis   _____

6. -rrhea   _____

7. -pexy   _____

8. -malacia   _____

9. -plasty   _____

10. -scopy   _____

11. -ectasis   _____

12. -phobia   _____

Exercise 7

ADVANCED RECALL

Match each combining form with its meaning.

scler/o   retin/o   pupill/o
corne/o   ir/o   conjunctiv/o

Meaning   **Combining Form**

1. colored muscular part of the eye   _____

2. innermost layer of the eye   _____

3. opening in the middle of the iris   _____

4. mucous membrane that lines the eyelids   _____

5. tough outer layer of the eye   _____

6. outer covering of the anterior portion of the eye   _____

Exercise 8

TERM CONSTRUCTION

Using the given combining form and a word part learned previously, build a medical term for the meaning given.

Combining Form	Meaning of Medical Term	Medical Term
conjunctiv/o	inflammation of the conjunctiva	1. _____
dipl/o	double vision	2. _____
blephar/o	drooping of the eyelid	3. _____
pupill/o	instrument for measuring the pupil	4. _____
phot/o	extreme sensitivity to light	5. _____
retin/o	disease of the retina	6. _____
irid/o	paralysis of the iris	7. _____
kerat/o	surgical repair of the cornea	8. _____
scler/o	incision into the sclera	9. _____
ophthalm/o	one specialized in the study of the eye	10. _____

Exercise 9

TERM CONSTRUCTION

For each term, first write the meaning of the term. Then write the meaning of the word parts in that term.

1. ophthalmoscope   _____

   ophthalm/o   _____

   -scope   _____

2. optometry   _____

   opt/o   _____

   -metry   _____

3. blepharospasm   _____

   blephar/o   _____

   -spasm   _____

4. dacryorrhea   _____

   dacry/o   _____

   -rrhea   _____

5. presbyopia _____

presby/o _____

-opia _____

6. retinopexy _____

retin/o _____

-pexy _____

7. corectasia _____

cor/e _____

-ectasia _____

8. iritis _____

ir/o _____

-itis _____

9. tonometer _____

ton/o _____

-meter _____

10. keratopathy _____

kerat/o _____

-pathy _____

■ MEDICAL TERMS RELATED TO THE EYE

Adjectives and Other Related Terms

Term	Pronunciation	Meaning
accommodation	ă-kom′ŏ-dā′shŭn	ability of the eye to adjust focus on near objects
binocular	bin-ok′yū-lăr	pertaining to both eyes
blepharal	blef′ă-răl	pertaining to the eyelid
conjunctival	kon′jŭnk-tī′văl	pertaining to the conjunctiva
corneal	kōr′nē-ăl	pertaining to the cornea
intraocular	in′tră-ok′yū-lăr	within or inside the eye

(continued)

Adjectives and Other Related Terms *(continued)*

Term	Pronunciation	Meaning
iridal, iridial	ĭ′ri-dăl, ir′i-dăl, ī-rid′ē-ăl	pertaining to the iris
lacrimal	lak′ri-măl	pertaining to tears
ocular, *syn.* ophthalmic	ok′yū-lăr, of-thal′mik	pertaining to the eye
optic	op′tik	pertaining to vision
pupillary	pyū′pi-lār′ē	pertaining to the pupil
retinal	ret′i-năl	pertaining to the retina
scleral	sklē′răl	pertaining to the sclera

■ Exercises: Adjectives and Other Related Terms

SIMPLE
RECALL

Exercise 10

Write the meaning of the term given.

1. ocular _____

2. lacrimal _____

3. optic _____

4. intraocular _____

5. iridal _____

6. conjunctival _____

7. ophthalmic _____

8. scleral _____

9. accommodation _____

ADVANCED
RECALL

Exercise 11

Match each medical term with its meaning.

retinal	pupillary	intraocular	iridial
blepharal	binocular	corneal	optic

Meaning	Term
1. within the eye	_____
2. pertaining to both eyes	_____

3. pertaining to the eyelids _____

4. pertaining to the pupil _____

5. pertaining to the retina _____

6. pertaining to vision _____

7. pertaining to the cornea _____

8. pertaining to the iris _____

ADVANCED
RECALL

Exercise 12

Circle the term that is most appropriate for the meaning of the sentence.

1. Mrs. Santos was suffering from (*binocular, dacryocyst, ophthalmic*) pain in her right eye.

2. The red spots in the patient's eye were due to a(n) (*lacrimal, conjunctival, optic*) hemorrhage, or a hemorrhage in the mucous membrane that lines the outer surface of the eyeball.

3. Mr. Kendrick's vision was blurred due to inflammation of his (*iridial, binocular, optic*) nerve.

4. The physician checked the patient's (*intraocular, lacrimal, blepharal*) pressure, or the pressure within each eye.

5. After the wind blew sand into Mr. Lin's eye, he suffered a (*corneal, retinal, lacrimal*) abrasion on the outside surface of the eye.

6. The child's left eyelid was red and swollen due to a (*corneal, blepharal, papillary*) infection.

7. The physician used a (*retinal, corneal, binocular*) microscope to make it possible for both her eyes to focus on the specimen.

Symptoms and Medical Conditions

Term	Pronunciation	Meaning
amblyopia	am′blē-ō′pē-ă	poor vision, usually in only one eye, caused by abnormal development of the visual areas; also known as "lazy eye"
astigmatism	ă-stig′mă-tizm	distorted, blurry vision caused by abnormal curvature of the cornea or lens
blepharitis	blef′ă-rī′tis	inflammation of the eyelid
blepharoptosis	blef′ă-rop′tō-sis	drooping of the eyelids; also shortened to ptosis (Fig. 13-3)
blepharospasm	blef′ă-rō-spazm	contraction of the muscles surrounding the eye, which causes uncontrolled blinking
cataract	kat′ă-rakt	clouding of the lens of the eye, which causes poor vision (Fig. 13-4, Fig. 13-8B)

(continued)

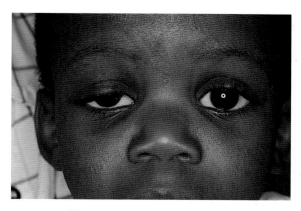

Figure 13-3 Blepharoptosis.

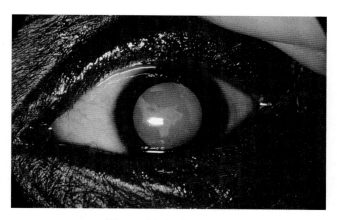

Figure 13-4 Cataract.

Symptoms and Medical Conditions *(continued)*

Term	Pronunciation	Meaning
chalazion, *syn.* meibomian cyst	ka-lā′zē-on, mī-bō′mē-ăn sist	obstruction of an oil gland in the eye (Fig. 13-5)
color blindness	kŭl′ŏr blīnd′nes	deficiency in distinguishing some colors
conjunctivitis	kon-jŭnk′ti-vī′tis	highly contagious inflammation of the conjunctiva; commonly known as pinkeye
dacryoadenitis	dak′rē-ō-ad′ĕ-nī′tis	inflammation of a lacrimal gland
dacryocystitis	dak′rē-ō-sis-tī′tis	inflammation of the lacrimal sac
dacryolith	dak′rē-ō-lith	stone in the lacrimal sac or ducts
dacryorrhea	dak′rē-ō-rē′ă	excessive discharge of tears
detached retina	dē-tacht′ ret′i-nă	separation of the retina from the choroid in the back of the eye; can be caused by injury, tumor, or hemorrhage (Fig. 13-6)

(continued)

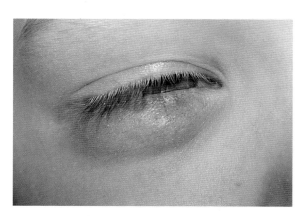

Figure 13-5 Chalazion.

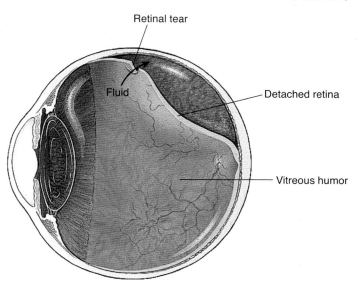

Figure 13-6 Detached retina.

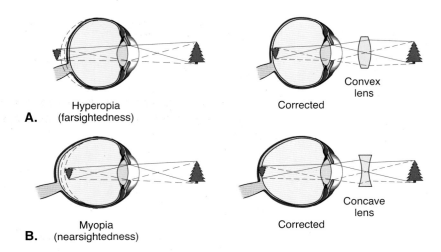

Figure 13-7 Deviations and corrections of vision. **A.** Hyperopia. **B.** Myopia.

Symptoms and Medical Conditions *(continued)*

Term	Pronunciation	Meaning
diabetic retinopathy	dī'ă-bet'ik ret'i-nop'ă-thē	degenerative changes of the retina caused by diabetes mellitus; may lead to blindness (Fig. 13-8C)
diplopia	di-plō'pē-ă	double vision
exophthalmos, *syn.* exophthalmus	eks'of-thal'mos, eks'of-thal'mŭs	abnormal protrusion of one or both eyeballs
glaucoma	glaw-kō'mă	group of diseases of the eye characterized by increased intraocular pressure that damages the optic nerve (Fig. 13-8D)
hordeolum	hōr-dē'ō-lŭm	infection of an oil gland of the eyelid; commonly called a sty
hyperopia	hī'pĕr-ō'pē-ă	farsightedness (Fig. 13-7)
iridomalacia	ir'i-dō-mă-lā'shē-ă	softening of the iris
iridoplegia	ir'i-dō-plē'jē-ă	paralysis of the iris
iritis	ī-rī'tis	inflammation of the iris
keratitis	ker'ă-tī'tis	inflammation of the cornea
keratomalacia	ker'ă-tō-mă-lā'shē-ă	softening of the cornea, usually associated with severe vitamin A deficiency
macular degeneration	mak'yū-lăr dē-jen'ĕr-ā'shŭn	deterioration of the macula (the central part of the retina), causing impaired central vision; most commonly related to advancing age (Fig. 13-8E)
myopia	mī-ō'pē-ă	nearsightedness (Fig. 13-7)

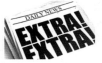

YOUR MATURING LENS As your eyes age so does the shape of the lens. In infancy, the lens is more spherical and tends to become flatter in the elderly. This flattening of the lens leads to the need for prescription lenses.

nyctalopia	nik-tă-lō'pē-ă	poor vision in reduced light or at night; commonly called night blindness

(continued)

A. Normal vision

B. Cataract
(hazy vision)

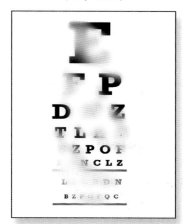

C. Diabetic retinopathy
(retinal damage leads to blind spots)

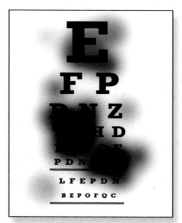

D. Glaucoma
(loss of peripheral vision)

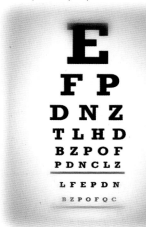

E. Macular degeneration
(loss of central vision)

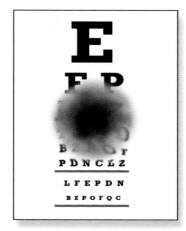

Figure 13-8   Simulated vision abnormalities. **A.** Normal vision. **B.** Cataract. **C.** Diabetic retinopathy. **D.** Glaucoma. **E.** Macular degeneration.

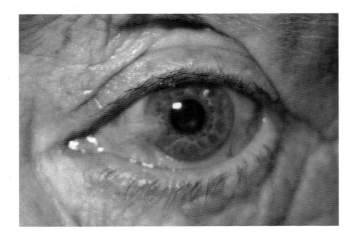

Figure 13-9   Pterygium.

Symptoms and Medical Conditions *(continued)*

Term	Pronunciation	Meaning
nystagmus	nis-tag′mŭs	involuntary rhythmic movements of the eye
ophthalmalgia	of′thal-mal′jē-ă	pain in the eye
ophthalmia	of-thal′mē-ă	condition of the eye characterized by severe conjunctivitis
ophthalmopathy	of′thal-mop′ă-thē	disease of the eye(s)
ophthalmoplegia	of-thal′mō-plē′jē-ă	paralysis of the eye muscle(s)
photophobia	fō′tō-fō′bē-ă	extreme sensitivity to light
presbyopia	prez′bē-ō′pē-ă	impaired vision caused by old age
pterygium	tĕ-rij′ē-ŭm	growth of conjunctival tissue over the cornea; usually associated with prolonged exposure to ultraviolet light (Fig. 13-9)
retinitis pigmentosa	ret′i-nī′tis pig′men-to′să	hereditary progressive deterioration of the retina causing nyctalopia and impaired vision
retinopathy	ret′i-nop′ă-thē	any disease of the retina
scleritis	sklē-rī′tis	inflammation of the sclera
scleromalacia	sklē′rō-mă-lā′shē-ă	softening or thinning of the sclera
strabismus	stra-biz′mŭs	a condition of ocular misalignment caused by intraocular muscle imbalance
xerophthalmia	zē′rof-thal′mē-ă	condition involving dry eye(s)

■ Exercises: Symptoms and Medical Conditions

Exercise 13

SIMPLE
RECALL

Write the meaning of the term given.

1. nystagmus _____

2. retinopathy _____

3. iridomalacia _____

4. blepharitis _____

5. cataract _____

6. exophthalmos _____

7. dacryolith _____

8. xerophthalmia _____

9. glaucoma _____

10. ophthalmopathy _____

ADVANCED
RECALL

Exercise 14

Complete each sentence by writing in the correct medical term.

1. Distorted blurry vision caused by abnormal curvature of the cornea or lens is called

   _____ .

2. _____ is the medical term for farsightedness.

3. _____ is a deficiency in distinguishing some colors.

4. The medical term for poor vision, usually in one eye, commonly referred to as "lazy eye,"

   is _____ .

5. The medical term for double vision is _____ .

6. Vision impairment caused by old age is called _____ .

7. The term for poor vision in reduced light or at night (night blindness) is

   _____ .

8. _____ is the medical term for nearsightedness.

9. The term for deterioration of the macula causing impaired central vision, most commonly

   caused by aging, is _____ .

10. Extreme sensitivity to light is known as _____ .

11. The term _____ refers to a condition of the eye characterized by severe
    conjunctivitis.

Exercise 15

ADVANCED RECALL

Match each medical term with its meaning.

hordeolum   ophthalmoplegia   chalazion   dacryocystitis
detached retina   diabetic retinopathy   pterygium   dacryoadenitis
retinitis pigmentosa   strabismus

Meaning   **Term**

1. degenerative changes of the retina caused by
   diabetes mellitus   _____

2. paralysis of the eye muscle   _____

3. inflammation of a lacrimal gland   _____

4. obstruction of an oil gland in the eye   _____

5. inflammation of the tear sac   _____

6. infection of an oil gland of the eyelid   _____

7. growth of conjunctival tissue over the cornea   _____

8. hereditary deterioration of the retina   _____

9. condition of eye misalignment caused by
   intraocular muscle imbalance   _____

10. separation of the retina from the choroid   _____

Exercise 16

TERM CONSTRUCTION

Break the given medical term into its word parts and define each part. Then define the medical term.

For example:
   iritis   *word parts:*   ir/o   /   -itis
                         meanings: iris   /   inflammation
                         term meaning: inflammation of the iris

1. scleromalacia   *word parts:*   _____ / _____

                         meanings: _____ / _____

                         term meaning: _____

2. keratitis

word parts: _____ / _____

meanings: _____ / _____

term meaning: _____

3. iridoplegia

word parts: _____ / _____

meanings: _____ / _____

term meaning: _____

4. dacryorrhea

word parts: _____ / _____

meanings: _____ / _____

term meaning: _____

5. blepharospasm

word parts: _____ / _____

meanings: _____ / _____

term meaning: _____

6. scleritis

word parts: _____ / _____

meanings: _____ / _____

term meaning: _____

7. conjunctivitis

word parts: _____ / _____

meanings: _____ / _____

term meaning: _____

8. ophthalmalgia

word parts: _____ / _____

meanings: _____ / _____

term meaning: _____

9. blepharoptosis

word parts: _____ / _____

meanings: _____ / _____

term meaning: _____

10. keratomalacia

word parts: _____ / _____

meanings: _____ / _____

term meaning: _____

Tests and Procedures

Term	Pronunciation	Meaning
Diagnostic Procedures		
extraocular movement (EOM)	eks′tră-ok′yū-lăr mūv′mĕnt	movement of the upper eyelids and eyeballs through use of the extraocular muscles; assessed during clinical examination to screen for eye movement disorders

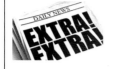 **DOCUMENTATION INVOLVING THE EYES** In a clinical examination, the physician checks the eyes as part of an overall review of the head, eyes, ears, neck, and throat (abbreviated as *HEENT*). Documentation of the physician's findings in the patient's medical record might look something like this:

EYES: Pupils equal, round, and reactive to light and accommodation. Conjunctivae are clear. Extraocular movements are intact bilaterally. Sclerae not icteric.

Term	Pronunciation	Meaning
fluorescein angiography	flōr-es′ē-in an′jē-og′ră-fē	visualization and photographic recording of the flow of an orange fluorescent dye through the blood vessels of the eye
keratometer	ker′ă-tom′ĕ-tĕr	instrument for measuring the curvature of the cornea
ophthalmoscope	of-thal′mō-skōp	instrument used for examining the interior of the eye through the pupil (Fig. 13-10)

(continued)

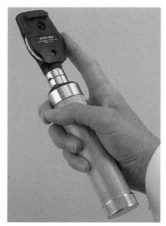
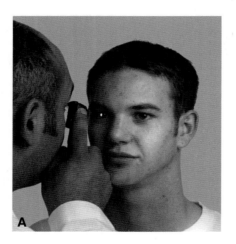

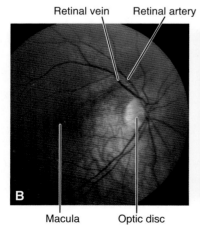
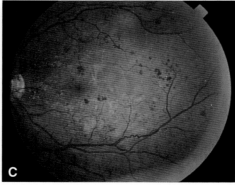
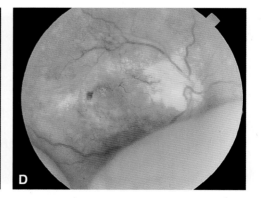

Retinal vein   Retinal artery

Macula   Optic disc

Figure 13-10   A. Using an ophthalmoscope to perform ophthalmoscopy. **B.** Normal retina. **C.** Aneurysms seen in diabetic retinopathy. **D.** Retinal detachment.

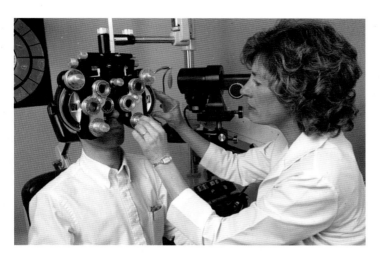

Figure 13-11   A manual refractor assists the physician in determining exact vision correction.

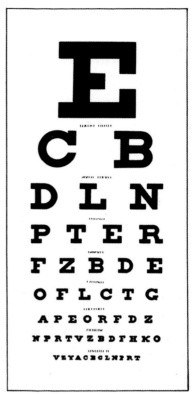

Figure 13-12   Snellen eye chart.

Tests and Procedures *(continued)*

Term	Pronunciation	Meaning
ophthalmoscopy	of′thal-mos′kŏ-pē	use of the ophthalmoscope to view the interior of the eye (Fig. 13-10)
pupillometer	pyū′pi-lom′ĕ-tĕr	instrument for measuring the diameter of the pupil
pupillometry	pyū′pi-lom′ĕ-trē	measurement of the pupil
refraction	rē-frak′shŭn	test using a manual refractor to determine an exact vision prescription (Fig. 13-11)
retinoscopy	ret′i-nos′kŏ-pē	examination of the retina
Snellen chart	snel′ĕn chart	chart containing symbols that is used in the testing of visual acuity (Fig. 13-12)
tonometer	tō-nom′ĕ-tĕr	instrument for measuring pressure within the eye
tonometry	tō-nom′ĕ-trē	use of the tonometer to measure intraocular pressure within the eye; done to diagnose glaucoma
visual acuity (VA) testing	vizh′yū-ăl ă-kyū′i-tē test′ing	testing for the sharpness (clarity) of distant vision, usually with a Snellen chart; normal visual acuity is 20/20
visual field (VF) testing	izh′ū-ăl fĕld test′ing	assessment of the range (area) visible to one eye without movement

■ Exercises: Tests and Procedures

Exercise 17

SIMPLE
RECALL

Write the meaning of the term given.

1. tonometer _____

2. ophthalmoscope _____

3. retinoscopy _____

4. keratometer _____

5. pupillometry _____

Exercise 18

ADVANCED
RECALL

Match each medical term with its meaning.

visual field testing   pupillometry   extraocular movement assessment
Snellen chart   refraction   fluorescein angiography

Meaning   **Term**

1. measurement of the range of one eye   _____

2. chart used to test visual acuity   _____

3. measurement of the pupil   _____

4. recording of the flow of a dye through the blood
   vessels of the eye   _____

5. test to determine how to correct vision   _____

6. assessment of the extraocular muscles working together _____

Exercise 19

ADVANCED
RECALL

Circle the term that is most appropriate for the meaning of the sentence.

1. The physician performed (*tonometry, pupillometry, fluorescein angiography*), a procedure that allowed him to record the flow of fluorescent dye through the blood vessels in the patient's eye.

2. Mrs. Rina's retinal tear was diagnosed using (*tonometry, retinoscopy, pupillometry*).

3. The nurse asked Mr. Ketson to read a (*tonometer, refraction, Snellen chart*) so that she could test his visual acuity.

4. Dr. Pujabi performed (*retinoscopy, refraction, pupillometry*) to measure the degree of refractive errors and determine how to correct Mrs. Frank's vision.

5. The physician measured the amount of pressure in Mr. Johannson's eye using a(n) (*ophthalmoscope, keratometer, tonometer*) to rule out glaucoma.

6. The optometrist used a Snellen chart to measure the patient's (*visual acuity, visual field, extraocular movements*).

TERM CONSTRUCTION

Exercise 20

Break the given medical term into its word parts and define each part. Then define the medical term.

For example:

iritis	*word parts:*	ir/o / -itis
	meanings:	iris / inflammation
	term meaning:	inflammation of the iris

1. pupillometer   *word parts:* _____ / _____

  meanings: _____ / _____

  term meaning: _____

2. tonometry   *word parts:* _____ / _____

  meanings: _____ / _____

  term meaning: _____

3. ophthalmoscopy   *word parts:* _____ / _____

  meanings: _____ / _____

  term meaning: _____

4. keratometer   *word parts:* _____ / _____

  meanings: _____ / _____

  term meaning: _____

5. retinoscopy   *word parts:* _____ / _____

  meanings: _____ / _____

  term meaning: _____

6. ophthalmoscope   *word parts:* _____ / _____

  meanings: _____ / _____

  term meaning: _____

Surgical Interventions

Term	Pronunciation	Meaning
blepharoplasty	blef'ă-ro-plast'tē	surgical repair of the eyelid
cataract extraction	kat'ă-rakt eks-trak'shŭn	surgical removal of a cataract
cryoretinopexy	krī'ō-ret'i-nō-pek'sē	surgical fixation of a detached retina or retinal tear by using extreme cold (freezing) to seal the tear
dacryocystotomy	dak'rē-ō-sis-tot'ŏ-mē	incision into the tear sac
enucleation	ē-nū'klē-ā'shŭn	removal of an eyeball
intraocular lens (IOL) implant	in'tră-ok'yū-lăr lenz im'plant	implantation of an artificial lens to replace a defective natural lens
iridectomy	ir'i-dek'tŏ-mē	excision of part of the iris
iridotomy	ir'i-dot'ŏ-mē	incision into the iris, usually with a laser, to allow drainage of aqueous humor in therapy for narrow-angle glaucoma
keratoplasty	ker'ă-tō-plas'tē	surgical repair of the cornea; corneal transplantation
laser-assisted in situ keratomileusis (LASIK)	lā'zĕr ă-sis'-ted in sī'tū ker'ă-tō-mī-lū'sis	procedure that uses a laser to create a corneal flap and reshape the corneal tissue; used to correct vision problems such as myopia, hyperopia, and astigmatism
phacoemulsification	fak'ō-ē-mŭl'si-fi-kā'shŭn	use of ultrasound to shatter and break up a cataract, followed by aspiration and removal
photorefractive keratectomy (PRK)	fō'tō-rē-frak'tiv ker'ă-tek'tŏ-mē	procedure using a laser to reshape the cornea to correct vision
retinal photocoagulation	ret'i-năl fō'tō-kō-ag'yū-lā'shŭn	repair of a retinal detachment or tear by using a laser beam to coagulate the tissues to allow a seal to form
scleral buckling	sklē'răl bŭk-ling	repair of a retinal detachment by attaching a band (buckle) around the sclera to keep the retina from pulling away (Fig. 13-13)

(continued)

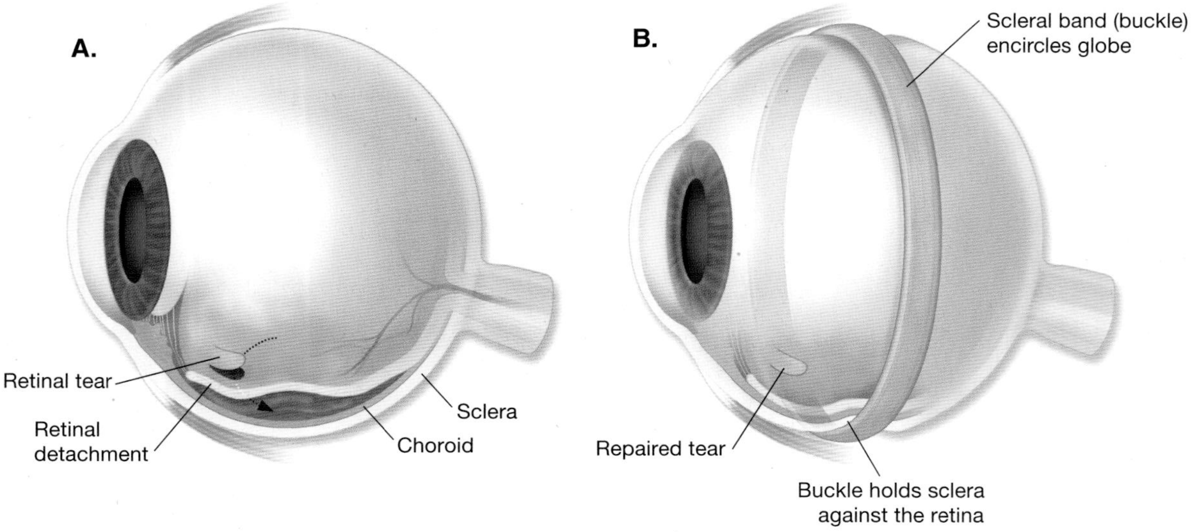

Figure 13-13   A. Detached retina. The *arrow* shows the movement of fluid. **B.** Scleral buckling. Repair of a retinal tear by attaching a band (buckle) around the sclera to keep the retina from pulling away.

Surgical Interventions *(continued)*

Term	Pronunciation	Meaning
sclerotomy	sklē-rot'ŏ-mē	incision into the sclera
trabeculectomy	tră-bek'yū-lek'tŏ-mē	surgical procedure to create a drain to reduce pressure within the eye
vitrectomy	vi-trek'tŏ-mē	removal of all or part of the vitreous humor

■ Exercises: Surgical Interventions

SIMPLE
RECALL

Exercise 21

Write the correct medical term for the definition given.

1. removal of an eyeball

   _____

2. repair of a detached retina using extreme cold

   _____

3. removal of all or part of the vitreous humor

   _____

4. laser vision correction by reshaping the cornea

   _____

5. surgical removal of a cataract

   _____

6. repair of a retinal detachment or tear using a laser beam

   _____

7. laser vision correction by creating a corneal flap and
   reshaping the corneal tissue

   _____

ADVANCED
RECALL

Exercise 22

Complete each sentence by writing in the correct medical term.

1. _____ is the use of ultrasound to shatter and break up a cataract, followed

   by aspiration and removal.

2. The surgical procedure that creates a drain in the eye to reduce pressure within it is a(n)

   _____.

3. Making an incision into the tear sac is called _____.

4. When a physician repairs a retinal detachment by attaching a band around the sclera to keep

   it from pulling away, he or she is performing _____.

5. Corneal transplantation and repairing a cornea to alter its shape are both called

   _____.

6. The procedure to repair a drooping eyelid is _____.

7. A(n) _____ replaces a defective natural lens with an artificial one.

Exercise 23

TERM CONSTRUCTION

Write the remainder of the term for the meaning given.

1. incision into the sclera   sclero _____

2. surgical repair of the eyelid   _____ plasty

3. excision of part of the iris   irid _____

4. surgical repair of the cornea   _____ plasty

5. removal of the vitreous humor   vitr _____

6. incision into the iris   _____ tomy

Medications and Drug Therapies

Term	Pronunciation	Meaning
corticosteroid	kŏr'ti-kō-ster'oyd	drug that reduces inflammation; used to treat swelling and itching of the eye
hypotonic	hī'pō-ton'ik	drug used to relieve dry irritated eyes
miotic	mī-ot'ik	drug used to constrict the pupil
mydriatic	mi-drē-at'ik	drug used to dilate the pupil
prostaglandin	pros'tă-glan'děn	drug that relaxes muscles in the eye's interior structure to allow better outflow of fluids

■ Exercise: Medications and Drug Therapies

Exercise 24

SIMPLE RECALL

Write the correct medication or drug therapy term for the definition given

1. dilates the pupil   _____

2. treats swelling and itching of the eye   _____

3. relaxes muscles in the eye's interior   _____

4. constricts the pupil   _____

5. relieves dry irritated eyes   _____

Specialties and Specialists

Term	Pronunciation	Meaning
optician	op-tish′ăn	one who fills prescriptions for corrective lenses
optometry	op-tom′ĕ-trē	medical specialty concerned with the measurement of vision and prescription of corrective treatment or lenses
optometrist	op-tom′ĕ-trist	one who practices optometry
ophthalmology	of′thal-mol′ŏ-jē	medical specialty concerned with the study of the eye, its diseases, and refractive errors
ophthalmologist	of′thal-mol′ŏ-jist	physician who specializes in ophthalmology

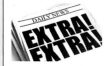 **OPTOMETRIST VS. OPHTHALMOLOGIST** What is the difference between an optometrist and an ophthalmologist? An optometrist is an O.D., a Doctor of Optometry. Optometrists can evaluate vision problems, diagnose some eye conditions, and prescribe corrective treatments such as exercises or corrective lenses. Because optometrists are not medical doctors, however, they cannot perform eye surgery and are limited in the medical treatments they may render. An ophthalmologist is an M.D., a Doctor of Medicine, who has completed medical school. Ophthalmologists can diagnose and treat any eye disease or vision problem as well as perform eye surgery.

■ Exercise: Specialties and Specialists

Exercise 25

ADVANCED RECALL

Match each medical term with its meaning.

ophthalmologist optometrist optician
optometry ophthalmology

Meaning **Term**

1. specialty in the measurement of vision and prescription of treatment _____

2. specialty in the study of the eye and its diseases _____

3. one who fills prescriptions for corrective lenses _____

4. specialist in the study and treatment of eyes _____

5. one who specializes in measuring vision _____

Abbreviations

Abbreviation	Meaning
EOM	extraocular movement
IOL	intraocular lens

(continued)

Abbreviations *(continued)*

Abbreviation	Meaning
IOP	intraocular pressure
LASIK	laser-assisted in situ keratomileusis
OD	right eye (oculus dexter)
OS	left eye (oculus sinister)
OU	each eye or both eyes (oculus uterque)

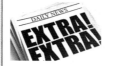 **DANGEROUS ABBREVIATIONS RELATED TO THE EYE** The abbreviations OD, OS, and OU are included on the list of "Error-Prone Abbreviations, Symbols, and Dose Designations" published by the Institute for Safe Medication Practices. According to the ISMP, these abbreviations are frequently confused for each other or for the abbreviations for right ear (AD), left ear (AS), or both ears (AU), which can lead to errors in patient care. If you encounter these abbreviations in practice, use special care to ensure proper interpretation.

PRK	photorefractive keratectomy
VA	visual acuity
VF	visual field

■ Exercises: Abbreviations

Exercise 26

SIMPLE RECALL

Write the meaning of each abbreviation.

1. OU _____

2. EOM _____

3. IOL _____

4. OS _____

5. VF _____

Exercise 27

ADVANCED RECALL

Write the meaning of each abbreviation used in these sentences.

1. The patient's **VA** was 20/40 in the right eye without corrective lenses.

_____

2. Mr. Friedman expressed interest in having **LASIK** surgery to correct his astigmatism.

_____

3. The physician instructed Ms. Herrera to instill two drops of the ophthalmic drops **OD** for 5 days as therapy for her conjunctivitis.

_____

4. Mr. Hall's vision was corrected using a laser to reshape his cornea, a process known as **PRK.**

_____

5. Dr. Morgan's patient is scheduled to undergo a trabeculectomy to minimize the **IOP** in his left eye.

_____

■ ANATOMY AND PHYSIOLOGY OF THE EAR

Functions

- ■ To provide hearing by translating sound waves into nerve impulses that are carried to the brain
- ■ To assist the body in maintaining equilibrium or balance

Organs and Structures

- ■ The ear consists of three parts: the outer ear, middle ear, and inner ear.
- ■ The outer ear consists of the pinna, external auditory meatus, and tympanic membrane. The tympanic membrane separates the outer ear from the middle ear.
- ■ The middle ear consists of the pharyngotympanic tube and the auditory ossicles: the malleus, incus, and stapes.
- ■ The inner ear, also known as the labyrinth, consists of the cochlea, semicircular canals, and vestibule.

Terms Related to the Ear (Fig. 13-14)

Term	Pronunciation	Meaning
Outer Ear		
auricle, *syn.* pinna	aw'ri-kl, pin'ă	external portion of the ear
external auditory meatus, *syn.* external auditory canal	eks-ter'năl aw'di-tōr-ē mē-ā'tŭs, kă-nal'	canal that extends from the auricle to the tympanic membrane
cerumen	sĕ-rū'men	waxy substance created by glands of the external auditory meatus; earwax
tympanic membrane (TM)	tim-pan'ik mem'brān	eardrum; a semitransparent membrane that vibrates to transmit sound waves to the ossicles; separates the external auditory meatus from the middle ear cavity
Middle Ear		
mastoid bone and cells	mas'toyd bōn and selz	bone located behind the ear that is filled with air cavities and encloses the middle ear
pharyngotympanic tube, *syn.* eustachian tube, auditory tube	fă-ring'gō-tim-pan'ik tūb, yū-stā'shăn tūb, aw'di-tōr-ē tūb	tubular channel that runs from the middle ear cavity to the pharynx

(continued)

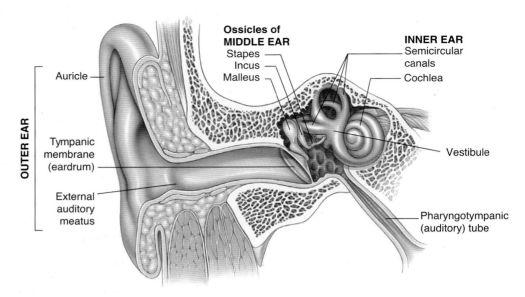

Figure 13-14   Structures of the outer, middle, and inner ear.

Terms Related to the Ear (continued)

Term	Pronunciation	Meaning
auditory ossicles	aw'di-tōr-ē os'i-kĕlz	middle ear bones contained in the tympanic cavity that transmit sound vibrations (Fig. 13-15)
malleus	mal'ē-ŭs	auditory ossicle shaped like a hammer or club
incus	ing'kŭs	auditory ossicle shaped like an anvil
stapes	stā'pēz	auditory ossicle shaped like a stirrup

(continued)

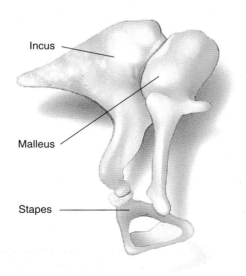

Figure 13-15   Ossicles of the middle ear.

Terms Related to the Ear *(continued)*

Term	Pronunciation	Meaning
Inner Ear		
labyrinth	lab'i-rinth	inner ear, which is made up of a series of semicircular canals, the vestibule, and the cochlea
cochlea	kok'lē-ă	a snail-shaped organ that contains the organ of hearing
spiral organ, *syn.* organ of Corti	spī'răl ōr'găn, ōr'găn of kōr'tē	receptor for hearing located within the cochlea; the organ of hearing
vestibule	ves'ti-byŭl	anatomic chamber such as that found in the inner ear
semicircular canals and ducts	sem'ē-sir'kyū-lăr kă-nal'z and dŭktz	small tubes in the labyrinth that contain receptors that assist the body in maintaining balance

■ Exercises: Anatomy and Physiology of the Ear

SIMPLE
RECALL

Exercise 28

Write the meaning of the anatomic structure given.

1. stapes   _____

2. spiral organ   _____

3. external auditory meatus   _____

4. incus   _____

5. pinna   _____

6. malleus   _____

7. auditory ossicles   _____

8. cerumen   _____

9. labyrinth   _____

ADVANCED
RECALL

Exercise 29

Match each anatomic structure with its meaning.

vestibule	cochlea	tympanic membrane
auricle	auditory ossicles	pharyngotympanic tube
semicircular canals	mastoid bone	external auditory canal

Meaning   **Term**

1. chamber such as that found in the inner ear   _____

2. small tubes in the labyrinth that help with balance   _____

3. middle ear bones   _____

4. eardrum   _____

5. tube that leads from the middle ear to the pharynx   _____

6. bone behind the ear that is filled with air cavities   _____

7. external portion of the ear   _____

8. snail-shaped organ that contains the organ of hearing   _____

9. canal that leads from the auricle to the eardrum   _____

Exercise 30

ADVANCED
RECALL

Complete each sentence by writing in the correct medical term.

1. The middle ear bones are known as the _____ .

2. The bone located behind the ear that is filled with air cavities is the _____ .

3. The _____ is the name for the inner ear that is made up of semicircular canals, the vestibule, and the cochlea.

4. A waxy substance created by glands in the external auditory meatus (commonly known as earwax) is called _____ .

5. The organ of hearing is known as the _____ .

6. The _____ are the small tubes in the labyrinth that help a person maintain balance.

7. A chamber, such as that of the inner ear, is called a(n) _____ .

8. The tubular channel that leads from the middle ear to the pharynx is the _____ .

9. The semitransparent membrane that vibrates to transmit sound waves is called the

_____ .

■ WORD PARTS FOR THE EAR

Combining Forms

Combining Form	Meaning
acous/o	hearing, sound
audi/o	hearing
aur/i, aur/o, ot/o	ear
cochle/o	cochlea

(continued)

Combining Forms *(continued)*

Combining Form	Meaning
labyrinth/o	labyrinth, inner ear
mastoid/o	mastoid bone
myring/o, tympan/o	tympanic membrane, eardrum
scler/o	hard, sclera
staped/o	stapes
vestibul/o	vestibule

Prefix

Prefix	Meaning
dys-	painful, difficult, abnormal

Suffixes

Suffix	Meaning
-acousis, -acusis	hearing
-algia	pain
-ectomy	excision, surgical removal
-stomy	surgical opening

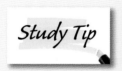

myring/o vs. tympan/o: When trying to decide whether to use *myring/o* or *tympan/o* for the tympanic membrane (eardrum), remember this hint: *Myring/o* usually refers only to the tympanic membrane. *Tympan/o*, however, usually refers to the tympanic membrane and/or the middle ear space. The space behind the tympanic membrane is referred to as the middle ear space or the tympanic cavity.

■ Exercises: Word Parts for the Ear

SIMPLE RECALL

Exercise 31

Write the meaning of the word part given.

1. -acousis _____

2. -algia _____

3. vestibul/o _____

4. aur/i _____

5. acous/o _____

6. scler/o _____

7. dys- _____

8. cochle/o _____

ADVANCED
RECALL

Exercise 32

Match each word part with its meaning.

-stomy	dys-	-ectomy
labyrinth/o	scler/o	ot/o

Meaning   **Term**

1. labyrinth, inner ear _____

2. excision, surgical removal _____

3. surgical opening _____

4. hard _____

5. painful, difficult, abnormal _____

6. ear _____

TERM
CONSTRUCTION

Exercise 33

Considering the meaning of the combining form from which the medical term is made, write the meaning of the medical term.

Combining Form	Meaning	Medical Term	Meaning of Term
labyrinth/o	inner ear	labyrinthitis	**1.** _____
tympan/o	middle ear	tympanostomy	**2.** _____
mastoid/o	mastoid bone	mastoiditis	**3.** _____
ot/o	ear	otorrhea	**4.** _____
audi/o	hearing	audiometer	**5.** _____
myring/o	eardrum	myringotomy	**6.** _____
staped/o	stapes	stapedectomy	**7.** _____

TERM CONSTRUCTION

Exercise 34

Using the given combining form, build a medical term for the meaning given.

Combining Form	Meaning of Medical Term	Medical Term
vestibul/o	incision into the vestibule	1._____
aur/i	pertaining to the ear	2._____
acous/o	pertaining to hearing or sound	3._____
cochle/o	inflammation of the cochlea	4._____
scler/o	abnormal condition of hardness	5._____
ot/o	pain in the ear	6._____
myring/o	inflammation of the eardrum	7._____

■ MEDICAL TERMS RELATED TO THE EAR

Adjectives and Other Related Terms

Term	Pronunciation	Meaning
acoustic	ă-kūs′tik	pertaining to hearing or sound
auditory	aw′di-tōr-ē	pertaining to hearing
aural, *syn.* otic	aw′răl, ō′tik	pertaining to the ear
cochlear	kok′lē-ăr	pertaining to the cochlea
labyrinthine	lab′i-rin′thīn	pertaining to the labyrinth or inner ear
mastoid	mas′toyd	pertaining to the mastoid bone and cells
tympanic	tim-pan′ik	pertaining to the tympanic membrane or tympanic cavity
vestibular	ves-tib′yū-lăr	pertaining to a vestibule

■ Exercises: Adjectives and Other Related Terms

SIMPLE RECALL

Exercise 35

Write the meaning of the term given.

1. otic _____

2. acoustic _____

3. aural _____

4. tympanic _____

5. vestibular _____

6. auditory _____

7. cochlear _____

Exercise 36

ADVANCED
RECALL

Match each medical term with its meaning.

| vestibular | aural | labyrinthine |
| acoustic | tympanic | mastoid |

Meaning	**Term**

1. pertaining to the ear _____

2. pertaining to the vestibule _____

3. pertaining to the tympanic membrane _____

4. pertaining to sound _____

5. pertaining to the labyrinth _____

6. pertaining to the mastoid cells _____

Exercise 37

ADVANCED
RECALL

Circle the term that is most appropriate for the meaning of the sentence.

1. The school nurse used a(n) (*aural, mastoid, acoustic*) thermometer to take the child's temperature in his ear.

2. Mrs. Gallo had an inner ear or (*acoustic, mastoid, labyrinthine*) infection.

3. Helen is a(n) (*auditory, otic, tympanic*) learner, so she does best in school when she listens to lectures.

4. The physician showed Timmy's mother how to put (*labyrinthine, acoustic, otic*) drops in his ears.

5. The (*auditory, mastoid, vestibular*) infection was in the bone behind the patient's left ear.

6. Fluid had accumulated in the middle ear behind the (*acoustic, otic, tympanic*) membrane.

Symptoms and Medical Conditions

Term	Pronunciation	Meaning
acoustic neuroma	ă-kūs′tik nū-rō′mă	a benign tumor that develops on the acoustic nerve (the eighth cranial nerve that connects the ear to the brain) and causes hearing loss
cerumen impaction	sĕ-rū′men im-pak′shŭn	excessive buildup of earwax
cholesteatoma	kō′les-tē′ă-tō′mă	cystlike tumor of skin in the middle ear behind the tympanic membrane usually caused by chronic otitis media
conductive hearing loss	kon′dŭk-tiv′ hēr′ing los	hearing loss due to obstruction or lesion in the outer and/or middle ear
dysacousia	dis-ă-kyū′zē-ă	impairment of hearing involving difficulty in the processing of sound
labyrinthitis	lab′i-rin-thī′tis	inflammation of the inner ear
mastoiditis	mas′toy-dī′tis	inflammation of the mastoid bone
Ménière disease, *syn.* Ménière syndrome	men-ē-ār′ di-zēz′	a chronic condition of the inner ear characterized by dizziness, tinnitus, hearing loss, and a sensation of pressure in the ear
myringitis	mir′in-jī′tis	inflammation of the tympanic membrane
otalgia	ō-tal′jē-ă	pain in the ear
otitis externa (OE)	ō-tī′tis eks-ter′nă	inflammation of the external auditory meatus; also known as "swimmer's ear"
otitis media (OM)	ō-tī′tis mē′dē-ă	inflammation of the middle ear (Fig. 13-16)
otomycosis	ō′tō-mī-kō′sis	fungal infection in the ear
otopyorrhea	ō-tō-pī′ō-rē′ă	discharge of pus from the ear
otorrhea	ō-tō-rē′ă	discharge from the ear
otosclerosis	ō′tō-sklĕ-rō′sis	hardening of the ossicles, particularly the stapes
presbycusis	prez′bē-kū′sis	impaired hearing caused by old age
sensorineural hearing loss	sen′sŏ-rē nū′răl hēr′ing los	hearing loss caused by damage to the inner ear or the auditory nerve
tinnitus	tin′i-tŭs	noises in the ear, such as ringing, buzzing, or humming
tympanic membrane perforation	tim-pan′ik mem′brān per′fō-rā′shŭn	a hole in or rupture of the eardrum
vertigo	ver-ti′gō	a spinning sensation; commonly used to mean dizziness

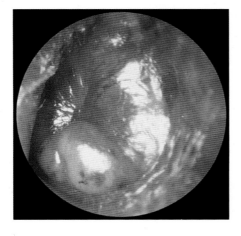

Figure 13-16   Otitis media.

■ Exercises: Symptoms and Medical Conditions

SIMPLE
RECALL

Exercise 38

Write the correct medical term for the definition given.

1. fungal infection in the ear   _____

2. hardening of the ossicles, particularly the stapes   _____

3. noises within the ear   _____

4. cystlike tumor of skin in the middle ear   _____

5. excessive buildup of earwax   _____

6. age-related hearing loss   _____

7. spinning sensation, dizziness   _____

8. a tumor that develops on the acoustic nerve   _____

ADVANCED
RECALL

Exercise 39

Match each medical term with its meaning.

presbycusis   conductive hearing loss   otitis externa
otitis media   sensorineural hearing loss   dysacousia

Meaning   **Term**

1. inflammation of the middle ear   _____

2. hearing loss due to damage to the inner ear   _____

3. age-related hearing loss   _____

4. inflammation of the external auditory meatus   _____

5. hearing loss due to obstruction or lesion in the outer
   and/or middle ear   _____

6. impairment of hearing involving difficulty in the
   processing of sound   _____

ADVANCED
RECALL

Exercise 40

Complete each sentence by writing in the correct medical term.

1. Hearing loss caused by damage to the inner ear or auditory nerve is called _____.

2. _____ is inflammation of the external auditory meatus.

3. Hearing loss due to an obstruction or lesion in the outer and/or middle ear is called _____ .

4. _____ is a discharge of pus from the ear.

5. A chronic condition of the ear known as _____ is characterized by dizziness, tinnitus, hearing loss, and a sensation of pressure.

6. A hole or rupture of the eardrum is called a(n) _____ .

7. Inflammation of the middle ear is called _____ .

TERM
CONSTRUCTION

Exercise 41

Build the correct medical term for the meaning given. Write the term in the blank indicating the word parts (CF = combining form, S = suffix).

1. pain in the ear

   _____ / _____
   CF   S

2. inflammation of the inner ear

   _____ / _____
   CF   S

3. discharge from the ear

   _____ / _____
   CF   S

4. inflammation of the mastoid bone

   _____ / _____
   CF   S

5. inflammation of the tympanic membrane

   _____ / _____
   CF   S

Tests and Procedures

Term	Pronunciation	Meaning
Diagnostic Procedures		
audiogram	aw'dē-ō-gram	record of hearing (presented in graph form) (Fig. 13-21)
audiometer	aw'dē-om'ĕ-ter	instrument for measuring hearing
audiometry	aw'dē-om'ĕ-trē	measurement of hearing (Fig. 13-17)
decibel (dB)	des'i-bel	unit for expressing the intensity of sound

NOISE-INDUCED HEARING LOSS Sound is measured in decibels (dB). Noises that are greater than 80 decibels are considered dangerous to your hearing. Exposure to this level of sound can cause permanent hearing damage. Examples of noises greater than 80 dB are chain saws, leaf blowers, loud car stereos, and airplanes at the point of takeoff. The use of earbuds with MP3 players is a potential hazard to hearing if the volume is kept too high.

Term	Pronunciation	Meaning
electronystagmography (ENG)	ē-lek'trō-nis'tag-mog'ră-fē	recording of eye movements in response to electrical impulses to diagnose balance problems

(continued)

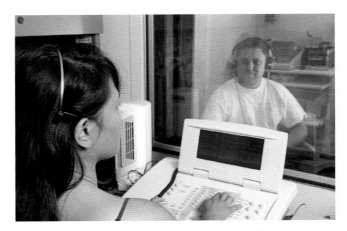

Figure 13-17　Patient undergoing audiometry.

Tests and Procedures *(continued)*

Term	Pronunciation	Meaning
hertz (Hz)	herts	unit of measure of frequency or pitch of sound
otoscope	ō'tō-skōp	instrument for examining the ear (Fig. 13-18)
otoscopy	ō-tos'kŏ-pē	use of an otoscope to examine the external auditory canal and tympanic membrane
tympanogram	tim'pă-nō-gram	record of middle ear function (presented in graph form)
tympanometer	tim'pă-nom'ĕ-tĕr	instrument for measuring middle ear function
tympanometry	tim'pă-nom'ĕ-trē	measurement of middle ear function

ANIMATION

Learn more about the measurement of hearing by viewing the *Audiometry* video on the Student Resources.

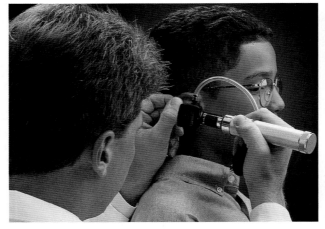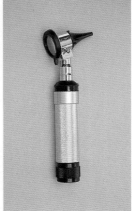

Figure 13-18　Using an otoscope to perform otoscopy.

■ Exercises: Tests and Procedures

Exercise 42

SIMPLE
RECALL

Write the meaning of the term given.

1. hertz _____

2. audiogram _____

3. otoscopy _____

4. tympanometry _____

5. decibel _____

6. tympanogram _____

Exercise 43

ADVANCED
RECALL

Circle the term that is most appropriate for the meaning of the sentence.

1. The physician used a(n) (*otoscope, audiometer, decibel*) to assess the patient's hearing.

2. Mr. Vladimir was referred to the (*tympanometry, electronystagmography, audiometry*) department to get a measurement of his hearing.

3. The results of Mrs. James' (*tympanogram, audiogram, electronystagmogram*) indicated that she had significant hearing loss in her right ear.

4. Dr. Davies measured Mrs. MacDonald's middle ear function using a(n) (*audiometer, otoscope, tympanometer*).

Exercise 44

TERM
CONSTRUCTION

Using the given combining form, build a medical term for the meaning given.

Combining Form	Meaning of Medical Term	Medical Term
ot/o	instrument for examining the ear	**1.** _____
tympan/o	record of middle ear function	**2.** _____
audi/o	instrument for measuring hearing	**3.** _____
ot/o	use of an otoscope to examine the ear	**4.** _____
tympan/o	measurement of middle ear function	**5.** _____
audi/o	record of hearing	**6.** _____

A.

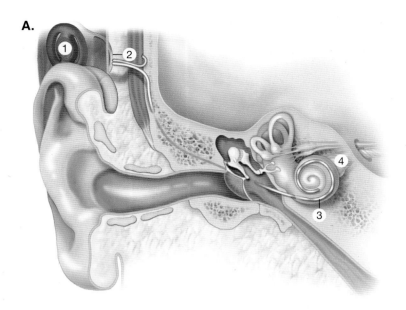

B.

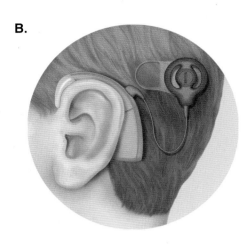

1. External speech processor captures sound and converts it into digital signals

2. Processor sends digital signal to internal implant

3. Internal implant converts signals into electrical energy, sending it to an electrode array inside the cochlea

4. Electrodes stimulate hearing nerve, bypassing damaged hair cells, and the brain perceives signals to hear sound

Figure 13-19   **A.** Function of a cochlear implant. **B.** Side view showing placement of external speech processor.

Surgical Interventions and Therapeutic Procedures

Term	Pronunciation	Meaning
cochlear implant	kok′lē-ăr im′plant	an electronic device implanted in the cochlea to stimulate the auditory nerve and provide hearing sensations for the profoundly deaf (Fig. 13-19)
ear lavage	ēr lă-vahzh′	irrigation of the ear to remove cerumen buildup
labyrinthectomy	lab′i-rin-thek′tŏ-mē	excision of part of the labyrinth
mastoidectomy	mas′toy-dek′tŏ-mē	excision of part of the mastoid bone
mastoidotomy	mas′toyd-ot′ ŏ-mē	incision into the mastoid bone
myringotomy, *syn.* tympanostomy	mir′in-got′ŏ-mē, tim′pan-os′tŏ-mē	surgical incision (opening) into the tympanic membrane to drain fluid from the middle ear (usually done with subsequent tympanostomy tube placement) (Fig. 13-20)
otoplasty	ō′tō-plas′tē	surgical repair of the external ear
stapedectomy	stā′pĕ-dek′tŏ-mē	removal of the stapes and replacement with a prosthesis; done to correct hearing loss from otosclerosis
tympanoplasty	tim′pă-nō-plas′tē	surgical repair of the tympanic membrane and/or middle ear
tympanostomy tube placement	tim′pan-os′tŏ-mē tūb plās′mĕnt	placement of a tube in the tympanic membrane to relieve symptoms caused by fluid buildup

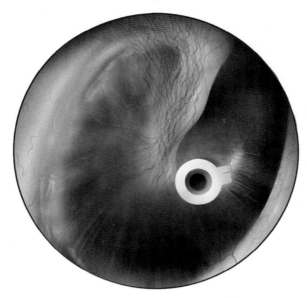

Figure 13-20   Tympanic membrane with tympanostomy tube in place, as viewed through otoscope.

■ Exercises: Surgical Interventions and Therapeutic Procedures

SIMPLE
RECALL

Exercise 45

Write the correct medical term for the definition given.

1. excision of part of the labyrinth _____

2. incision into the mastoid bone and cells _____

3. removal of the stapes bone _____

4. irrigation of the ear to remove cerumen _____

5. surgical repair of the external ear _____

ADVANCED
RECALL

Exercise 46

Complete each sentence by writing in the correct medical term.

1. Sammy was profoundly deaf so the otologist recommended a(n) _____,
   which is an electronic device that stimulates the hearing nerves to provide hearing sensations.

2. Dr. Cole drained the fluid out of Kara's middle ear with a procedure called a(n)
   _____, in which he made an incision into her tympanic membrane.

3. Jenny had chronic otitis media, so the physician recommended a(n) _____
   to create an opening into the middle ear and _____ with placement of a
   tube into the tympanic membrane to prevent further buildup of fluid.

4. Mr. Douglas's tympanic membrane perforation would not heal, so the physician performed a(n) _____ to repair the tympanic membrane.

5. The surgeon performed a(n) _____ to remove part of the mastoid bone.

TERM
CONSTRUCTION

Exercise 47

Using the given suffix, build a medical term for the meaning given.

Suffix	Meaning of Medical Term	Medical Term
-tomy	incision into the mastoid	1. _____
-ectomy	removal of the stapes	2. _____
-stomy	surgical opening into tympanic membrane	3. _____
-plasty	surgical repair of the tympanic membrane	4. _____

Medications and Drug Therapies

Term	Pronunciation	Meaning
antibiotic	an'tē-bī-ot'ik	drug that acts against susceptible microorganisms; used to treat otitis media and other ear diseases caused by bacteria
ceruminolytic	sĕ-rū'mi-nō-lit'ik	a substance instilled into the external auditory canal to soften earwax
otic	ō'tik	any medication that can be instilled into the ear drop by drop

SIMPLE
RECALL

Exercise 48

Write the correct medication or drug therapy term for the definition given.

1. medication that can be instilled into the ear drop by drop   _____

2. drug used to treat ear diseases caused by bacteria   _____

3. medication used to soften earwax   _____

Specialties and Specialists

Term	Pronunciation	Meaning
audiology	aw'dē-ol'ō-jē	medical specialty concerned with the study and treatment of hearing disorders and fitting of hearing aids
audiologist	aw'dē-ol'ō-jist	one who specializes in audiology
otology	ō-tol'ŏ-jē	medical specialty concerned with the study of the ears and treatment of ear disease
otologist	ō-tol'ŏ-jist	physician who specializes in otology
otorhinolaryngology	ō'tō-rī'nō-lar-in-gol'ŏ-jē	medical specialty concerned with diseases of the ear, nose, and throat
otorhinolaryngologist	ō'tō-rī'nō-lar-in-gol'ŏ-jist	physician who specializes in otorhinolaryngology

■ Exercise: Specialties and Specialists

Exercise 49

SIMPLE
RECALL

Write the correct medical term for the definition given.

1. medical specialty concerned with the study of the ears and treatment of ear diseases _____

2. one who specializes in audiology _____

3. medical specialty concerned with diseases of the ear, nose, and throat _____

4. medical specialty concerned with the study and treatment of hearing disorders and fitting of hearing aids _____

5. physician who specializes in otology _____

6. physician who specializes in otorhinolaryngology _____

Abbreviations

Abbreviation	Meaning
AD	right ear (auris dexter)
AS	left ear (auris sinister)
AU	each ear, both ears (auris utraque)

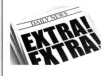 **DANGEROUS ABBREVIATIONS RELATED TO THE EAR** The Institute on Safe Medication Practices includes the abbreviations AD, AS, and AU on their list of "Error-Prone Abbreviations, Symbols, and Dose Designations" and recommends that they not be used in any medical communications. See the box entitled "Dangerous Abbreviations" on p. xx for more information.

dB	decibel
EENT	eyes, ears, nose, and throat
ENG	electronystagmography
ENT	ears, nose, and throat
Hz	hertz
OE	otitis externa
OM	otitis media
TM	tympanic membrane

■ Exercises: Abbreviations

Exercise 50

SIMPLE RECALL

Write the definition of each abbreviation.

1. EENT _____

2. AU _____

3. Hz _____

4. OM _____

5. dB _____

6. AD _____

Exercise 51

ADVANCED RECALL

Write the definition of each abbreviation used in these sentences.

1. Sara's mother took her to an **ENT** physician because of her chronic otitis media.

_____

2. The patient is a surfer and frequently suffers from **OE**.

_____

3. Mr. Malach has severe hearing loss **AS**.

_____

4. Ms. Tasara's physician recommended **ENG** to diagnose the cause of her vertigo.

_____

5. The otologist diagnosed a ruptured **TM** as the cause of the patient's otalgia and otorrhea.

_____

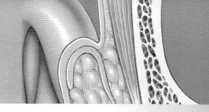

Chapter Review

Review of Terms for Anatomy and Physiology

VISUAL

Exercise 52

Write the correct terms on the blanks for the anatomic structures indicated.

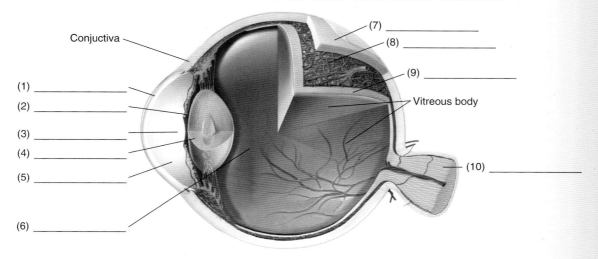

Conjuctiva

(1) _____
(2) _____
(3) _____
(4) _____
(5) _____
(6) _____

(7) _____
(8) _____
(9) _____
Vitreous body
(10) _____

VISUAL

Exercise 53

Write the correct terms on the blanks for the anatomic structures indicated.

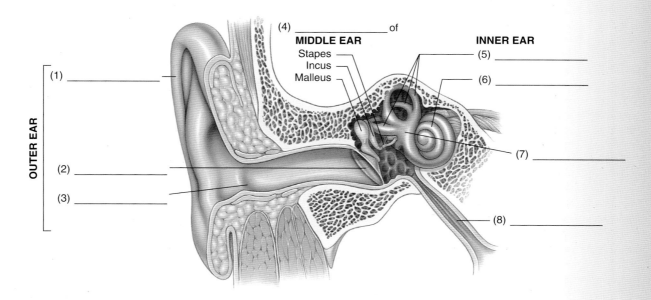

(4) _____ of
MIDDLE EAR   **INNER EAR**
Stapes
Incus
Malleus

(1) _____
(2) _____
(3) _____

OUTER EAR

(5) _____
(6) _____
(7) _____
(8) _____

Understanding Term Structure

TERM
CONSTRUCTION

Exercise 54

Break the given medical term into its word parts and define each part. Then define the medical term.

For example:

mastoiditis	*word parts:*	mastoid/o / -itis	
	meanings:	mastoid bone / inflammation of	
	term meaning:	inflammation of the mastoid bone	

1. ophthalmic   *word parts:* _____ / _____

               meanings: _____ / _____

               term meaning: _____

2. audiometer   *word parts:* _____ / _____

               meanings: _____ / _____

               term meaning: _____

3. blepharitis   *word parts:* _____ / _____

               meanings: _____ / _____

               term meaning: _____

4. tympanostomy   *word parts:* _____ / _____

               meanings: _____ / _____

               term meaning: _____

5. iridomalacia   *word parts:* _____ / _____

               meanings: _____ / _____

               term meaning: _____

6. labyrinthitis   *word parts:* _____ / _____

               meanings: _____ / _____

               term meaning: _____

7. retinopathy   *word parts:* _____ / _____

               meanings: _____ / _____

               term meaning: _____

8. acoustic   *word parts:*   _____ / _____

              meanings: _____ / _____

              term meaning: _____

9. pupillometer   *word parts:*   _____ / _____

              meanings: _____ / _____

              term meaning: _____

10. stapedectomy   *word parts:*   _____ / _____

              meanings: _____ / _____

              term meaning: _____

11. tonometer   *word parts:*   _____ / _____

              meanings: _____ / _____

              term meaning: _____

12. vestibular   *word parts:*   _____ / _____

              meanings: _____ / _____

              term meaning: _____

13. sclerotomy   *word parts:*   _____ / _____

              meanings: _____ / _____

              term meaning: _____

14. otoscopy   *word parts:*   _____ / _____

              meanings: _____ / _____

              term meaning: _____

Exercise 55

TERM
CONSTRUCTION

For each term, first write the meaning of the term. Then write the meaning of the word parts in that term.

1. otorrhea   _____

   ot/o   _____

   -rrhea   _____

2. ophthalmoscopy _____

ophthalm/o _____

-scopy _____

3. optometry _____

opt/o _____

-metry _____

4. myringitis _____

myring/o _____

-itis _____

5. otopyorrhea _____

ot/o _____

py/o _____

-rrhea _____

6. dacryorrhea _____

dacry/o _____

-rrhea _____

7. aural _____

aur/o _____

-al _____

8. presbyopia _____

presby/o _____

-opia _____

9. audiogram _____

audi/o _____

-gram _____

10. mastoidectomy _____

mastoid/o _____

-ectomy _____

11. conjunctivitis _____

    conjunctiv/o _____

    -itis _____

12. tympanometry _____

    tympan/o _____

    -metry _____

13. keratoplasty _____

    kerat/o _____

    -plasty _____

14. presbycusis _____

    presby/o _____

    -cusis _____

Comprehension Exercises

Exercise 56

COMPREHENSION

Match each medical specialist with the description of the specialty in which he or she works.

audiologist   optometrist   otologist
ophthalmologist   otorhinolaryngologist

1. diseases of the ears, nose, and throat _____

2. measurement of vision and prescription of corrective treatment or lenses _____

3. study and treatment of hearing disorders _____

4. study of the ears and treatment of ear disease _____

5. study of the eye, its diseases, and refractive errors _____

Exercise 57

COMPREHENSION

Fill in the blank with the correct term.

1. The snail-shaped organ that contains the spiral organ is the _____.

2. The _____ are the auditory bones that include the malleus, incus, and stapes.

3. The part of the eye that contains the vision receptors is the _____.

4. A buildup of a waxy substance created by the glands in the external auditory meatus is called a(n) _____.

5. The _____ lubricate the eyes by producing tears.

6. _____ is a chronic condition of the inner ear causing dizziness, tinnitus, and hearing loss.

7. The medical term for an inflammation of the external auditory canal, often referred to as "swimmer's ear," is _____.

8. _____ is blurry or distorted vision due to abnormal curvature of the cornea.

9. _____ is hearing loss that is related to aging.

10. An ophthalmologist might use _____ drops to dilate the pupils.

11. Medication used to relieve dry irritated eyes is called a(n) _____.

12. _____ is the term for separation of the retina from the choroid in the back of the eye.

13. The procedure that uses a laser to reshape the cornea to correct vision problems is called _____.

14. The term for dry eye is _____.

15. A photographic recording of the flow of a fluorescent dye through the blood vessels of the eye is called _____.

16. The procedure for irrigating the ear to remove earwax buildup is called _____.

17. A(n) _____ is a chart containing symbols that is used to test visual acuity.

18. A(n) _____ is done to correct otosclerosis by removing the stapes bone and replacing it with a prosthesis.

19. _____ are medications that relax muscles in the eye's interior structure to facilitate better fluid outflow.

20. _____ is the procedure in which extreme cold is used to repair a retinal tear.

Exercise 58

COMPREHENSION **Write a short answer for each question.**

1. What is the clinical term for nearsightedness? _____

2. Define vertigo. _____

_____

3. What symptom would an elderly patient with presbyopia experience? _____

_____

4. What is the medical term for "seeing double"? _____

5. A patient asks you to dim the lights because she states that they are "too bright." What

condition might this patient have? _____

6. How does hyperopia differ from myopia? _____

_____

7. Why would a patient be given a ceruminolytic?_____

8. Which procedure is usually followed by placement of a tympanostomy tube? _____

_____

Exercise 59

COMPREHENSION **Circle the letter of the best answer in the following questions.**

1. A chalazion involves obstruction of which of these?

    A. lacrimal glands
    B. ossicles
    C. tarsal glands
    D. dacryocyst

2. A clinical test used to diagnose glaucoma is:

    A. tonometry
    B. pupillometry
    C. audiometry
    D. tympanometry

3. A person who has difficulty driving at night due to poor vision in reduced light probably has:

    A. diplopia
    B. amblyopia
    C. presbyopia
    D. nyctalopia

4. Which of the following is located within the cochlea?

    A. pharyngotympanic tube
    B. mastoid bone
    C. spiral organ
    D. vestibule

5. A patient with a hole in her or his eardrum has a ruptured:

    A. cochlea
    B. retina
    C. pinna
    D. tympanic membrane

6. A construction worker who is out in the sun all day might develop a growth of conjunctival tissue over his cornea known as a:

    A. pterygium
    B. dacryolith
    C. hordeolum
    D. cataract

7. The medical term for earwax is:

    A. auricle
    B. cerumen
    C. vestibule
    D. cholesteatoma

8. A stapedectomy might be performed for which condition?

    A. otosclerosis
    B. cholesteatoma
    C. acoustic neuroma
    D. otomycosis

9. Which of these is *not* an ossicle?

    A. incus
    B. stapes
    C. labyrinth
    D. malleus

10. Patients with diabetes mellitus are at increased risk of blindness due to:

    A. glaucoma
    B. presbyopia
    C. conjunctivitis
    D. diabetic retinopathy

11. Children with poor vision in one eye have a condition commonly called "lazy eye." In clinical terms, this condition is called:

    A. photophobia
    B. amblyopia
    C. myopia
    D. retinitis pigmentosa

12. Removal of a lesion from the middle ear might relieve which condition?

    A. sensorineural hearing loss
    B. conductive hearing loss
    C. presbycusis
    D. otopyorrhea

13. Which condition is usually caused by chronic otitis media?

    A. otitis externa
    B. acoustic neuroma
    C. otomycosis
    D. cholesteatoma

14. Which of the following conditions is caused by the aging process?

    A. diabetic retinopathy
    B. retinitis pigmentosa
    C. exophthalmos
    D. macular degeneration

15. What condition involves the eighth cranial nerve that connects the ear to the brain?

    A. acoustic neuroma
    B. cholesteatoma
    C. tympanic membrane perforation
    D. cerumen impaction

16. The condition that is known to be hereditary is:

    A. hyperopia
    B. retinitis pigmentosa
    C. macular degeneration
    D. detached retina

17. The structure that runs from the middle ear space to the pharynx is called the:

    A. ossicle
    B. semicircular canal
    C. vestibule
    D. pharyngotympanic tube

18. The test that might be performed to diagnose semicircular canal and duct problems is called:

    A. Weber test
    B. electronystagmography
    C. tympanometry
    D. Rinne test

19. Children who appear "cross-eyed" have a condition of ocular misalignment called:

    A. retinopathy
    B. strabismus
    C. amblyopia
    D. nystagmus

20. Which of these is *not* a procedure to repair a torn or detached retina?

    A. trabeculectomy
    B. cryoretinopexy
    C. scleral buckling
    D. retinal photocoagulation

Application and Analysis

CASE REPORTS

Exercise 60

APPLICATION

Read the case reports and circle the letter of your answer choice for the questions that follow.

CASE 13-1

Mr. Larson was working with a compressor when the hose broke loose and he was injured from the blast of air pressure that was released near the right side of his head. He suddenly could not hear out of his right ear. He was sent to an otorhinolaryngologist for evaluation. Mr. Larson described symptoms of vertigo as well as right-sided hearing loss. An audiogram revealed pronounced hearing loss at between 4,000 and 8,000 Hz (Fig. 13-21). The diagnosis was sensorineural hearing loss due to blast injury with accompanying tinnitus.

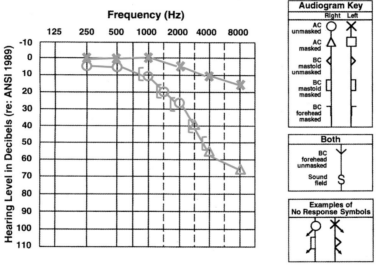

Figure 13-21 Audiogram revealing sensorineural hearing loss on the right side.

1. An otorhinolaryngologist, such as the one seen by Mr. Larson, specializes in:

A. eyes
B. ears, nose, and throat
C. vision
D. hearing aids

2. Vertigo refers to which of these symptoms?

A. hearing loss
B. pressure sensation in the ears

C. noise in the ears
D. spinning sensation, dizziness

3. Tinnitus is defined as the perception of various noises in the ear, such as:

A. ringing
B. buzzing
C. humming
D. all of the above

4. The audiogram was a recording of:

A. eardrum movement
B. the middle ear space
C. hearing measurement
D. eye movements in response to electrical stimulation

5. Hz is the abbreviation for a:

A. unit of measure of sound frequency
B. hearing test
C. unit for expressing the intensity of sound
D. two-pronged steel bar whose vibrations produce pure tones

CASE 13-2

Mrs. Holtzinger failed the eye test when she tried to renew her driver's license. She went to an ophthalmologist for evaluation of her vision problem. Visual acuity testing was performed using a Snellen chart. Ophthalmoscopy was also performed. The diagnosis was cataracts in both eyes (OU). It was recommended that she be scheduled for phacoemulsification and lens replacement.

6. An ophthalmologist specializes in:

A. ears, nose, and throat
B. eyes
C. hearing
D. making of corrective lenses

7. Visual acuity testing is the testing for:

A. sharpness of vision
B. ability to hear
C. pressure in the eyes
D. chalazions

8. An ophthalmoscopy is an:

A. examination of the eye
B. examination of the pupil

C. examination of the interior of the eye
D. examination of the sclera

9. A cataract is:

A. increased pressure in the eye
B. clouding of the lens of the eye
C. detachment of the retina
D. hemorrhage of the choroid

10. In phacoemulsification, a cataract is removed by:

A. enucleation
B. cryoretinopexy
C. LASIK
D. breaking up the lens by vibration using a needle probe

MEDICAL RECORD ANALYSIS

MEDICAL RECORD 13-1

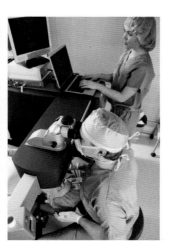

You are the ophthalmic technologist for Dr. Brunner. Patient Nikita Stewart is here for a postoperative refraction after undergoing LASIK surgery 2 weeks ago. The operative report for her LASIK surgery, during which you served as Dr. Brunner's assistant, is as follows:

An ophthalmic technologist assists an ophthalmologist performing LASIK surgery.

Medical Record

LASIK SURGERY REPORT

Preoperative Diagnosis: Myopia, right eye
Postoperative Diagnosis: Myopia, right eye
Operation: LASIK, right eye
Surgeon: Thomas Brunner, M.D.

Refraction and preoperative testing was performed 2 weeks ago. At that time, the patient underwent computerized topographic analysis via video keratography to map the surface of the eye. Corneal thickness and corneal surface elevations were measured. Tonometry revealed normal intraocular pressure. Slitlamp biomicroscopy was performed to ensure that there were no contraindications for the procedure. The retina appeared normal. The patient signed an informed consent for the procedure after the risks and benefits were explained in detail. Patient was given Valium for preoperative sedation to be taken 30 minutes prior to surgery.

On arrival today, topographic analysis was repeated to confirm all measurements. Measurements were then entered into the laser's computer. Patient was brought into the operating room and placed in a supine position on the table. Ophthalmic anesthetic drops were instilled into the right eye, and the eye was disinfected. A speculum was placed in the right eye for lid retraction. Reference marks were made for laser alignment.

A suction ring was applied to the eye, and the cornea was flattened. A small incision was made using the microkeratome to create a flap. The flap was lifted to reveal the underlying stromal tissue. Using the excimer laser, the cornea was contoured to the predetermined measurements. The eye was then irrigated, and the flap was repositioned. The suction ring and speculum were removed.

The patient tolerated the procedure well. Postoperative instructions and medications were given to the patient and she was discharged home in the care of her husband. She is to return in 2 weeks for postoperative follow-up and refraction.

Exercise 61

APPLICATION   **Read the medical report and circle the letter of your answer choice for the following questions.**

1. The term myopia means that the patient:

   A. is farsighted
   B. has presbyopia
   C. is nearsighted
   D. has macular degeneration

2. The test done to measure the patient's intraocular pressure was:

   A. tonometry
   B. refraction
   C. topographic analysis
   D. keratography

3. The term that means the patient's refractive errors were measured is:

   A. keratography
   B. refraction
   C. tonometry
   D. topographic analysis

Exercise 62

APPLICATION

Write the appropriate medical terms used in this medical record on the blanks after their definitions. Note that not all the terms appear in the chapter, but you should be able to identify these terms based on word parts that are included in this chapter.

1. relating to the cornea   _____

2. inside the eye   _____

3. instrument for making small cuts in the cornea   _____

4. process of recording the cornea   _____

Bonus Question

5. The term that describes an instrument that opens a body part for examination or procedures is

_____ .

MEDICAL RECORD 13-2

You are an audiologist working in an otorhinolaryngology office. One month ago, a child was referred to your office by his pediatrician for an ear problem. You performed the audiometry test to assess the patient's hearing loss.

Medical Record

OTORHINOLARYNGOLOGY CONSULTATION REPORT

Thank you for your kind referral of Kenny Mason. Kenny was seen today because of a right tympanic membrane perforation noted by you on recent examination. Kenny previously had a perforation of the right ear in February of 2007, after he had been hit on the ear with a ladder. This perforation healed spontaneously in several weeks. He had no postinjury infections or complications.

On questioning today, Kenny admits that he was hit in the right ear with a soccer ball about one and a half weeks ago and has had some tinnitus and dysacousis in the right ear since that time.

Past medical history is unremarkable with the exception of bilateral tympanostomies with insertion of tympanostomy tubes at age three and a tonsillectomy at age ten. He is otherwise in good health.

Examination today is unremarkable with the exception of an anterior superior tympanic membrane perforation with purulent otorrhea in the right ear. Audiometry done in the office revealed a significant conductive hearing loss in the right ear. The left ear was normal.

I prescribed otic antibiotic drops to be instilled in the right ear q.i.d. I instructed Kenny's mother to make sure that his ear stays dry at all times. We will adopt an expectant attitude toward this perforation. I think that there is a good chance that it will heal on its own. I will see Kenny back for a recheck in 1 month. If it has not healed at that time, we will schedule him for a right tympanoplasty.

Thank you for referring this pleasant young man to me. I will keep you updated as to his status.

Exercise 63

APPLICATION **Write the appropriate medical terms used in this medical record on the blanks after their definitions.**

1. measurement of hearing _____

2. discharge from the ear _____

3. pertaining to the ear _____

4. surgical repair of the eardrum _____

5. condition of impaired hearing _____

6. hole in the eardrum _____

7. pertaining to the tympanic membrane or cavity _____

8. ringing noise in the ear _____

9. surgical opening in the eardrums _____

10. hearing loss due to blockage of sound transmission through the external and middle ear _____

Bonus Questions

11. The record indicates that the patient has an *anterior superior* tympanic membrane perforation. Based on what you have learned previously, describe the location of the perforation on the tympanic membrane. _____

_____

12. What did the results of Kenny's audiometry reveal? _____

_____

Pronunciation and Spelling

AUDITORY

Exercise 64

Review the Chapter 13 terms in the Dictionary/Audio Glossary in the Student Resources and practice pronouncing each term, referring to the pronunciation guide as needed.

SPELLING

Exercise 65

Circle the correct spelling of each term.

1. tarsel	tarsal	tarrsal
2. koroid	choroyd	choroid
3. vitreous	vitrious	vitreus
4. corneal	cornial	korneal
5. opthalmology	ophthalmology	ophtholmology
6. chalazion	kalazion	calazion
7. diploplia	diplopea	diplopia
8. glawcoma	gluacoma	glaucoma
9. nystagmus	nistagmus	nystagmis
10. presbiopia	presbyopia	presbyopea
11. pterygium	pterigium	pterygeum
12. strabismus	strabysmus	strabismis
13. florescien	flurescien	fluorescein
14. refraction	refracshun	refraktion
15. Snellin	Snelen	Snellen
16. pupilometry	pupillometry	pupellometry
17. aquity	acuwity	acuity
18. catarect	catarract	cataract
19. midreatic	mydriatic	midriatic
20. optishun	optician	optishian

Media Connection

STUDENT
RESOURCES

Exercise 66

Complete each of the following activities available with the Student Resources. Check off each activity as you complete it, and record your score for the Chapter Quiz in the space provided.

Chapter Exercises

____ Flash Cards

____ Concentration

____ Abbreviation Match-Up

____ Roboterms

____ Word Builder

____ Fill the Gap

____ Break It Down

____ True/False Body Building

____ Quiz Show

____ Complete the Case

____ Medical Record Review

____ Look and Label

____ Image Matching

____ Spelling Bee

____ **Chapter Quiz**   *Score:* _____%

Additional Resources

____ Video: Audiometry

____ Dictionary/Audio Glossary

____ Health Professions Careers: Ophthalmic Technologist

____ Health Professions Careers: Audiologist

Musculoskeletal System

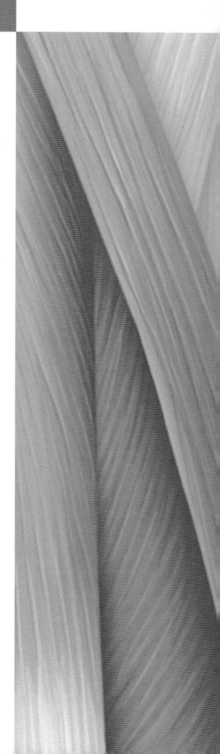

Chapter Outline

Objectives

After completion of this chapter you will be able to:

1. Describe the location of key bones and muscles in the body.

2. Define terms related to bone structure, joints, joint movements, and muscles.

3. Define combining forms, prefixes, and suffixes related to the musculoskeletal system.

4. Define common medical terminology related to the musculoskeletal system, including adjectives and related terms, symptoms and conditions, tests and procedures, surgical interventions and therapeutic procedures, medications and drug therapies, and specialties.

5. Explain abbreviations for terms related to the musculoskeletal system.

6. Successfully complete all chapter exercises.

7. Explain terms used in medical records and case studies involving the musculoskeletal system.

8. Successfully complete all pronunciation and spelling exercises, and complete all interactive exercises included with the companion Student Resources.

■ ANATOMY AND PHYSIOLOGY

Functions

- ■ To give shape and structure to the body and provide support
- ■ To allow movement
- ■ To protect internal organs
- ■ To store calcium and other minerals (bones)
- ■ To produce certain blood cells (bone marrow)
- ■ To produce heat (muscles)

Structures

- ■ The body has 206 bones, divided into the axial skeleton and appendicular skeleton.
- ■ The body has more than 600 muscles.
- ■ Bones articulate (meet) at joints where muscles allow for different types of joint movements.

Terms Related to Bone Structure (Fig. 14-1)

Term	Pronunciation	Meaning
bone marrow	bōn ma'rō	soft tissue within bone, with multiple functions including production of blood cells
cancellous bone, *syn.* spongy bone	kan'sě-lŭs bōn; spŏn'jē bōn	meshlike bone tissue (Fig. 14-2)
compact bone	kŏm-pakt' bōn	harder, denser bone (Fig. 14-2)
diaphysis	dī-af'i-sis	the shaft of a long bone
endosteum	en-dos'tē-ŭm	membrane within medullary cavity
epiphysis	e-pif'i-sis	the wider ends of a long bone
epiphysial plate	ep'i-fiz'ē-ăl plāt	the growth area of a long bone
medullary cavity	med'ŭ-lar'ē kav'i-tē	space within long bone shaft filled with bone marrow
metaphysis	mě-taf'i-sis	the flared section of a long bone between the diaphysis and epiphysis
os, *pl.* ossa	os, os'ă	bone
osteoblast	os'tē-ō-blast	bone-forming cell
osteoclast	os'tē-ō-klast	a cell that helps remove osseous (bony) tissue
osteocyte	os'tē-ō-sīt	bone cell
periosteum	per'ē-os'tē-ŭm	membrane surrounding a bone

Terms Related to the Skeleton and Bones (Fig. 14-3)

Term	Pronunciation	Meaning
The Skeleton		
axial skeleton	ak'sē-ăl skel'ě-tŏn	bones of the skull, spine, and chest
appendicular skeleton	ap'ěn-dik'yŭ-lăr skel'ě-tŏn	bones of the upper and lower limbs, shoulder, and pelvis
thorax	thō'raks	the chest

(continued)

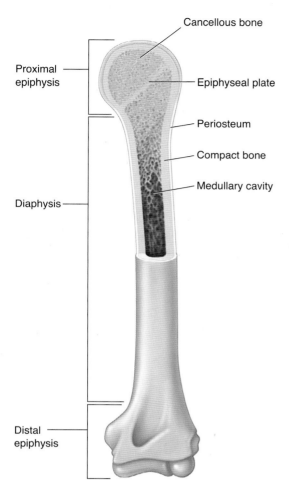

Figure 14-1 The external and internal composition of a long bone.

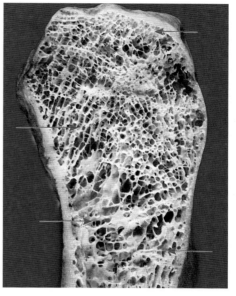

Figure 14-2 Types of bone tissue. Cancellous bone makes up most of the epiphysis of this long bone (*arrows*). A thin layer of compact bone is seen at the surface.

Terms Related to the Skeleton and Bones *(continued)*

Term	Pronunciation	Meaning
Bones		
acetabulum	as-ĕ-tab′yū-lŭm	the socket of the pelvic bone where the femur articulates
acromion	ă-krō′mē-on	lateral upper section of the scapula
calcaneus	kal-kā′nē-ŭs	bone of the heel
carpal bones	kahr′păl bōnz	the eight bones of the wrist
clavicle	klav′i-kĕl	collarbone
cranium	krā′nē-ŭm	the skull; composed of eight bones
femur	fē′mŭr	bone of the upper leg
fibula	fib′yū-lă	smaller, outer bone of the lower leg
humerus	hyū′mĕr-ŭs	bone of the upper arm
hyoid	hī′oyd	bone beneath the mandible
lamina	lam′i-nă	posterior section of a vertebra
mandible	man′di-bĕl	lower bone of the jaw

(continued)

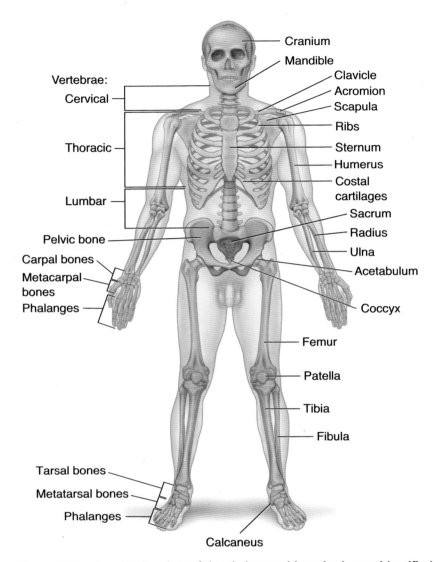

Figure 14-3   An anterior view of the skeleton with major bones identified.

Terms Related to the Skeleton and Bones *(continued)*

Term	Pronunciation	Meaning
maxilla	mak-sil′ă	upper bone of the jaw
metacarpal bones	met′ă-kahr′păl bōnz	the five bones of the palm of the hand
metatarsal bones	met′ă-tahr′săl bōnz	the five bones of the foot
patella	pă-tel′ă	kneecap
pelvic bone	pel′vik bōn	the hip bone, composed of three fused bones on each side
ischium	is′kē-ŭm	posterior lower section of the pelvic bone
ilium	il′ē-ŭm	upper section of the pelvic bone
pubis	pyū′bis	anterior lower section of pelvic bone; pubic bone
phalanges	fă-lan′-jēz	the bones of the fingers and toes; 14 in each hand or foot

(continued)

Terms Related to the Skeleton and Bones *(continued)*

Term	Pronunciation	Meaning
radius	rā′dē-ŭs	the outer of two bones of the lower arm
ribs	ribz	long curved bones that form the bony wall of the chest
scapula	skap′yū-lă	shoulder blade
sternum	stĕr′nŭm	anterior bone of thorax; breast bone
tarsal bones	tahr′săl bōnz	the seven bones of the ankle
tibia	tib′ē-ă	larger inner bone of the lower leg
ulna	ŭl′nă	the more inner of two bones of the lower arm
vertebra	vĕr′tĕ-bră	a bone of the spine (Fig. 14-4)
cervical vertebrae (C1–C7)	sĕr′vi-kăl vĕr′tĕ-brā	bones of neck
thoracic vertebrae (T1–T12)	thōr-as′ik vĕr′tĕ-brā	bones of midspine
lumbar vertebrae (L1–L5)	lŭm′bahr vĕr′tĕ-brā	bones of lower back
sacrum	sā′krŭm	five fused vertebrae below the lumbar spine
coccyx	kok′siks	four fused vertebrae at the lower end of the spine, below the sacrum; the tailbone
xiphoid process	zī′foyd pros′es	lower section of the sternum

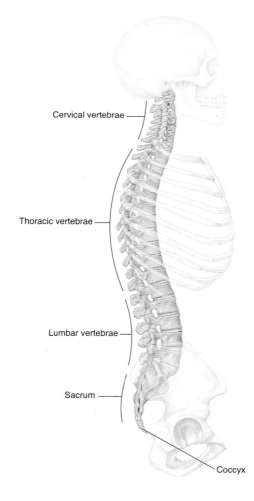

Cervical vertebrae

Thoracic vertebrae

Lumbar vertebrae

Sacrum

Coccyx

Figure 14-4 The vertebral column showing the types of vertebrae.

ANIMATION

View the *Vertebral Disk* video on the electronic Student Resources to learn more about the structure of the bones of the spine.

Joints and Joint Movements

- Joints occur wherever bones come together.
- Joints are categorized by the movements they perform.
- Terms for joint movements are based on the type and direction of movement.

Terms Related to Joints and Joint Movements

Term	Pronunciation	Meaning
Joints		
articulation	ahr-tik′yū-lā′shŭn	the site where bones come together
bursa	bŭr′să	a fluid-filled fibrous sac within some joints
cartilage	kahr′ti-lăj	dense connective tissue attached to bone in many joints
synovial joint, *syn.* diarthrosis	si-nō′vē-ăl joynt, dī′ahr-thrō′sis	a joint that moves freely; the joint cavity contains synovial fluid (Fig. 14-5)
intervertebral disk (or disc)	in′tĕr-vĕr′tĕ-brăl disk	platelike structure of connective tissue between vertebrae
ligament	lig′ă-mĕnt	band of strong connective tissue joining bones

(continued)

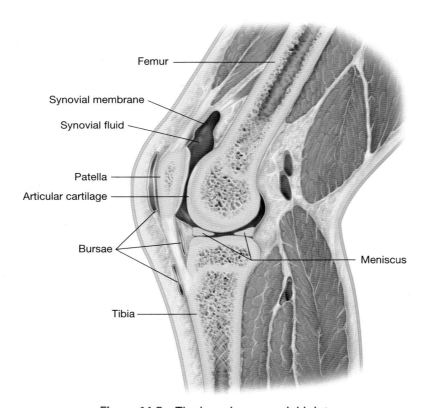

Femur

Synovial membrane

Synovial fluid

Patella

Articular cartilage

Bursae

Meniscus

Tibia

Figure 14-5   The knee is a synovial joint.

Terms Related to Joints and Joint Movements *(continued)*

Term	Pronunciation	Meaning
meniscus	mĕ-nis′kŭs	cartilage structure in the knee
suture	sū′chŭr	an immovable joint, such as that which joins the bones of the skull

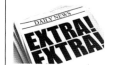 **SUTURE** When we think of joints, we think of those joints that move. Your skull also has joints, but the joints of the skull do not move. These joints, called *sutures*, hold the bones of the skull together, just as surgical sutures (or "stitches") hold two surfaces together.

symphysis	sim′fi-sis	a joint that moves only slightly
synovial fluid	si-nō′vē-ăl flū′id	lubricating fluid in a freely moving joint
tendon	ten′dŏn	band of fibrous connective tissue attaching a muscle to a bone

Joint Movements (Fig. 14-6)		
abduction	ab-dŭk′shŭn	moving away from the midline
adduction	ă-dŭk′shŭn	moving toward the midline
circumduction	sĭr′kŭm-dŭk′shŭn	moving in a circular manner
inversion	in-vĕr′zhŭn	turning inward
eversion	ē-vĕr′zhŭn	turning outward
dorsiflexion	dōr-si-flek′shŭn	bending foot upward
plantar flexion	plan′tahr flek′shŭn	bending foot downward
extension	eks-ten′shŭn	motion that increases the joint angle
flexion	flek′shŭn	motion that decreases the joint angle
pronation	prō-nā′shŭn	turning downward (palm of hand or sole of foot)
supination	sū′pi-nā′shŭn	turning upward (palm of hand or sole of foot)
rotation	rō-tā′shŭn	moving in circular direction around an axis

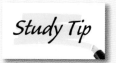 **Adduction, abduction:** When distinguishing abduction from adduction, remember the common word abduct, meaning to take *away*. Adduction has the word "add," meaning to bring *to*.

 View the animation entitled *Muscle Extension and Flexion* for a demonstration of muscles at work.

ANIMATION

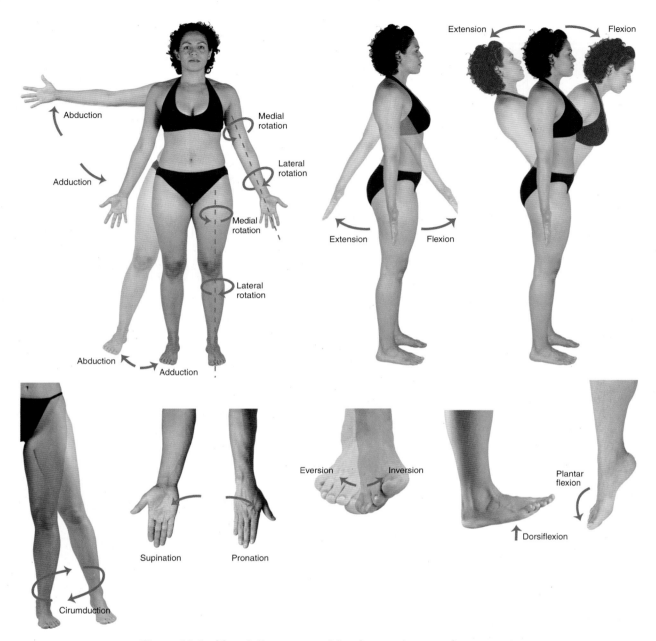

Figure 14-6 Most joints are capable of several types of movement.

Muscles

- The three types of muscle tissue in the body are skeletal muscle, smooth muscle, and cardiac muscle.
- Muscles are composed of bundles of muscle fibers along with other tissues.
- Tendons attach muscles to bones in or near joints.

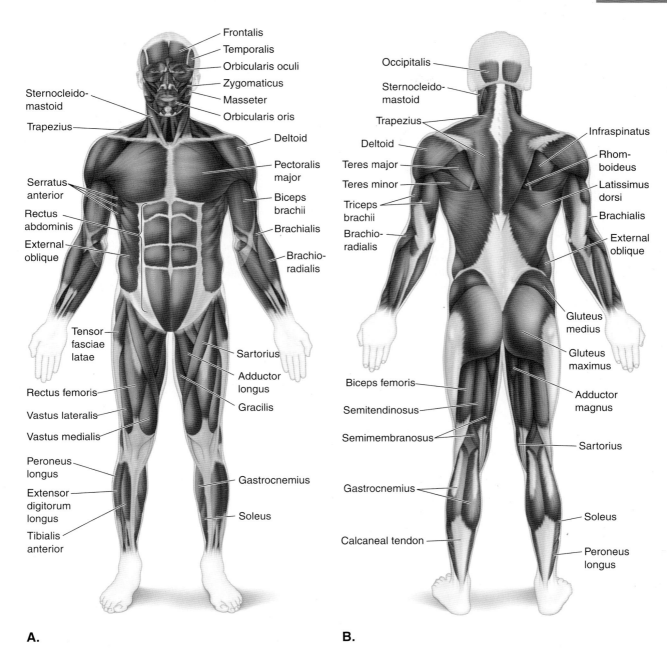

Figure 14-7   Skeletal muscles of the body. **A.** Anterior view. **B.** Posterior view.

Terms Related to Muscles (Fig. 14-7)

Term	Pronunciation	Meaning
agonist	ag'ŏn-ist	skeletal muscle that creates a movement by contracting; prime mover
antagonist	an-tag'ŏ-nist	skeletal muscle that opposes an agonist muscle and relaxes when the agonist contracts
cardiac muscle	kahr'dē-ak mŭs'ĕl	heart muscle (Fig. 14-8)
fascia	fash'ē-ă	sheet of connective tissue covering a muscle
fascicle	fas'i-kĕl	bundle of muscle fibers (Fig. 14-10)

(continued)

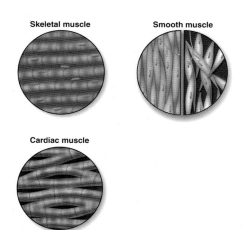

Figure 14-8 Muscles have varying internal characteristics depending on their function.

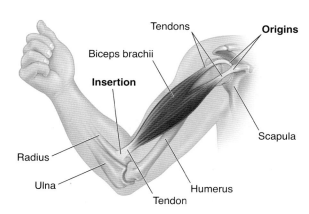

Figure 14-9 Muscles are attached to bones by tendons.

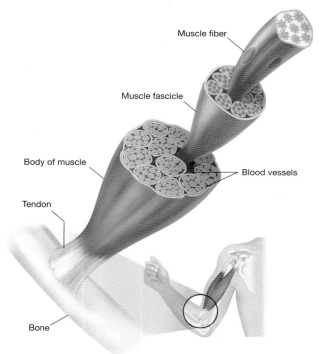

Figure 14-10 The structure of a skeletal muscle.

Terms Related to Muscles *(continued)*

Term	Pronunciation	Meaning
insertion of muscle	in-sĕr'shŭn mŭs'ĕl	end of muscle attached to bone that moves during contraction (Fig. 14-9)
origin of muscle	ōr'i-jin mŭs'ĕl	end of muscle attached to bone that does not move during contraction
smooth muscle, *syn.* unstriated muscle	smūth mŭs'ĕl, ŭn-strī'āt-ĕd mŭs'ĕl	type of muscle not under voluntary control; present in internal organs (Fig. 14-8)
skeletal muscle, *syn.* striated muscle	skel'ĕ-tăl mŭs'ĕl, strī'āt-ĕd mŭs'ĕl	type of muscle under voluntary control ("striated" refers to light and dark bands in muscle fibers) (Fig. 14-10, also Fig. 14-8)
tonus	tō'nŭs	muscle tone

■ Exercises: Anatomy and Physiology

SIMPLE
RECALL

Exercise 1

Write the correct anatomic structure for the definition given.

1. bone of upper arm   _____

2. bones of the palm   _____

3. shoulder blade   _____

4. breast bone   _____

5. shaft of long bone   _____

6. attaches muscle to bone   _____

7. bundle of muscle fibers   _____

8. bone of the heel   _____

9. bones of the skull, spine, chest   _____

10. a bone of the spine   _____

SIMPLE
RECALL

Exercise 2

Write the meaning of the term given.

1. abduction   _____

2. ligament   _____

3. articulation   _____

4. dorsiflexion   _____

5. acetabulum   _____

6. cranium   _____

7. mandible   _____

8. synovial joint   _____

9. maxilla   _____

10. cartilage   _____

11. epiphysial plate   _____

12. ossa   _____

Exercise 3

SIMPLE
RECALL

Circle the term that is most appropriate for the meaning of the sentence.

1. A severe injury to the kneecap may involve a fractured (*cerebellum, patella, scapula*).

2. The cartilage structure in the knee is called the (*synovium, meniscus, bursa*).

3. Muscle tissue present in internal organs is (*unstriated, agonist, fascial*).

4. (*Synovial fluid, Endosteum, Fascia*) is a sheet of connective tissue covering a muscle.

5. The smaller bone in the lower leg is the (*femur, ulna, fibula*).

6. The (*epiphysis, ilium, patella*), or upper section of the pelvic bone, connects with the ischium and pubis.

7. The (*tibia, sacrum, lamina*) is a part of each vertebra.

8. The (*clavicle, metaphysis, radius*) articulates with the acromion at one end and the top of the sternum at the other end.

9. Between the diaphysis and the epiphysis of a long bone is the (*metaphysis, meniscus, diarthrosis*).

10. The large inner bone of the lower leg is the (*tibia, ulna, radius*).

11. A (*tendon, fascia, bursa*) is a fluid-filled fibrous sac within some joints.

12. The (*ischium, ilium, pubis*) is the posterior lower section of the pelvic bone, whereas the (*ischium, ilium, pubis*) is the anterior lower section of the pelvic bone.

13. The plural of vertebra is (*vertebrum, vertebras, vertebrae*).

14. The metatarsal bones are just distal to the (*tarsal, carpal, phalangeal*) bones.

15. Movement that decreases the joint angle is termed (*extension, flexion, inversion*).

Exercise 4

ADVANCED
RECALL

Match each medical term with its meaning.

| cancellous bone | ulna | carpal bones | endosteum | sacrum |
| intervertebral disk | radius | compact bone | ossa | osteocyte |

Meaning   **Term**

1. membrane within medullary cavity   _____

2. strong solid bone tissue   _____

3. outer bone in lower arm   _____

4. eight bones of wrist   _____

5. spongy bone   _____

6. composed of fused vertebrae   _____

7. connective tissue between vertebrae _____

8. inner bone in lower arm   _____

9. bones   _____

10. bone cell   _____

ADVANCED
RECALL

Exercise 5

Complete each sentence by writing in the correct medical term.

1. A patient with a broken collarbone has a fracture of the _____.

2. A fracture of the upper arm bone, the _____, is generally painful.

3. Bone tissue that is spongy and meshlike is called _____ bone.

4. A(n) _____ is a band of strong connective tissue that joins bones together at a joint.

5. The end of a muscle attached to bone that moves with contraction is called the _____ of the muscle.

6. A(n) _____ is a skeletal muscle that opposes a prime mover.

7. Skeletal muscle is _____, whereas smooth muscle is _____.

8. A freely moving joint is lubricated by _____ fluid.

9. The movement of turning the foot outward is called _____.

10. The type of immovable joint connecting skull bones is a(n) _____.

11. Bones in many types of joint are joined by _____, a dense connective tissue.

12. Just above the coccyx is the spinal structure called the _____.

■ WORD PARTS

Note that some word parts that have been introduced earlier in the book may not be repeated here.

Combining Forms

Combining Form	Meaning
ankyl/o	stiff
arthr/o, articul/o	joint
burs/o	bursa
carp/o	carpal bones
chondr/o	cartilage
clavic/o, clavicul/o	clavicle
cervic/o	neck
cost/o	rib
crani/o	cranium, skull

(continued)

Combining Forms *(continued)*

Combining Form	Meaning
disk/o	disk or disc
fasci/o	fascia, band
femor/o	femur
fibul/o	fibula
humer/o	humerus
ili/o	ilium
ischi/o	ischium
kinesi/o, kinet/o	movement
kyph/o	humpback
lei/o	smooth
lamin/o	lamina
lord/o	curved, bent
lumb/o	lumbar region, lower back
mandibul/o	mandible
maxill/o	maxilla
menisc/o	meniscus
my/o, myos/o, muscul/o	muscle
myel/o	bone marrow, spinal cord
oste/o	bone
patell/o	patella
pelv/i, pelv/o	pelvis, pelvic cavity
phalang/o	phalanges
pub/o	pubis
rachi/o	spine
radi/o	radius
rhabd/o	striated muscle
sacr/o	sacrum
scapul/o	scapula
scoli/o	crooked, twisted
stern/o	sternum
synovi/o	synovial joint or fluid
tars/o	tarsal bones
ten/o, tend/o, tendin/o	tendon
thorac/o	thorax, chest
ton/o	tone, tension
uln/o	ulna
vertebr/o, spondyl/o	vertebra

Prefixes

Prefix	Meaning
inter-	between
intra-	within
supra-	above
sub-	below, beneath
sym-, syn-	together, with

Suffixes

Suffix	Meaning
-algia	pain
-asthenia	weakness
-centesis	puncture to aspirate
-clasia, -clasis, -clast	to break
-desis	surgical fixation, binding
-ectomy	excision, surgical removal
-itis	inflammation
-osis	abnormal condition
-physis	growth
-plasty	surgical repair, reconstruction
-porosis	pore, passage
-rrhaphy	suture
-schisis	to split
-trophy	development, nourishment

■ Exercises: Word Parts

SIMPLE
RECALL

Exercise 6

Write the meaning of the combining form given.

1. crani/o _____

2. lumb/o _____

3. scoli/o _____

4. oste/o _____

5. stern/o _____

6. maxill/o _____

7. chondr/o _____

8. carp/o _____

9. ten/o, tend/o _____

10. spondyl/o _____

11. fasci/o _____

12. my/o, myos/o _____

13. mandibul/o _____

14. sacr/o _____

15. femor/o _____

SIMPLE
RECALL

Exercise 7

Write the correct combining form(s) for the meaning given.

1. rib _____

2. tarsal bones _____

3. smooth _____

4. fibula _____

5. bursa _____

6. joint _____

7. pelvis _____

8. chest _____

9. ischium _____

10. collarbone _____

11. lamina _____

12. neck _____

13. meniscus _____

14. phalanges _____

SIMPLE
RECALL

Exercise 8

Write the meaning of the prefix or suffix given.

1. -plasty _____

2. -asthenia _____

3. sub- _____

4. -desis _____

5. -ectomy _____

6. -physis _____

7. -rrhaphy _____

8. sym- _____

9. -schisis _____

10. -clasis _____

ADVANCED
RECALL

Exercise 9

Considering the meaning of the combining form from which the medical term is made, write the meaning of the medical term. (You have not yet learned many of these terms but can build their meaning from the word parts.)

Combining Form	Meaning	Medical Term	Meaning of Term
oste/o	bone	osteitis	1. _____
lord/o	bent (forward)	lordosis	2. _____
my/o	muscle	myalgia	3. _____
burs/o	bursa	bursitis	4. _____
maxill/o	maxilla	maxillitis	5. _____
scapul/o	scapula	subscapular	6. _____
pelv/i	pelvis	pelvic	7. _____
tend/o	tendon	tendonitis	8. _____
vertebr/o	vertebra	intervertebral	9. _____
arthr/o	joint	arthroplasty	10. _____

ADVANCED RECALL

Exercise 10

Using the given combining form and a word part from the earlier tables, build a medical term for the meaning given.

Combining Form	Meaning of Medical Term	Medical Term
myos/o	inflammation of muscle	1. _____
crani/o	surgical repair of skull	2. _____
patell/o	excision of patella	3. _____
ten/o	suture of tendon	4. _____
arthr/o	pain in a joint	5. _____
crani/o	pertaining to within the skull	6. _____
tars/o	excision of tarsal bone	7. _____
menisci/o	inflammation of a meniscus	8. _____
disk/o	excision of intervertebral disk	9. _____
chondr/o	surgical repair of cartilage	10. _____

■ MEDICAL TERMS

Adjectives and Other Related Terms

Term	Pronunciation	Meaning
carpal	kahr′păl	pertaining to the carpal bones
costovertebral	kos′tō-vĕr′tĕ-brăl	pertaining to the ribs and thoracic vertebrae
cranial	krā′nē-ăl	pertaining to the skull
femoral	fem′ŏr-ăl	pertaining to the femur
humeral	hyū′mĕr-ăl	pertaining to the humerus
iliofemoral	il′ē-ō-fem′ŏr-ăl	pertaining to the ilium and femur
intercostal	in′tĕr-kos′tăl	pertaining to the area between the ribs
intervertebral	in′tĕr-vĕr′tĕ-brăl	pertaining to the area between vertebrae
intracranial	in-tră-krā′nē-ăl	pertaining to the area within the skull
ischiofemoral	is′kē-ō-fem′ŏr-ăl	pertaining to the ischium and femur
lumbar	lŭm′bahr	pertaining to the lower back
lumbocostal	lŭm′bō-kos′tăl	pertaining to the lumbar vertebrae and ribs

(continued)

Adjectives and Other Related Terms *(continued)*

Term	Pronunciation	Meaning
lumbosacral	lŭm′bō-sā′krăl	pertaining to the lumbar vertebrae and sacrum
osseous	os′ē-ŭs	pertaining to bone
pelvic	pel′vik	pertaining to the pelvis or pelvic cavity
sacral	sā′krăl	pertaining to the sacrum
sacrovertebral	sā′krō-vĕr′tĕ-brăl	pertaining to the sacrum and the vertebrae above
sternoclavicular	stĕr′nō-klă-vik′yū-lăr	pertaining to the sternum and clavicle
sternoid	stĕr′noyd	resembling the sternum
subcostal	sŭb-kos′tăl	pertaining to the area below a rib or the ribs
submandibular	sŭb′man-dib′yū-lăr	pertaining to the area below the mandible
submaxillary	sŭb-mak′si-lar-ē	pertaining to the area below the maxilla
subscapular	sŭb-skap′yū-lăr	pertaining to the area below the scapula
substernal	sŭb-stĕr′năl	pertaining to the area below the sternum
suprapatellar	sū′pră-pă-tel′ăr	pertaining to the area above the patella
suprascapular	sū′pră-skap′yū-lăr	pertaining to the area above the scapula
synovial	si-nō′vē-ăl	pertaining to, containing, or consisting of synovial fluid

■ Exercises: Adjectives and Other Related Terms

SIMPLE
RECALL

Exercise 11

Circle the term that is most appropriate for the meaning of the sentence.

1. An (*iliofemoral, ischiopubic, intercostal*) wound is located between the ribs.

2. A broken upper leg bone is called a (*humeral, cranial, femoral*) fracture.

3. A herniated (*intervertebral, carpal, sternoclavicular*) disk involves an injury to the disks between the vertebrae.

4. The (*ischiofemoral, lumbocostal, subscapular*) area includes both the ischium and femur.

5. Diagnosing a knee condition may require a needle puncture to draw (*submaxillary, sternoid, synovial*) fluid for testing.

6. A(n) (*substernal, pelvic, osseous*) examination includes all of the organs in the pelvis.

7. The area below the shoulder blade is called the (*subcostal, pubofemoral, subscapular*) region.

8. A wrist injury may involve a (*carpal, subcostal, sternoid*) fracture.

Exercise 12

Match each medical term with its meaning.

substernal	costovertebral	intracranial	intervertebral
lumbar	submandibular	suprapatellar	sacral
humeral	lumbosacral	intercostal	cranial

Meaning   **Term**

1. pertaining to the humerus   _____

2. pertaining to the area between ribs   _____

3. pertaining to the area below the sternum   _____

4. pertaining to the area above the patella   _____

5. pertaining to the skull   _____

6. pertaining to the sacrum   _____

7. pertaining to the area between vertebrae   _____

8. pertaining to the area within the skull   _____

9. pertaining to the lower back   _____

10. pertaining to the ribs and thoracic vertebrae   _____

11. pertaining to the area below the mandible   _____

12. pertaining to the lumbar vertebrae and sacrum _____

Symptoms and Medical Conditions

Term	Pronunciation	Meaning
ankylosing spondylitis	ang′ki-lōs-ing spon′di-lī′tis	arthritis of the spine
ankylosis	ang′ki-lō′sis	abnormal condition of stiffening or fixation of a joint
arthralgia	ahr-thral′jē-ă	condition of pain in a joint
arthritis	ahr-thrī′tis	inflammation of a joint (Fig. 14-11)
arthrochondritis	ahr′thrō-kon-drī′tis	inflammation of an articular cartilage
atrophy	at′rŏ-fē	a wasting of tissue or an organ
bradykinesia	brad′ē-kin-ē′sē-ă	condition of decreased movement
bunion	bŭn′yŏn	swelling at metatarsophalangeal joint caused by inflammatory bursa
bursitis	bŭr-sī′tis	inflammation of a bursa
bursolith	bŭr′sō-lith	a calculus (stone) formed in a bursa

(continued)

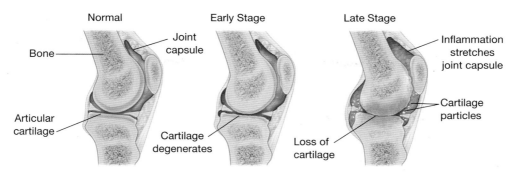

Figure 14-11   Progressive joint changes in arthritis of the knee.

Symptoms and Medical Conditions *(continued)*

Term	Pronunciation	Meaning
carpal tunnel syndrome (CTS)	kahr′păl tŭn′ĕl sin′drŏm	nerve entrapment syndrome in the wrist, causing pain
carpoptosis, *syn.* wrist-drop	kar′pop-tō′sis, rist drop	paralysis of wrist and finger muscles
chondromalacia	kon′drō-mă-lā′shē-ă	softening of a cartilage
cranioschisis	krā′nē-os′ki-sis	congenital incomplete closure of the skull
curvature of the spine	kŭr′vă-chŭr spīn	abnormal curving of the spine in one or more directions (Fig. 14-12)
kyphosis	kī-fō′sis	abnormal forward curvature; humpback
lordosis	lōr-dō′sis	abnormal backward curvature
scoliosis	skō′lē-ō′sis	abnormal lateral curvature
dyskinesia	dis′ki-nē′sē-ă	difficulty performing voluntary movements

(continued)

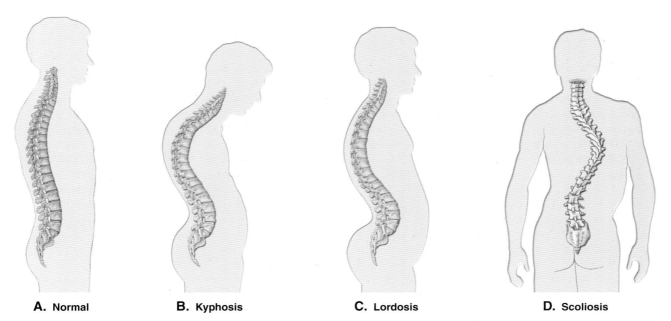

A. Normal   **B.** Kyphosis   **C.** Lordosis   **D.** Scoliosis

Figure 14-12   Curvatures of the spine can cause pain and disfigurement.

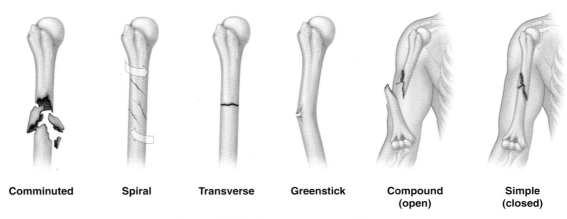

| Comminuted | Spiral | Transverse | Greenstick | Compound (open) | Simple (closed) |

Figure 14-13 Common types of fractures.

Symptoms and Medical Conditions *(continued)*

Term	Pronunciation	Meaning
dystrophy	dis'trŏ-fē	abnormal development or growth of a tissue or organ often resulting from nutritional deficiency
exostosis	eks'os-tō'sis	bony projection that develops from cartilage
fibromyalgia	fī'brō-mī-al'jē-ă	condition of chronic aching and stiffness of muscles and soft tissues of unknown cause
fracture (fx)	frak'shŭr	a break in a bone or cartilage (Figs. 14-13 and 14-14)
gout	gowt	metabolic disorder involving painful deposits of crystals in connective tissue and articular cartilage

(continued)

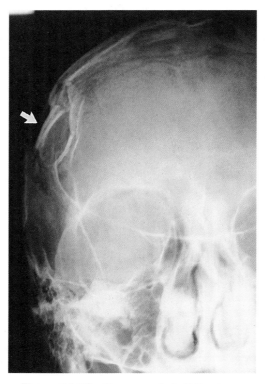

Figure 14-14 Depressed skull fracture.

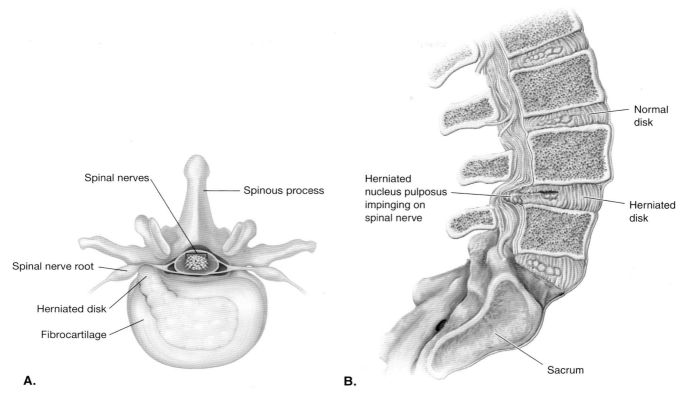

Figure 14-15   Protrusion of a herniated disk through the fibrocartilage. **A.** Cross-section view. **B.** Lateral view.

Symptoms and Medical Conditions *(continued)*

Term	Pronunciation	Meaning
herniated disk (or disc)	hĕr'nē-ā-tĕd disk	protrusion of a degenerated or fragmented intervertebral disk (Fig. 14-15)
hyperkinesia	hī'pĕr-ki-nē'zē-ă	condition of excessive muscular movements
hypertrophy	hī-pĕr'trŏ-fē	increased development of a part or organ not caused by a tumor
maxillitis	mak'si-lī'tis	inflammation of the maxilla
meniscitis	men-i-sī'tis	inflammation of a meniscus
muscular dystrophy (MD)	mŭs'kyū-lăr dis'trŏ-fē	hereditary condition causing progressive degeneration of skeletal muscles

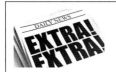 **MUSCULAR DYSTROPHY** While there are several variations of muscular dystrophy, there are two prominent types. They are called Becker and Duchenne. Both of these are X-linked, which means the mother can pass along this genetic mutation to the children. However, muscular dystrophy affects more boys than girls.

myalgia	mī-al'jē-ă	condition of muscular pain
myasthenia gravis (MG)	mī-as-thē'nē-ă gra'vis	condition of neuromuscular disorder causing weakness and fatigue of voluntary muscles
myositis	mī-ō-sī'tis	inflammation of a muscle
osteitis	os-tē-ī'tis	inflammation of bone

(continued)

Symptoms and Medical Conditions *(continued)*

Term	Pronunciation	Meaning
osteoarthritis (OA)	os′tē-ō-ahr-thrī′tis	arthritis involving erosion and inflammation of articular cartilage
osteochondritis	os′tē-ō-kon-drī′tis	inflammation of a bone and its articular cartilage
osteomalacia	os′tē-ō-mă-lā′shē-ă	condition of softening of bones
osteomyelitis	os′tē-ō-mī-ĕ-lī′tis	inflammation of bone marrow
osteonecrosis	os′tē-ō-nĕ-krō′sis	condition or process of bone tissue death
osteoporosis	os′tē-ō-pŏr-ō′sis	age-related disorder of decreased bone mass and weakening (Fig. 14-16)
polymyositis	pol′ē-mī′ō-sī′tis	inflammation of multiple voluntary muscles
rachischisis	ră-kis′ki-sis	embryologic failure of vertebral arches to fuse
rheumatoid arthritis (RA)	rū′mă-toyd ahr-thrī′tis	disease causing progressive destructive changes and inflammation in multiple joints, especially in the hands and feet (Fig. 14-17)
rickets	rik′ĕts	disease caused by vitamin D deficiency, involving skeletal deformities and muscular weakness
spondylarthritis	spon′dil-ahr-thrī′tis	inflammation of intervertebral articulations
sprain	sprān	injury of a ligament caused by abnormal or excessive forces on a joint
strain	strān	injury of a muscle caused by overuse or improper use
tendonitis, tendinitis	ten′dŏ-nī′tis, ten′di-nī′tis	inflammation of a tendon
tenodynia	ten-ō-din′ē-ă	condition of pain in a tendon
tenosynovitis	ten′ō-sin-ō-vī′tis	inflammation of a tendon and its sheath

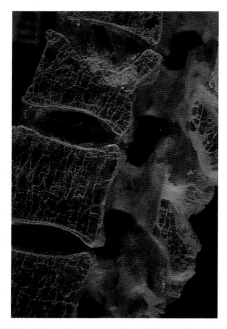

Figure 14-16 Bone becomes less dense in osteoporosis.

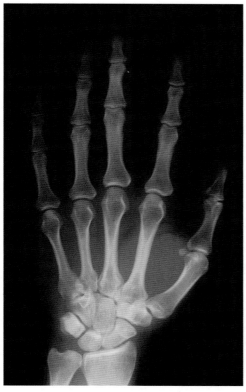

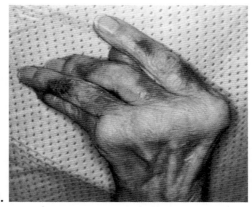

A.   **B.**

Figure 14-17   The changes of severe rheumatoid arthritis. **A.** X-ray of normal hand. **B.** Hand severely deformed from rheumatoid arthritis.

■ Exercises: Symptoms and Medical Conditions

SIMPLE
RECALL

Exercise 13

Write the correct medical term for the definition given.

1. abnormal lateral curvature of spine   _____

2. inflamed tendon   _____

3. break in a bone   _____

4. softening of cartilage   _____

5. inflamed bursa   _____

6. decreased bone mass   _____

7. disease caused by vitamin D deficiency   _____

8. pain in a tendon   _____

9. inflamed intervertebral articulations   _____

10. arthritis of the spine   _____

11. abnormal forward curvature of spine _____

12. pain in a joint _____

13. inflammation of a joint _____

14. softening of bone _____

Exercise 14

ADVANCED
RECALL

Circle the term that is most appropriate for the meaning of the sentence.

1. Mrs. Jones presented with weakness and fatigue in her voluntary muscles, and, after clinical study, her physician diagnosed her condition as (*myasthenia, myalgia, myositis*) gravis.

2. Mr. Carelton was seen in follow-up for his condition of inflammation of multiple voluntary muscles, also called (*polymyositis, carpal tunnel syndrome, atrophy*).

3. Dr. Gonzalez informed Mr. Lawson that when (*gout, fibromyalgia, osteitis*) occurs, crystals are deposited in connective tissue and articular cartilage.

4. Young Bridget LaRoux suffered a(n) (*sprain, strain, atrophy*) to her calf muscle and a(n) (*sprain, strain, atrophy*) to one of her ligaments.

5. Mrs. Anderson suffers from progressive destructive changes in multiple joints caused by (*muscular dystrophy, rheumatoid arthritis, myasthenia gravis*).

6. After spending years in chronic pain without a known cause, the patient was diagnosed with (*fibromyalgia, gout, hypertrophy*).

7. After his x-ray report showed a stone in his elbow area, the patient was told that he had a(n) (*bunion, bursolith, exostosis*).

8. Mrs. Gabai had (*atrophy, hypertrophy, dystrophy*) of her lower limbs after spending many years in a wheelchair.

9. The physician diagnosed Ms. Allen with (*carpal, metacarpal, tarsal*) tunnel syndrome after she complained of pain in her wrist after many years of repetitive work.

10. Mr. Kowalski suffered from (*osteitis, dyskinesia, exostosis*) after his stroke.

11. After reporting pain in his left throwing arm, the baseball player was diagnosed with inflammation of a tendon and its sheath, also called (*tenosynovitis, tenodynia, osteochondritis*).

Exercise 15

TERM
CONSTRUCTION

Build a medical term from an appropriate combining form and suffix, given their meanings.

Use Combining Form for	Use Suffix for	Term
1. joint	inflammation	_____
2. joint	pain	_____

3. spine   split   _____

4. maxilla   inflammation   _____

5. tendon   pain   _____

6. bursa   inflammation   _____

7. muscle   pain   _____

8. joint and cartilage   inflammation   _____

9. bone   softening   _____

TERM
CONSTRUCTION

Exercise 16

Break the given medical term into its word parts and define each part. Then define the medical term. (Note: This exercise uses some suffixes learned previously.)

For example:
arthritis   _word parts:_   arthr/o / -itis
                   meanings: joint / inflammation
                   term meaning: inflammation of a joint

1. hypertrophy   _word parts:_   _____ / _____

                      meanings: _____ / _____

                      term meaning: _____

2. scoliosis   _word parts:_   _____ / _____

                      meanings: _____ / _____

                      term meaning: _____

3. cranioschisis _word parts:_   _____ / _____

                      meanings: _____ / _____

                      term meaning: _____

4. carpoptosis   _word parts:_   _____ / _____

                      meanings: _____ / _____

                      term meaning: _____

5. ankylosis   _word parts:_   _____ / _____

                      meanings: _____ / _____

                      term meaning: _____

6. bursolith   *word parts:* _____ / _____

                      meanings: _____ / _____

                      term meaning: _____

7. atrophy   *word parts:* _____ / _____

                      meanings: _____ / _____

                      term meaning: _____

8. osteitis   *word parts:* _____ / _____

                      meanings: _____ / _____

                      term meaning: _____

9. bradykinesia   *word parts:* _____ / _____ / _____

                      meanings: _____ / _____ / _____

                      term meaning: _____

10. polymyositis   *word parts:* _____ / _____ / _____

                      meanings: _____ / _____ / _____

                      term meaning: _____

Tests and Procedures

Term	Pronunciation	Meaning
Laboratory Tests		
creatine kinase (CK)	krē'ă-tin kī'nās	test for the presence of the enzyme creatine kinase in the blood that may indicate conditions that can cause muscle weakness or pain
erythrocyte sedimentation rate (ESR)	ĕ-rith'rŏ-sīt sed'i-mĕn-tā'shŭn rāt	time measurement of red blood cells settling in a test tube over 1 hour; used to assess for inflammatory or necrotic conditions
rheumatoid factor (RF)	rū'mă-toyd fak'tŏr	blood test used to help diagnose rheumatoid arthritis
synovial fluid analysis	si-nō'vē-ăl flū'id ă-nal'i-sis	test for the presence of crystals caused by some conditions, such as arthritis, and also signs of joint infection
uric acid	yūr'ik as'id	test for elevated presence of uric acid in the blood, indicating gout
Diagnostic Procedures		
arthrography	ahr-throg'ră-fē	x-ray imaging of a joint using a contrast agent
arthroscopy	ahr-thros'kŏ-pē	endoscopic examination of the interior of a joint (Fig. 14-18)
bone densitometry	dens'i-tom'ĕ-trē	x-ray technique for determining density of bone
bone scan	bōn skan	nuclear medicine imaging of bone to diagnose bone disorders (Fig. 14-19)

(continued)

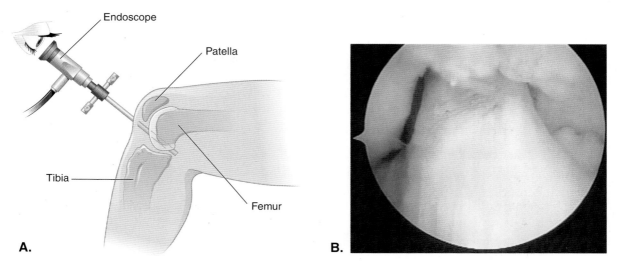

Figure 14-18 **A.** Arthroscopic examination of the knee. **B.** Endoscopic view of joint interior.

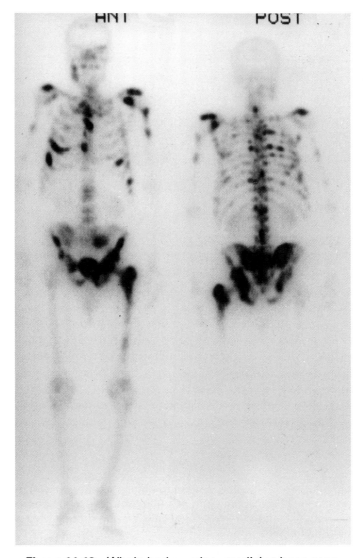

Figure 14-19 Whole body nuclear medicine bone scan.

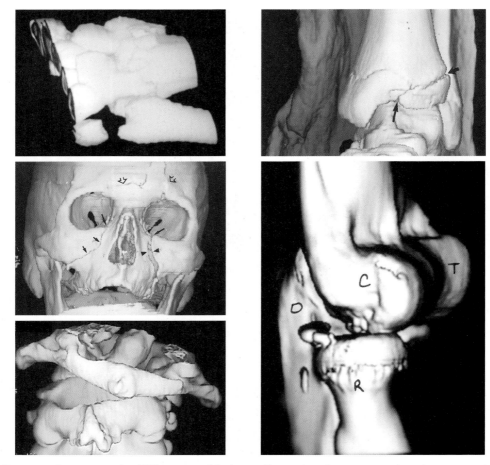

Figure 14-20   Computed tomography (CT) scans with three-dimensional reconstruction demonstrating different types of fractures.

Tests and Procedures *(continued)*

Term	Pronunciation	Meaning
computed tomography (CT)	kŏm-pyū'tĕd tŏ-mog'ră-fē	x-ray technique producing computer-generated cross-sectional images; used to evaluate disorders of and injuries to the musculoskeletal system (Fig. 14-20)
electromyogram (EMG)	ĕ-lek'trō-mī'ō-gram	diagnostic test producing graphic record of electric currents associated with muscular action (Fig. 14-21)
magnetic resonance imaging (MRI)	mag-net'ik rez'ŏ-năns im'ăj-ing	imaging technique that uses magnetic fields and radiofrequency waves to visualize anatomic structures; often used for diagnosing joint disorders (Fig. 14-22)
radiography	rā'dē-og'ră-fē	examination of any part of the body by x-ray
range of motion (ROM) testing	rănj mō'shŭn	measurement of the amount of movement allowed in a joint

DAILY NEWS
EXTRA!
EXTRA!

Range of motion testing is done to assess a patient's joint motion, and range of motion exercises are used to preserve or increase the amount of movement allowed in a joint. An instrument called a goniometer measures the range of motion of a joint.

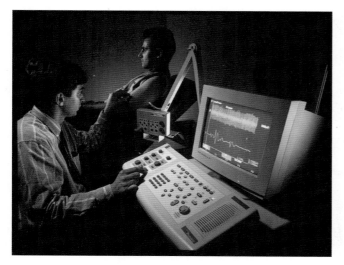

Figure 14-21   Electromyography.

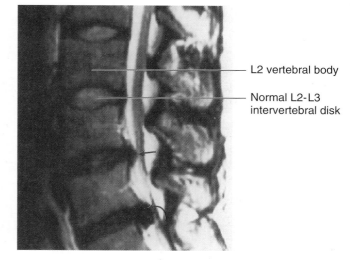

— L2 vertebral body

— Normal L2-L3 intervertebral disk

Figure 14-22   Magnetic resonance imaging (MRI) of a herniated intervertebral disk (*arrows*).

■ Exercises: Tests and Procedures

Exercise 17

ADVANCED RECALL

Circle the term that is most appropriate for the meaning of the sentence.

1. Wanting a cross-sectional view of the lateral meniscus, the orthopedist ordered a procedure using (*computed tomography, arthroscopy, range of motion testing*).

2. A record of the electrical currents associated with muscular action is called a(n) (*arthrogram, radiograph, electromyogram*).

3. (*Magnetic resonance imaging, Arthroscopy, Arthrography*) is a radiographic technique for imaging a joint, usually after administering a contrast agent.

4. A bone scan is produced with (*nuclear medicine imaging, endoscopy, arthrography*).

5. The examination of any part of the body by x-ray is called (*radiography, electromyography, computed tomography*).

6. The laboratory test for (*creatine kinase, rheumatoid factor, uric acid*) may help diagnose conditions that cause muscle weakness and pain.

7. (*Rheumatoid factor, Uric acid, Creatine kinase*) is the laboratory test that indicates gout.

8. The laboratory test that will help determine the presence of rheumatoid arthritis is called (*erythrocyte sedimentation rate, uric acid, rheumatoid factor*).

Exercise 18

ADVANCED RECALL

Complete each sentence by writing in the correct medical term.

1. The radiographic technique used to determine bone density is called _____.

2. The amount of movement a joint allows can be determined by _____.

3. The use of nuclear medicine imaging of bone to diagnose bone disorders is called a(n) _____ .

4. An interior joint space can be viewed through an endoscope in _____ .

5. The diagnostic modality based on the effects of a magnetic field on body tissues is called _____ .

6. The laboratory test that can indicate inflammation in the body is called _____ .

7. The laboratory test that may detect crystals caused by certain conditions and also signs of joint infection is called _____ .

Surgical Interventions and Therapeutic Procedures

Term	Pronunciation	Meaning
arthrocentesis	ahr'thrō-sen-tē'sis	needle puncture to remove fluid from a joint (Fig. 14-23)
arthroclasia	ahr'thrō-klā'zē-ă	surgical breaking of adhesions in ankylosis
arthrodesis	ahr-throd'ĕ-sis	surgical artificial stiffening of a joint
arthroplasty	ahr'thrō-plas-tē	surgical restoration of joint function or creation of an artificial joint (such as a total hip or knee replacement)
bursectomy	bŭr-sek'tŏ-mē	excision of a bursa
carpectomy	kahr-pek'tŏ-mē	excision of part or all of the carpal bones
chondrectomy	kon-drek'tŏ-mē	excision of cartilage
chondroplasty	kon'drō-plas-tē	surgical repair of cartilage
costectomy	kos-tek'tŏ-mē	excision of a rib
cranioplasty	krā'nē-ō-plas-tē	surgical repair of the skull
craniotomy	krā'nē-ot'ŏ-mē	surgical creation of an opening (incision) into the skull
diskectomy	disk-ek'tŏ-mē	excision of part or all of an intervertebral disk (Fig. 14-24)
laminectomy	lam'i-nek'tŏ-mē	excision of a vertebral lamina
laminotomy, *syn.* rachiotomy	lam-i-not'ŏ-mē, rā'kē-ot'ŏ-mē	enlargement of the intervertebral foramen by excision of a portion of the lamina
maxillotomy	mak'si-lot'ŏ-mē	surgical resection of the maxilla

(continued)

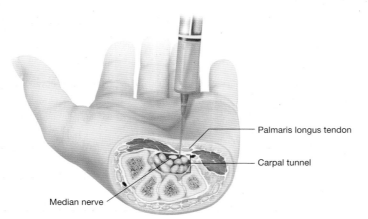

Median nerve — Palmaris longus tendon — Carpal tunnel

Figure 14-23 In arthrocentesis, synovial fluid is aspirated from the wrist joint to reduce inflammation.

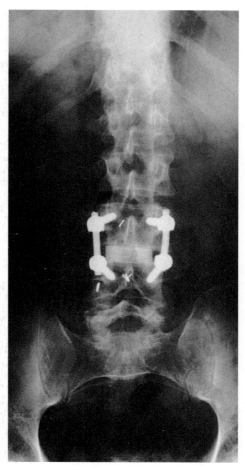

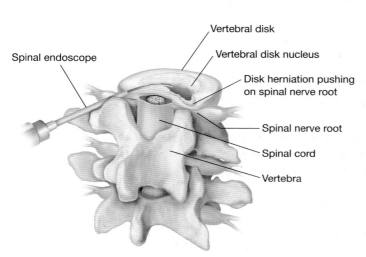

Spinal endoscope

Vertebral disk

Vertebral disk nucleus

Disk herniation pushing
on spinal nerve root

Spinal nerve root

Spinal cord

Vertebra

Figure 14-24 Surgical excision of a tissue from a herniated disk (diskectomy).

Figure 14-25 Surgical fixation is done to produce spinal fusion (spondylosyndesis) and limit patient movement.

Surgical Interventions and Therapeutic Procedures *(continued)*

Term	Pronunciation	Meaning
meniscectomy	men′i-sek′tŏ-mē	excision of a meniscus, usually from the knee joint
myoplasty	mī′ō-plas-tē	surgical repair of muscular tissue
myorrhaphy	mī-ōr′ă-fē	suture of a muscle
open reduction, internal fixation (ORIF)	ō′pĕn rĕ-duk′shŭn, in-tĕr′năl fik-sā′shŭn	surgical repair of a fracture by making an incision into the skin and muscle at the site of the fracture, manually moving the bones into alignment, and fixing the bones in place with surgical wires, screws, pins, rods, or plates
ostectomy	os-tek′tŏ-mē	excision of bone tissue
osteoclasis	os-tē-ok′lă-sis	intentional fracture of a bone to correct deformity
osteoclast	os′tē-ō-klast	surgical instrument used to fracture a bone to correct a deformity
patellectomy	pat-ĕ-lek′tŏ-mē	excision of the patella
phalangectomy	fal-an-jek′tŏ-mē	excision of one or more phalanges of the hand or foot

(continued)

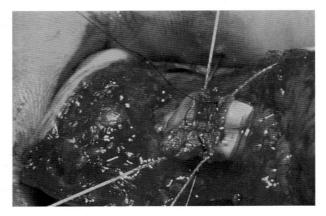

Figure 14-26   Suturing a torn tendon (tenorrhaphy).

Surgical Interventions and Therapeutic Procedures *(continued)*

Term	Pronunciation	Meaning
reduction	rĕ-dŭk′shŭn	manipulative or surgical procedure to restore a part to its normal position, such as by reducing a fracture (putting bone ends back in place)
spondylosyndesis	spon′di-lō-sin-dē′sis	surgical procedure to create ankylosis between two or more vertebrae (Fig. 14-25); also called spinal fusion
synovectomy	sin′ō-vek′tŏ-mē	excision of part or all of a joint's synovial membrane
tarsectomy	tahr-sek′tŏ-mē	excision of part or all of the tarsal bones
tenorrhaphy	te-nōr′ă-fē	suture of the divided ends of a tendon (Fig. 14-26)
traction	trak′shŭn	a pulling force exerted on a limb or other part of the body to maintain a desired position for healing (Fig. 14-27)

(continued)

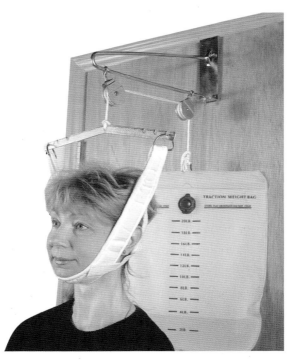

Figure 14-27   Cervical traction.

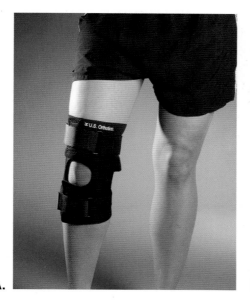
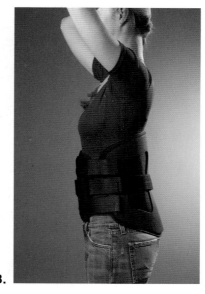

A.   **B.**

Figure 14-28   Orthopedic devices (orthoses). **A.** Knee brace. **B.** Back brace.

Surgical Interventions and Therapeutic Procedures *(continued)*

Term	Pronunciation	Meaning
		Related Terms
orthosis	ōr-thō′sis	external orthopedic device, such as a brace or splint (Fig. 14-28)
prosthesis	pros-thē′sis	fabricated substitute for a damaged or missing part of the body

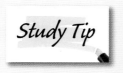

Study Tip

Osteoclast: "Osteoclast" has two meanings in medicine: (i) a body cell that helps remove osseous tissue and (ii) a surgical instrument used to fracture a bone to correct a deformity. The correct definition depends on the context in which it is used. For example, the first definition might be used in a laboratory report, and the second definition might be used in an operative report.

■ Exercises: Surgical Interventions and Therapeutic Procedures

SIMPLE
RECALL

Exercise 19

Write the correct medical term for the definition given.

1. excision of some or all of a synovial membrane _____

2. putting bone ends back in their proper place _____

3. suture of a muscle _____

4. excision of cartilage _____

5. surgical breaking of adhesions in ankylosis _____

6. excision of an intervertebral disk   _____

7. pulling force exerted on a limb   _____

8. surgical repair of skull   _____

9. spinal fusion   _____

10. intentional fracture to correct bone deformity   _____

11. excision of the patella   _____

12. surgical instrument used to break a bone   _____

13. surgical repair of cartilage   _____

14. excision of a meniscus   _____

15. surgical resection of the maxilla   _____

16. surgical creation of an artificial joint   _____

ADVANCED
RECALL

Exercise 20

Circle the term that is most appropriate for the meaning of the sentence.

1. Mrs. Yin required a(n) (*cranioplasty, arthrodesis, ostectomy*) to excise a cancerous bone growth.

2. Mr. Behringer had a very painful bursa but was, nonetheless, reluctant to undergo (*arthroplasty, bursectomy, laminectomy*) to remove it.

3. The first step of surgery for Ms. Barbosa's brain tumor was a (*craniotomy, cranioplasty, costectomy*).

4. Following surgical removal of a sarcoma that had spread through his vastus medialis muscle, Mr. McCarty required extensive (*tenorrhaphy, myoplasty, arthrodesis*) to repair the muscle.

5. To brace her leg and provide support while healing occurred, Mrs. Ahern needed to wear a custom (*osteoclasis, arthrodesis, orthosis*) at all times.

6. After breaking her arm, Mrs. Latta had a(n) (*meniscectomy; open reduction, internal fixation; osteoclast*) to repair the fracture.

7. Mr. Karposky's surgery for a herniated intervertebral disk included (*carpectomy, tarsectomy, laminectomy*).

8. During surgery for the skier's injured knee, Dr. Tanaka discovered a tendon that had completely divided and had to perform (*phalangectomy, tenorrhaphy, arthroclasia*).

9. With (*arthrocentesis, arthrodesis, chondrectomy*), the orthopedic surgeon aspirated synovial fluid from Mrs. Updike's severely swollen shoulder joint.

10. Within months of the emergency amputation of her gangrenous left leg, Ms. Pappas was adapting well to walking using a (*spondylosyndesis, prosthesis, traction*).

Exercise 21

Using the given suffix, build a medical term for the meaning given.

Suffix	Meaning of Medical Term	Medical Term
-plasty	surgical repair of muscle	1._____
-ectomy	excision of cartilage	2._____
-desis	surgical fixation or binding of a joint	3._____
-rrhaphy	suture of divided ends of a tendon	4._____
-tomy	incision into the skull	5._____

Exercise 22

Break the given medical term into its word parts and define each part. Then define the medical term.

For example:

arthritis	*word parts:*	arthr/o / -itis
	meanings:	joint / inflammation
	term meaning:	inflammation of a joint

1. osteoclasis

word parts: _____ / _____

meanings: _____ / _____

term meaning: _____

2. myorrhaphy

word parts: _____ / _____

meanings: _____ / _____

term meaning: _____

3. arthroplasty

word parts: _____ / _____

meanings: _____ / _____

term meaning: _____

4. phalangectomy

word parts: _____ / _____

meanings: _____ / _____

term meaning: _____

5. rachiotomy

word parts: _____ / _____

meanings: _____ / _____

term meaning: _____

6. diskectomy   *word parts:*   _____ / _____

                          meanings: _____ / _____

                          term meaning: _____

7. chondroplasty   *word parts:*   _____ / _____

                          meanings: _____ / _____

                          term meaning: _____

8. arthrocentesis   *word parts:*   _____ / _____

                          meanings: _____ / _____

                          term meaning: _____

9. synovectomy   *word parts:*   _____ / _____

                          meanings: _____ / _____

                          term meaning: _____

10. ostectomy   *word parts:*   _____ / _____

                          meanings: _____ / _____

                          term meaning: _____

Medications and Drug Therapies

Term	Pronunciation	Meaning
analgesic	an'ăl-jē'zik	a drug that relieves pain without producing anesthesia
corticosteroid	kōr'ti-kō-ster'oyd	a drug that reduces inflammation around joints
nonsteroidal anti-inflammatory drug (NSAID)	non'ster-oy'dăl an'tī-in-flam'ă-tōr-ē drŭg	drug with anti-inflammatory action (and usually analgesic and antipyretic effects as well); used to treat joint and muscle conditions
skeletal muscle relaxant	skel'ĕ-tăl mŭs'ĕl rē-lak'sănt	a drug that relaxes skeletal muscle spasms and spasticity

■ Exercise: Medications and Drug Therapies

SIMPLE
RECALL

Exercise 23

Write the correct medication or drug therapy term for the definition given.

1. relaxes skeletal muscles   _____

2. relieves pain without anesthesia   _____

3. reduces inflammation around joints _____

4. reduces inflammation without the use of steroids _____

Specialties and Specialists

Term	Pronunciation	Meaning
chiropractic	kī′rō-prak′tik	health care discipline involving physical manipulation of musculoskeletal structures
chiropractor	kī′rō-prak′tŏr	one who specializes in chiropractic
orthopedics, orthopaedics	ōr′thō-pē′diks	medical specialty focusing on diagnosis and treatment of disorders of the musculoskeletal system
orthopedist, orthopaedist	ōr′thō-pē′dist	physician who specializes in orthopedics
orthotics	ōr-thot′iks	the science of making and fitting orthopedic devices
orthotist	ōr-thŏt′ist	one who makes and fits orthopedic appliances
osteopathy	os′tē-op′ă-thē	school of medicine emphasizing manipulative measures in addition to techniques of conventional medicine
osteopath	os′tē-ō-path	physician who specializes in osteopathy
podiatry	pō-dī′ă-trē	medical specialty focusing on diagnosis and treatment of disorders of the foot
podiatrist	pō-dī′ă-trist	physician who specializes in podiatry
rheumatology	rū′mă-tol′ŏ-jē	medical specialty focusing on the study, diagnosis, and treatment of joint conditions
rheumatologist	rū′mă-tol′ŏ-jist	physician who specializes in rheumatology

■ Exercise: Specialties and Specialists

ADVANCED
RECALL

Exercise 24

Match each medical specialist with the description of the specialty.

podiatrist   chiropractor   orthopedist
rheumatologist   osteopath   orthotist

Description   **Term**

1. physical manipulation of
   musculoskeletal structures   _____

2. diagnosis and treatment of foot disorders   _____

3. making and fitting orthopedic devices   _____

4. school of medicine emphasizing
   manipulative measures   _____

5. diagnosis and treatment of joint conditions   _____

6. diagnosis and treatment of disorders of the
   musculoskeletal system   _____

Abbreviations

Abbreviation	Meaning
C1 to C7	cervical vertebrae 1 to 7
CK	creatine kinase
CT	computed tomography
CTS	carpal tunnel syndrome
EMG	electromyogram
ESR	erythrocyte sedimentation rate
fx	fracture
L1 to L5	lumbar vertebrae 1 to 5
MD	muscular dystrophy
MG	myasthenia gravis
MRI	magnetic resonance imaging
NSAID	nonsteroidal anti-inflammatory drug
OA	osteoarthritis
ORIF	open reduction, internal fixation
RA	rheumatoid arthritis
RF	rheumatoid factor
ROM	range of motion
T1 to T12	thoracic vertebrae 1 to 12

■ Exercises: Abbreviations

Exercise 25

ADVANCED
RECALL

Write the definition of each abbreviation used in these sentences.

1. Mr. de la Cruz had an **MRI** to assist with the diagnosis of a herniated intervertebral disk.

   _____

2. Because of her **MG**, Ms. Hart frequently felt fatigued after walking even a short distance.

   _____

3. After her car accident, Mrs. Stegner was found on radiography to have a fracture of **C2**.

   _____

4. **MD** is a hereditary degenerative disease.

   _____

5. Because of pain resulting from severe osteoarthritis, Mr. Springer has limited **ROM** in his shoulder.

_____

6. An **ORIF** was performed to repair Mr. Harrell's fracture of the femur.

_____

7. An **EMG** was obtained to help diagnose the nerve damage in Mr. Dura's arm.

_____

8. Ms. Dhalaya told her orthopedist that she was sure her **CTS** resulted from all the typing she did at work.

_____

9. Mr. Murphy's medical record indicated **RA** diagnosed at age 55.

_____

10. Mrs. Helmsley's physician wanted her to try a **NSAID** for her arthritis before prescribing a different drug.

_____

11. To test for musculoskeletal problems, Mr. Kapur was scheduled for the following lab tests: **ESR**, **RF**, and **CK**.

_____

Exercise 26

ADVANCED RECALL

Match each abbreviation with the appropriate description.

| CT | OA | T4 |
| L3 | fx | MRI |

1. fourth thoracic vertebra   _____

2. injury of osseous tissue   _____

3. radiographic cross-section   _____

4. located well below the ribs   _____

5. imaging of magnetic effects   _____

6. involving articular cartilage _____

Review of Terms for Anatomy and Physiology

VISUAL

Exercise 27

Write the appropriate combining forms on the blanks for the bones indicated.

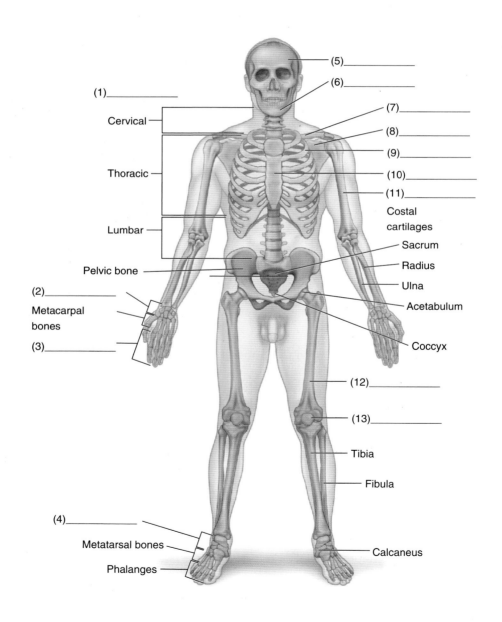

(1)_____

Cervical

Thoracic

Lumbar

Pelvic bone

(2)_____

Metacarpal bones

(3)_____

(4)_____

Metatarsal bones

Phalanges

(5)_____

(6)_____

(7)_____

(8)_____

(9)_____

(10)_____

(11)_____

Costal cartilages

Sacrum

Radius

Ulna

Acetabulum

Coccyx

(12)_____

(13)_____

Tibia

Fibula

Calcaneus

Exercise 28

Fill in the blanks as appropriate for the structures illustrated.

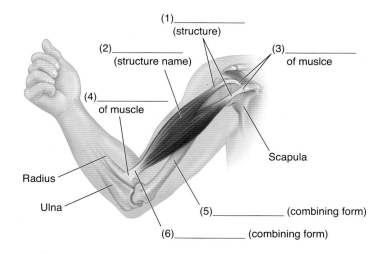

(1)_____
(structure)

(2)_____
(structure name)

(3)_____
of muslce

(4)_____
of muscle

Scapula

Radius

Ulna

(5)_____ (combining form)

(6)_____ (combining form)

Understanding Term Structure

Exercise 29

Break the given medical term into its word parts and define each part. Then define the medical term. (Note: you may need to use word parts from other chapters.)

For example:
  arthritis   *word parts:*   arthr/o / -itis
                     meanings: joint / inflammation
                     term meaning: inflammation of a joint

1. ankylosis   *word parts:*   _____ / _____

                     meanings: _____ / _____

                     term meaning: _____

2. carpoptosis   *word parts:*   _____ / _____

                     meanings: _____ / _____

                     term meaning: _____

3. electromyogram *word parts:*   _____ / _____ / _____

                     meanings: _____ / _____ / _____

                     term meaning: _____

4. myositis

word parts: _____ / _____

meanings: _____ / _____

term meaning: _____

5. kyphosis

word parts: _____ / _____

meanings: _____ / _____

term meaning: _____

6. intracranial

word parts: _____ / _____ / _____

meanings: _____ / _____ / _____

term meaning: _____

7. polymyositis

word parts: _____ / _____ / _____

meanings: _____ / _____ / _____

term meaning: _____

8. suprapatellar

word parts: _____ / _____ / _____

meanings: _____ / _____ / _____

term meaning: _____

9. tenodynia

word parts: _____ / _____

meanings: _____ / _____

term meaning: _____

10. arthrocentesis

word parts: _____ / _____

meanings: _____ / _____

term meaning: _____

11. chondrectomy

word parts: _____ / _____

meanings: _____ / _____

term meaning: _____

12. costovertebral

word parts: _____ / _____ / _____

meanings: _____ / _____ / _____

term meaning: _____

13. submandibular   *word parts:*   _____ / _____ / _____

                           meanings: _____ / _____ / _____

                           term meaning: _____

14. osteoarthritis   *word parts:*   _____ / _____ / _____

                           meanings: _____ / _____ / _____

                           term meaning: _____

15. myorrhaphy   *word parts:*   _____ / _____

                           meanings: _____ / _____

                           term meaning: _____

16. osteomalacia   *word parts:*   _____ / _____

                           meanings: _____ / _____

                           term meaning: _____

17. arthroscopy   *word parts:*   _____ / _____

                           meanings: _____ / _____

                           term meaning: _____

18. myalgia   *word parts:*   _____ / _____

                           meanings: _____ / _____

                           term meaning: _____

19. spondylarthritis   *word parts:*   _____ / _____ / _____

                           meanings: _____ / _____ / _____

                           term meaning: _____

Comprehension Exercises

Exercise 30

COMPREHENSION   **Fill in the blank with the correct term.**

1. Movement of an appendage toward the midline of the body is called _____ .

2. _____ is the science of making and fitting orthopedic devices.

3. The general term for the surgical restoration of joint function or creation of an artificial joint is _____ .

4. A(n) _____ is one who specializes in the diagnosis and treatment of disorders of the foot.

5. An artificial leg is an example of a(n) _____ .

6. _____ is caused by nerve entrapment in the wrist that produces pain.

7. The type of bone tissue that is solid and strong is called _____ bone.

8. The abnormal development or growth of a tissue or organ, often resulting from nutritional deficiency, is called _____ .

9. _____ is a condition of chronic aching and stiffness of muscles and soft tissues of unknown cause.

10. _____ is a direction of movement that increases the joint angle.

11. Nuclear medicine imaging can produce an image of the body's bones, called a(n) _____, to diagnose possible bone disorders.

12. Muscular _____ is a hereditary condition causing progressive degeneration of skeletal muscles.

13. Progressive destructive changes in multiple joints, especially in the hands and feet, may be caused by _____ .

14. The amount of movement allowed in a joint is termed its _____ .

15. Excessive muscular activity is termed _____ .

16. _____ is a nonmedical specialty involving physical manipulation of musculoskeletal structures.

17. _____ is the joint movement that bends the foot upward.

18. The medical specialty focusing on diagnosis and treatment of disorders of the musculoskeletal system is _____ .

Exercise 31

COMPREHENSION

Write a short answer for each question.

1. What kind of joint is a suture? _____

_____

2. A ligament attaches what structures together?_____

3. Where in the body are the metacarpal bones?_____

4. What does it mean to say a tissue is osseous?_____

_____

5. How is the practice of an osteopath different from that of other physicians?_____

_____

6. In what situation might a tenorrhaphy be performed?_____

_____

7. Rickets may result from a deficiency of what?_____

8. Arthrodesis performed during spinal surgery does what to a spinal joint?_____

_____

9. What is deposited in a joint's tissues that causes pain in someone with gout?_____

10. What kind of diagnostic image is produced with arthrography?_____

_____

11. Which end of a muscle is its insertion?_____

_____

12. Where is the xiphoid process located?_____

_____

13. In addition to skeletal and unstriated muscle tissue, what other type of muscle tissue is found

in the body? _____

14. What is another term for a laminotomy?_____

Exercise 32

COMPREHENSION   **Circle the letter of the best answer in the following questions.**

1. The term that most specifically applies to inflammation of an articular cartilage is:

A. osteitis
B. chondritis
C. arthrochondritis
D. arthritis

2. The clavicle articulates with the:

A. femur
B. fibula
C. ilium
D. sternum

3. A diarthrosis:

   A. moves freely
   B. causes pain
   C. requires surgery
   D. is herniated

4. An exostosis may develop from:

   A. bone marrow
   B. a sarcoma
   C. a herniated disk
   D. cartilage

5. Hypertrophy of an organ means it is:

   A. abnormally large
   B. malignant
   C. gouty
   D. necrotic

6. Dyskinesia generally refers to difficulty in:

   A. hyperextending the wrist
   B. embryonic fusing of vertebra
   C. obtaining a clear radiographic image
   D. performing voluntary movements

7. Even if you had never heard of this condition, you might assume that chondromalacia refers to:

   A. hardening of cartilage
   B. softening of cartilage
   C. hardening of bone
   D. softening of bone

8. An example of circumduction is:

   A. movement at the shoulder joint when the arm is moved in circles
   B. movement at cervical spinal joints when the head is turned right and left
   C. movement at the wrist when the hand is turned from palm down to palm up
   D. movement at the wrist when the hand is turned from palm up to palm down

9. A patient with ankylosing spondylitis is most likely to feel pain when:

   A. typing at a computer keyboard
   B. bending down to tie their shoes
   C. waving hello to someone at a distance
   D. chewing gum

10. A traumatic injury that fractures the patella might also injure which other structure?

    A. the humerus
    B. a suture
    C. the pubis
    D. a meniscus

11. Which of the following vertebrae is closest to the sacrum?

    A. L5
    B. T12
    C. T1
    D. C7

12. Which kind of tissue is in closest proximity to periosteal tissue?

    A. bone
    B. muscle
    C. ligament
    D. bone marrow

13. Tenodynia is most likely to occur with:

    A. rickets
    B. tarsectomy
    C. tenosynovitis
    D. bursitis

14. In scoliosis, the spine curves:

    A. from side to side
    B. from forward to backward in the lumbar area
    C. from forward to backward in the cervical area
    D. from backward to forward

Application and Analysis

Exercise 33

APPLICATION

Read the case reports and circle the letter of your answer choice for the questions that follow each case.

CASE 14-1

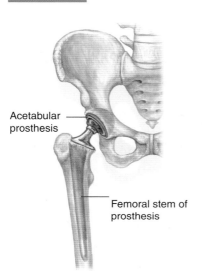

Acetabular prosthesis

Femoral stem of prosthesis

Figure 14-29 Total hip replacement with the prosthesis in place.

Because of severe osteoarthritis, Mr. Hughes is undergoing total hip replacement. During this surgery the proximal end of his femur will be resected, and the stem of a metal prosthesis will be inserted in the femur. Damaged bone in the acetabulum will be excised, and a plastic cup-shaped prosthetic piece cemented into the bone. The ball on top of the femoral prosthesis fits within this cup. Together these components will compose his new hip joint (Fig. 14-29).

1. The acetabulum is part of what bone?

  A. the pelvic bone
  B. the femur
  C. the coccyx
  D. the ilium

2. The new hip is called a prosthesis because it is:

  A. a surgical correction
  B. inside the body
  C. an orthopedic device
  D. a fabricated replacement part

3. Resection of the proximal end of the femur means:

  A. it is filed down to a smooth surface
  B. it is surgically removed
  C. a new osseous section will be transplanted there
  D. surgical reconstruction

4. The stem of the femoral prosthesis will extend down into:

  A. the pubis
  B. the patella
  C. the femur's medullary cavity
  D. the epiphysis of the tibia

5. In Mr. Hughes' new hip, the metallic femoral ball will articulate with:

  A. the ischium
  B. the acetabular prosthesis
  C. the femoral periosteum
  D. cancellous bone

6. This total hip replacement is an example of a(n):

  A. chondroplasty
  B. diskectomy
  C. arthroplasty
  D. arthroclasia

CASE 14-2

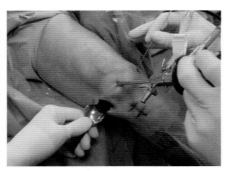

Mr. Bhatnagar suffered a tear of his anterior cruciate ligament (ACL) during a football game, causing significant pain and instability of the joint. The diagnosis was made with x-rays, MRI scans, and a stress test of the ligament. Arthroscopic reconstructive surgery of the knee joint is to be performed. The ACL will be reconstructed using a harvested section of the central third of the patellar tendon in a graft. The entire procedure will be performed arthroscopically (Fig. 14-30).

Figure 14-30   Arthroscopic knee surgery.

7. The ACL joins:

   A. muscle to muscle
   B. muscle to bone
   C. bone to muscle
   D. bone to bone

8. An arthroscope is an instrument that:

   A. allows viewing inside a joint
   B. forms an image based on tissue effects of magnetism
   C. is used to create radiographic images
   D. involves administration of radionuclides

9. Which suffix most likely is used in the term for the procedure for creating an opening into the knee joint?

   A. -physis
   B. -desis

   C. -clasia
   D. -tomy

10. The patellar tendon harvested for use in the graft normally joins:

   A. muscle to muscle
   B. muscle to bone
   C. bone to ligament
   D. bone to bone

11. If the grafted tendon section is sutured to a section of the torn ligament, which suffix is most likely used in the term for that procedure?

   A. -rrhaphy
   B. -physis
   C. -ectomy
   D. -centesis

MEDICAL RECORD ANALYSIS

MEDICAL RECORD 14-1

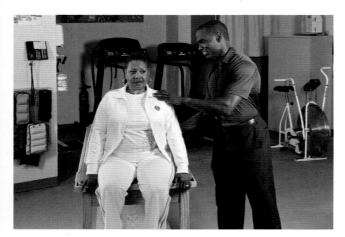

You are a physical therapy assistant working in a physical therapy clinic. It is your job to help assess patients and develop individualized treatment programs under the guidance of the physical therapist. Ms. Jackson was referred to your clinic by her primary physician because of a history of chronic back pain. You review this medical record from her physician so you may assist in her care.

Physical therapy assistant working with a patient.

Medical Record

LOW BACK PAIN

SUBJECTIVE: The patient came to my office with chief complaints of chronic back pain radiating down to the right more than left buttock and the thigh area. This pain increases with walking, standing, and rotating the back. She is taking Ambien and etodolac at this time. She is a known hypertensive with low back pain and left foot pain. She denies any new family or social history. She was on Vioxx and stopped when changed to etodolac. On review of systems, she reports some weight loss. She denies any heart pain, skin problems, eye problems, ear problems, hearing problems, swallowing problems, abdominal problems, diarrhea, constipation, or bowel/bladder incontinence.

OBJECTIVE: On examination the patient is a moderately built, well-nourished female. She appears to be comfortable. Her blood pressure is 136/69, heart rate 63, temperature 98.6. Her current weight is 200 pounds. She is awake, alert, and oriented. Pupils are equal and reacting. Sclerae are anicteric. Oropharynx is clear. The neck is supple. Carotid pulses are felt well. Trachea is midline. Breath sounds are heard. The abdomen is soft. The breath sounds are easily heard. The heart has a regular rate and rhythm. Upper extremity sensation reveals motor power within normal limits. The back has an old surgical scar. There is severe myofascial tenderness noted, paraspinal region in the lower lumbar and upper sacral area. Lower extremities are symmetrical. There is mild edema noted, more so in the ankles. There is decreased range of motion in the hips secondary to pain. Sensation is intact to light touch. Gait is slow and stable. She walks with a single-point cane. Sensation is intact.

ASSESSMENT: This is a patient with chronic low back pain, bilateral total knee replacement, and a prior low back surgery. She continues to have pain.

PLAN: The previous injection significantly helped the patient with her pain for about 3 months. I will consider her for a repeat L5-S1 foraminal block under fluoroscopy in the next 2 to 3 weeks. I have advised the patient to continue the current medications and have ordered a physical therapy consultation.

Exercise 34

APPLICATION

Write the appropriate medical terms used in this medical record on the blanks after their definitions. Note that not all the terms appear in the chapter, but you should be able to identify these terms based on word parts that are included in this chapter.

1. pertaining to area beside or around the spine   _____

2. pertaining to fused vertebrae below lumbar vertebrae   _____

3. pertaining to muscle and fascia   _____

4. amount of movement in a joint   _____

Bonus Question

5. Where has this patient had arthroplasty in the past?

_____

MEDICAL RECORD 14-2

Mrs. Formosa, a patient who suffers from rheumatoid arthritis, has returned to the physician's office where you work as a phlebotomist. You are responsible for drawing blood samples from Mrs. Formosa to be used for the CBC and sedimentation rate tests ordered by the physician.

Medical Record

RHEUMATOID ARTHRITIS FOLLOW-UP NOTE

HISTORY OF PRESENT ILLNESS: The patient is a 38-year-old woman who has an illness of about 3 to 4 years, characterized by myalgias, (1)_____, and arthritis located in the MCP joints, PIP joints, wrists, and ankles. In addition, the patient has had intermittent Raynaud, mild hair loss, and a transient rash located on the face and the neck. Other problems are sleep abnormalities and problems with equilibrium that are under evaluation by neurology. In our initial evaluation, we considered that the patient may have an undifferentiated connective tissue disease, and the possibilities were rheumatoid arthritis, lupus, or scleroderma. A trial of prednisone 15 mg was initiated. Two days after the patient started taking prednisone, she felt an impressive improvement that she describes as a miracle. The chronic sensation of fatigue was almost eliminated, and the (2)_____ is very mild, as well as the arthritis. The patient has not had episodes of (3)_____ since. The patient has been unusually active at work with energy and is able to do gardening. There is no significant change in morning stiffness, and this is still about 30 minutes in duration.

PERTINENT PHYSICAL FINDINGS: The general examination is benign. There is no hair loss. There is very mild erythema on the neck with fine telangiectasis that was mentioned before. There are no other skin lesions, and there are no mucosal lesions either. Musculoskeletal examination shows a motor power of 5/5 in all four extremities, (4)_____ is normal in all joints, and there is no evidence of synovitis at any level.

X-rays of hands show only mild osteopenia around the MCP and PIP joints. There are no erosions.

ASSESSMENT/PLAN: The patient is a 38-year-old woman with an undifferentiated inflammatory polyarthritis. Considering the family history of a father and a brother with rheumatoid arthritis, it is possible that the patient is at the stage of an early (5)_____, which is seronegative. Given the presence of Raynaud and fine telangiectasis, we have to keep in mind the possibility of this illness evolving to scleroderma. We do not have serologic evidence of lupus, and there is no biochemical evidence of myositis. Our plan at the moment will be to initiate high-dose chloroquine at 400 mg once daily, evaluation by an ophthalmologist, and a slow reduction of prednisone to 10 mg in 1 month and then 1 mg per week. We are scheduling an appointment in 2 months and requesting a CBC and sedimentation rate for the next visit.

APPLICATION

Exercise 35

Fill in the blanks in the medical record above with the correct medical terms. The definitions of the missing terms are listed below.

1. joint pain

2. muscle pain

3. joint inflammation

4. amount of movement in a joint

5. disease causing progressive destructive changes in multiple joints

Bonus Question

6. Although this chapter does not define the term "polyarthritis" used in the Assessment/Plan section of the record, you should be able to define it from its word parts:

_____

Pronunciation and Spelling

Exercise 36

AUDITORY **Review the Chapter 14 terms in the Dictionary/Audio Glossary in the Student Resources and practice pronouncing each term, referring to the pronunciation guide as needed.**

Exercise 37

SPELLING **Circle the correct spelling of each term.**

1. laminetomy	laminotomy	lamanotomy
2. ostoarthritis	ostioarthritis	osteoarthritis
3. rheumatology	rhuematology	rheumetology
4. tenodyne	tenodyna	tenodynia
5. osseis	osseous	oseous
6. clavicle	clavicel	clavecle
7. myorhaphy	myorrhapphy	myorrhaphy
8. vertebrea	vertebrae	vertabrae
9. fibromyalgia	fibrilmyalgia	fibromyolgia
10. dorseflexion	dorsaflexion	dorsiflexion
11. ankelosis	ankylosis	ankylesis
12. polimyositis	polymyositis	polymiositis

13. faisca	fasckia	fascia
14. osteoporosis	ostioporosis	osteoporesis
15. intervertebrel	intervertabral	intervertebral

Media Connection

STUDENT
RESOURCES

Exercise 38

Complete each of the following activities available with the Student Resources. Check off each activity as you complete it, and record your score for the Chapter Quiz in the space provided.

Chapter Exercises

____ Flash Cards

____ Concentration

____ Abbreviation Match-Up

____ Roboterms

____ Word Builder

____ Fill the Gap

____ Break It Down

____ True/False Body Building

____ Quiz Show

____ Complete the Case

____ Medical Record Review

____ Look and Label

____ Image Matching

____ Spelling Bee

____ **Chapter Quiz**   *Score:* _____%

Additional Resources

____ Video: Vertebral Disk

____ Animations: Muscle Flexion and Extension; Bone Growth

____ Dictionary/Audio Glossary

____ Health Professions Careers: Physical Therapy Assistant

____ Health Professions Careers: Phlebotomist

Endocrine System

15

Chapter Outline

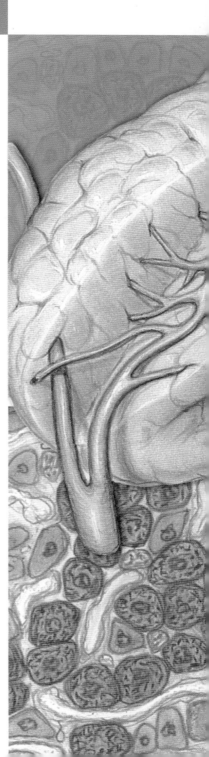

Objectives

After completion of this chapter you will be able to:

1. Describe the location of main structures in the endocrine system.

2. Define terms related to the anatomy and physiology of the endocrine system.

3. Define combining forms, prefixes, and suffixes related to the endocrine system.

4. Define common medical terminology related to the endocrine system, including adjectives and related terms, symptoms and conditions, tests and procedures, surgical interventions, medications and drug therapies, and specialties.

5. Explain abbreviations for terms related to the endocrine system.

6. Successfully complete all chapter exercises.

7. Explain terms used in case studies and medical records involving the endocrine system.

8. Successfully complete all pronunciation and spelling exercises, and complete all interactive exercises included with the companion Student Resources.

■ ANATOMY AND PHYSIOLOGY

Functions

- To produce, store, and release hormones directly into the bloodstream, which are then used by other organs to control and coordinate functions such as metabolism, reproduction, growth, and development

Organs and Structures

- Endocrine glands are ductless glands that secrete hormones directly into the bloodstream.
- Glands include the adrenal glands, islets of Langerhans in the pancreas, ovaries, parathyroid glands, pineal gland, pituitary gland, testes, thymus gland, and thyroid gland.

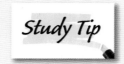

Study Tip

Endocrine: The word endocrine comes from the prefix *endo-*, meaning in or within, and the word root *crin*, meaning to secrete. The endocrine glands secrete directly into the bloodstream rather than through a channel of ducts.

Terms Related to the Endocrine System (Fig. 15-1)

Term	Pronunciation	Function
Organs		
adrenal glands, *syn.* suprarenal glands	ă-drē′năl glandz, sū′pră-rē′năl glandz	pair of glands located on top of the kidneys that secrete hormones that aid in metabolism, electrolyte balance, and stress reactions; each gland consists of an outer portion, called the adrenal cortex, and an inner portion, called the adrenal medulla
hypothalamus	hī′pō-thal′ă-mŭs	part of the brain located near the pituitary gland that controls the release of hormones by the pituitary gland
islets of Langerhans	ī′lets ov lahng′ĕr-hahnz	endocrine cells inside the pancreas that secrete hormones that aid carbohydrate and glucose metabolism (Fig. 15-2)
ovaries	ō′vă-rēz	female reproductive glands attached to the uterus that produce hormones and release eggs
parathyroid glands	par′ă-thī′royd glandz	four small glands located behind the thyroid that regulate calcium and phosphorus levels in the bloodstream and bones
pineal gland, *syn.* pineal body	pin′ē-ăl gland, pin′ē-ăl bod′ē	small, cone-shaped gland located in the brain that secretes melatonin, which affects sleep-wake cycles and reproduction

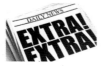

PINEAL GLAND The pineal gland sits deep inside the brain and was once thought to be the center of the soul. As research emerged, it was found that the only hormone secreted by the pineal gland is melatonin. Melatonin is instrumental in the circadian or sleep-wake cycle in the body. As we age, the amount of melatonin secreted from the pineal gland decreases. However, when we are young, large amounts of melatonin are secreted. This may explain why some younger people can sleep until noon or later!

(continued)

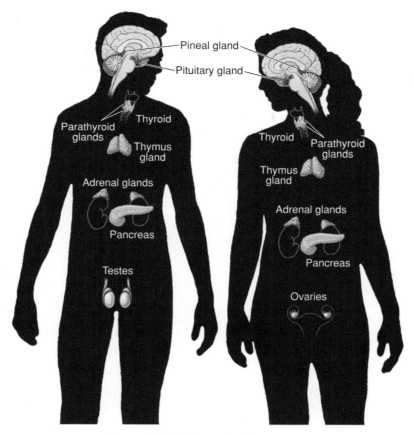

Figure 15-1   The endocrine system.

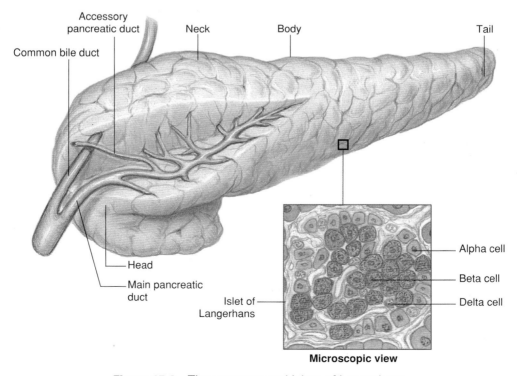

Microscopic view

Figure 15-2   The pancreas and islets of Langerhans.

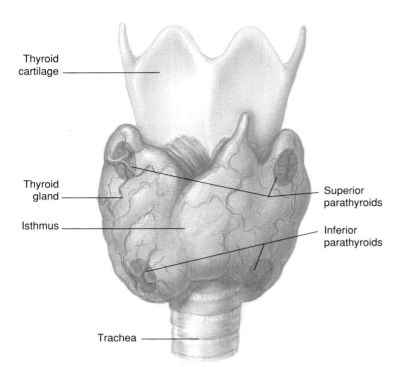

Figure 15-3   The thyroid gland and adjacent structures.

Labels: Thyroid cartilage, Thyroid gland, Isthmus, Trachea, Superior parathyroids, Inferior parathyroids

Terms Related to the Endocrine System *(continued)*

Term	Pronunciation	Function
pituitary gland	pi-tū'i-tār'ē gland	pea-sized gland located at the base of the brain that secretes hormones that stimulate the function of other endocrine glands; also known as the "master gland"; divided into anterior and posterior lobes
testes, *syn.* testicles	tes'tēz, tes'tĭ-kĕlz	male reproductive glands located in the scrotum, which produce sperm and testosterone
thymus gland	thī'mŭs gland	gland in the mediastinum that secretes a hormone that regulates the immune system
thyroid gland	thī'royd gland	gland located below the larynx that secretes a hormone that is needed for cell metabolism and energy; the largest endocrine gland; has two lobes connected by a tissue called the isthmus (Fig. 15-3)

Hormones

pituitary gland—anterior lobe

adrenocorticotropic hormone (ACTH)	ă-drē'nō-kōr'ti-kō-trō'pik hōr'mōn	stimulates the adrenal cortex
follicle-stimulating hormone (FSH)	fol'i-kĕl-stim'yū-lā'ting hōr'mōn	regulates the ovaries and testicles; stimulates secretion of estrogen in females and sperm production in males
growth hormone (GH)	grōth hōr'mōn	regulates body growth
luteinizing hormone (LH)	lū'tē-in-ī-zing hōr'mōn	stimulates secretion of progesterone in females and testosterone in males
prolactin	prō-lak'tin	stimulates milk production
thyroid-stimulating hormone (TSH)	thī'royd-stim'yū-lā'ting hōr'mōn	stimulates the thyroid gland

Terms Related to the Endocrine System *(continued)*

Term	Pronunciation	Function
pituitary gland—posterior lobe		
antidiuretic hormone (ADH)	an'tē-dī-yū-ret'ik hōr'mōn	stimulates water absorption by the kidneys
oxytocin	ok'sē-tō'sin	stimulates uterine contractions
pineal gland		
melatonin	mel'ă-tōn'in	affects sleep-wake cycles and reproduction
thyroid gland		
thyroxine (T_4)	thī-rok'sēn	regulates metabolism
triiodothyronine (T_3)	trī'ī-ō'dō-thī'rō-nēn	regulates metabolism
parathyroid glands		
parathyroid hormone (PTH)	par'ă-thī'royd hōr'mōn	regulates calcium and phosphorus levels in blood and bones
islets of Langerhans		
insulin	in'sŭ-lin	regulates blood glucose levels
thymus gland		
thymosin	thī'mō-sin	regulates immune responses
adrenal cortex		
aldosterone	al-dos'tĕr-ōn	regulates electrolyte levels
cortisol	kōr'ti-sol	aids in metabolism and also aids the body during stress
adrenal medulla		
epinephrine and norepinephrine	ep'i-nef'rin, nōr'ep-i-nef'rin	aid body during stress by raising heart rate, blood pressure, and respiration
ovaries		
estrogen and progesterone	es'trō-jen, prō-jes'tĕr-ōn	affect the development of female sexual organs and secondary sexual characteristics; regulate menstrual cycle and pregnancy
testes		
testosterone	tes-tos'tĕ-rōn	affects development of sexual organs in males and secondary sexual characteristics

■ Exercises: Anatomy and Physiology

SIMPLE RECALL

Exercise 1

Write the correct organ for the meaning given.

1. pea-sized gland at the base of the brain   _____

2. glands on top of the kidneys   _____

3. endocrine cells inside the pancreas   _____

4. largest endocrine gland located near the larynx _____

5. four small glands behind the thyroid _____

6. cone-shaped gland in the brain _____

7. part of the brain that controls the release of hormones by the pituitary gland _____

8. gland that affects the immune system _____

9. glands that secrete estrogen and progesterone _____

Exercise 2

ADVANCED RECALL

Match each medical term with its meaning.

thyroxine	prolactin	aldosterone
growth hormone	oxytocin	melatonin
parathyroid hormone	insulin	follicle-stimulating hormone

Meaning   **Term**

1. regulates body growth _____

2. regulates metabolism _____

3. regulates ovaries and testicles _____

4. regulates calcium levels in blood _____

5. stimulates milk production _____

6. stimulates uterine contractions _____

7. regulates electrolyte levels _____

8. regulates sleep-wake cycles _____

9. regulates blood glucose levels _____

Exercise 3

ADVANCED RECALL

Complete each sentence by writing in the correct medical term.

1. The hormone that regulates calcium and phosphorus levels in the blood and bones is

   _____.

2. _____, the hormone secreted by the thymus gland, regulates immune responses.

3. The _____ hormone stimulates the adrenal cortex.

4. The secretion of progesterone in females and testosterone in males is stimulated by

_____, the hormone secreted by the anterior lobe of the pituitary gland.

5. The thyroid gland is stimulated by _____.

6. _____ and _____ are produced by the thyroid gland and

help regulate metabolism.

7. The posterior lobe of the pituitary gland secretes _____, the hormone
that stimulates the kidneys to absorb water.

8. Testosterone is secreted by the _____.

9. The glands that produce the hormones that aid in regulating the menstrual cycle are the

_____.

10. The adrenal cortex produces _____, which aids the body during stress.

■ WORD PARTS

Note that some word parts that have been introduced earlier in the book may not
be repeated here.

Combining Forms

Combining Form	Meaning
acr/o	extremity, tip
aden/o	gland
adren/o, adrenal/o	adrenal glands
calc/i	calcium
cortic/o	cortex
crin/o	to secrete
dips/o	thirst
endocrin/o	endocrine
gluc/o, glucos/o, glyc/o, glycos/o	glucose, sugar
hormon/o	hormone
kal/i	potassium
natr/i	sodium
pancreat/o	pancreas
parathyroid/o	parathyroid glands
thym/o	thymus gland
thyr/o, thyroid/o	thyroid gland

Prefixes

Prefix	Meaning
eu-	good, normal
hyper-	above, excessive
hypo-	below, deficient
poly-	many, much

Suffixes

Suffix	Meaning
-al, -ic	pertaining to
-emia	blood (condition of)
-ism	condition of
-megaly	enlargement
-oid	resembling
-osis	abnormal condition
-penia	deficiency
-uria	urine, urination

■ Exercises: Word Parts

SIMPLE
RECALL

Exercise 4

Write the meaning of the combining form given.

1. glucos/o _____

2. cortic/o _____

3. thyr/o _____

4. kal/i _____

5. crin/o _____

6. dips/o _____

7. gluc/o _____

8. natr/i _____

Exercise 5

ADVANCED RECALL

Considering the meaning of the suffix used in the medical term, write the meaning of the medical term.

Suffix	Meaning	Medical Term	Meaning of Term
-ectomy	excision, surgical removal	adrenalectomy	1. _____
-penia	deficiency	calcipenia	2. _____
-al	pertaining to	hormonal	3. _____
-megaly	enlargement	acromegaly	4. _____
-tomy	incision	thyroidotomy	5. _____
-itis	inflammation	thymitis	6. _____
-ectomy	excision, surgical removal	parathyroidectomy	7. _____
-logist	one who specializes in	endocrinologist	8. _____

Exercise 6

TERM CONSTRUCTION

For each term, first write the meaning of the term. Then write the meaning of the word parts in that term.

1. hypothyroidism _____

    hypo- _____

    thyroid/o _____

    -ism _____

2. pancreatic _____

    pancreat/o _____

    -ic _____

3. euthyroid _____

    eu- _____

    thyr/o _____

    -oid _____

4. glycosuria _____

  glyc/o _____

  -uria _____

5. hyperglycemia _____

  hyper- _____

  glyc/o _____

  -emia _____

6. adrenopathy _____

  adren/o _____

  -pathy _____

7. polydipsia _____

  poly- _____

  dips/o _____

  -ia _____

8. adenosis _____

  aden/o _____

  -osis _____

■ MEDICAL TERMS

Adjectives and Other Related Terms

Term	Pronunciation	Meaning
cortical	kōr′ti-kăl	pertaining to the cortex
endogenous	en-doj′ĕ-nŭs	produced inside the body
euthyroid	yū′thī i-royd	normal thyroid
exogenous	eks-oj′ĕ-nŭs	produced outside of the body
metabolism	mĕ-tab′ō-lizm	all physical and chemical changes that occur in tissue
pancreatic	pan′rē-at′ik	pertaining to the pancreas
thymic	thī′mik	pertaining to the thymus gland

■ Exercises: Adjectives and Other Related Terms

Exercise 7

SIMPLE
RECALL

Write the correct medical term for the meaning given.

1. pertaining to the cortex   _____

2. produced outside of the body   _____

3. pertaining to the pancreas   _____

4. pertaining to the thymus gland   _____

5. produced inside the body   _____

Exercise 8

ADVANCED
RECALL

Complete each sentence by writing in the correct medical term.

1. The term that denotes a normal thyroid is _____.

2. A disease that is related to the pancreas is considered to be _____.

3. All physical and chemical changes that occur in tissues are called _____.

4. A hormonal change related to the thymus is _____.

5. Hormones that are not produced by the body are _____ hormones.

Exercise 9

TERM
CONSTRUCTION

Write the combining form used in the medical term, followed by the meaning of the combining form.

Term	Combining Form	Combining Form Meaning
1. thymic	_____	_____
2. cortical	_____	_____
3. adrenal	_____	_____
4. euthyroid	_____	_____
5. pancreatic	_____	_____
6. hormonal	_____	_____

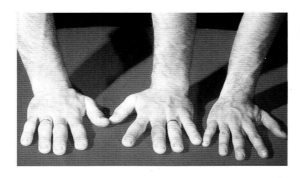

Figure 15-4 Comparison of patient with normal hand (right) and hands of a patient with acromegaly.

Symptoms and Medical Conditions

Term	Pronunciation	Meaning
acidosis	as'i-dō'sis	abnormal accumulation of acidic waste products in the blood
acromegaly	ak'rō-meg'ă-lē	enlargement of the extremities caused by excessive production of growth hormone (Fig. 15-4)
Addison disease	ad'i-sŏn di-zēz'	disease caused by deficiency of cortisol production by the adrenal glands; characterized by darkening of the skin, weakness, and loss of appetite
adenalgia	ad'ě-nal'jē-ă	pain in a gland
adenitis	ad'ě-nī'tis	inflammation of a gland
adenomegaly	ad'ě-nō-meg'ă-lē	enlargement of a gland
adrenalitis	ă-drē-năl-ī'tis	inflammation of an adrenal gland
adrenomegaly	ă-drē-nō-meg'ă-lē	enlargement of an adrenal gland
adrenopathy	a-dren-op'ă-thē	disease of the adrenal gland
calcipenia	kal'si-pē'nē-ă	deficiency of calcium
congenital hypothyroidism	kon-jen'i-tăl hī'pō-thī'royd-izm	condition caused by absence or atrophy of the thyroid gland present at birth characterized by mental deficiency and dwarfism (formerly known as cretinism)
Cushing syndrome	kush'ing sin'drōm	disease caused by excessive cortisol production by the adrenal glands characterized by fat pads in the chest and abdomen, moon-shaped face, and skin pigmentation (Fig. 15-5)

(continued)

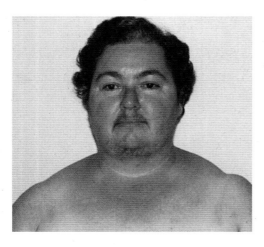

Figure 15-5 Patient with Cushing syndrome.

Symptoms and Medical Conditions *(continued)*

Term	Pronunciation	Meaning
diabetes insipidus (DI)	dī'ă-bē'tēz in-sip'i-dŭs	disorder caused by deficiency of antidiuretic hormone production by the pituitary gland resulting in excessive urination and excessive thirst
diabetes mellitus (DM)	dī-ă-bē'tēz mel'i-tŭs	disorder caused by deficiency of insulin and/or insulin resistance causing poor carbohydrate metabolism and high blood glucose levels
Type 1 diabetes mellitus	tīp 1 dī-ă-bē'tēz mel'i-tŭs	diabetes caused by a total lack of insulin production; usually develops in childhood, and patients require insulin replacement therapy to control the disorder
Type 2 diabetes mellitus	tīp 2 dī-ă-bē'tēz mel'i-tŭs	diabetes caused by either a lack of insulin or the body's inability to use insulin efficiently; usually develops in middle-aged or older adults, and patients usually do not require insulin replacement therapy to control the disorder

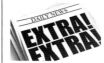

DIABETES MELLITUS The World Health Organization (WHO) calls the incidence of diabetes mellitus (DM) an epidemic and estimates that the number of people diagnosed with DM worldwide will double by the year 2030. In the United States, the high incidence of Type 2 DM is linked to an increase in obesity. The American Diabetes Association (ADA) recommends screening for DM for people with risk factors for Type 2 DM, which include:

- Obesity
- Age 45 years or older
- Family history of diabetes mellitus (parents or siblings with diabetes)
- Race/ethnicity (Black, Hispanic, Asian, Native American, Pacific Islanders)
- History of gestational diabetes
- Inactivity
- Smoking
- Cardiovascular disease
- Hypertension

Term	Pronunciation	Meaning
diabetic ketoacidosis (DKA)	dī'ă-bet'ik kē'tō-as'i-dō'sis	excessive ketones in blood due to breakdown of stored fats for energy; a complication of diabetes mellitus; if left untreated, can lead to coma and death
endocrinopathy	en'dō-kri-nop'ă-thē	disease of an endocrine gland
exophthalmos	ek'sof-thal'mos	protruding or bulging eyes (Fig. 15-6)
gigantism	jī-gan'tizm	condition of excessive body growth caused by overproduction of growth hormone by the pituitary gland
glucosuria, glycosuria	glū'kō-syū'rē-ă, glī'kō-syū'rē-ă	glucose in the urine
goiter	goy'tĕr	enlargement of the thyroid gland (Fig. 15-7)

(continued)

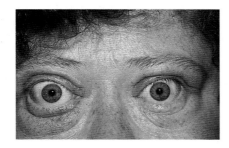

Figure 15-6 Patient with exophthalmos.

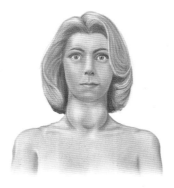
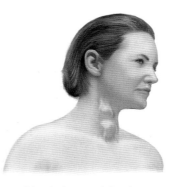
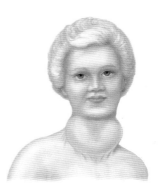

Toxic goiter (Graves disease)   Simple (nontoxic) goiter   Nodular goiter

Figure 15-7   Goiter.

Symptoms and Medical Conditions *(continued)*

Term	Pronunciation	Meaning
Graves disease	grāvz di-zēz′	condition of excessive secretion of thyroid hormone causing goiter and exophthalmos
Hashimoto thyroiditis, *syn.* Hashimoto disease	hah-shē-mō′tō thī′roy-dī′tis, hah-shē-mō′tō di-zēz′	autoimmune disease causing chronic thyroiditis
hirsutism	hĭr′sū-tizm	excessive hair growth or hair growth in unusual places (e.g., beard growth on a woman)
hypercalcemia	hī′pĕr-kal-sē′mē-ă	high levels of calcium in the blood
hyperglycemia	hī′pĕr-glī-sē′mē-ă	high levels of glucose or sugar in the blood
hyperkalemia	hī′pĕr-kă-lē′mē-ă	high levels of potassium in the blood
hypernatremia	hī′per-nă-trē′mē-ă	high levels of sodium in the blood
hyperparathyroidism	hī′pĕr-par′ă-thī′royd-izm	excessive hormone production by the parathyroid glands
hyperthyroidism	hī-per-thī′royd-izm	excessive hormone production by the thyroid gland
hypocalcemia	hī′pō-kal-sē′mē-ă	low levels of calcium in the blood
hypoglycemia	hī′pō-glī-sē′mē-ă	low levels of glucose or sugar in the blood
hypokalemia	hī′pō-ka-lē′mē-ă	low levels of potassium in the blood
hyponatremia	hī′pō-nă-trē′mē-ă	low levels of sodium in the blood
hypoparathyroidism	hī′pō-par′ă-thī′royd-izm	deficient hormone production by the parathyroid glands
hypothyroidism	hī′pō-thī′royd-izm	deficient hormone production by the thyroid gland
ketosis	kē-tō′sis	excessive ketones in the blood
myxedema	miks′e-dē′mă	severe hypothyroidism in an adult characterized by pale dry skin, brittle hair, and sluggishness
pancreatitis	pan′krē-ă-tī′tis	inflammation of the pancreas
polydipsia	pol′ē-dip′sē-ă	excessive thirst
polyuria	pol′ē-yū′rē-ă	excessive and frequent urination

(continued)

Symptoms and Medical Conditions *(continued)*

Term	Pronunciation	Meaning
tetany	tet'ă-nē	spasms of nerves and muscles due to low levels of calcium in the blood caused by deficient production of parathyroid hormone
thyroiditis	thī'roy-dī'tis	inflammation of the thyroid gland
thyromegaly	thī'rō-meg'ă-lē	enlargement of the thyroid gland
thyrotoxicosis	thī'rō-tok'si-kō'sis	condition of excessively high levels of thyroid hormone (either endogenous or exogenous)

ANIMATION

For a more in-depth look at diabetes, view the animation *Diabetes Mellitus* on the Student Resources.

■ Exercises: Symptoms and Medical Conditions

SIMPLE
RECALL

Exercise 10

Write the correct medical term for the meaning given.

1. excessive thirst   _____

2. autoimmune disease causing chronic thyroiditis   _____

3. protruding eyes   _____

4. abnormal accumulation of acidic waste   _____

5. excessively high levels of thyroid hormone   _____

6. excessive hair growth or growth of hair in
   unusual places   _____

7. excessive ketones in the blood   _____

8. disorder caused by total lack of insulin   _____

9. severe hypothyroidism causing dry skin
   and hair   _____

10. excessive urination   _____

11. enlargement of a gland   _____

12. excessive production of thyroid hormone   _____

13. disorder caused by body's inability to use
    insulin efficiently   _____

Exercise 11

SIMPLE
RECALL

Circle the term that is most appropriate for the meaning of the sentence.

1. Excessive body growth due to overproduction of growth hormone by the pituitary gland can result in a condition called (*goiter, gigantism, tetany*).

2. (*Cushing syndrome, Diabetes insipidus, Addison disease*) is caused by a deficiency of adrenal gland hormone production.

3. Congenital absence of the thyroid gland can cause a condition known as (*myxedema, hirsutism, congenital hypothyroidism*).

4. Enlargement of the extremities is known as (*goiter, hypokalemia, acromegaly*).

5. A blood test that shows low levels of thyroid hormone in the blood indicates that the patient has (*hypernatremia, hypokalemia, hypothyroidism*).

6. Excessive hormone production by the thyroid causing goiter and exophthalmos can result in a condition known as (*Graves disease, Cushing syndrome, gigantism*).

7. A patient with polyuria and polydipsia may have (*Cushing syndrome, diabetes insipidus, thyrotoxicosis*).

8. (*Hashimoto disease, Addison disease, Diabetic ketoacidosis*) is a condition where there are excessive ketones in the blood due to breakdown of fats stored for energy.

9. A patient with fat pads on the chest and abdomen and a moon-shaped face may have (*myxedema, Hashimoto disease, Cushing syndrome*).

10. Inflammation of the adrenal gland is known as (*hyperthyroidism, adrenalitis, adenitis*).

11. (*Adenitis, Goiter, Ketosis*) is the name for enlargement of the thyroid gland.

12. Spasms of nerves and muscles caused by deficient parathyroid hormone production leads to a condition called (*Graves disease, Addison disease, tetany*).

Exercise 12

ADVANCED
RECALL

Match each medical term with its meaning.

hypercalcemia	polydipsia	hyponatremia
glycosuria	calcipenia	hyperkalemia
polyuria	hyperglycemia	hypocalcemia

Meaning   **Term**

1. low levels of sodium in the blood   _____

2. high levels of potassium in the blood   _____

3. high levels of calcium in the blood   _____

4. excessive urination

_____

5. glucose in the urine

_____

6. high levels of glucose in the blood

_____

7. deficiency of calcium

_____

8. excessive thirst

_____

9. low levels of calcium in the blood

_____

TERM
CONSTRUCTION

Exercise 13

Build a medical term from an appropriate combining form and suffix, given their meanings.

Use Combining Form for	Use Suffix for	Term
1. glucose, sugar	urine, urination	_____
2. endocrine gland	disease	_____
3. gland	pain	_____
4. adrenal gland	enlargement	_____
5. thyroid gland	inflammation	_____
6. gland	inflammation	_____
7. pancreas	inflammation	_____
8. calcium	deficiency	_____
9. adrenal gland	disease	_____
10. thyroid gland	enlargement	_____

TERM
CONSTRUCTION

Exercise 14

Write the meaning of the word parts used in each of the medical terms in the correct blanks (P = prefix, CF = combining form, S = suffix).

1. hyperparathyroidism   _____/_____/_____
                                            P   CF   S

2. hypoparathyroidism   _____/_____/_____
                                            P   CF   S

3. hypercalcemia   _____/_____/_____
                                     P   CF   S

4. hypocalcemia

_____ / _____ / _____
P   CF   S

5. hyperglycemia

_____ / _____ / _____
P   CF   S

6. hypoglycemia

_____ / _____ / _____
P   CF   S

7. hypernatremia

_____ / _____ / _____
P   CF   S

8. hyponatremia

_____ / _____ / _____
P   CF   S

9. hyperkalemia

_____ / _____ / _____
P   CF   S

10. hypokalemia

_____ / _____ / _____
P   CF   S

Tests and Procedures

Term	Pronunciation	Meaning
Laboratory Tests		
blood glucose, _syn._ blood sugar	blŭd glū'kōs, blŭd shug'ăr	test to measure the amount of glucose in the blood (Fig. 15-8)
electrolyte panel	ĕ-lek'trō-līt pan'ĕl	blood test to measure the amount of sodium, potassium, chloride, and carbon dioxide in the blood

(continued)

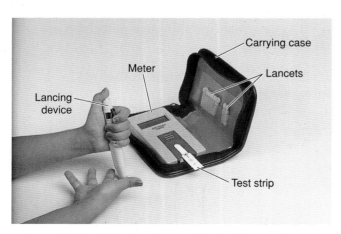

Figure 15-8 Materials for monitoring blood glucose.

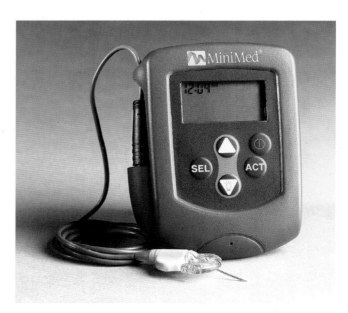

Figure 15-9 Glucometer.

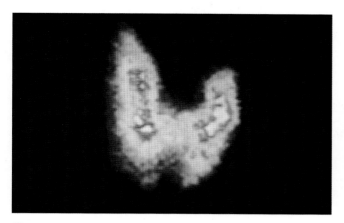

Figure 15-10 Image of an abnormal thyroid using radioactive iodine uptake test (RAIU). The right lobe (on the left) appears brighter and larger than the left, indicating it has higher activity.

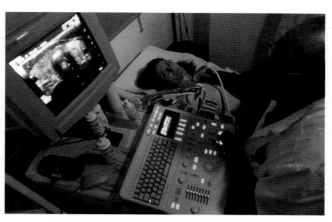

Figure 15-11 Ultrasound of the thyroid.

Tests and Procedures *(continued)*

Term	Pronunciation	Meaning
fasting blood glucose (FBG)	fast'ing blŭd glū'kōs	blood test that measures the amount of glucose in the blood after fasting for at least 8 hours
glucometer	glū-kom'ĕ-ter	device for measuring blood glucose levels from a drop of blood obtained by a fingerstick (Fig. 15-9)
glucose tolerance test (GTT)	glū'kos tol'ĕr-ăns test	blood test that measures the amount of glucose in the blood after administering a dose of glucose to the patient; used to gauge the body's ability to metabolize glucose
glycosylated hemoglobin	glī-kō'si-lāt-ĕd hē'mō-glō-bin	blood test that indicates the amount of glucose in the blood over the previous few months; used to indicate how well diabetes mellitus is being controlled
thyroid function tests	thī'royd fŭnk'shŭn testz	blood tests that measure thyroid hormone levels in the blood
thyroid-stimulating hormone level	thī'royd-stim'yū-lā'ting hōr'mōn lev'ĕl	blood test that measures the amount of thyroid-stimulating hormone in the blood; used to diagnosis hyperthyroidism or to monitor thyroid replacement therapy
thyroxine level	thī-rok'sēn lev'ĕl	blood test that measures the amount of thyroxine in the blood to diagnose hyperthyroidism or hypothyroidism
Diagnostic Procedures		
radioactive iodine uptake test (RAIU), *syn.* ^{131}I uptake test	rā'dē-ō-ak'tiv ī'ō-dīn ŭp'tăk test	test of thyroid function by measuring the uptake of iodine by the thyroid (Fig. 15-10)
thyroid scan	thī'royd skan	scan of the thyroid gland using a radioactive substance, ultrasound, or computed tomography to show the size, shape, and position of the thyroid gland (Fig. 15-11)

■ Exercises: Tests and Procedures

Exercise 15

SIMPLE
RECALL

Write the correct medical term for the meaning given.

1. instrument for measuring blood glucose level from a drop of blood _____

2. measures thyroid hormone levels in the blood _____

3. test measuring glucose in the blood after administration of a dose of glucose _____

4. test of thyroid function by measuring thyroid's uptake of iodine _____

5. scan that shows size, shape, and position of thyroid _____

6. test that measures the amount of TSH in the blood _____

Exercise 16

ADVANCED
RECALL

Match each medical term with its meaning.

glycosylated hemoglobin   electrolyte panel   fasting blood glucose
thyroxine level   blood glucose   glucose tolerance test

Meaning	Term
1. measures amount of thyroxine in the blood	_____
2. measures body's ability to metabolize glucose	_____
3. measures amount of glucose in the blood	_____
4. measures glucose in the blood after a period of fasting	_____
5. measures sodium, potassium, chloride and carbon dioxide in blood	_____
6. measures how well diabetes is being controlled	_____

Surgical Interventions

Term	Pronunciation	Meaning
adenectomy	ad'ĕ-nek'tŏ-mē	excision of a gland
adrenalectomy	ă-drē-năl-ek'tŏ-mē	excision of an adrenal gland
pancreatectomy	pan'krē-ă-tek'tŏ-mē	excision of the pancreas
parathyroidectomy	par'ă-thī-royd-ek'tŏ-mē	excision of a parathyroid gland
thymectomy	thī-mek'tŏ-mē	excision of the thymus gland
thyroidectomy	thī'roy-dek'tŏ-mē	excision of the thyroid gland
thyroidotomy	thī'roy-dot'ŏ-mē	incision into a thyroid gland
thyroparathyroidectomy	thī'rō-par'ă-thī'roy-dek'tŏ-mē	excision of the thyroid and parathyroid glands

■ Exercises: Surgical Interventions

SIMPLE
RECALL

Exercise 17

Write the meaning of the term given.

1. thyroidectomy _____

2. adrenalectomy _____

3. thymectomy _____

4. thyroparathyroidectomy _____

ADVANCED
RECALL

Exercise 18

Circle the term that is most appropriate for the meaning of the sentence.

1. Mrs. Riley was hospitalized for a thyroidectomy, which involves removal of her (*thymus, thyroid, parathyroid*).

2. Mr. Ling has been diagnosed with a tumor on his adrenal gland and will require a (*thyroidectomy, adenectomy, adrenalectomy*).

3. Part of Ms. Williamson's surgery will include a thyroidotomy, which is a(n) (*excision, removal, incision*) of her thyroid gland.

4. The surgeon performed a thyroparathyroidectomy, which includes excision of the (*thymus, thyroid, thyroxine*) gland.

TERM
CONSTRUCTION

Exercise 19

Write the combining form used in the medical term, followed by the meaning of the combining form.

Term	Combining Form	Combining Form Meaning
1. pancreatectomy	_____	_____
2. thyroidotomy	_____	_____
3. adenectomy	_____	_____
4. parathyroidectomy	_____	_____
5. thymectomy	_____	_____

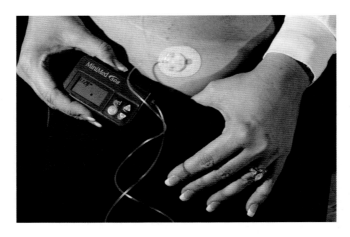

Figure 15-12 Continuous subcutaneous insulin infusion (CSII) insulin pump.

Medications and Drug Therapies

Term	Pronunciation	Meaning
antidiabetic	an'tē-dī-ă-bet'ik	drug used to treat diabetes mellitus by lowering glucose levels in the blood
antithyroid	an'tē-thī'royd	drug used to treat overproduction of thyroid hormone
continuous subcutaneous insulin infusion (CSII), *syn.* insulin pump	kon-tin'yū-ŭs sŭb'kyū-tā'nē-ŭs in'sŭ-lin in-fyū'zhŭn, in'sŭ-lin pŭmp	infusion of insulin to subcutaneous tissues by a device worn on the body (Fig. 15-12)
insulin therapy	in'sŭ-lin thār'ă-pē	method used to treat diabetes mellitus by replacing natural insulin
hormone replacement therapy	hōr'mōn rě-plās'měnt thār'ă-pē	method used to replace a hormone normally produced by the body

■ Exercise: Medications and Drug Therapies

SIMPLE RECALL

Exercise 20

Write the correct medication or drug therapy term for the meaning given.

1. used to replace natural insulin _____

2. used to treat overproduction of thyroid hormone _____

3. used to replace a hormone _____

4. used to lower glucose levels in the blood _____

5. device worn on the body to infuse insulin _____

Specialties and Specialists

Term	Pronunciation	Meaning
endocrinology	en'dō-kri-nol'ŏ-jē	medical specialty concerned with diagnosis and treatment of disorders of the endocrine system
endocrinologist	en'dō-kri-nol'ŏ-jist	physician who specializes in endocrinology

■ Exercise: Specialties and Specialists

Exercise 21

SIMPLE RECALL

Write the correct medical term for the meaning given.

1. specialty concerned with the endocrine system   _____

2. specialist in the endocrine system   _____

Abbreviations

Abbreviation	Meaning
ACTH	adrenocorticotropic hormone
ADH	antidiuretic hormone
CSII	continuous subcutaneous insulin infusion
DI	diabetes insipidus
DKA	diabetic ketoacidosis
DM	diabetes mellitus
FBG	fasting blood glucose
FSH	follicle-stimulating hormone
GH	growth hormone
GTT	glucose tolerance test
LH	luteinizing hormone
PTH	parathyroid hormone
RAIU	radioactive iodine uptake
T_3	triiodothyronine
T_4	thyroxine
TSH	thyroid-stimulating hormone

■ Exercises: Abbreviations

SIMPLE
RECALL

Exercise 22

Write the meaning of each abbreviation.

1. DI _____

2. TSH _____

3. FBG _____

4. ADH _____

5. PTH _____

6. GTT _____

7. RAIU _____

8. T_3 _____

Exercise 23

ADVANCED
RECALL

Match each abbreviation with the appropriate description.

DI	DM	CSII
DKA	LH	T_4
GH	FSH	ACTH

1. hormone that stimulates the adrenal cortex _____

2. disorder caused by deficiency of insulin _____

3. regulates the ovaries and testicles _____

4. regulates metabolism _____

5. excessive ketones in the blood that can lead to coma or death _____

6. device worn by patient to administer insulin subcutaneously _____

7. disorder caused by deficiency of antidiuretic hormone _____

8. regulates body growth _____

9. stimulates secretion of progesterone in females _____

Chapter Review

Review of Terms for Anatomy and Physiology

VISUAL

Exercise 24

Write the correct terms on the blanks for the anatomic structures indicated.

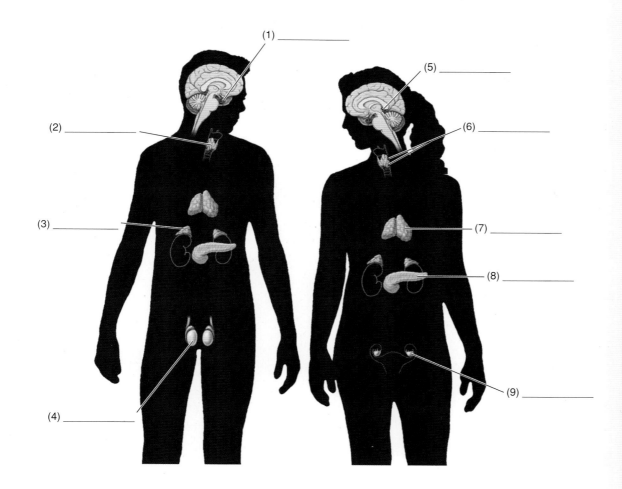

(1) _____

(2) _____

(3) _____

(4) _____

(5) _____

(6) _____

(7) _____

(8) _____

(9) _____

Understanding Term Structure

TERM CONSTRUCTION

Exercise 25

Break the given medical term into its word parts and define each part. Then define the medical term.

For example:

thymitis	*word parts:*	thym/o / -itis
	meanings:	thymus / inflammation
	term meaning:	inflammation of the thymus gland

1. pancreatic   *word parts:*   _____ / _____

                      meanings: _____ / _____

                      term meaning: _____

2. adrenalitis   *word parts:*   _____ / _____

                      meanings: _____ / _____

                      term meaning: _____

3. glucosuria   *word parts:*   _____ / _____

                      meanings: _____ / _____

                      term meaning: _____

4. acromegaly   *word parts:*   _____ / _____

                      meanings: _____ / _____

                      term meaning: _____

5. cortical   *word parts:*   _____ / _____

                      meanings: _____ / _____

                      term meaning: _____

6. calcipenia   *word parts:*   _____ / _____

                      meanings: _____ / _____

                      term meaning: _____

7. thyroidotomy   *word parts:*   _____ / _____

                      meanings: _____ / _____

                      term meaning: _____

TERM
CONSTRUCTION

Exercise 26

Write the combining form used in the medical term, followed by the meaning of the combining form.

Term	Combining Form	Combining Form Meaning
1. thymic	_____	_____
2. thyromegaly	_____	_____
3. hypokalemia	_____	_____
4. adrenalectomy	_____	_____
5. hypernatremia	_____	_____
6. endocrinopathy	_____	_____
7. adenalgia	_____	_____
8. polydipsia	_____	

Comprehension Exercises

COMPREHENSION

Exercise 27

Fill in the blank with the correct term.

1. Excessive production of the T_3 and T_4 hormones can lead to a condition called _____.

2. The test that measures the glucose levels in the blood after administering a dose of glucose is called the _____.

3. A patient who has the surgical procedure known as a(n) _____ is no longer able to produce the hormone cortisol.

4. The hormone that keeps the body from accumulating excess water is called the

   _____.

5. _____ are endocrine cells that aid in glucose metabolism.

6. The opposite of anuria is _____.

7. The term for a thyroid with no functional problems is _____.

8. A patient who was born without a thyroid gland has _____.

9. The disease that includes symptoms of both polydipsia and polyuria is _____.

10. A physician specializing in all types of thyroid disorders is called a(n) _____.

Exercise 28

COMPREHENSION **Circle the letter of the best answer in the following questions.**

1. A patient who has hypothyroidism does not have enough thyroxine that is:

   A. endogenous
   B. euthyroid
   C. exogenous
   D. cortical

2. The blood test used to measure how well diabetes is being controlled over a period of months is:

   A. thyroid function tests
   B. thyroid scan
   C. fasting blood sugar
   D. glycosylated hemoglobin

3. The condition caused by severely deficient hormone production by the thyroid gland is called:

   A. tetany
   B. myxedema
   C. Cushing syndrome
   D. Graves disease

4. An autoimmune disease that causes chronic inflammation of the thyroid is:

   A. Graves disease
   B. Cushing syndrome
   C. Addison disease
   D. Hashimoto disease

5. Excessive hair growth on the face of a woman might be diagnosed as:

   A. hirsutism
   B. myxedema
   C. acromegaly
   D. hyperkalemia

6. The test that measures the hormone made by the thyroid that helps to regulate metabolism is the:

   A. radioactive iodine uptake test
   B. thyroxine level test
   C. glycosylated hemoglobin test
   D. thyroid function test

7. A hormone that might be used to induce labor is called:

   A. insulin
   B. oxytocin
   C. luteinizing hormone
   D. thymosin

8. A patient with diabetes mellitus tests blood sugar level using a(n):

   A. electrolyte panel
   B. glucometer
   C. ketosis
   D. hirsutism

9. A patient with fat pads on the chest, pigmented skin, and a moon-shaped face may have:

   A. Hashimoto thyroiditis
   B. thyrotoxicosis
   C. Cushing syndrome
   D. goiter

10. Enlargement of the largest endocrine gland is called:

   A. acromegaly
   B. goiter
   C. hyperglycemia
   D. myxedema

Application and Analysis

Exercise 29

APPLICATION   **Read the case reports and circle the letter of your answer choice for the questions that follow.**

CASE 15-1

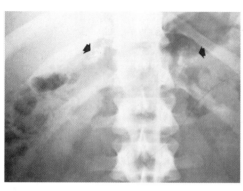

Mrs. Brewer presented to the office today for a complaint of significant weight loss, worsening fatigue, anorexia, lethargy, and irregular menses. Examination revealed hyperpigmentation of her skin. A review of the patient's record from the previous visit reveals a weight loss of 20 pounds over the past 4 months. A blood glucose level test was done and revealed hypoglycemia. Lab tests were ordered including an FBG, electrolytes, and ACTH hormone levels. A CT scan of the adrenal glands was also ordered (Fig. 15-13). The patient will return after testing for follow-up.

Figure 15-13   Computed tomography scan of a patient with Addison disease. The adrenal glands (*arrows*) appear small and with dense calcification.

1. The test that will measure the levels of sodium, potassium, chloride, and CO_2 in the patient's blood is:

    A. CT scan
    B. blood glucose
    C. electrolytes
    D. FBG

2. The term that describes low blood glucose is:

    A. anorexia
    B. hypoglycemia
    C. hyperpigmentation
    D. lethargy

3. The ACTH hormone level test will measure the amount of hormone produced by the:

    A. thyroid
    B. adrenal glands
    C. ovaries
    D. thymus

4. Based on the patient's symptoms and the workup ordered by the physician, which disease is most likely being considered for this patient?

    A. Addison disease
    B. Cushing syndrome
    C. Hashimoto thyroiditis
    D. Graves disease

CASE 15-2

Ms. Ramirez returned to her physician, Dr. Doray, for a followup visit for hyperthyroidism and a repeat of her thyroid tests. The results show that her TSH level remains suppressed below 0.04. Free T_4 and total T_4 remain in the upper limit of normal. A thyroid scan and uptake show predominantly active uptake in the left lobe. Based on these findings, Dr. Doray indicated that a diagnosis of multinodular toxic goiter was more likely than Graves disease. She discussed possible treatment options, including surgery, with the patient. Ms. Ramirez is inclined to undergo radioactive iodine treatment and understands that she will need to receive lifelong hormone replacement.

5. The term hyperthyroidism refers to _____ production of thyroid hormone.

   A. inefficient
   B. deficient
   C. excessive
   D. unacceptable

6. The abbreviation T_4 stands for:

   A. thyroid
   B. thyroxine
   C. triiodothyronine
   D. tetany

7. A goiter is an enlargement of the:

   A. parathyroid gland
   B. endocrine gland
   C. adrenal gland
   D. thyroid gland

8. A thyroid scan can indicate a thyroid's size, shape, and:

   A. functionality
   B. position
   C. color
   D. fullness

MEDICAL RECORD ANALYSIS

MEDICAL RECORD 15-1

You are a nurse practitioner specializing in diabetes care. You have been asked to see Ms. Hayes to discuss her newly diagnosed diabetes mellitus and are reviewing the medical record from her physician prior to meeting with her.

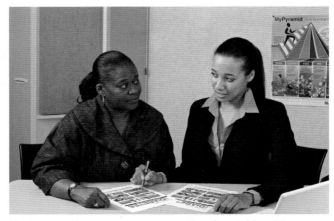

Nurse practioners manage a patient's total health care, including treatment of chronic conditions such as diabetes or high blood pressure.

Medical Record

NEW ONSET DIABETES MELLITUS

SUBJECTIVE: The patient is seen today for complaints of an unusually large appetite as well as polydipsia and polyuria. She is concerned because she has had a significant weight loss over the past few months despite her increased appetite. On questioning, she admits to increased fatigue as well as some irritability. The patient takes exogenous thyroxine for hypothyroidism. Past medical history reveals a single episode of pancreatitis 3 years ago. It is otherwise noncontributory with the exception of gestational diabetes during her second pregnancy. Family history is positive for a mother and sister with diabetes mellitus. Her sister is under treatment with a continuous subcutaneous insulin infusion.

OBJECTIVE: General exam reveals an obese female in no acute distress. Blood pressure is elevated at 150/95. Physical exam was unremarkable. Inspection of skin was negative for rashes, lesions, or ulcerations. Snellen testing revealed 20/20 vision in both eyes.

Urinalysis was performed and revealed slight glycosuria. Blood glucose testing revealed a glucose level of 260 two hours postprandial.

ASSESSMENT: My impression is new-onset diabetes mellitus with a family history of DM.

PLAN: Laboratory testing has been ordered to include a GTT, electrolytes, glycosylated hemoglobin, and lipid panel. The patient has been counseled regarding dietary considerations. She was advised of the importance of blood glucose control and regular exercise. The patient was counseled at length about the risks associated with diabetes, including diabetic nephropathy, retinopathy, and peripheral vascular disease.

Patient will be referred to endocrinologist, Tom Hong, for further evaluation and workup as soon as insurance authorization can be procured. A copy of her laboratory results will be forwarded to Dr. Hong on completion.

Exercise 30

APPLICATION

Write the appropriate medical terms used in this medical record on the blanks after their meanings.

1. produced inside the body   _____

2. excessive urination   _____

3. test of blood glucose level   _____

4. inflammation of the pancreas   _____

5. glucose in the urine   _____

Exercise 31

APPLICATION **Read the medical report and circle the letter of your answer choice for the following questions.**

1. What test did the physician perform on the patient to check her vision?

   A. urinalysis
   B. glycosylated hemoglobin
   C. Snellen
   D. continuous subcutaneous insulin infusion

2. The glycosylated hemoglobin test that was ordered will test for:

   A. blood levels of thyroid hormone
   B. blood glucose levels over the past few months
   C. blood levels of calcium
   D. blood levels of thyroxine

3. The physician's impression is that the patient has a deficiency and/or resistance to insulin, which is called:

   A. diabetes mellitus
   B. nephropathy
   C. peripheral vascular disease
   D. diabetes insipidus

4. The symptom polydipsia means that the patient is excessively:

   A. overweight
   B. hungry
   C. thirsty
   D. tired

5. The abbreviation GTT stands for a test that measures:

   A. blood levels of potassium
   B. blood levels of glucose after administration of a measured dose of glucose
   C. blood levels of thyroxine
   D. amount of thyroid-stimulating hormone in the blood

MEDICAL RECORD 15-2

Mirinda Maloney was admitted for a thyroidectomy after being diagnosed with hyperthyroidism. As a surgical technologist, you assisted in this patient's surgery by maintaining supplies, counting materials, and assisting in suturing. The resulting operative report is as follows:

Medical Record

OPERATIVE REPORT: THYROIDECTOMY

Preoperative Diagnosis: Primary (1)_____
Postoperative Diagnosis: Left thyroid tumor
Operation: Minimally invasive thyroidectomy
Surgeon: Joel Sugiwara, M.D.
Assistant Surgeon: Tom Hansen, M.D.
Anesthesia: General

INDICATIONS: The patient is a 54-year-old female with a history of weight loss, fatigue,
(2)_____, and (3)_____. A thyroxine level test revealed excessive

levels of thyroxine and a(n) (4)_____ showed a nodule in the left thyroid. The patient is brought to the operating room for minimally invasive (5) _____.

PROCEDURE: The patient was taken to the operating room and placed in a supine position on the operating table. After satisfactory induction of general endotracheal anesthesia, the patient was positioned and draped for the procedure. The patient's recurrent laryngeal nerves were monitored throughout the operating using electromyography.

A small horizontal incision was made in the lower neck. Flaps were raised superiorly and inferiorly. The left thyroid was identified and separated from surrounding tissues. The blood supply to the left thyroid gland was clamped off. The gland was removed from the neck. The mass was sent for frozen section diagnosis and was determined to be nodular thyroid gland tissue. Hemostasis was obtained using bipolar cautery.

A Penrose drain was placed, and the wound was closed using layered closure. The patient was awakened from anesthesia.

Exercise 32

APPLICATION

Fill in the blanks in the medical record above with the correct medical terms. The meanings of the missing terms are listed below.

1. excessive hormone production by a thyroid gland

2. enlargement of the thyroid gland

3. bulging eyes

4. scan showing the size, shape, and position of the thyroid

5. excision of a thyroid gland

Bonus Questions

6. What term used in this record means to stop bleeding? _____

7. The patient was placed in the supine position. Describe this position. _____
_____

Pronunciation and Spelling

Exercise 33

AUDITORY

Review the Chapter 15 terms in the Dictionary/Audio Glossary in the Student Resources and practice pronouncing each term, referring to the pronunciation guide as needed.

Exercise 34

SPELLING

Check the spelling of each term. If it is correct, check off the correct box. If incorrect, write the correct spelling on the line.

1. pituitery   ☐   _____

2. pancrease   ☐   _____

3. antidiuretic   ☐   _____

4. metabolism   ☐   _____

5. uthyroyd   ☐   _____

6. diabeties   ☐   _____

7. exopthalmos   ☐   _____

8. hirutism   ☐   _____

9. hyperkalemia   ☐   _____

10. glycosuria   ☐   _____

11. mixedema   ☐   _____

12. thyromegaly   ☐   _____

13. polydipsia   ☐   _____

14. glycosilated   ☐   _____

15. glucose   ☐   _____

Media Connection

Exercise 35

STUDENT
RESOURCES

Complete each of the following activities available with the Student Resources. Check off each activity as you complete it, and record your score for the Chapter Quiz in the space provided.

Chapter Exercises

____ 🔘 Flash Cards

____ 🔘 Concentration

____ 🔘 Abbreviation Match-Up

____ 🔘 Roboterms

____ 🔘 Word Builder

____ 🔘 Fill the Gap

____ 🔘 Break It Down

____ 🔘 True/False Body Builder

____ 🔘 Quiz Show

____ 🔘 Complete the Case

____ 🔘 Medical Record Review

____ 👁 Look and Label

____ 👁 Image Matching

____ 🔘 Spelling Bee

____ **Chapter Quiz**   *Score:* _____%

Additional Resources

____ 👁 Animation: Diabetes Mellitus

____ 👂 Dictionary/Audio Glossary

____ Health Professions Careers: Nurse Practitioner

____ Health Professions Careers: Surgical Assistant

Oncology and Cancer Terms

Chapter Outline

Objectives

After completion of this chapter you will be able to:

1. Define combing forms, prefixes, and suffixes related to oncology and cancer.

2. Define general terms related to oncology and cancer.

3. Define terms related to cancers of different body systems.

4. Define common medical terminology related to tests and procedures, surgical interventions and therapeutic procedures, medications and drug therapies, and specialties used to evaluate and identify cancer and cancer progression.

5. Explain abbreviations for terms related to oncology and cancers of various body systems.

6. Successfully complete all chapter exercises.

7. Explain terms used in case studies and medical records involving cancers of the various body systems.

8. Successfully complete all pronunciation and spelling exercises, and complete all interactive exercises included with the companion Student Resources.

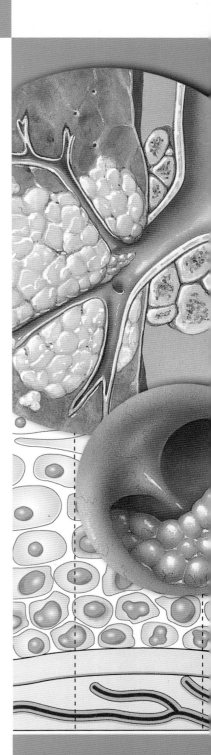

■ WORD PARTS

Note that some word parts that have been introduced earlier in the book may not be repeated here.

Combining Forms

Combining Form	Meaning
ablat/o	to take away
bi/o	life
cancer/o, carcin/o	cancer
chem/o	chemical, drug
cry/o	cold
cyt/o	cell
kary/o	nucleus
lapar/o	abdomen
lei/o	smooth
leuk/o	white
melan/o	black, dark
onc/o	tumor
path/o	disease
plas/o	growth, formation
radi/o	x-rays, radiation
rhabd/o	striated muscle
sarc/o	connective tissue, flesh
squam/o	scalelike structure

Prefixes

Prefix	Meaning
dys-	painful, difficult, abnormal
intra-	within
mal-	bad, poor
meta-	change, beyond
neo-	new
para-	beside
trans-	across, through

Suffixes

Suffix	Meaning
-gen	origin, production
-genic	originating, producing
-oma	tumor
-opsy	process of viewing
-scopy	process of examining, examination

■ Exercises: Word Parts

Exercise 1

Write the meaning of the combining form given.

1. path/o _____

2. carcin/o _____

3. onc/o _____

4. cancer/o _____

5. cry/o _____

6. melan/o _____

7. leuk/o _____

8. sarc/o _____

9. radi/o _____

10. lapar/o _____

Exercise 2

Write the correct combining form for the meaning given.

1. cell _____

2. nucleus _____

3. chemical, drug _____

4. smooth _____

5. striated muscle _____

6. scalelike structure _____

7. growth, formation _____

8. life _____

9. to take away _____

10. flesh _____

Exercise 3

SIMPLE
RECALL

Write the meaning of the prefix or suffix given.

1. meta- _____

2. -scopy _____

3. -oma _____

4. -gen _____

5. intra- _____

6. mal- _____

7. -opsy _____

8. neo- _____

9. dys- _____

10. -genic _____

11. para- _____

12. trans- _____

Exercise 4

ADVANCED
RECALL

Considering the meaning of the combining form(s) from which the medical term is made, write the meaning of the medical term (You have not yet learned many of these terms but can build their meaning from the word parts).

Combining Form(s)	Meaning(s)	Medical Term	Meaning of Term
oste/o	bone	osteoma	**1.** _____
chondr/o	cartilage	chondroma	**2.** _____
lei/o, my/o	smooth, muscle	leiomyoma	**3.** _____

carcin/o	cancer	carcinoma	4. _____
leuk/o	white	leukemia	5. _____
bi/o	life	biopsy	6. _____
my/o	muscle	myoma	7. _____
duct/o	duct	ductal	8. _____

Exercise 5

TERM
CONSTRUCTION

Using the given combining form(s) and a word part from the earlier tables, build a medical term for the meaning given.

Combining Form(s)	Meaning of Medical Term	Medical Term
cyt/o	study of cells	1. _____
squam/o	pertaining to a scalelike structure	2. _____
lei/o, my/o	tumor of smooth muscle	3. _____
sarc/o	tumor of connective tissue	4. _____
aden/o	tumor of glandular tissue	5. _____
lymph/o	tumor of lymphoid tissue	6. _____
myel/o	tumor of the bone marrow	7. _____
nephr/o	tumor of the kidney	8. _____
angi/o	tumor consisting of a mass of blood vessels	9. _____
neur/o	tumor of nervous tissue	10. _____

■ MEDICAL TERMS

General Terms Related to Oncology and Cancer

Term	Pronunciation	Meaning
		General Terms
benign	bĕ-nīn′	nonmalignant form of a neoplasm
cancer (CA)	kan′sĕr	general term for a group of diseases characterized by an abnormal, uncontrolled growth of cells

(continued)

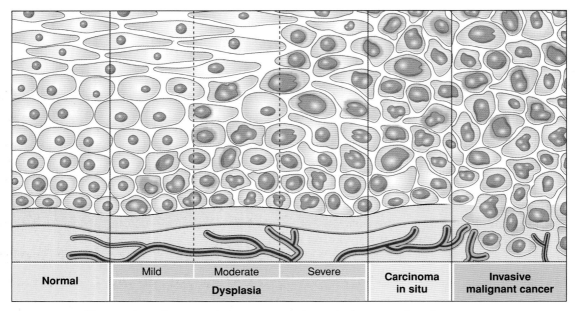

Normal	Mild	Moderate	Severe	Carcinoma in situ	Invasive malignant cancer
	Dysplasia				

Figure 16-1 Examples of tissue showing cell changes related to cancer.

General Terms Related to Oncology and Cancer *(continued)*

Term	Pronunciation	Meaning
cancerous	kan'sĕr-ŭs	pertaining to cancer
carcinogen	kahr-sin'ŏ-jen	any cancer-causing substance or organism
differentiation	dif'ĕr-en'shē-ā'shŭn	determination of how developed, or mature, the cancer cells are in a tumor
dysplasia	dis-plā'zē-ă	abnormal growth of tissue (Fig. 16-1)
in situ	in sī'tū	in the original place or site without any expansion or spread (Fig. 16-1)
invasion	in-vā'zhŭn	the direct migration and penetration by cancerous cells into neighboring tissues
lesion	lē'zhŭn	a pathologic change in tissue resulting from disease or injury
malignant	mă-lig'nănt	having the properties of locally invasive and destructive growth and metastasis (Fig. 16-1)
metastasis	mě-tas'tă-sis	spread of a disease process from one part of the body to another (Fig. 16-2)
oncogenes	ong'kō-jenz	mutated forms of genes that cause normal cells to grow out of control and become cancer cells
oncogenic	ong'kō-jen'ik	causing or being suitable for the development of a tumor
recurrence	rē-kŭr'ĕns	the return of cancer after all visible signs of it had been eradicated previously
remission	rē-mish'ŭn	lessening in severity of disease symptoms; the period of time when a cancer is responding to treatment or is under control

(continued)

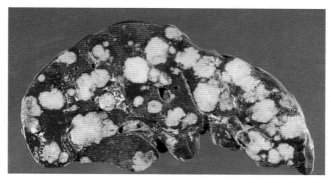

Figure 16-2 Metastatic carcinoma to the liver. The original cancer site was located elsewhere in the body.

General Terms Related to Oncology and Cancer *(continued)*

Term	Pronunciation	Meaning
Types of Tumors (Fig. 16-3)		
adenocarcinoma	ad'ĕ-nō-kahr'si-nō'mă	malignant neoplasm composed of glandular tissue (Fig. 16-4)

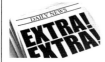 **UNDERSTANDING TUMORS** Most cancers involve the formation of tumors, meaning that they are adenocarcinomas. For example, approximately 95% of prostate cancer is classified as adenocarcinoma of the prostate and many breast cancers are determined to be adenocarcinoma of the breast.

Term	Pronunciation	Meaning
adenoma	ad'ĕ-nō'mă	benign neoplasm composed of glandular tissue
carcinoma	kahr'si-nō'mă	malignant neoplasm of any epithelial tissue
fibroma	fī-brō'mă	benign neoplasm of fibrous connective tissue
fibrosarcoma	fī'brō-sahr-kō'mă	malignant neoplasm of deep fibrous tissue
lipoma	li-pō'mă	benign neoplasm of adipose (fat) tissue
liposarcoma	lip'ō-sahr-kō'mă	malignant neoplasm of adipose (fat) tissue
malignant neoplasm	mă-lig'nănt nē'ō-plazm	tumor that invades surrounding tissue and is usually capable of metastasizing; can be located in any organ or tissue in the body
melanoma	mel'ă-nō'mă	tumor characterized by a dark appearance; most commonly occurs in the skin or in the eye
neoplasm, *syn.* tumor	nē'ō-plazm, tū'mŏr	abnormal growth of new tissue into a mass; can be benign or malignant
neuroma	nūr-ō'mă	tumor derived from nervous tissue
myeloma	mī'ĕ-lō'mă	tumor composed of cells derived from bone marrow
sarcoma	sahr-kō'mă	malignant neoplasm of connective tissue

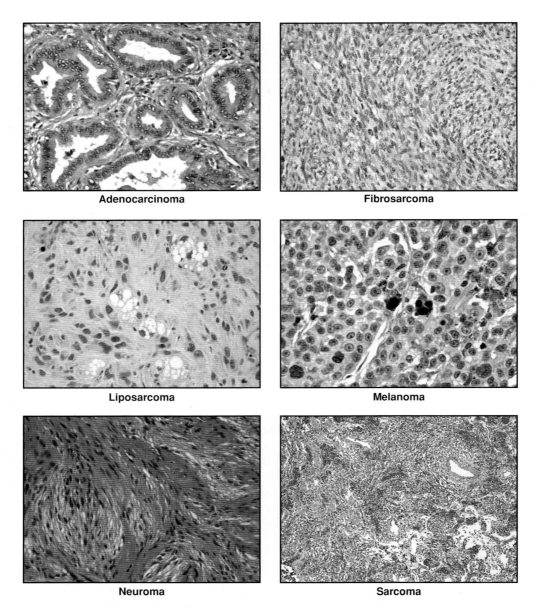

Figure 16-3   Types of tumors seen under the microscope.

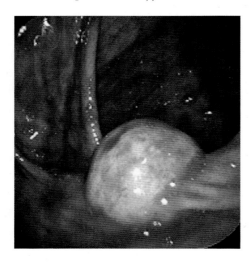

Figure 16-4   Adenocarcinoma
of the rectum.

■ Exercises: General Terms Related to Oncology and Cancer

SIMPLE
RECALL

Exercise 6

Circle the term that is most appropriate for the meaning of the sentence.

1. A nonmalignant tumor is (*oncogenic, benign, invasive*).

2. A liposarcoma is different from a lipoma in that it is a(n) (*malignant, benign, oncogenic*) neoplasm.

3. Tumors that derive from cells in the bone marrow are called (*lipomas, sarcomas, myelomas*).

4. A tumor characterized by a dark appearance is called a (*sarcoma, melanoma, myeloma*).

5. An adenocarcinoma is composed of (*squamous cells, nerve cells, glandular tissue*).

6. Something that is responsible for causing the development of a tumor is described as (*malignant, oncogenic, recurrent*).

7. Cancer that has returned after being eradicated previously is known as a (*promotion, progression, recurrence*).

8. A tumor derived from nervous tissue is called a (*nucleus, recurrence, neuroma*).

9. A tumor that is locally invasive and characterized by destructive growth and metastasis is referred to as (*benign, malignant, oncogenic*).

10. A benign neoplasm derived from fatty tissue is referred to as a (*neuroma, lipoma, fibroma*).

11. A tumor that invades surrounding tissue and is usually capable of producing metastasis is known as a(n) (*malignant neoplasm, adenoma, carcinoma*).

ADVANCED
RECALL

Exercise 7

Match each medical term with its meaning.

| dysplasia | lesion | in situ | invasion | benign |
| cancer | metastasis | tumor | carcinoma | |

Meaning	**Term**
1. malignant neoplasm of any epithelial tissue	_____
2. nonmalignant form of a neoplasm	_____
3. pathological change in tissue	_____
4. abnormal growth of tissue	_____
5. abnormal growth of new tissue into a mass	_____
6. general term for a group of diseases characterized by an abnormal, uncontrolled growth of cells	_____

7. in the original place or site   _____

8. direct migration of cancerous cells to   _____
   neighboring tissues

9. spread of disease from one part of the body   _____
   to another

TERM
CONSTRUCTION

Exercise 8

Build a medical term from the appropriate combining form(s) and suffix, given
their meanings.

Use Combining Form(s) for	Use Suffix for	Term
1. gland	tumor	_____
2. fiber	tumor	_____
3. life	process of viewing	_____
4. fatty tissue	tumor	_____
5. connective tissue	tumor	_____
6. bone marrow	tumor	_____
7. cancer	pertaining to	_____
8. fiber; connective tissue	tumor	_____

Selected Types of Cancer by Body System

Note that the table that follows describes specific cancers other than
adenocarcinomas such as carcinoma of the prostate and carcinoma of the breast.

Term	Pronunciation	Meaning
Integumentary System (Fig. 16-5)		
basal cell carcinoma (BCC)	bā′săl sel kahr′si-nō′mă	a cancer that begins in the lowest layer of the epidermis of the skin
Kaposi sarcoma	kap-ŏ′zē sahr-kō′mă	type of cancer found in the tissues under the skin or mucous membranes that line the mouth, nose, and anus; most commonly seen in patients with acquired immunodeficiency syndrome (AIDS)

(continued)

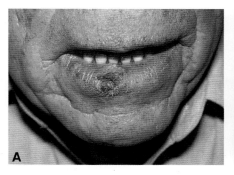
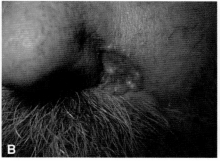
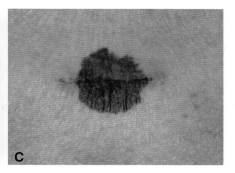

Figure 16-5   Types of skin cancer. **A.** Squamous cell carcinoma. **B.** Basal cell carcinoma. **C.** Melanoma.

Term	Pronunciation	Meaning
melanoma of the skin	mel′ă-nō′mă	a malignant skin cancer that arises from the melanocytes in the epidermis, usually caused by exposure to ultraviolet radiation

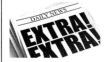

ABCD SIGNS OF MELANOMAS   UVA and UVB rays are the two types of ultraviolet rays from the sun that cause our skin to age prematurely and make us more susceptible to melanomas. The American Cancer Society encourages people to check their skin at least once a month to check for signs of melanomas. These signs can be remembered with the acronym *ABCD:*

- *A* is for *asymmetry.* Look for any areas of skin, pigmentation, or moles that are not the same all around.
- *B* stands for *border.* Check to be sure that any suspicious areas do not have a ragged border.
- *C* is for *color.* If an area is changing in color or is not the same color throughout, this is a clear sign that the area needs to be checked.
- *D* is for the *diameter.* Check for spots that are the size of a pencil eraser or larger.

The American Academy of Dermatology adds a fifth sign, *E,* that stands for *evolving.* A dermatologist should examine an area of skin, a mole, or any pigmentation that changes in any way from one skin check to the next.

squamous cell carcinoma (SCC)	skwā′mŭs sel kahr′si-nō′mă	a cancer that begins in the squamous cells located in the upper levels of the epidermis of the skin
Digestive System		
gastrointestinal stromal tumor (GIST)	gas′trō-in-tes′ti-năl strō′măl tū′mŏr	a very rare cancer affecting the digestive tract or nearby structures within the abdomen
Urinary System		
malignant neoplasm of the bladder	mă-lig′nănt nē′ō-plazm blad′ĕr	cancerous tumor of the bladder
nephroma	ne-frō′mă	tumor of the kidney
urothelial carcinoma, *syn.* transitional cell carcinoma	yūr′ō-thē′lē-ăl kahr′si-nō′mă, tran-zish′ŭn-ăl sel kahr′si-nō′mă	cancer arising in the urothelium lining the urinary tract
Wilms tumor	vilmz tū′mŏr	rare type of kidney cancer that affects children (Fig. 16-6)

(continued)

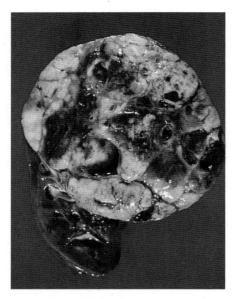

Figure 16-6   Wilms tumor.

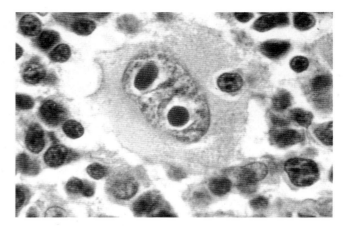

Figure 16-7   Reed-Sternberg cells as seen in Hodgkin disease.

Term	Pronunciation	Meaning
Blood and Immune System		
Hodgkin disease	hoj′kin di-zēz′	abnormal malignant enlargement of lymph nodes, spleen, and liver; indicated by the presence of Reed-Sternberg cells (Fig. 16-7)
leukemia	lū-kē′mē-ă	cancer of the blood indicated by malignant increase in the number of white blood cells
lymphangioma	lim-fan′jē-ō′mă	mass or tumor of lymph vessels
lymphoma	lim-fō′mă	tumor of lymphoid tissue, including lymphocytes and plasma cells
non-Hodgkin lymphoma (NHL)	non-hoj′kin lim-fō′mă	lymphoma other than Hodgkin disease
Respiratory System		
bronchogenic carcinoma	brong′kō-jen′ik kahr′si-nō′mă	carcinoma that arises from the mucosa of the large bronchi

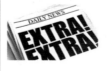 **TOBACCO USE AND CANCERS** Tobacco use, which is the most preventable cause of cancer, can be linked to at least 15 different types of cancers. These include bronchogenic carcinoma and other cancers of the lung, as well as pancreatic, uterine, mouth, nose, throat, larynx, stomach, kidney, and bladder cancers.

mesothelioma	mez′ō-thē-lē-ō′mă	a carcinoma of the mesothelium lining of the lungs or heart, usually associated with exposure to asbestos dust
oat cell carcinoma	ōt sel kahr′si-nō′mă	highly malignant form of lung or bronchogenic cancer in which cells appear small and rounded under a microscope (Fig. 16-8)

(continued)

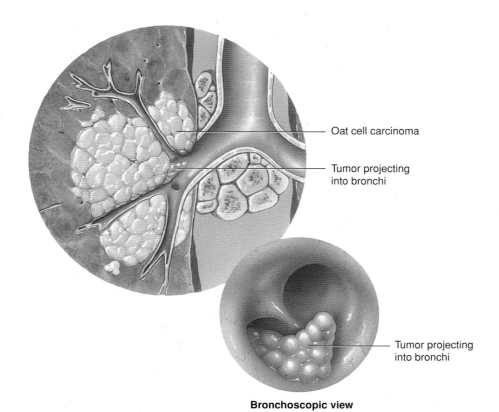

Oat cell carcinoma

Tumor projecting
into bronchi

Tumor projecting
into bronchi

Bronchoscopic view

Figure 16-8   Oat cell carcinoma.

Term	Pronunciation	Meaning
Female Reproductive System		
ductal carcinoma in situ (DCIS)	dŭk′tăl kahr′si-nō′mă in sĭ′tū	a breast cancer that is confined to the ducts and has not spread into the tissue of the breast (Fig. 16-9)
germ cell tumor	jĕrm sel tū′mŏr	cancer that begins in the egg-producing cells of the ovaries
stromal cell tumor	strō′măl sel tū′mŏr	cancer that begins in the cells of the ligaments of the ovaries
Nervous System		
astrocytoma	as′trō-sī-tō′mă	a tumor that arises from small, star-shaped cells in the brain and spinal cord
glioma	glī-ō′mă	cancer that arises from the glial cells of the nervous system
medulloblastoma	mĕ-dŭl′ō-blas-tō′mă	cancer that develops from the primitive nerve cells in the cerebellum
meningioma	mĕ-nin′jē-ō′mă	benign and slow-growing tumor of the meninges
neuroblastoma	nūr′ō-blas-tō′mă	a cancer of the nervous system

(continued)

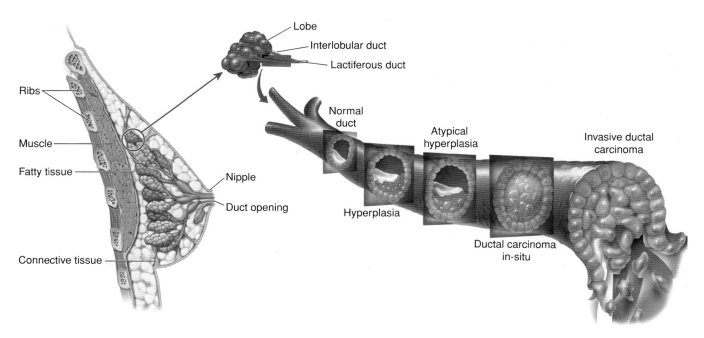

Figure 16-9 Progression to ductal carcinoma in situ and invasive ductal carcinoma of the breast.

Term	Pronunciation	Meaning
Sensory Systems		
glomus tumor	glō′mŭs tū′mŏr	a benign but locally invasive tumor arising out of glomus tissue found in the middle ear, jugular bulb, and carotid artery
intraocular melanoma	in′tră-ok′yū-lăr mel′ă-nō′mă	a malignant cancer that forms in the tissues of the eye
retinoblastoma	ret′i-nō-blas-tō′mă	a malignant ocular tumor of retinal cells
Musculoskeletal System		
chondroma	kon-drō′mă	a common benign tumor arising from cartilage cells
chondrosarcoma	kon′drō-sahr-kō′mă	a large malignant tumor arising from cartilage cells
Ewing tumor, *syn.* Ewing sarcoma	ū′ing tū′mŏr, ū′ing sahr-kō′mă	a malignant tumor found in bone or soft tissue
giant cell tumor	jī′ănt sel tū′mŏr	a tumor of the tendon sheath that can be either benign or malignant
leiomyoma	lī′ō-mī-ō′mă	benign tumor of smooth (nonstriated) muscle
leiomyosarcoma	lī′ō-mī′ō-sahr-kō′mă	malignant tumor of smooth (nonstriated) muscle
liposarcoma	lip′ō-sahr-kō′mă	a malignant tumor of adipose (fat) tissue; occurs in the retroperitoneal tissues and the thigh

(continued)

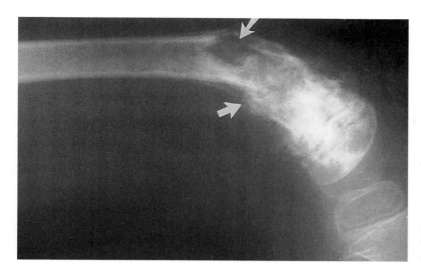

Figure 16-10 Radiograph of a 5-year-old girl with an osteosarcoma of the left femur showing an acute fracture (*arrows*).

Term	Pronun ciation	Meaning
osteofibroma	os'tē-ō-fī-brō'mă	benign lesion of bone consisting chiefly of fairly dense, moderately cellular, fibrous connective tissue
osteosarcoma	os'tē-ō-sahr-kō'mă	a fast-growing malignant type of bone cancer that develops in the osteoblast cells that form the outer covering of bone (Fig. 16-10)
rhabdomyoma	rab'dō-mī-ō'mă	benign tumor of striated muscle
rhabdomyosarcoma	rab'dō-mī'ō-sahr-kō'mă	a highly malignant tumor of striated muscle
Endocrine System		
multiple endocrine neoplasia (MEN)	mŭl'ti-pĕl en'dō-krin nē-ō-plā'zē-ă	a group of disorders characterized by functioning tumors in more than one endocrine gland
pheochromocytoma	fē'ō-krō'mō-sī-tō'mă	a vascular tumor of the adrenal gland (Fig. 16-11)
pituitary adenoma	pi-tū'i-tar-ē ad'ĕ-nō'mă	a benign tumor arising in the pituitary gland

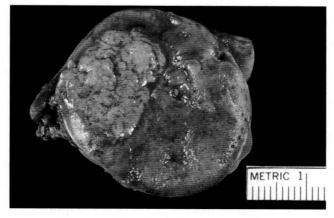

Figure 16-11 Pheochromocytoma.

■ Exercises: Selected Types of Cancer by Body System

Exercise 9

Write the correct medical term for the meaning given.

1. tumor of lymphoid tissue _____

2. tumor of mucosa of the bronchi _____

3. benign tumor of smooth muscle _____

4. benign tumor of cartilage cells _____

5. malignant tumor arising from bone-forming cells _____

6. malignant tumor of fat cells _____

7. tumor of lymph vessels _____

8. a rare type of kidney cancer _____

9. skin cancer usually caused by UV radiation _____

10. tumor of the glial cells _____

11. benign, fibrous tumor of bone _____

12. tumor of the tendon sheath _____

13. benign tumor of striated muscle _____

14. tumor of the mesothelium lining of the lungs or heart _____

15. tumor in the middle ear _____

Exercise 10

Circle the term that is most appropriate for the meaning of the sentence.

1. (*Cytopenia, Leukemia, Liposarcoma*) is cancer of the blood.

2. A(n) (*GIST, SCC, DCIS*) tumor is typically found in the gastrointestinal tract.

3. A type of kidney cancer that affects children is known as a(n) (*Ewing, Kaposi, Wilms*) tumor.

4. The presence of Reed-Sternberg cells signifies (*non-Hodgkin, Hodgkin, Ewing*) disease.

5. A vascular tumor of the adrenal gland is known as a(n) (*adrenal adenoma, pheochromocytoma, vascular adenoma*).

6. Ewing sarcoma is a malignant tumor found in (*skin, bone, cartilage*) or soft tissue.

7. A(n) (*osteofibroma, leiomyoma, chondrosarcoma*) is a malignant tumor arising from cartilage cells.

8. A (*giant cell tumor, GIST, sarcoma*) involves the tendon sheaths.

9. A(n) (*adenoma, leiomyosarcoma, retinoblastoma*) could eventually lead to blindness.

10. A (*myoma, squamous cell carcinoma, meningioma*) grows from the meninges.

ADVANCED
RECALL

Exercise 11

Match each medical term with its meaning.

| neuroblastoma | stromal cell tumor | basal cell carcinoma | Kaposi sarcoma |
| medulloblastoma | oat cell carcinoma | squamous cell carcinoma | |

Meaning   **Term**

1. cancer from the primitive nerve cells in the cerebellum   _____

2. cancer in the cells of the ligaments of the ovaries   _____

3. highly malignant form of lung cancer   _____

4. a cancer in the upper layer of the epidermis   _____

5. a cancer in the lowest layer of the epidermis   _____

6. a cancer of the nervous system   _____

7. cancer most commonly seen in patients with AIDS   _____

TERM
CONSTRUCTION

Exercise 12

Build a medical term for each meaning, using one or more of the listed combining forms and one of the listed suffixes (Note: Combining forms and suffixes may be used more than once.)

Combining Forms		**Suffixes**
my/o	gli/o	-oma
lei/o	sarc/o	-emia
aden/o	astr/o	
cyt/o	carcin/o	
rhabd/o	lymph/o	
nephr/o	leuk/o	

1. tumor of the kidney   _____

2. tumor of lymphoid tissue   _____

3. cancer of the blood   _____

4. tumor of glial cells   _____

5. tumor of a gland _____

6. benign tumor of smooth (nonstriated) muscle _____

7. malignant tumor of smooth (nonstriated) muscle _____

8. tumor arising from starlike cells _____

9. malignant neoplasm of epithelial tissue _____

10. malignant tumor of nonsmooth (striated) muscle _____

Laboratory Tests

Term	Pronunciation	Meaning
alpha fetoprotein (AFP)	al′fă fē′tō-prō′tēn	blood test for substance produced by tumor cells in the body; found in elevated levels in patients with ovarian cancer
estrogen receptors	es′trō-jen rĕ-sep′tŏrz	blood test for a type of protein present on some breast cancer cells to which estrogen attaches
human chorionic gonadotropin (hCG) test	hyū′măn kōr′ē-on′ik gō-nad′ō-trō′pin	blood test for the substance that, in elevated levels, may indicate cancer in the testis, ovary, liver, stomach, pancreas, or lung
Papanicolaou (Pap) test	pa-pă-ni′kō-lō (pap) test	microscopic examination of cells collected from the vagina and cervix to detect abnormal changes (e.g., cancer)
prostate-specific antigen (PSA)	pros′tăt-spĕ-sif′ik an′ti-jen	blood test for substance produced only by the prostate; elevated levels may indicate prostate cancer in its early stages
tumor marker test	tū′mŏr mahr′kĕr test	various blood tests for specific substances produced by certain types of tumors

Diagnostic Procedures

Term	Pronunciation	Meaning
General Diagnostic Procedures		
biopsy	bī′op-sē	the process of removing tissue from living patients for diagnostic examination
fine needle aspiration (FNA)	fīn nē′dĕl as-pir-ā′shŭn	procedure of withdrawing cells from a lesion for examination with a fine needle on a syringe (Fig. 16-12)
radionuclide scan	rā′dē-ō-nū′klīd skan	imaging scan in which a small amount of radioactive substance is injected into the vein; a machine measures levels of radioactivity in certain organs, which may indicate abnormal areas or tumors
sentinel lymph node biopsy	sen′ti-nĕl limf nōd bī′op-sē	removal and examination of the sentinel nodes, which are the first lymph nodes to which cancer cells are likely to spread from a primary tumor

(continued)

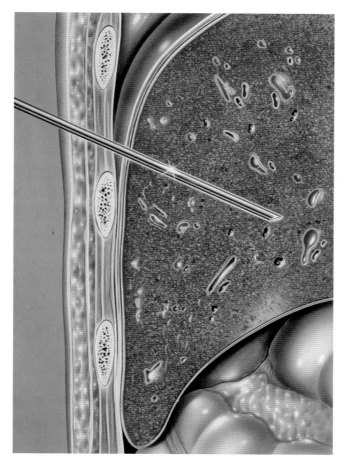

Figure 16-12 Fine needle aspiration of the liver.

Diagnostic Procedures *(continued)*

Term	Pronunciation	Meaning
single photon emission computed tomography (SPECT) scan	sing'gĕl fō'ton ē-mi'shŭn kŏm-pyūt'ĕd tŏ-mog'ră-fē skan	type of nuclear imaging test that shows how blood flows to tissues and organs; can help identify certain types of tumors
Related to the Integumentary System		
punch biopsy	pŭnch bī'op-sē	removal of a small oval core of skin for laboratory analysis using a sharp, hollow instrument
shave biopsy	shav bī'op-sē	removal of a sample of skin for laboratory analysis using a scalpel to slice the specimen from the site
Related to the Digestive System		
cholescintigraphy, *syn.* hepatobiliary iminodiacetic acid (HIDA) scan	kō'lē-sin-tig'ră-fē, hĕ-pat'ō-bil'ē-ar-ē i'mĕ-nō-dī-ă-sē'tik as'id skan	imaging test used to examine the function of the liver, gallbladder, and bile ducts
endoscopic retrograde cholangiopancreatography (ERCP)	en'dō-skop'ik ret'rō-grād kō-lan'jē-ō-pan'krē-ă-tog'ră-fē	procedure using x-ray and injectable dye to examine disorders in the bile ducts, gallbladder, and pancreas

(continued)

Diagnostic Procedures *(continued)*

Term	Pronunciation	Meaning
endoscopic ultrasound (EUS)	en'dō-skop'ik ŭl'tră-sownd	procedure using an ultrasound imaging device on the tip of an endoscope for evaluation of the bowel wall and adjacent structures
magnetic resonance cholangiopancreato-graphy (MRCP)	mag-net'ik rez'ŏ-năns kō-lan'jē-ō-pan'krē-ă-tog'ră-fē	procedure using magnetic resonance imaging and an injectable dye to examine problems in the bile ducts, gallbladder, and pancreas
Related to the Lymph System		
lymph node biopsy	limf nōd bī'op-sē	removal of lymph node tissue for pathologic evaluation
Related to the Blood and Immune System		
bone marrow aspiration	bōn mar'ō as-pir-ā'shŭn	removal of a small amount of fluid and cells from inside the bone with a needle and syringe
bone marrow biopsy	bōn mar'ō bī'op-sē	removal and evaluation of a small amount of bone along with fluid and cells from inside the bone
lumbar puncture (LP)	lŭm'bahr pungk'shŭr	the process of inserting a needle into the subarachnoid space of the lumbar spine to obtain cerebrospinal fluid for analysis; used to determine if leukemic cells are present
Related to the Respiratory System		
thoracoscopy, *syn.* pleuroscopy	thōr-ă-kos'kŏ-pē, plŭr-os'kŏ-pē	endoscopic examination of the thorax made through a small opening in the chest wall
Related to the Male Reproductive System		
prostate biopsy	pros'tāt bī'op-sē	a procedure in which tissue samples are removed from the body for examination under a microscope to determine whether cancerous or other abnormal cells are present
transrectal ultrasound (TRUS)	trans-rek'tăl ŭl'tră-sownd	ultrasound imaging of the prostate done through the rectum; used to diagnose prostate cancer

(continued)

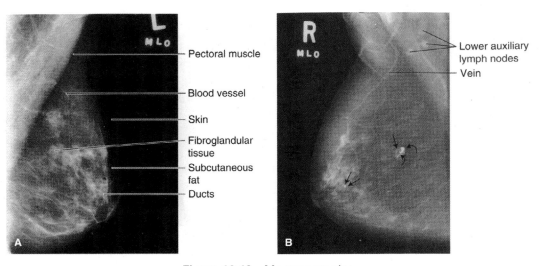

Figure 16-13 Mammography.

Diagnostic Procedures *(continued)*

Term	Pronunciation	Meaning
Related to the Female Reproductive System		
cervical conization, *syn.* cone biopsy	sĕr'vi-kăl kon'i-zā'shŭn, kōn bī'op-sē	biopsy of the cervix in which a cone-shaped sample of tissue is removed from the cervix
colposcopy	kol-pos'kŏ-pē	visual examination of the tissues of the cervix and vagina using a lighted microscope (colposcope) to identify abnormal cell growth and, if necessary, remove a tissue sample for biopsy
endometrial biopsy	en'dō-mē'trē-ăl bīop-sē	procedure whereby a sample of the endometrium of the uterus is removed from the body and examined under a microscope; used to check for uterine cancer
mammography	mă-mog'ră-fē	an x-ray examination of the breasts; used to detect breast tumors (Fig. 16-13)

■ Exercises: Laboratory Tests and Diagnostic Procedures

SIMPLE
RECALL

Exercise 13

Circle the term that is most appropriate for the meaning of the sentence.

1. A scan that measures levels of radioactivity in certain organs is called a (*single photon emission computed tomography scan, radionuclide scan, cholescintigraphy*).

2. (*Endoscopic retrograde cholangiopancreatography, Magnetic resonance imaging, Magnetic resonance cholangiopancreatography*) is a procedure using x-ray and injectable dye.

3. A gallbladder function problem may be diagnosed by a(n) (*endometrial biopsy, pleuroscopy, cholescintigraphy*).

4. A (*transrectal ultrasound, lumbar puncture, fine needle aspiration*) withdraws cells from a lesion for examination with a fine needle on a syringe.

5. To help determine if leukemic cells are present in the cerebrospinal fluid, a patient may undergo a (*lumbar puncture, bronchoscopy, colonoscopy*).

6. An examination of cells obtained from the cervix is called a (*prostate biopsy, prostate-specific antigen, Pap test*).

7. Various blood tests for specific substances produced by certain types of tumors are called (*tumor markers, progesterone receptors, estrogen receptors*).

8. To investigate carcinoma of the lung, a surgeon may make a small opening in the chest wall to perform a (*bone marrow biopsy, hepatobiliary iminodiacetic acid scan, thoracoscopy*).

9. To help identify certain types of tumors, a physician may order a test that shows an image of blood flow to tissues and organs, called a (*mammography, single photon emission computed tomography scan, computed tomography scan*).

10. The blood test for the substance that, in elevated levels, may indicate cancer in the testis, ovary, liver, stomach, pancreas, or lung is abbreviated (*SPECT, hCG, AFP*).

Exercise 14

ADVANCED RECALL

Complete each sentence by writing in the correct medical term.

1. Removal and examination of the first lymph node to which cancer cells are likely to spread from a primary tumor is called a(n) _____.

2. A(n) _____ is a blood test for a substance produced by tumor cells found in elevated levels in patients with ovarian cancer.

3. A blood test for a substance made only by the prostate, elevated levels of which may indicate prostate cancer in its early stages, is called _____.

4. A type of protein present on some breast cancer cells to which estrogen attaches is called _____.

5. The removal of a sample of skin for laboratory analysis using a scalpel to slice the specimen from the site is called a(n) _____.

6. A(n) _____ is the removal of a sample of skin using a hollow instrument.

7. A procedure using an ultrasound imaging device on the tip of an endoscope for evaluation of bowel wall and adjacent structures is known as a(n) _____.

8. An x-ray examination of the breasts used to detect breast tumors is called _____.

9. A(n) _____ is a diagnostic test that uses ultrasound to visualize the prostate gland.

10. A(n) _____ is a visual examination of the tissues of the cervix and vagina using a lighted instrument.

Exercise 15

TERM CONSTRUCTION

Build a medical term from the appropriate combining form and suffix, given their meanings.

Use Combining Form for	Use Suffix for	Term
1. vagina	process of examining	_____
2. life	process of viewing	_____
3. thorax, chest	process of examining	_____
4. breast	process of recording	_____

Surgical Interventions

Term	Pronunciation	Meaning
General Surgical Interventions		
brachytherapy, *syn.* seed implantation	brak′ē-thăr′ă-pē, sēd im′plan-tā′shŭn	procedure by which radioactive "seeds" are placed inside cancerous tissue and positioned to kill nearby cancer cells
cryosurgery	krī′ō-sŭr′jĕr-ē	the use of freezing temperatures to destroy tissue
debulking surgery	dē-bŭlk′ing sŭr′jĕr-ē	excision of a major part of a tumor that cannot be completely removed
palliative surgery	pal′ē-ă-tiv sŭr′jĕr-ē	surgery that is performed to relieve pain or other symptoms but not to cure the cancer or prolong a patient's life
radiofrequency ablation (RFA)	rā′dē-ō-frē′kwĕn-sē ab-lā′shŭn	procedure in which a surgical oncologist uses a small probe to deliver heat from radiofrequency energy to kill cancerous tissue; used primarily to treat liver, prostate, renal, bone, and breast cancer
reconstructive surgery	rē′kon-strŭk′tiv sŭr′jĕr-ē	surgery performed to return function and appearance to a specific area of the body after removal of a tumor
Related to the Integumentary System		
Mohs surgery	mōz sŭr′jĕr-ē	surgical procedure that involves removing and examining a piece of tumor in the skin bit by bit until the entire lesion is removed
Related to the Digestive System		
colectomy	kŏ-lek′tŏ-mē	excision of all or part of the colon
esophagectomy	ĕ-sof-ă-jek′tŏ-mē	excision of the diseased portion of the esophagus and all associated tissues that might contain cancer
gastrectomy, *syn.* Billroth operation I and II	gas-trek′tŏ-mē, bil′rōt op-ĕr-ā′shŭn	excision of part or all of the stomach
pancreaticoduodenectomy, *syn.* Whipple operation	pan′krē-at′ĭ-kō-dū-od′en-ek′tŏ-mē, wip′ĕl op-ĕr-ā′shŭn	partial excision of the stomach, complete excision of the gallbladder, a portion of the bile duct, head of the pancreas, portions of the small intestine, and regional lymph nodes to stop the spread of cancer in these areas
Related to the Urinary System		
cystectomy	sis-tek′tŏ-mē	surgical removal of part or all of the bladder
fulguration	ful′gŭr-ā′shŭn	destruction of tissue by means of high-frequency electric current; commonly used to remove tumors from inside the bladder
nephrectomy	ne-frek′tŏ-mē	excision of a kidney
transurethral resection of bladder tumor (TURB)	trans-yŭr-ē′thrăl rē-sek′shŭn of blad′ĕr tū′mŏr	excision of a tumor from the bladder through the urethra using a resectoscope

(continued)

Surgical Interventions *(continued)*

Term	Pronunciation	Meaning
Related to the Lymph System		
lymphadenectomy	lim-fad'ĕ-nek'tŏ-mē	excision of a lymph node
Related to the Blood and Immune System		
bone marrow transplant (BMT)	bōn ma'rō trans'plant	transfer of bone marrow from one person to another
peripheral stem cell transplant	pĕr-if'ĕr-ăl stem sel trans'plant	the collection and freezing of stem cells from the blood, which are then reintroduced into the patient after chemotherapy
Related to the Respiratory System		
lobectomy	lō-bek'tŏ-mē	excision of a lobe (of the lung)
pneumonectomy	nū'mō-nek'tŏ-mē	excision of the lung
wedge resection	wej rē-sek'shŭn	excision of part of a lobe of the lung (Fig. 16-14)
Related to the Male Reproductive System		
prostatectomy, *syn.* transurethral resection of the prostate (TURP)	pros'tă-tek'tŏ-mē, trans-yŭr-ē'thrăl rē-sek'shŭn of pros'tāt	removal of prostate tissue through the urethra using a resectoscope
Related to the Female Reproductive System		
loop electrosurgical excision procedure (LEEP)	lūp ĕ-lek'trō-sĭr'jik-ăl ek-sizh'ŭn prŏ-sē'jŭr	gynecologic procedure that uses a thin, low-voltage electrified wire loop to cut out cancerous tissue in the cervix
mastectomy	mas-tek'tŏ-mē	excision of a breast to remove a malignant tumor
modified radical mastectomy	mod'i-fīd rad'i-kăl mas-tek'tŏ-mē	excision of a breast along with some of the underlying muscle and lymph nodes in the adjacent armpit (Fig. 16-15B)

(continued)

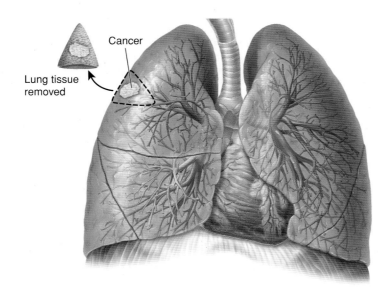

Cancer

Lung tissue removed

Figure 16-14 Wedge resection of the lung.

Surgical Interventions *(continued)*

Term	Pronunciation	Meaning
radical mastectomy	rad′i-kăl mas-tek′tŏ-mē	excision of the breast as well as the underlying muscles and lymph nodes in the adjacent armpit (Fig. 16-15C)
simple mastectomy	simp′ĕl mas-tek′tŏ-mē	excision of a breast, leaving the underlying muscles and the lymph nodes intact (Fig 16-15A)
myomectomy	mī′ō-mek′tŏ-mē	excision of myomas
Related to the Nervous System		
craniectomy	krā′nē-ek′tŏ-mē	excision of part of the cranium to access the brain
stereotactic radiosurgery	ster′ē-ō-tak′tik rā′dē-ō-sŭr′jĕr-ē	radiation therapy technique for treating brain tumors by aiming high-dose radiation beams directly at the tumors
Related to the Sensory System		
enucleation	ē-nū′klē-ā′shŭn	removal of an eyeball
iridectomy	ir′i-dek′tŏ-mē	excision of part of the iris (for very small melanomas)
laryngectomy	lar′in-jek′tŏ-mē	excision of all or part of the larynx, usually to treat cancer of the larynx
Related to the Musculoskeletal System		
amputation	amp′yū-tā′shŭn	surgical removal of an entire limb
limb salvage surgery	lim salvăj sŭr′jĕr-ē	surgical procedure in which only the cancerous section of bone is removed but nearby muscles, tendons, and other structures are left intact
Related to the Endocrine System		
parathyroidectomy	par′ă-thī-roy-dek′tŏ-mē	excision of a parathyroid gland
thyroidectomy	thī′roy-dek′tŏ-mē	excision of the thyroid gland
transsphenoidal resection	tranz-sfē-noy′dăl rē-sek′shŭn	excision of a pituitary adenoma by making an incision through the nose to the bottom of the skull where the pituitary gland is located

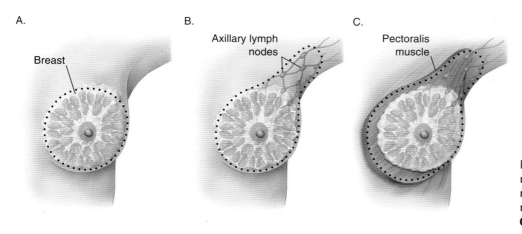

A.
Breast

B.
Axillary lymph nodes

C.
Pectoralis muscle

Figure 16-15 Types of mastectomies. **A.** Simple mastectomy. **B.** Modified radical mastectomy. **C.** Radical mastectomy.

Therapeutic Procedures

Term	Pronunciation	Meaning
external beam radiation	eks-tĕr'năl bēm rā'dē-ā'shŭn	procedure by which a beam of high-energy radiation is applied externally directly to the tumor to minimize damage to other tissues
radiation therapy	rā'dē-ā'shŭn thăr'ă-pē	the use of high-energy x-rays or other particles to kill cancer cells

■ Exercises: Surgical Interventions and Therapeutic Procedures

SIMPLE RECALL

Exercise 16

Write the correct medical term for the meaning given.

1. use of heat from radiofrequency energy to kill cancerous tissue _____

2. use of high-energy x-rays or other particles to kill cancer cells _____

3. excision of a breast to remove a malignant tumor _____

4. transfer of bone marrow from one person to another _____

5. use of an electrified wire loop to cut out cancerous tissue in the cervix _____

6. surgical removal of an entire limb _____

7. destruction of tissue using high-frequency electric current to remove tumors from the bladder _____

8. process of removing and examining a piece of tumor in the skin bit by bit until the entire lesion is removed _____

9. excision of a major part of a tumor that can not be completely removed _____

10. collection and freezing of stem cells from the blood and then reintroducing them into the patient after chemotherapy _____

ADVANCED RECALL

Exercise 17

Circle the term that is most appropriate for the meaning of the sentence.

1. The patient underwent a (*TURP, TURB, LEEP*) procedure to remove a tumor from her bladder.

2. Although her cancer could not be cured, Mrs. Johnson underwent (*reconstructive, debulking, palliative*) surgery to relieve her pain and symptoms.

3. The patient is a 51-year-old woman with recently diagnosed colon cancer who recently underwent a subtotal (*colectomy, iridectomy, myomectomy*).

4. The patient had a (*Billroth, Whipple, Mohs*) operation to stop the spread of cancer to various digestive organs and lymph nodes.

5. Mr. McDowell has had no bone pain since his (*thyroidectomy, limb salvage surgery, craniectomy*) for metastatic cancer of the femur.

6. Mrs. Elias was scheduled for a (*thyroidectomy, parathyroidectomy, transsphenoidal resection*) for removal of a pituitary adenoma.

7. The surgeon performed a (*pneumonectomy, wedge resection, lobectomy*) to remove the small tumor located in the lobe of the patient's lung.

8. Because of the malignant nature of Mrs. Harmon's cancer, the surgeon removed the breast as well as the underlying muscles and lymph nodes in the adjacent armpit; this procedure is known as a (*simple, modified radical, radical*) mastectomy.

9. The patient underwent (*wedge resection, transsphenoidal resection, stereotactic radiosurgery*) to treat his brain tumor.

10. Mr. O'Malley had small pellets of radioactive material applied directly to a cancer lesion during a procedure called (*radiation therapy, reconstructive surgery, brachytherapy*).

TERM
CONSTRUCTION

Exercise 18

Using the given suffix, build a medical term for the meaning given.

Suffix	Meaning of Medical Term	Medical Term
-ectomy	excision of all or part of the esophagus	1. _____
-ectomy	excision of the thyroid gland	2. _____
-ectomy	excision of all or part of the stomach	3. _____
-ectomy	excision of a breast	4. _____
-ectomy	excision of one or both kidneys	5. _____
-ectomy	excision of a lymph node	6. _____
-ectomy	excision of myomas	7. _____
-ectomy	excision of a lobe (of the lung)	8. _____

TERM
CONSTRUCTION

Exercise 19

Break the given medical term into its word parts and define each part. Then define the medical term.

For example:

laparotomy	*word parts:*	lapar/o / -tomy
	meanings:	abdomen / incision
	term meaning:	incision into the abdomen

1. pneumonectomy *word parts:* _____ / _____

 meanings: _____ / _____

 term meaning: _____

2. colectomy *word parts:* _____ / _____

 meanings: _____ / _____

 term meaning: _____

3. cystectomy *word parts:* _____ / _____

 meanings: _____ / _____

 term meaning: _____

4. thyroidectomy *word parts:* _____ / _____

 meanings: _____ / _____

 term meaning: _____

5. laryngectomy *word parts:* _____ / _____

 meanings: _____ / _____

 term meaning: _____

6. iridectomy *word parts:* _____ / _____

 meanings: _____ / _____

 term meaning: _____

7. craniectomy *word parts:* _____ / _____

 meanings: _____ / _____

 term meaning: _____

8. gastrectomy   *word parts:*   _____ / _____

                           meanings: _____ / _____

                           term meaning: _____

Medications and Drug Therapies

Term	Pronunciation	Meaning
aromatase inhibitors	ă-rō′mă-tās in-hib′i-tŏrz	group of drugs designed to reduce estrogen levels in a woman's body and stop the growth of cancer cells that depend on estrogen to live and grow
chemoprevention	kē′mō-prē-ven′shŭn	the use of natural or synthetic products to keep cancer at bay or to stop the disease process before it becomes invasive
chemotherapy	kē′mō-thār′ă-pē	regimen of therapy that uses chemicals to treat cancer (Fig. 16-16)
adjuvant chemotherapy	ad′jū-vănt kē′mō-thār′ă-pē	chemotherapy given in addition to surgery, to destroy remaining residual tumor or to reduce the risk of recurrence

(continued)

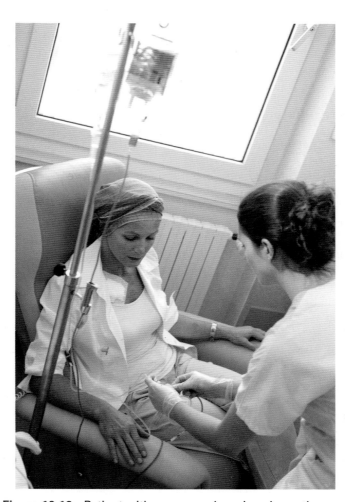

Figure 16-16 Patient with cancer undergoing chemotherapy.

Surgical Interventions *(continued)*

Term	Pronunciation	Meaning
interstitial chemotherapy	in'tĕr-stish'ăl kē'mō-thār'ă-pē	placement of chemotherapy drugs directly into a tumor
intrathecal chemotherapy	in'tră-thē'kăl kē'mō-thār'ă-pē	delivery of chemotherapy drugs into the spinal canal
palliative chemotherapy	pal'ē-ă-tiv kē'mō-thār'ă-pē	chemotherapy that is given to relieve pain or other symptoms of cancer but not to cure it
epidermal growth factor receptor (EGFR) inhibitor therapy	ep'i-dĕr'măl grōth fak'tŏr rĕ-sep'tŏr in-hib'i-tŏr thār'ă-pē	drugs that interfere with the growth of individual cancer cells
hormonal therapy	hôr-mōn'ăl thār'ă-pē	use of hormones to stop a tumor from growing, to relieve symptoms caused by a tumor, or to replace the hormone that is needed by the body to function properly after a body part is removed due to cancer
immunotherapy, *syn.* biologic therapy	im'yū-nō-thār'ă-pē, bī'ŏ-loj'ik thār'ă-pē	method of boosting the body's natural defenses to fight cancer by using materials made either by the body or in a laboratory to bolster, target, or restore immune system function

■ Exercise: Medications and Drug Therapies

SIMPLE
RECALL

Exercise 20

Write the correct medication or drug therapy term for the meaning given.

1. chemotherapy given in addition to surgery   _____

2. use of hormones to stop a tumor from growing or relieve symptoms caused by a tumor   _____

3. delivery of chemotherapy drugs into the spinal canal   _____

4. group of drugs designed to reduce estrogen levels in a woman's body and stop the growth of cancer cells   _____

5. method of boosting the body's natural defenses to fight cancer   _____

6. chemotherapy given to relieve pain only   _____

7. regimen of therapy that uses chemicals to kill cancer cells   _____

8. use of natural or synthetic products to keep cancer at bay or to derail the disease process before it becomes invasive   _____

9. use of drugs that interfere with the growth of individual cancer cells   _____

10. placement of chemotherapy drugs directly into a tumor   _____

Specialties and Specialists

Term	Pronunciation	Meaning
gynecologic oncology	gī′nĕ-kŏ-loj′ik ong-kol′ŏ-jē	medical specialty concerned with the diagnosis and treatment of cancers of the female reproductive system
gynecologic oncologist	gī′nĕ-kŏ-loj′ik ong-kol′ŏ-jist	physician who specializes in the care and treatment of women with gynecologic cancers
medical oncology	med′i-kăl ong-kol′ŏ-jē	medical specialty concerned with the use of medical and chemotherapeutic treatments of cancer
medical oncologist	med′i-kăl ong-kol′ŏ-jist	physician who specializes in treating cancer with chemotherapy
oncology	ong-kol′ŏ-jē	medical specialty concerned with the physical, chemical, and biologic properties and features of cancers
oncologist	ong-kol′ŏ-jist	physician who specializes in the science of oncology
pediatric oncology	pē-dē-at′rik ong-kol′ŏ-jē	medical specialty concerned with the diagnosis and treatment of childhood cancers and blood diseases
pediatric oncologist	pē-dē-at′rik ong-kol′ŏ-jist	physician who specializes in the treatment of childhood cancers and blood diseases
radiation oncology	rā′dē-ā′shŭn ong-kol′ŏ-jē	radiologic specialty concerned with radiation treatment as the main mode of treatment for cancer
radiation oncologist	rā′dē-ā′shŭn ong-kol′ŏ-jist	physician who specializes in treating cancer with high-energy x-rays to destroy cancerous cells
surgical oncology	sŭr′ji-kăl ong-kol′ŏ-jē	surgical specialty concerned with the surgical aspects of cancer
surgical oncologist	sŭr′ji-kăl ong-kol′ŏ-jist	physician who specializes in the surgical aspects of cancer, including biopsy and tumor staging and resection

■ Exercises: Specialties and Specialists

ADVANCED RECALL

Exercise 21

Match each type of medical specialty or specialist with its description.

medical oncology	surgical oncology	radiation oncology
pediatric oncology	gynecologic oncology	surgical oncologist
radiation oncologist	medical oncologist	pediatric oncologist
gynecologic oncologist		

Description   **Term**

1. medical specialty concerned with the diagnosis and treatment of   _____
   cancers of the female reproductive system

2. radiologic specialty concerned with radiation treatment as the   _____
   main mode of treatment for cancer

3. surgical specialty concerned with the surgical management of   _____
   malignant tumors

4. medical specialty concerned with the diagnosis and treatment of childhood cancers and blood diseases _____

5. physician who specializes in the care and treatment of women with gynecologic cancers _____

6. physician who specializes in treating cancer with chemotherapy _____

7. medical specialty concerned with the use of medical and chemotherapeutic treatments of cancer _____

8. physician who specializes in the treatment of childhood cancers and blood diseases _____

9. physician who specializes in treating cancer with high-energy x-rays to destroy cancer cells _____

10. physician who specializes in the surgical aspects of cancer, including biopsy and tumor staging and resection _____

Abbreviations

Abbreviation	Meaning
AFP	alpha fetoprotein
BCC	basal cell carcinoma
BMT	bone marrow transplant
CA	cancer
DCIS	ductal carcinoma in situ
EGFR	epidermal growth factor receptor
ERCP	endoscopic retrograde cholangiopancreatography
EUS	endoscopic ultrasound
FNA	fine needle aspiration
GIST	gastrointestinal stromal tumor
hCG	human chorionic gonadotropin
HIDA	hepatobiliary iminodiacetic acid
LEEP	loop electrosurgical excision procedure
LP	lumbar puncture
MEN	multiple endocrine neoplasia
MRCP	magnetic resonance cholangiopancreatography
NHL	non-Hodgkin lymphoma
PSA	prostate-specific antigen
RFA	radiofrequency ablation
SCC	squamous cell carcinoma
SPECT	single photon emission computed tomography
TRUS	transrectal ultrasound
TURB	transurethral resection of bladder tumor
TURP	transurethral resection of prostate

■ Exercises: Abbreviations

SIMPLE
RECALL

Exercise 22

Write the meaning of each abbreviation used in these sentences.

1. A **GIST** tumor is one of the most common tumors found in the gastrointestinal tract.

   _____

2. One form of breast cancer is called **DCIS.**

   _____

3. A patient who has prostate cancer may undergo treatment with a **TURP.**

   _____

4. A **HIDA** scan is a type of imaging study called a nuclear medicine scan that tracks the flow of bile from the liver.

   _____

5. A **BMT** is used to treat patients whose bone marrow has been destroyed by chemotherapy.

   _____

6. In an **RFA** procedure, the physician applies heat from radiofrequency energy directly onto the tumor to kill cancerous tissue.

   _____

7. A **TRUS** is ultrasound imaging of the prostate done through the rectum.

   _____

8. **EGFRs** are drugs that interfere with the growth of individual cancer cells.

   _____

9. A procedure using MRI and injectable dye to examine problems in the bile ducts, gallbladder, and pancreas is called **MRCP.**

   _____

10. An **EUS** is a procedure using an ultrasound imaging device on the tip of an endoscope for evaluation of bowel wall and adjacent structures.

    _____

11. SPECT is a type of nuclear imaging test that shows how blood flows to tissues and organs.

_____

12. The substance produced by tumor cells in the body found in elevated levels in patients with ovarian cancer is **AFP.**

_____

Exercise 23

ADVANCED
RECALL

Match each abbreviation with the appropriate description.

CA	TURB	FNA	BCC
PSA	LP	LEEP	MEN
ERCP	SCC	NHL	hCG

1. procedure to remove cerebrospinal fluid from the spinal cord   _____

2. procedure that uses a needle to aspirate material for examination   _____

3. general term for a group of diseases characterized by an abnormal uncontrolled growth of cells   _____

4. surgical treatment for bladder cancer   _____

5. procedure using x-ray and injectable dye to examine disorders in the bile ducts, gallbladder, and pancreas   _____

6. use of a low-voltage wire loop to remove cancerous tissue   _____

7. blood test for prostate cancer   _____

8. the most common form of skin cancer   _____

9. elevated levels may indicate cancer in the testis, ovary, liver, stomach, pancreas, or lung   _____

10. a group of disorders characterized by functioning tumors in more than one endocrine gland   _____

11. lymphoma other than Hodgkin disease   _____

12. a cancer that begins in the squamous cells   _____

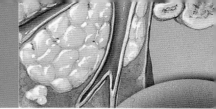

Chapter Review

Understanding Term Structure

TERM CONSTRUCTION

Exercise 24

Break the given medical term into its word parts and define each part. Then define the medical term. (Note: You may need to use word parts from other chapters.)

For example:

laparotomy *word parts:* lapar/o / -tomy
 meanings: abdomen / incision
 term meaning: incision into the abdomen

1. rhabdomyosarcoma *word parts:* _____ / _____ / _____ / _____

  meanings: _____ / _____ / _____ / _____

  term meaning: _____

2. myoma *word parts:* _____ / _____

  meanings: _____ / _____

  term meaning: _____

3. nephroma *word parts:* _____ / _____

  meanings: _____ / _____

  term meaning: _____

4. bronchoscopy *word parts:* _____ / _____

  meanings: _____ / _____

  term meaning: _____

5. meningioma *word parts:* _____ / _____

  meanings: _____ / _____

  term meaning: _____

6. endoscopy *word parts:* _____ / _____

  meanings: _____ / _____

  term meaning: _____

665

7. osteosarcoma   *word parts:* _____ / _____ / _____

    meanings: _____ / _____ / _____

    term meaning: _____

8. neuroma   *word parts:* _____ / _____

    meanings: _____ / _____

    term meaning: _____

9. iridectomy   *word parts:* _____ / _____

    meanings: _____ / _____

    term meaning: _____

10. laparoscopy   *word parts:* _____ / _____

    meanings: _____ / _____

    term meaning: _____

Comprehension Exercises

COMPREHENSION

Exercise 25

Fill in the blank with the correct term.

1. The common sites for gastrointestinal tract cancer are the colon and rectum; together, these are referred to as _____ cancer.

2. A technique used to destroy cancer cells using extreme cold is _____.

3. During a(n) _____, a physician is able to view both the urethra and the bladder using a lighted scope.

4. When a tumor is nonmalignant, it is said to be _____.

5. Too much exposure to the sun can result in a(n) _____, the most dangerous type of skin cancer.

6. A(n) _____ is another name for a pancreaticoduodenectomy.

7. To remove a tumor in the bladder, a surgeon may perform _____ at the tumor site, which is the use of high-frequency electric current to destroy tissue.

8. A(n) _____ involves use of a scalpel to remove skin for examination.

9. A radiologist analyzes the images in a(n) _____ for signs of early breast cancer.

10. A(n) _____ is a fast-growing malignant tumor of the bone-forming cells of the body.

Exercise 26

COMPREHENSION   **Write a short answer for each question.**

1. What is the difference between a simple mastectomy and radical mastectomy? _____

_____

2. What is the difference between Hodgkin lymphoma and non-Hodgkin lymphoma? _____

_____

3. What is the name of the procedure used to surgically reduce the size of a tumor that cannot

be completely removed by removing as much of it as possible? _____

4. What is the purpose of palliative surgery? _____

_____

5. Which type of brain cancer starts from small, star-shaped cells? _____

6. What is the difference between a chondroma and a chondrosarcoma? _____

_____

7. What is the function of oncogenes? _____

_____

8. How is external beam radiation delivered to treat a tumor? _____

_____

9. How do aromatase inhibitors stop the growth of cancer cells? _____

_____

10. Are sarcomas benign or malignant? _____

Exercise 27

COMPREHENSION   **Circle the letter of the best answer to the following questions.**

1. Which of the following are mismatched?

    A. bladder cancer — cystectomy
    B. lymphoma — lymphadenectomy
    C. melanoma — mastectomy
    D. pancreatic cancer — Whipple procedure

2. *Benign* is another word for:

    A. harmful
    B. nonmalignant
    C. invasive
    D. brightly colored

3. What is another name for the Billroth operations I and II?

    A. colectomy
    B. Mohs surgery
    C. endoscopy
    D. gastrectomy

4. A retinoblastoma is a cancerous tumor involving the:

    A. cornea
    B. iris
    C. retina
    D. sclera

5. A procedure used to remove the prostate as a cancer treatment is called:

    A. LEEP
    B. TURB
    C. TURP
    D. EGFR

6. A tumor of the kidney is referred to as a:

    A. nephroma
    B. melanoma
    C. myoma
    D. leukemia

7. A Wilms tumor is a rare type of cancer that affects:

    A. the elderly
    B. children
    C. fetuses
    D. young men

8. Which type of surgery returns the function and appearance of an area of the body after a tumor has been removed?

    A. palliative surgery
    B. reconstructive surgery
    C. debulking surgery
    D. cryosurgery

9. Chemotherapy given in addition to surgery is called:

    A. adjuvant
    B. chemoprevention
    C. interstitial
    D. intrathecal

10. The specialist who treats cancers only in women is called a(n):

    A. pediatric oncologist
    B. oncologist
    C. gynecologic oncologist
    D. radiation oncologist

Application and Analysis

CASE REPORTS

Exercise 28

APPLICATION   **Read the case reports and circle the letter of your answer choice for the questions that follow each case.**

CASE 16-1

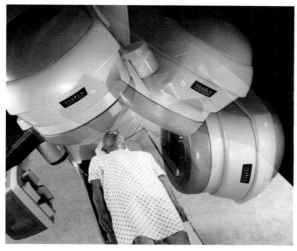

Figure 16-17 Patient undergoing radiation therapy.

Ms. Kumar has come in for her regularly scheduled clinic visit. She was previously diagnosed with metastatic left breast cancer and underwent a left mastectomy. She then received a 5-year course of aromatase inhibitor therapy. She had recurrence of the cancer along with a suspicious left intramammary lymph node and the presence of multiple bony metastases. She recently underwent a course of palliative radiation therapy (Fig. 16-17) for bony metastasis. She will be rescheduled for follow-up. In addition, a PET scan has been ordered for the patient, which will be completed next week.

1. What kind of imaging study is the patient going to undergo?

   A. aromatase inhibitor therapy
   B. PET
   C. palliative radiation therapy
   D. none of the above

2. What treatment did the patient receive for her bony metastases?

   A. therapy that uses chemicals to treat cancer
   B. placement of chemotherapy drugs directly into a tumor
   C. the use of high-energy x-rays or other particles to kill cancer
   D. drugs designed to reduce estrogen levels in a woman's body

3. How long did the patient take aromatase inhibitors?

   A. 5 years
   B. 2 years

   C. 1 week
   D. 1 year

4. What kind of radiation therapy did the patient receive?

   A. reconstructive
   B. systemic
   C. adjuvant
   D. palliative

5. What surgical treatment did the patient receive for her breast cancer?

   A. lumpectomy
   B. colectomy
   C. mastectomy
   D. adenectomy

CASE 16-2

Mr. Able came into the clinic for a regularly scheduled follow-up visit for squamous cell cancer of the base of the tongue. He is 5 years postop with no recurrence found. He speaks covering his tracheostomy and is easily understood. His tracheostomy site was found to be clean, dry, and intact. His neck was edematous and firm. The temporomandibular joint (TMJ) was tender to palpation. His oropharynx was not examined due to patient's inability to open his mouth. His abdomen has a left

J feeding tube. He seems to be doing very well. An x-ray of his jaw was ordered to evaluate his TMJ symptoms.

6. Where is the TMJ located?

A. in the chest
B. in the face
C. in the neck
D. in the abdomen

7. How long has the patient been cancer free?

A. 2 years
B. 4 years
C. 5 years
D. patient is not cancer free

8. A tracheostomy is defined as a(n):

A. excision of part of the trachea
B. creation of an artificial opening in the trachea

C. incision into the trachea
D. excision of all of the trachea

9. The return of cancer after all visible signs of it had been eradicated previously is called:

A. recurrence
B. remission
C. metastasis
D. post-operative

10. What does the term *edematous* mean?

A. hydrated
B. stiff
C. red
D. swollen

MEDICAL RECORD ANALYSIS

MEDICAL RECORD 16-1

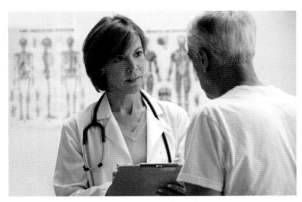

You are a physician's assistant working in a surgical oncology clinic. Mr. Lowe is a patient who is being seen for a carcinoma of the nose with subsequent evaluation of that lesion. You are reviewing the record of his visit to assist in his postoperative care.

A physician's assistant works closely with the physician and can perform various medical tasks.

Medical Record

CLINIC NOTE

SUBJECTIVE: The patient is a 50-year-old male with a 10-year history of a nasal lesion. He initially described it as being a possible infection of his hair follicle that progressed. The patient never did seek medical attention for this and over the course of these years, he has noticed that his nose has slowly started to disappear. He has recently been using a self-made nasal prosthesis made out of silicone. The patient does have a history of sun exposure as a child but no significant occupational exposure. He also has no history of smoking. He was seen by an outside physician and had a biopsy of his lesion performed, which was consistent with basal cell carcinoma.

OBJECTIVE: Temperature 99.6, pulse 96, respirations 16. He is alert and oriented, in no apparent distress. What remains of the nose shows only some septal cartilage and nasal bones with skin covering; otherwise he has no ala and no lower or upper lateral cartilages. He does have an ulcerative lesion along the nasolabial fold on the left side. There is surrounding skin and mucosal ulceration and some friable tissue that bleeds with any extensive manipulation.

Anterior rhinoscopy demonstrates no obvious masses.

ASSESSMENT: Basal cell carcinoma of the nose.

PLAN: At this time, the patient is a candidate for a total rhinectomy as well as possible skin graft, possible lip resection, possible primary lip repair, possible nasolabial flap. We would like to have the patient admitted to the hospital postoperatively. The patient was informed about the risks and benefits of the procedure, which include but are not limited to bleeding, infection, pain, nasal obturator stenosis, cosmetic defect, recurrence, need for additional surgery, psychosocial impact, lip and oral incompetence, and numbness. Despite this, informed consent was obtained today.

Exercise 29

APPLICATION

Write the appropriate medical terms used in this medical record on the blanks after their meanings. Note that not all the terms appear in the chapter, but you should be able to identify these terms based on word parts that are included in this chapter.

1. narrowing of a canal or orifice   _____

2. the formation of an ulcer   _____

3. process of examining the nose   _____

4. malignant cancer of epithelial tissue _____

5. surgical removal of the nose   _____

MEDICAL RECORD 16-2

Ms. Collins was admitted to the hospital last week for definitive surgical treatment of her left breast cancer. You, as an oncology nurse, are reviewing her record in anticipation of talking to the patient about future chemotherapy.

Medical Record

OPERATIVE REPORT

PREOPERATIVE DIAGNOSIS: Recurrent infiltrative poorly differentiated ductal carcinoma of the breast.

POSTOPERATIVE DIAGNOSIS: Recurrent infiltrative poorly differentiated ductal carcinoma of the breast.

OPERATION: Left simple mastectomy.

INDICATIONS FOR PROCEDURE: The patient is a 46-year-old female with history of left breast carcinoma diagnosed at an outside hospital. She then underwent excisional biopsy with chemotherapy and radiation therapy. The patient was referred for evaluation of continuously enlarging left breast mass; biopsy performed revealed recurrent infiltrative poorly differentiated ductal carcinoma with features of metastatic carcinoma. It was recommended that the patient undergo a left simple mastectomy. The patient agreed to the procedure and signed the consent.

DESCRIPTION OF PROCEDURE: The patient was taken to the operating room and placed in supine position on the operating table. The left breast and arm were prepped and draped in the standard sterile surgical fashion. An elliptic incision was made to encompass the entire right breast. This incision extended from the sternum in the direction to the axilla up to the lateral margin of the left breast. The knife was used to cut down the dermis and then Bovie electrocautery was used to take this incision down to the breast tissue. Meticulous hemostasis was achieved throughout. Flaps were raised medially to the sternum, laterally to the pectoralis major lateral border, inferiorly to the mammary crease, and superior to the clavicle. The dissection was carried down to the level of the pectoralis fascia. At that time, the pectoralis minor was dissected from the overlying breast tissue, and this proceeded in a medial to lateral dissection. The dissection continued laterally, freeing up the edge of the pectoralis minor muscle.

After meticulous hemostasis was achieved, a #10 J-P drain was placed. The skin was closed in 2 layers, one with interrupted 4-0 Maxon sutures for the dermis, and the skin was closed with 4-0 Vicryl in a subcuticular fashion. Dry dressings were applied. The patient was revived from anesthesia, extubated, and transferred to the recovery room in stable condition.

ADVANCED
RECALL

Exercise 30

Read the medical report and circle the letter of your answer choice for the following questions.

1. What type of biopsy did the patient undergo during an earlier procedure?

   A. incisional
   B. excisional
   C. fine needle aspiration
   D. punch biopsy

2. What was used to access the breast tissue during the operation?

   A. J-P drains
   B. Bovie electrocautery
   C. Flaps
   D. A knife

3. What type of mastectomy did the patient undergo?

   A. radical
   B. simple
   C. suprapubic
   D. modified radical

4. What kind of carcinoma was found in the patient's left breast?

   A. benign
   B. simple
   C. ductal
   D. lymph-dependent

5. What type of sutures were used to close the uppermost layer of skin?

   A. Maxon
   B. catgut
   C. Vicryl
   D. Both Maxon and Vicryl

6. What type of surgery might the patient have in the future to improve the appearance of her chest?

   A. debulking surgery
   B. reconstructive surgery
   C. chemotherapy
   D. brachysurgery

Bonus Question

7. What is the main difference in the type of breast cancer that this patient has and ductal
carcinoma in situ (DCIS) defined earlier in the chapter? _____

_____

Pronunciation and Spelling

AUDITORY

Exercise 31

**Review the Chapter 16 terms in the Dictionary/Audio Glossary in the Student
Resources and practice pronouncing each term, referring to the pronunciation
guide as needed.**

SPELLING

Exercise 32

Circle the correct spelling of each term.

1. cranectomy   craniectomy   crenectomy

2. fulguration   fulgeration   fuljuration

3. rabdomyoma   rhabdomioma   rhabdomyoma

4. thiroidectomy   thyroidectomy   thyrodectomy

5. condrosarcoma   chondrosarcoma   chondrasacoma

6. criosurgery   cyrosurjery   cryosurgery

7. gleoma   glioma   glyoma

8. leiomyosarcoma   liomyosarcoma   leomiosarcoma

9. mamography   mammographe   mammography

10. feochromocytoma   pheochromocytoma   pheocrhomcitoma

11. brakytherapy   brachytherapy   brachytherape

12. cholescintigraphy colescintriphy   cholesintrigraphy

13. lipomma   lipoma   lypoma

14. nefrectome   nephrectomy   nephrictomy

15. palliative   paliative   pallative

Media Connection

STUDENT
RESOURCES

Exercise 33

Complete each of the following activities available with the Student Resources. Check off each activity as you complete it, and record your score for the Chapter Quiz in the space provided.

Chapter Exercises

_____ Flash Cards

_____ Concentration

_____ Abbreviation Match-Up

_____ Roboterms

_____ Word Builder

_____ Fill the Gap

_____ Break It Down

_____ True/False Body Building

_____ Quiz Show

_____ Complete the Case

_____ Medical Record Review

_____ Look and Label

_____ Image Matching

_____ Spelling Bee

_____ **Chapter Quiz**   _Score:_ _____%

Additional Resources

_____ Dictionary/Audio Glossary

_____ Health Professions Careers: Physician's Assistant

_____ Health Professions Careers: Oncology Nurse

Glossary of Combining Forms, Prefixes, and Suffixes

Word Part	Meaning
a-	without, not
ab-	away from
abdomin/o	abdomen
ablat/o	to take away
-ac	pertaining to
acous/o	hearing, sound
-acousis, -acusis	hearing
acr/o	extremity, tip
ad-	to, toward
aden/o	gland
adenoid/o	adenoids
adip/o	fat
adren/o, adrenal/o	adrenal glands
-al	pertaining to
albumin/o	albumin
-algia	pain
aliment/o	nutrition
alveol/o	alveolus
amni/o, amnion/o	amnion
an-	without, not
an/o	anus
andr/o	male
angi/o	vessel, duct
ankyl/o	stiff
ante-	before
anter/o	front
anti-	opposing, against
anxi/o	anxiety
aort/o	aorta
appendic/o	appendix
-ar	pertaining to
-arche	beginning
arteri/o	artery

Word Part	Meaning
arthr/o, articul/o	joint
-ary	pertaining to
-ase	enzyme
aspir/o	to breathe in or suck in
-asthenia	weakness
atel/o	incomplete
ather/o	fatty paste
atri/o	atrium
audi/o	hearing
aur/i, aur/o	ear
ausculat/o	listening
auto-	self, same
bacteri/o	bacteria
balan/o	glans penis
basi-, baso-	base
bi-, bin-	two, twice
bi/o, bio-	life
bil/o	bile
blast/o	immature cell
blephar/o	eyelid
brachi/o	arm
brady-	slow
bronchi/o, bronch/o	bronchus
bucc/o	cheek
burs/o	bursa
calc/i	calcium
cancer/o	cancer
capn/o, capn/i	carbon dioxide
carcin/o	cancer
cardi/o	heart
carp/o	carpal bones
caud/o	tail
cec/o	cecum

(continued)

Word Part	Meaning
-cele	herniation, protrusion
-centesis	puncture to aspirate
cephal/o	head
cerebell/o	cerebellum (little brain)
cerebr/o	brain, cerebrum
cervic/o	neck, cervix (neck of uterus)
cheil/o	lip
chem/o	chemical, drug
chlor/o	green
chol/e	gall, bile
cholecyst/o	gallbladder
chondr/o	cartilage
chori/o	chorion
chrom/o, chromat/o	color
chyl/o	juice
circum-	around
-clasia, -clasis, -clast	to break
clavic/o, clavicul/o	clavicle
cochle/o	cochlea
col/o, colon/o	colon
colp/o	vagina
conjunctiv/o	conjunctiva
contra-	opposing, against
cor/e, cor/o	pupil
corne/o	cornea
coron/o	circle or crown
cortic/o	cortex
cost/o	rib
crani/o	cranium, skull
crin/o	to secrete
cry/o	cold
crypt-	hidden
cutane/o	skin
cyan/o	blue
cyst/o	urinary bladder
cyt/o	cell
-cyte	cell
dacry/o	tears or tear ducts
de-	away from, cessation, without

Word Part	Meaning
dent/o	tooth
derm/o, dermat/o	skin
-derma	skin condition
-desis	surgical fixation, binding
di-	two, twice
diaphragmat/o	diaphragm
dipl/o	double, two
dips/o	thirst
dis-	separate, remove
disk/o	disk or disc
diverticul/o	diverticulum
dors/o	back
duoden/o	duodenum
dur/o	hard, dura mater
-dynia	pain
dys-	painful, difficult, abnormal
-eal	pertaining to
ec-	out of, away from
-ectasia	dilation, stretching
ecto-	outer, outside
-ectomy	excision, surgical removal
electr/o	electric, electricity
em-	in
embry/o, embryon/o	embryo; immature form
-emesis	vomiting
-emia	blood (condition of)
en-, end-, endo-	in, within
encephal/o	entire brain
endocrin/o	endocrine
enter/o	small intestine
enur/o	to urinate
epi-	on, following
epididym/o	epididymis
epiglott/o	epiglottis
episi/o	vulva
epitheli/o	epithelium (type of tissue)
erythr/o	red
-esis	condition of
esophag/o	esophagus

(continued)

Word Part	Meaning
esthesi/o	sensation
eu-	good, normal
ex-	out of, away from
exo-	outer, outside
fasci/o	fascia, band
femor/o	femur
fet/o	fetus
fibr/o	fiber
fibul/o	fibula
fund/o	fundus
galact/o	milk
gangli/o, ganglion/o	ganglion
gastr/o	stomach
-gen	origin, production
-genic, -genesis	originating, producing
gestat/o	from conception to birth
gli/o	neuroglia, glue
glomerul/o	glomerulus
gluc/o, glucos/o, glyc/o, glycos/o	glucose, sugar
-gram	record, recording
granul/o	granules
-graph	instrument for recording
-graphy	process of recording
gravid/o	pregnancy
gyn/o, gynec/o	woman
hallucin/o	to wander in one's mind
hem/o, hemat/o	blood
hemi-	half
hepat/o	liver
herni/o	hernia
hetero-	other, different
hidr/o	sweat
hist/o	tissue
homo-, homeo-	same, alike
hormon/o	hormone
humer/o	humerus
hydr/o	water, fluid
hyper-	above, excessive
hypn/o	sleep, hypnosis

Word Part	Meaning
hypo-	below, deficient
hyster/o	uterus
-ia	condition of
-iasis	condition of
-iatrist	one who specializes in
-ic	pertaining to
-icle	small
-ictal	seizure
ide/o	idea, ideation
ile/o	ileum
ili/o	ilium
im-	not
immun/o	immune, safe
in-	not
infer/o	below
infra-	below, beneath
inguin/o	groin
inter-	between
intra-	within
ir/o, irid/o	iris
ischi/o	ischium
-ism	condition of
iso-	equal, alike
-ist	one who specializes in
-itis	inflammation
-ium	tissue, structure
jejun/o	jejunum
kal/i	potassium
kary/o	nucleus
kerat/o	cornea, hard
kin/o, kin/e, kinesi/o, kinet/o	movement
kyph/o	humpback
labi/o	lip
labyrinth/o	labyrinth, inner ear
lacrim/o	tears or tear ducts
lact/o	milk
lamin/o	lamina
lapar/o	abdomen
laryng/o	larynx

(continued)

Word Part	Meaning
later/o	side
lei/o	smooth
-lepsy	seizure
leuk/o	white
lingu/o	tongue
lip/o	fat
-lith	stone, calculus
lith/o	stone, calculus
lob/o	lobe
-logist	one who specializes in
-logy	study of
lord/o	curved, bent
lumb/o	lumbar region, lower back
lymph/o	lymph
-lysis	destruction, breakdown, separation
-lytic	pertaining to destruction, breakdown, separation
macro-	large, long
mal-	bad, poor
-malacia	softening
mamm/o	breast, mammary gland
mandibul/o	mandible
-mania	excited state, obsession
mast/o	breast, mammary gland
mastoid/o	mastoid bone
maxill/o	maxilla
meat/o	meatus
medi/o	middle
mediastin/o	mediastinum
mega-, megalo-	large, oversize
-megaly	enlargement
melan/o	black, dark
men/o	menstruation
mening/o, meningi/o	meninges
menisc/o	meniscus
menstru/o	menstruation
ment/o	mind, mental
meta-	change, beyond
-meter	instrument for measuring
metr/o, metri/o	uterus

Word Part	Meaning
-metry	measurement of
micro-	small
mono-	one
morph/o	form, shape
muc/o	mucus
multi-	many
muscul/o	muscle
my/o, myos/o	muscle
myc/o	fungus
myel/o	bone marrow, spinal cord
myring/o	tympanic membrane, eardrum
narc/o	stupor, unconsciousness
nas/o	nose
nat/o	birth
natr/i	sodium
necr/o	death
neo-	new
nephr/o	kidney
neur/o	nerve
neutr/o	neutral
noct/i	night
non-	not
normo-	normal
nucle/o	nucleus
nulli-	none
ocul/o	eye
odont/o	tooth
-oid	resembling
-ole	small
olig/o	scanty, few
-oma	tumor
omphal/o	umbilicus, navel
onc/o	tumor
onych/o	nail
oophor/o	ovary
ophthalm/o	eye
-opia, -opsia	vision
-opsy	process of viewing
opt/o	vision, eye

(continued)

Word Part	Meaning
or/o	mouth
orch/o, orchi/o, orchid/o	testis, testicle
-osis	abnormal condition
oste/o	bone
ot/o	ear
-ous	pertaining to
ovari/o	ovary
ox/o, ox/a	oxygen
pachy/o	thick
palat/o	palate
pan-	all, entire
pancreat/o	pancreas
para-	beside
parathyroid/o	parathyroid glands
-paresis	slight paralysis
-partum	childbirth, labor
patell/o	patella
path/o	disease
-pathy	disease
pector/o	chest
ped/o	foot
pelv/i, pelv/o	pelvis, pelvic cavity
-penia	deficiency
peps/o	digestion
per-	through
peri-	around, surrounding
perine/o	perineum
-pexy	surgical fixation
phag/o	eat, swallow
-phagia	to eat
phalang/o	phalanges
pharyng/o	pharynx
phas/o	speech
-philia	attraction for
phleb/o	vein
-phobia	abnormal fear, aversion to, sensitivity to
phon/o	sound, voice
-phonia	condition of the voice
phot/o	light

Word Part	Meaning
phren/o	diaphragm; mind, mental
-phrenia	the mind
-physis	growth
plas/o	formation, growth
-plasia	formation, growth
-plasty	surgical repair, reconstruction
-plegia	paralysis
pleur/o	pleura
-pnea	breathing
pneum/o, pneumat/o, pneumon/o	lung, air
pod/o	foot
-poiesis	production, formation
poli/o	gray
poly-	many, much
polyp/o	polyp
-porosis	pore, passage
post-	after, behind
poster/o	back
-prandial	meal
pre-	before (in time or space)
presby/o	related to aging
pro-	before, promoting
proct/o	rectum and anus
prostat/o	prostate
proxim/o	near the point of origin
pseudo-	false
psych/o	mind, mental
-ptosis	prolapse, drooping, sagging
pub/o	pubis
pulmon/o	lung
pupill/o	pupil
py/o	pus
pyel/o	renal pelvis
pylor/o	pylorus
quadri-	four
rachi/o	spine
radi/o	radius; x-rays, radiation
radicul/o	nerve root
re-	again, backward

(continued)

Word Part	Meaning	Word Part	Meaning
rect/o	rectum	-stenosis	stricture, narrowing
ren/o	kidney	stern/o	sternum
retin/o	retina	steth/o	thorax, chest
retro-	backward, behind	stomat/o	mouth
rhabd/o	striated muscle	-stomy	surgical opening
rhin/o	nose	sub-	below, beneath
rhytid/o	wrinkle	super-	above
-rrhage, -rrhagia	flowing forth	super/o	above
-rrhaphy	suture	supra-	above
-rrhea	flow, discharge	sym-, syn-	together, with
sacr/o	sacrum	synovi/o	synovial joint or fluid
salping/o	salpinx, fallopian tube	tachy-	rapid, fast
sarc/o	flesh	tars/o	tarsal bones
scapul/o	scapula	tel-	end
-schisis	to split	ten/o, tend/o, tendin/o	tendon
schiz/o	split	test/o, testicul/o	testis, testicle
scler/o	hard, sclera	thalam/o	thalamus
scoli/o	crooked, twisted	thorac/o	thorax, chest
-scope	instrument for examination	thromb/o	blood clot
-scopy	process of examining, examination	thym/i, thym/o	mind, soul, emotion
seb/o	sebum	thym/o	thymus gland
semi-	half	thyr/o, thyroid/o	thyroid gland
sept/o	septum	-tic	pertaining to
sial/o	saliva	-tion	process
sigmoid/o	sigmoid colon	toc/o	labor, birth
sinus/o	sinus	-tome	instrument used to cut
-sis	condition, process	-tomy	incision
soci/o	social, society	ton/o	tension, pressure
somn/o, somn/i	sleep	tonsill/o	tonsil
son/o	sound, sound waves	trache/o	trachea
-spasm	involuntary movement	trans-	across, through
sperm/o, spermat/o	sperm, spermatozoon	tri-	three
sphygm/o	pulse	trich/o	hair
spin/o	spine	-tripsy	crushing
spir/o	breathe	troph/o	nourishment
spondyl/o	vertebra	-trophia	to turn
squam/o	scalelike structure	-trophy	development, nourishment
staped/o	stapes	tympan/o	tympanic membrane, eardrum
-stasis	stopped, standing still	-ule	small

(continued)

Word Part	Meaning
uln/o	ulna
ultra-	excess, beyond
uni-	one
ur/o	urine, urinary system/tract
ureter/o	ureter
urethr/o	urethra
-uria	urine, urination
urin/o	urine, urinary system/tract
uter/o	uterus
vagin/o	vagina
valv/o, valvul/o	valve
varic/o	swollen or twisted vein
vas/o	duct, vessel, vas deferens

Word Part	Meaning
vascul/o	vessel, duct
ven/i, ven/o	vein
ventr/o	belly
ventricul/o	ventricle
vertebr/o	vertebra
vesicul/o, vesic/o	fluid-filled sac (urinary bladder, seminal vesicle)
vestibul/o	vestibule
viscer/o	internal organs
vulv/o	vulva
xanth/o	yellow
xer/o	dry
-y	condition of

Word Part Lookup by Meaning

Meaning	Word Part(s)
abdomen	lapar/o, abdomin/o
abnormal	dys-
abnormal condition	-iasis, -osis
abnormal fear	-phobia
above	hyper-, super/o, supra-, super-
across	trans-
adenoids	adenoid/o
adrenal glands	adren/o, adrenal/o
after	post-
again	re-
against	anti-, contra-
aging, related to	presby/o
air	pneum/o, pneumat/o, pneumon/o
albumin	albumin/o
alike	homo-, homeo-, iso-
all	pan-
alveolus	alveol/o
amnion	amni/o, amnion/o
anus	an/o
anus and rectum	proct/o
anxiety	anxi/o
aorta	aort/o
appendix	appendic/o
arm	brachi/o
around	circum-, peri-
artery	arteri/o
atrium	atri/o
attraction for	-philia, -phile
aversion to	-phobia
away from	ab-, de-, ec-, ex-
back	dors/o, poster/o
backward	re-, retro-
bacteria	bacteri/o

Meaning	Word Part(s)
bad	mal-
band	fasci/o
base	basi-, baso-
before	ante-, pre-, pro-
beginning	-arche
behind	post-, retro-
belly	ventr/o
below	hypo-, infer/o, infra-, sub-
beneath	sub-, infra-
bent, curved	lord/o
beside	para-
between	inter-
beyond	meta-, ultra-
bile	bil/o, chol/e
birth	nat/o, toc/o
black, dark	melan/o
blood	hem/o, hemat/o
blood (condition of)	-emia
blood clot	thromb/o
blue	cyan/o
bone	oste/o
bone marrow	myel/o
brain (cerebrum)	cerebr/o
breakdown	-lysis
breast	mamm/o, mast/o
breathe	spir/o
breathing	-pnea
bronchus	bronchi/o, bronch/o
bursa	burs/o
calcium	calc/i
cancer	cancer/o, carcin/o
carbon dioxide	capn/o, capn/i
carpal bones	carp/o

(continued)

Meaning	Word Part(s)
cartilage	chondr/o
cecum	cec/o
cell	cyt/o, -cyte
cerebellum (little brain)	cerebell/o
cerebrum	cerebr/o
cervix	cervic/o
cessation	de-
change	meta-
cheek	bucc/o
chemical	chem/o
chest	pector/o
childbirth	-partum
chorion	chori/o
circle	coron/o
clavicle	clavic/o, clavicul/o
cochlea	cochle/o
cold	cry/o
colon	col/o, colon/o
color	chrom/o, chromat/o
condition of	-ism, -ia, -iasis, -esis, -y
condition of the voice	-phonia
condition, process	-sis
conjunctiva	conjunctiv/o
cornea	corne/o, kerat/o
cortex	cortic/o
cranium	crani/o
crooked, twisted	scoli/o
crown	coron/o
crushing	-tripsy
curved, bent	lord/o
dark	melan/o
death	necr/o
deficiency	-penia
deficient	hypo-
destruction	-lysis
development	-trophy
diaphragm	diaphragmat/o, phren/o
different	hetero-
difficult	dys-

Meaning	Word Part(s)
digestion	peps/o
dilation, stretching	-ectasia, -ectasis
discharge	-rrhea
disease	path/o, -pathy
disk or disc	disk/o
diverticulum	diverticul/o
double	dipl/o
drooping	-ptosis
drug	chem/o
dry	xer/o
duct	vas/o
duodenum	duoden/o
dura mater	dur/o
ear	aur/i, aur/o, ot/o
eat	phag/o
electric, electricity	electr/o
embryo	embry/o, embryon/o
emotion	thym/i, thym/o
end	tel-
endocrine	endocrin/o
enlargement	-megaly
entire	pan-
entire brain	encephal/o
enzyme	-ase
epididymis	epididym/o
epiglottis	epiglott/o
epithelium	epitheli/o
equal	iso-
esophagus	esophag/o
examination	-scopy
excess	ultra-
excessive	hyper-
excision, surgical removal	-ectomy
excited state	-mania
extremity	acr/o
eye	ocul/o, ophthalm/o
eyelid	blephar/o
fallopian tube	salping/o
fascia, band	fasci/o

(continued)

Meaning	Word Part(s)
fast	tachy-
fat	lip/o, adip/o
fatty paste	ather/o
femur	femor/o
fetus	fet/o
few	olig/o
fiber	fibr/o
fibula	fibul/o
flesh	sarc/o
flow	-rrhea
flowing forth	-rrhage, -rrhagia
fluid-filled sac (seminal vesicle or urinary bladder)	vesicul/o, vesic/o
following	epi-
foot	ped/o, pod/o
form, shape	morph/o
formation	plas/o, -plasia, -poiesis
four	quad-, quadri-
from conception to birth	gestat/o
front	anter/o
fundus	fund/o
fungus	myc/o
gall	chol/e
gallbladder	cholecyst/o
ganglion	gangli/o, ganglion/o
gland	aden/o
glans penis	balan/o
glomerulus	glomerul/o
glucose, sugar	gluc/o, glucos/o, glyc/o, glycos/o
glue	gli/o
good	eu-
granules	granul/o
gray	poli/o
green	chlor/o
groin	inguin/o
growth	plas/o, -plasia, -physis
hair	trich/o
half	hemi-, semi-
hard	dur/o, kerat/o, scler/o

Meaning	Word Part(s)
head	cephal/o
hearing	acous/o, audi/o, -acousis, -acusis
heart	cardi/o
hernia	herni/o
herniation	-cele
hidden	crypt-
hormone	hormon/o
humerus	humer/o
humpback	kyph/o
hypnosis	hypn/o
idea, ideation	ide/o
ileum	ile/o
ilium	ili/o
immature cell	blast/o
immune, safe	immun/o
in	em-, en-, end-, endo-
incision	-tomy
incomplete	atel/o
inflammation	-itis
inner ear	labyrinth/o
instrument for examination	-scope
instrument for measuring	-meter
instrument for recording	-graph
instrument used to cut	-tome
internal organs	viscer/o
involuntary movement	-spasm
iris	ir/o, irid/o
ischium	ischi/o
jejunum	jejun/o
joint	arthr/o, articul/o
juice	chyl/o
kidney	nephr/o, ren/o
labor	-partum, toc/o
labyrinth	labyrinth/o
lamina	lamin/o
large	macro-, mega-, megalo-
larynx	laryng/o
life	bi/o, bio-

(continued)

Meaning	Word Part(s)
light	phot/o
lip	labi/o, cheil/o
listening	auscultat/o
liver	hepat/o
lobe	lob/o
long	macro-
lumbar region (lower back)	lumb/o
lung	pneum/o, pneumat/o, pneumon/o, pulmon/o
lymph	lymph/o
male	andr/o
mammary gland	mamm/o, mast/o
mandible	mandibul/o
many	multi-, poly-
mastoid bone	mastoid/o
maxilla	maxill/o
meal	-prandial
measurement of	-metry
meatus	meat/o
mediastinum	mediastin/o
meninges	mening/o, meningi/o
meniscus	menisc/o
menstruation	men/o, menstru/o
mental	ment/o, psych/o, phren/o
middle	medi/o
milk	lact/o, galact/o
mind	ment/o, psych/o, phren/o, thym/i, thym/o
mouth	or/o, stomat/o
movement	kin/o, kin/e, kinesi/o, kinet/o
much	poly-
mucus	muc/o
muscle	my/o, myos/o, muscul/o
nail	onych/o
near the point of origin	proxim/o
neck	cervic/o
nerve	neur/o
nerve root	radicul/o
neuroglia	gli/o

Meaning	Word Part(s)
neutral	neutr/o
new	neo-
night	noct/i
none	nulli-
normal	eu-, normo-
nose	nas/o, rhin/o
not	in-, im-, non-
nourishment	troph/o, -trophy
nucleus	kary/o, nucle/o
nutrition	aliment/o
obsession	-mania
on	epi-
one	mono-, uni-
one who specializes in	-logist, -ist, -iatrist
opposing	anti-, contra-
origin	-gen
originating	-genic, -genesis
other	hetero-
out of	ec-, ex-
outer, outside	ecto-, exo-
ovary	ovari/o, oophor/o
oversize	mega-, megalo-
oxygen	ox/o, ox/a
pain	-algia, -dynia
painful	dys-
palate	palat/o
pancreas	pancreat/o
paralysis	-plegia
parathyroid glands	parathyroid/o
passage	-porosis
patella	patell/o
pelvis, pelvic cavity	pelv/i, pelv/o
perineum	perine/o
pertaining to	-ac, -al, -ar, -ary, -eal, -ic, -ous, -tic
pertaining to destruction, breakdown, separation	-lytic
phalanges	phalang/o
pharynx	pharyng/o
pleura	pleur/o

(continued)

Meaning	Word Part(s)
polyp	polyp/o
poor	mal-
pore	-porosis
potassium	kal/i
pregnancy	gravid/o
process	-sis, -tion
process of examining, examination	-scopy
process of recording	-graphy
process of viewing	-opsy
producing	-genic, -genesis
production	-gen, -poiesis
prolapse	-ptosis
promoting	pro-
prostate	prostat/o
protrusion	-cele
pubis	pub/o
pulse	sphygm/o
puncture to aspirate	-centesis
pupil	cor/e, cor/o, pupill/o
pus	py/o
pylorus	pylor/o
radius	radi/o
rapid	tachy-
record, recording	-gram
rectum	rect/o
rectum and anus	proct/o
red	erythr/o
related to aging	presby/o
remove	dis-
renal pelvis	pyel/o
resembling	-oid
retina	retin/o
rib	cost/o
sacrum	sacr/o
safe	immun/o
sagging	-ptosis
saliva	sial/o
salpinx	salping/o
same	auto-, homo-, homeo-

Meaning	Word Part(s)
scalelike structure	squam/o
scanty	olig/o
scapula	scapul/o
sclera	scler/o
sebum	seb/o
seizure	-ictal, -lepsy
self	auto-
seminal vesicle	vesicul/o
sensation	esthesi/o
sensitivity to	-phobia
separate	dis-
separation	-lysis
septum	sept/o
shape	morph/o
side	later/o
sigmoid colon	sigmoid/o
sinus	sinus/o
skin	derm/o, dermat/o, cutane/o
skin condition	-derma
skull	crani/o
sleep	somn/o, somn/i, hypn/o
slight paralysis	-paresis
slow	brady-
small	micro-, -icle, -ole, -ule
small intestine	enter/o
smooth	lei/o
social, society	soci/o
sodium	natr/i
softening	-malacia
soul	thym/i, thym/o
sound	acous/o, son/o, phon/o
sound waves	son/o
speech	phas/o
sperm, spermatozoon	sperm/o, spermat/o
spinal cord	myel/o
spine	spin/o, rachi/o
split	schiz/o
stapes	staped/o
stretching	-ectasia, -ectasis

(continued)

Meaning	Word Part(s)
sugar	gluc/o, glucos/o, glyc/o, glycos/o
surgical removal	-ectomy
surrounding	peri-
swallow	phag/o
through	trans-
tip	acr/o
twisted, crooked	scoli/o

Meaning	Word Part(s)
two	dipl/o
urinary bladder	vesicul/o, vesic/o
vas deferens	vas/o
vertebra	spondyl/o, vertebr/o
vessel	vas/o
voice	phon/o
within	en-, end-, endo-
without	de-

■ ROUTINE URINALYSIS

Test	Normal Value	Clinical Significance
General Characteristics and Measurements		
Color	Pale yellow to amber	Color change can be due to concentration or dilution, drugs, metabolic or inflammatory disorders
Odor	Slightly aromatic	Foul odor typical of urinary tract infection, fruity odor in uncontrolled diabetes mellitus
Appearance (clarity)	Clear to slightly hazy	Cloudy urine occurs with infection or after refrigeration; may indicate presence of bacteria, cells, mucus, or crystals
Specific gravity	1.003–1.030 (first morning catch; routine is random)	Decreased in diabetes insipidus, acute renal failure, water intoxication; increased in liver disorders, heart failure, dehydration
pH	4.5–8.0	Acid urine accompanies acidosis, fever, high protein diet; alkaline urine in urinary tract infection, metabolic alkalosis, vegetarian diet
Chemical Determinations		
Glucose	Negative	Glucose present in uncontrolled diabetes mellitus, steroid excess
Ketones	Negative	Present in diabetes mellitus and in starvation
Protein	Negative	Present in kidney disorders, such as glomerulonephritis, acute kidney failure
Bilirubin	Negative	Breakdown product of hemoglobin; present in liver disease or in bile blockage
Urobilinogen	0.2–1.0 Ehrlich units /dL	Breakdown product of bilirubin; increased in hemolytic anemias and in liver disease; remains negative in bile obstruction
Blood (occult)	Negative	Detects small amounts of blood cells, hemoglobin, or myoglobin; present in severe trauma, metabolic disorders, bladder infections
Nitrite	Negative	Product of bacterial breakdown of urine; positive result suggests urinary tract infection and needs to be followed up with a culture of the urine

(continued)

Test	Normal Value	Clinical Significance
Microscopic		
Red blood cells	0–3 per high-power field	Increased because of bleeding within the urinary tract from trauma, tumors, inflammation, or damage within the kidney
White blood cells	0–4 per high-power field	Increased by kidney or bladder infection
Renal epithelial cells	Occasional	Increased number indicates damage to kidney tubules
Casts	None	Hyaline casts normal; large number of abnormal casts indicates inflammation or a systemic disorder
Crystals	Present	Most are normal; may be acid or alkaline
Bacteria	Few	Increased in urinary tract infection or contamination from infected genitalia
Others		Any yeasts, parasites, mucus, spermatozoa, or other microscopic findings would be reported here

■ COMPLETE BLOOD COUNT (CBC)

Test	Normal Value*	Clinical Significance
Red blood cell (RBC) count	Men: 4.2–5.4 million/μL Women: 3.6–5.0 million/mL	Decreased in anemia; increased in dehydration, polycythemia
Hemoglobin (Hb)	Men: 13.5–17.5 g/dL Women: 12–16 g/dL	Decreased in anemia, hemorrhage, and hemolytic reactions; increased in dehydration, heart and lung disease
Hematocrit (Hct) or packed cell volume (PCV)	Women: 37%–47%	Decreased in anemia; increased in polycythemia, dehydration
Red blood cell (RBC) indices (examples)	Men: 40%–50%	These values, calculated from the RBC count, Hb, and Hct, give information valuable in the diagnosis and classification of anemia
Mean corpuscular volume (MCV)	87–103 μL/red cell	Measures the average size or volume of each RBC: small size (microcytic) in iron-deficiency anemia; large size (macrocytic) typical of pernicious anemia
Mean corpuscular hemoglobin (MCH)	26–34 pg/red cell	Measures the weight of hemoglobin per RBC; useful in differentiating types of anemia in a severely anemic patient
Mean corpuscular hemoglobin concentration (MCHC)	31–37 g/dL	Defines the volume of hemoglobin per RBC; used to determine the color or concentration of hemoglobin per RBC
White blood cell (WBC) count	5,000–10,000/μL	Increased in leukemia and in response to infection, inflammation, and dehydration; decreased in bone marrow suppression
Platelets	150,000–350,000/μL	Increased in many malignant disorders; decreased in disseminated intravascular coagulation (DIC) or toxic drug effects; spontaneous bleeding may occur at platelet counts less than 20,000 μL

(continued)

Test	Normal Value*	Clinical Significance
Differential (peripheral blood smear)	40%–74%	A stained slide of the blood is needed to perform the differential. The percentages of the different WBCs are estimated, and the slide is microscopically checked for abnormal characteristics in WBCs, RBCs, and platelets.
WBCs		
Segmented neutrophils (SEGs, POLYs)	0%–3%	Increased in bacterial infections; low numbers leave person very susceptible to infection
Immature neutrophils (BANDs)	20%–40%	Increased when neutrophil count increases
Lymphocytes (LYMPHs)	2%–6%	Increased in viral infections; low numbers leave person dangerously susceptible to infection
Monocytes (MONOs)	1%–4%	Increased in specific infections
Eosinophils (EOs)	0.5%–1%	Increased in allergic disorders
Basophils (BASOs)		Increased in allergic disorders

*Values vary depending on instrumentation and type of test.

■ BLOOD CHEMISTRY TESTS

Test	Normal Value	Clinical Significance
Basic Panel: An Overview of Electrolytes, Waste Product Management, and Metabolism		
Blood urea nitrogen (BUN)	7–18 mg/dL	Increased in renal disease and dehydration; decreased in liver damage and malnutrition
Carbon dioxide (CO_2) (includes bicarbonate)	23–30 mmol/L	Useful to evaluate acid-base balance by measuring total carbon dioxide in the blood: elevated in vomiting and pulmonary disease; decreased in diabetic acidosis, acute renal failure, and hyperventilation
Chloride (Cl)	98–106 mEq/L	Increased in dehydration, hyperventilation, and congestive heart failure; decreased in vomiting, diarrhea, and fever
Creatinine	0.6–1.2 mg/dL	Produced at a constant rate and excreted by the kidney; increased in kidney disease
Glucose	Fasting: 70–110 mg/dL Random: 85–125 mg/dL	Increased in diabetes and severe illness; decreased in insulin overdose or hypoglycemia
Potassium (K)	3.5–5 mEq/L	Increased in renal failure, extensive cell damage, and acidosis; decreased in vomiting, diarrhea, and excess administration of diuretics or IV fluids
Sodium (Na)	101–111 mEq/L or 135–148 mEq/L (depending on test)	Increased in dehydration and diabetes insipidus; decreased in overload of IV fluids, burns, diarrhea, or vomiting

(continued)

Test	Normal Value	Clinical Significance
Additional Blood Chemistry Tests		
Alanine aminotransferase (ALT)	10–40 U/L	Used to diagnose and monitor treatment of liver disease and to monitor the effects of drugs on the liver; increased in myocardial infarction
Albumin	3.8–5.0 g/dL	Albumin holds water in blood; decreased in liver disease and kidney disease
Albumin-globulin ratio (A/G ratio)	Greater than 1	Low A/G ratio signifies a tendency for edema because globulin is less effective than albumin at holding water in the blood
Alkaline phosphatase (ALP)	20–70 U/L (varies by method)	Enzyme of bone metabolism; increased in liver disease and metastatic bone disease
Amylase	21–160 U/L	Used to diagnose and monitor treatment of acute pancreatitis and to detect inflammation of the salivary glands
Aspartate aminotransferase (AST)	0–41 U/L (varies)	Enzyme present in tissues with high metabolic activity; increased in myocardial infarction and liver disease
Bilirubin, total	0.2–1.0 mg/dL	Breakdown product of hemoglobin from red blood cells; increased when excessive red blood cells are being destroyed or in liver disease
Calcium (Ca)	8.8–10.0 mg/dL	Increased in excess parathyroid hormone production and in cancer; decreased in alkalosis, elevated phosphate in renal failure, and excess IV fluids
Cholesterol	120–220 mg/dL desirable range	Screening test used to evaluate risk of heart disease; levels of 200 mg/dL or greater indicate increased risk of heart disease and warrant further investigation
Creatine kinase (CK)	Men: 38–174 U/L Women: 96–140 U/L	Elevated enzyme level indicates myocardial infarction or damage to skeletal muscle. When elevated, specific fractions (isoenzymes) are tested for
Gamma-glutamyl transferase (GGT)	Men: 6–26 U/L Women: 4–18 U/L	Used to diagnose liver disease and to test for chronic alcoholism
Globulins	2.3–3.5 g/dL	Proteins active in immunity; help albumin keep water in blood
High-density lipoproteins (HDLs)	Men: 30–70 mg/dL Women: 30–85 mg/dL	Used to evaluate the risk of heart disease
Iron, serum (Fe)	Men: 75–175 mg/dL Women: 65–165 m/dL	Decreased in iron deficiency and anemia; increased in hemolytic conditions
Lactic dehydrogenase (LDH or LD)	95–200 U/L (normal ranges vary greatly)	Enzyme released in many kinds of tissue damage, including myocardial infarction, pulmonary infarction, and liver disease
Lipase	4–24 U/L (varies with test)	Enzyme used to diagnose pancreatitis
Low-density lipoproteins (LDLs)	80–140 mg/dL	Used to evaluate the risk of heart disease
Magnesium (Mg)	1.3–2.1 mEq/L	Vital in neuromuscular function; decreased levels may occur in malnutrition, alcoholism, pancreatitis, diarrhea

(continued)

Test	Normal Value*	Clinical Significance
Phosphorus (P) (inorganic)	2.7–4.5 mg/dL	Evaluated in response to calcium; main store is in bone: elevated in kidney disease; decreased in excess parathyroid hormone
Protein, total	6–8 g/dL	Increased in dehydration, multiple myeloma; decreased in kidney disease, liver disease, poor nutrition, severe burns, excessive bleeding
Serum glutamic oxalacetic transaminase (SGOT)		See aspartate aminotransferase (AST)
Serum glutamic pyruvic transaminase (SGPT)		See alanine aminotransferase (ALT)
Thyroid-stimulating hormone (TSH)	0.5–6 mU/L	Produced by pituitary to promote thyroid gland function; elevated when thyroid gland is not functioning
Thyroxin (T_4)	5–12.5 mg/dL (varies)	Screening test of thyroid function; increased in hyperthyroidism; decreased in myxedema and hypothyroidism
Triglycerides	Men: 40–160 mg/dL Women: 35–135 mg/dL	An indication of ability to metabolize fats; increased triglycerides and cholesterol indicate high risk of atherosclerosis
Triiodothyronine (T_3)	120–195 mg/dL	Elevated in specific types of hyperthyroidism
Uric acid	Men: 3.5–7.2 mg/dL Women: 2.6–6.0 mg/dL	Produced by breakdown of ingested purines in food and nucleic acids; elevated in kidney disease, gout, and leukemia

Adapted from Cohen, BJ. *Memmler's The Human Body in Health and Disease*, 11th ed. Baltimore: Lippincott Williams & Wilkins, 2009.

Abbreviation	Meaning
A&P resection	abdominoperineal resection
AB	abortion
Ab	antibody
ABG	arterial blood gas
ACB	aortocoronary bypass
ACS	acute coronary syndrome
ACTH	adrenocorticotropic hormone
ADH	antidiuretic hormone
ADHD	attention deficit hyperactivity disorder
ADL	activities of daily living
AFB	acid-fast bacilli
AFP	alpha fetoprotein
Ag	antigen
AIDS	acquired immunodeficiency syndrome
ALS	amyotrophic lateral sclerosis
ANA	antinuclear antibody test
AP	anteroposterior (from front to back)
ARDS	acute respiratory distress syndrome
ARF	acute renal failure
ARMD	age-related macular degeneration
ASHD	arteriosclerotic heart disease
AV	arteriovenous, atrioventricular
BAL	bronchoalveolar lavage
BCC	basal cell carcinoma
BE	barium enema
b.i.d.	twice a day
BM	bowel movement
BMA	bone marrow aspiration
BMT	bone marrow transplant
BOOP	bronchiolitis obliterans with organizing pneumonia
BP	blood pressure

Abbreviation	Meaning
BPH	benign prostatic hyperplasia; benign prostatic hypertrophy
BT	blood transfusion
BUN	blood urea nitrogen
Bx	biopsy
C	Celsius, centigrade (temperature)
C&S	culture and sensitivity
C1 to C7	cervical vertebrae 1 to 7
CA	cancer
CABG	coronary artery bypass graft
CAD	coronary artery disease
CAM	complementary and alternative medicine
cath	catheter; catheterize; catheterization
CBC	complete blood count
cc	cubic centimeter
CHF	congestive heart failure
CK	creatine kinase
cm	centimeter
CNS	central nervous system
COPD	chronic obstructive pulmonary disease
CP	cerebral palsy
CPAP	continuous positive airway pressure
CPR	cardiopulmonary resuscitation
creat	creatinine
CRF	chronic renal failure
CSF	cerebrospinal fluid
CSII	continuous subcutaneous insulin infusion
CT	computed tomography
CTS	carpal tunnel syndrome
CVA	cerebrovascular accident

(continued)

Abbreviation	Meaning
CVS	chorionic villus sampling
CXR	chest x-ray
D&C	dilation and curettage
DC	doctor of chiropractic medicine
DCIS	ductal carcinoma in situ
DDS	doctor of dental surgery
DI	diabetes insipidus
DKA	diabetic ketoacidosis
DM	diabetes mellitus
DOB	date of birth
DRE	digital rectal examination
DS	Doppler sonography
DTR	deep tendon reflex
DVT	deep venous thrombosis
Dx	diagnosis
EBV	Epstein-Barr virus
ECG or EKG	electrocardiography
ED	emergency department; erectile dysfunction
ED&C	electrodesiccation and curettage
EDC	estimated date of confinement
EDD	estimated date of delivery
EEG	electroencephalogram
EGD	esophagogastroduodenoscopy
EGFR	epidermal growth factor receptor
EMG	electromyogram
ENT	ears, nose, throat
EOM	extraocular movement
EPO	erythropoietin
ER	emergency room
ERCP	endoscopic retrograde cholangiopancreatography
ESR	erythrocyte sedimentation rate
ESRD	end stage renal disease
ESWL	extracorporeal shock wave lithotripsy
EUS	endoscopic ultrasound
F	Fahrenheit (temperature)
FBG	fasting blood glucose
Fe	iron

Abbreviation	Meaning
FNA	fine needle aspiration
FS	frozen section
FSH	follicle-stimulating hormone
fx	fracture
g or gm	gram
GERD	gastroesophageal reflux disease
GH	growth hormone
GI	gastrointestinal
GIST	gastrointestinal stromal tumor
GTT	glucose tolerance test
GU	genitourinary
GXT	graded exercise test
GYN	gynecology; gynecologist
H&P	history and physical (examination)
hCG	human chorionic gonadotropin
HCT, Hct, ht	hematocrit
HGB, Hb, Hgb	hemoglobin
HIDA	hepatobiliary iminodiacetic acid
HIV	human immunodeficiency virus
HM	Holter monitor
HPV	human papillomavirus
HRT	hormone replacement therapy
HSG	hysterosalpingogram
Ht	height
HTN	hypertension
Hx	history
I&D	incision and drainage
IBS	irritable bowel syndrome
ICU	intensive care unit
ILD	interstitial lung disease
IOL	intraocular lens
IOP	intraocular pressure
ITP	idiopathic thrombocytopenic purpura
IVF	in vitro fertilization
IVP	intravenous pyelogram; intravenous pyelography
IVU	intravenous urogram; intravenous urography
kg	kilogram

(continued)

Abbreviation	Meaning
KUB	kidneys, ureters, and bladder (x-ray)
L	liter
L1 to L5	lumbar vertebrae 1 to 5
lab	laboratory
LASIK	laser-assisted in situ keratomileusis
LEEP	loop electrosurgical excision procedure
LH	luteinizing hormone
LMP	last menstrual period
LP	lumbar puncture
m	meter
MD	doctor of medicine; muscular dystrophy
MEN	multiple endocrine neoplasia
mg	milligram
MG	myasthenia gravis
MI	myocardial infarction
mL	milliliter
mm	millimeter
MRA	magnetic resonance angiography
MRCP	magnetic resonance cholangiopancreatography
MRI	magnetic resonance imaging
MS	multiple sclerosis
MUGA	multiple uptake gated acquisition
NG	nasogastric
NHL	non-Hodgkin lymphoma
NICU	neonatal intensive care unit
noc	night
NPO	nothing by mouth (don't eat or drink)
NSAID	nonsteroidal anti-inflammatory drug
OA	osteoarthritis
OB	obstetrics; obstetrician
OB/GYN	obstetrics/gynecology
OCD	obsessive-compulsive disorder
OD	doctor of optometry; right eye (oculus dexter)
ORIF	open reduction, internal fixation
OS	left eye (oculus sinister)

Abbreviation	Meaning
OU	each eye or both eyes (oculus uterque)
oz	ounce
P	pulse rate
p.c.	after meals
p.r.n.	as needed
PA	physician's assistant
PAD	peripheral arterial disease
Peds	pediatrics
PET	positron emission tomography
PFTs	pulmonary function tests
PID	pelvic inflammatory disease
PLT	platelet or platelet count
POC	products of conception
postop, post-op	postoperative (after surgery)
PPD	purified protein derivative
preop, pre-op	preoperative (before surgery)
PRK	photorefractive keratectomy
PSA	prostate-specific antigen
pt	patient
PT	physical therapy; prothrombin time
PTCA	percutaneous transluminal coronary angioplasty
PTH	parathyroid hormone
PTSD	posttraumatic stress disorder
PUD	peptic ulcer disease
PVC	premature ventricular contraction
Px	prognosis
q.i.d.	four times a day
R	respiratory rate
RA	rheumatoid arthritis
RAD	reactive airway disease
RAIU	radioactive iodine uptake
RBC	red blood cell; red blood cell count
RF	rheumatoid factor; respiratory failure
RFA	radiofrequency ablation
RHD	rheumatic heart disease
ROM	range of motion
Rx	prescription

(continued)

Abbreviation	Meaning
SAB	spontaneous abortion
SCC	squamous cell carcinoma
SG	specific gravity
SLE	systemic lupus erythematosus
SPECT	single photon emission computed tomography
STAT	immediately
STD	sexually transmitted disease
SUI	stress urinary incontinence
Sx	symptom
T	temperature
T1 to T12	thoracic vertebrae 1 to 12
T_3	triiodothyronine
T_4	thyroxine
TAB	therapeutic abortion
TAH	total abdominal hysterectomy
TB	tuberculosis
TEE	transesophageal echocardiography
TIA	transient ischemic attack
TPN	total parenteral nutrition
Tr	treatment
TRUS	transrectal ultrasound

Abbreviation	Meaning
TSH	thyroid-stimulating hormone
TUIP	transurethral incision of the prostate
TURB	transurethral resection of bladder tumor
TURP	transurethral resection of the prostate
Tx	treatment
UA	urinalysis
UGI	upper gastrointestinal
URI	upper respiratory infection
UTI	urinary tract infection
VA	visual acuity
VATS	video-assisted thorascopic surgery
VCUG	voiding cystourethrogram; voiding cystourethrography
VD	venereal disease
VF	visual field
V/Q	ventilation-perfusion (scan)
VS	vital signs
vWD	von Willebrand disease
WBC	white blood cell; white blood cell count
Wt	weight

■ DANGEROUS ABBREVIATIONS, ACRONYMS, AND SYMBOLS

The Joint Commission (www.jointcommission.org) originally issued a list of dangerous abbreviations, acronyms, and symbols that should not be used in health care in 2004. This list was updated in 2005. Organizations that wish to be accredited by the Joint Commission must develop and implement a list of abbreviations not to be used.

Official "Do Not Use" List

Do Not Use	Potential Problem	Use Instead
U (unit)	Mistaken for 0 (zero), 4 (four), or cc	Write "unit".
IU (international unit)	Mistaken for IV (intravenous) or 10 (ten)	Write "international unit".
Q.D., QD, q.d., qd (daily)	Mistaken for each other.	Write "daily".
Q.O.D., QOD, q.o.d, qod (every other day)	Period after the Q mistaken for "I" and the "O" mistaken for "I"	Write "every other day".
Trailing zero (X.0 mg)*	Decimal point is missed.	Write "X mg".
Lack of leading zero (.X mg)		Write "0.X mg".
MS, MSO_4, and $MgSO_4$	Can mean morphine sulfate or magnesium sulfate; confused for one another.	Write "morphine sulfate". Write "magnesium sulfate".

*Exception: A trailing zero may be used only where required to demonstrate the level of precision of the value being reported, such as for laboratory results, imaging studies that report size of lesions, or catheter/tube sizes. It may not be used in medication orders or other medication-related documentation.

An abbreviation on the "do not use" list should not be used in any of its forms—upper or lower case, with or without periods (e.g., Q.D., QD, or qd). Any of those variations may be confusing and could be misinterpreted.

In addition, the Joint Commission has identified the following error-prone abbreviations for possible future inclusion on the official "do not use" list.

Additional Abbreviations, Acronyms and Symbols

Do Not Use	Potential Problem	Use Instead
> (greater than)	Mistaken for 7 (seven) or the letter "L"; confused for one another	Write "greater than".
< (less than)		Write "less than".
Abbreviations for drug names	Misinterpreted due to similar abbreviations for multiple drugs	Write drug names in full.
Apothecary units	Unfamiliar to many practitioners. Confused with metric units.	Use metric units.
@	Mistaken for 2 (two)	Write "at".
cc (for cubic centimeter)	Mistaken for U (units) when poorly written	Write "mL" or "ml" or "milliliters" ("mL" is preferred).
μg (for microgram)	Mistaken for mg (milligrams), resulting in 1,000-fold overdose	Write "mcg" or "micrograms".

Complementary and Alternative Medicine Terms

Term	Meaning
acupressure	A treatment involving the application of pressure to those areas of the body used in acupuncture.
acupuncture	A traditional Chinese therapeutic technique involving puncturing the skin with fine needles to influence the flow of *qi* (vital energy).
African medicine	Traditional African therapeutic techniques, based on naturopathic medicine, designed to treat the physical, mental, and spiritual causes of disease.
Alexander technique	A system of educational therapy involving the use of minimal effort for maximum movement to improve posture and alleviate pain.
allopathy	A term used to describe conventional, Western medicine, in contrast to alternative or complementary medicine.
Alpha Calm Therapy	A therapeutic technique involving guided imagery and hypnosis.
alternative medicine	A general term for therapeutic practices that fall outside the realm of evidence-based, mainstream medicine and are intended as replacements for conventional medical treatments. Alternative medical therapies fall into five main groups: complete medical systems (such as homeopathy and Chinese medicine), mind-body interventions (such as visualization and yoga), manipulative and body-based methods (such as chiropractic and massage), biologically based therapies (such as herbalism and macrobiotics), and energy therapies (such as qi gong and vibrational medicine).
Ama Deus	A South American Indian system of healing
apitherapy	Treatment of illness involving the administration of honeybee stings.
applied kinesiology	The use of muscle testing to identify illness. Applied kinesiology is based on the theory that weakness in certain muscles is associated with imbalances in the body.
aromatherapy	A form of treatment involving the use of concentrated oils from plants with healing properties.
art therapy	A therapy involving the use of artistic expression to promote emotional well-being.
Ayurveda (ī'yŭr-ved'dă)	A form of natural medicine, traditional in India, that provides an integrated approach to preventing and treating illness through lifestyle intervention and natural therapy. It involves *nadis* (canals) that carry *prana* (energy) throughout the body, *chakras* (centers of consciousness) that connect body and soul, and *marmas* (points on the body beneath which vital structures connect).
Bach flower therapy	A system of diagnosis and treatment, developed by British physician Edward Bach, that involves the use of flower essences.
biofeedback	A method of treatment that uses monitors to help patients recognize physiologic information of which they are normally unaware. Using this method, patients can learn to consciously control involuntary bodily processes such as blood pressure, temperature, gastrointestinal functioning, and brain wave activity.
bodywork	A group of therapeutic techniques that involve exercising or manipulating the body to produce healing.
Bowen technique	A form of bodywork developed by Australian Tom Bowen, in which certain body areas are lightly touched to stimulate energy flow.

(continued)

Term	Meaning
chelation therapy	The administration of *chelating agents* (drugs that bind and remove certain materials from the body) to treat or prevent illness.
Chinese medicine	An ancient health care system, traditional in China, based on the concept that disease results from disruption of *qi* (vital energy) and imbalance of *yin* (negative energy) and *yang* (positive energy). Chinese medicine encompasses several therapies, including herbal and nutritional therapy, restorative physical exercises, meditation, acupuncture, and massage.
chiropractic	A diagnostic and therapeutic system based on the concept that disease results from nervous system malfunction. Treatment involves manipulation and adjustment of body structures, particularly the spinal column, to relieve local and distant physical ailments.
complementary medicine	A general term for therapeutic techniques that are intended to accompany and support mainstream, evidence-based medical treatments.
craniosacral therapy	A diagnostic and therapeutic system in which the bones of the skull are manipulated to remove impediments to cerebrospinal fluid flow, with the goals of stress relief, pain alleviation, and overall health improvement.
cupping	A treatment that consists of attaching a cup to the skin and evacuating the air within to increase local blood flow.
curanderismo	A Mexican-American traditional form of medicine encompassing acupuncture and homeopathy. From the Spanish *curar* (to treat or cure).
Feldenkrais method	A form of bodywork, developed by Israeli physicist Moshe Feldenkrais, that includes private instruction (*Functional Integration*), and group instruction (*Awareness through Movement*).
Gerson therapy	A dietary therapy, by German physician Max Gerson, that involves sodium restriction, potassium supplementation, fat restriction, periodic protein restriction, and coffee enemas.
guided imagery	A technique in which patients imagine or visualize certain scenarios to improve health or promote healing.
herbal medicine	The practice of creating or prescribing plant-derived remedies for medical conditions.
holistic medicine	A general term for therapies, such as yoga, that emphasize the unity of body, mind, and spirit.
homeopathy	A therapeutic system based on the concept that a disease may be treated with minute doses of drugs that cause the same symptoms in healthy people as the disease itself. Substances are *potentized* (diluted) to prepare *remedies* (pharmacologic therapies) for patients. Homeopathic medicine is practiced in a holistic fashion, incorporating the elements of body, mind, and spirit.
hydrotherapy	The internal and external use of water for the treatment of disease.
hypnosis	The induction of trance to treat a wide variety of conditions such as substance addiction, pain, and phobias.
Kneipping	A system of natural healing developed by Dominican priest Sebastian Kneipp, based on the principles of hydrotherapy and herbalism.
Korean medicine	A form of medicine, traditional in Korea, that encompasses acupuncture and moxibustion.
macrobiotics	A vegetarian dietary therapy promoting health and longevity.
magnet therapy	A therapy in which magnetic fields are applied to the body using magnetic field‑generating machines, mattresses, or blankets.
massage therapy	A therapeutic system involving muscle manipulation to reduce tension and pain, promote relaxation, or diminish symptoms of muscular or neurologic diseases.
meridian therapy	A therapeutic method that involves rhythmic breathing, visualization, and moving one's hands along *meridians*, lines along the body that are said to represent channels through which *qi* (vital energy) flows.

(continued)

Term	Meaning
moxibustion	A traditional Chinese medical therapy that involves burning *moxa* (mugwort, or *Artemisia vulgaris*) and placing it at certain points on the body to stimulate *qi* (vital energy).
naturopathy	A therapeutic system involving the use of heat, water, light, air, and massage for treatment of disease. The discipline is composed of various alternative medical therapies, including homeopathy, herbal medicine, acupuncture, hydrotherapy, and manipulative therapy
orthomolecular medicine	A therapeutic modality and preventative medicine strategy involving the use of natural substances found in food, such as vitamins, amino acids, and minerals, to treat and prevent disease. Supplementation with relatively large doses of vitamins (*megavitamin therapy*) is sometimes used.
qigong	A component of Chinese medicine that uses physical movement, breathing regulation, and meditation to achieve optimum health. From the Mandarin *qi* (breath), and *gong* (work or technique).
reflexology	The practice of stimulating certain points on the body, most commonly on the feet, to improve health.
Reiki (rā' kē)	A therapy based on the theory that spiritual energy is channeled through a reek practitioner, healing the patient's body and spirit. From the Japanese *rein* (spirit or soul) and *kid* (energy or life force).
Rolfing	A form of myofascial massage, developed by American chemist Ida P. Rolf, that involves deep soft tissue manipulation to release stored tension and manually realign body structures.
shiatsu	A massage technique that originated in Japan, in which the thumbs, palms, fingers, and elbows are used to place pressure at certain points on the body.
tai chi	An ancient Chinese martial art involving a combination of intentional, leveraged movement and focused breathing to improve health and longevity.
Trager	A form of bodywork, developed by Milton Trager, M.D., that combines physical movement with meditation.
vibrational medicine	A general term for therapeutic modalities based on the concept that disease originates in subtle energy systems, which are affected by environmental, nutritional, spiritual, and emotional factors. Examples of vibrational medicine therapies include acupuncture, aromatherapy, homeopathy, crystal healing, and orthomolecular medicine.
yoga	A system of exercises for the improvement of physical and spiritual health, derived from Hindu tradition.

Rules for Forming Plurals

Some medical terms also add an -s (or -es) to make a plural, but many do not. They have special endings related to their origins in Greek or Latin. The following table shows some of the special plural endings common in medical terms.

Singular Ending	Example	Plural Ending	Example
a	vertebra	ae	vertebrae
en	lumen	ina	lumina
ex, ix, yx	index	ices	indices
is	testis	es	testes
on	spermatozoon	a	spermatozoa
um	diverticulum	a	diverticula
us	nucleus	i	nuclei
x, nx	phalanx	ges, nges	phalanges

Answers to Exercises

Chapter 1

Exercise 1
1. bone
2. disk
3. brain, cerebrum
4. lung
5. skin

Exercise 2
1. crani
2. cardi
3. gastr
4. col, colon
5. nephr, ren

Exercise 3
1. painful, difficult, abnormal
2. within
3. around, surrounding
4. after, behind
5. many, much

Exercise 4
1. pre-
2. inter-
3. a-, an-
4. supra-, super-
5. sub-, infra-

Exercise 5
1. -tomy
2. -ium
3. -gram
4. -al
5. -logy
6. -algia
7. -itis
8. -ectomy
9. -ism
10. -oma

Exercise 6
1. disk/o
2. gastr/o
3. nephr/o, ren/o
4. cardi/o
5. crani/o
6. oste/o
7. pulmon/o
8. cerebr/o
9. dermat/o
10. col/o, colon/o

Exercise 7
1. intracranial
2. subpulmonary
3. cardiogram
4. ostealgia
5. gastrotomy

Exercise 8
1. emboli
2. varicoses

3. aortae
4. larynges
5. ulcers

Exercise 9
Practice until your pronunciation matches that heard in the Audio Glossary in the Student Resources.

Exercise 10
1. arthr/o / -itis
   joint / inflammation
   inflammation of joint
2. pulmon/o / -ary
   lung / pertaining to
   pertaining to the lung
3. colon/o / -itis
   colon / inflammation
   inflammation of colon
4. oste/o / -al
   bone / pertaining to
   pertaining to bone
5. cardi/o / -tomy
   heart / incision
   incision into the heart

Exercise 11
1. dermatitis
2. pericardial
3. diskectomy
4. osteoma
5. renal

Exercise 12
1. below, beneath
2. osteoma
3. colonoscopy
4. skin
5. stomach
6. between
7. heart
8. lungs or lung
9. without, not
10. lymphoma

Exercise 13
1. D
2. B
3. A
4. D
5. B
6. B
7. A
8. B
9. C
10. B

Exercise 14
1. carditis
2. phenomena
3. pericardial
4. gastrectomy
5. nuclei

6. osteoarthritis
7. cardiography
8. vertebrae
9. dermatitis
10. cardiopulmonary

Chapter 2

Exercise 1
1. uni-, mono-
2. bi-, di-
3. tri-
4. quad-, quadri-
5. multi-, poly-

Exercise 2
1. half
2. half
3. double
4. one
5. four

Exercise 3
1. opposing, against
2. not
3. away from, cessation, without
4. without, not
5. separate, remove

Exercise 4
1. inter-
2. post-
3. per-, trans-
4. supra-
5. en-, end-, endo-, intra-

Exercise 5
1. outer, outside
2. away from
3. before
4. below, beneath
5. together, with

Exercise 6
1. hetero-
2. normo-
3. mega-, megalo-, macro-
4. oligo-
5. iso-, homo-, homeo-
6. micro-, oligo-

Exercise 7
1. dys-
2. eu-
3. hyper-
4. pan-
5. iso-
6. hypo-

Exercise 8
1. rapid
2. new
3. slow
4. again, backward
5. false

Exercise 9
1. enlarged
2. abnormal condition
3. condition of
4. condition of
5. condition of

Exercise 10
1. -algia
2. -itis
3. -rrhea
4. -emia
5. -oma
6. -pathy

Exercise 11
1. puncture to aspirate
2. excision, surgical removal
3. surgical opening
4. surgical repair, reconstruction

Exercise 12
1. -tomy
2. -rrhaphy
3. -stomy
4. -ectomy

Exercise 13
1. instrument for measuring
2. process of recording
3. pertaining to
4. pertaining to
5. record
6. pertaining to
7. study of
8. pertaining to

Exercise 14
1. -logist
2. -oid
3. -ium
4. -ole
5. -genic
6. -scope

Exercise 15
1. intensive care unit
2. red blood cell
3. pulse rate
4. history and physical
5. activities of daily living
6. emergency department
7. liter
8. treatment
9. ears, nose, and throat
10. laboratory

Exercise 16
1. Sx
2. VS
3. Dx
4. Ht
5. STAT
6. p.r.n.
7. R
8. BP
9. Rx
10. noc
11. PT
12. Hx

Exercise 17
1. im-
2. ad-
3. poly-

4. per-
5. intra-
6. exo-
7. hemi-
8. hetero-
9. hypo-
10. dys-

Exercise 18
1. -osis
2. -rrhaphy
3. -gram
4. -tomy
5. -emia
6. -pathy
7. -ar
8. -plasty
9. -graphy
10. -ium

Exercise 19
1. bisect
2. submandibular
3. cavitary
4. cardiotomy
5. psychology
6. endoscope
7. polyarthritis
8. thrombosis
9. panarthritis
10. semiconscious

Exercise 20
1. myositis
2. lobectomy
3. cardiopathy
4. intercostal
5. postnasal
6. microbiologist
7. lymphoma
8. dermatoid
9. cranioplasty
10. tenorrhaphy

Exercise 21
1. mononeural
2. hemiplegia
3. ectoderm
4. infrasonic
5. pericarditis
6. megalosplenia
7. oligodipsia
8. bradycardia
9. diarrhea
10. heterogenic
11. myalgia
12. cystorrhaphy
13. osteogenesis
14. edematous
15. gastrotomy

Exercise 22
Practice until your pronunciation matches that heard in the Audio Glossary in the Student Resources.

Chapter 3

Exercise 1
1. condition, process
2. death
3. muscle
4. tumor
5. water, watery

6. disease
7. nerve
8. blood
9. smooth
10. form, shape

Exercise 2
1. gluc/o
2. blast/o
3. viscer/o
4. hist/o
5. -pathy
6. -osis
7. oste/o
8. lip/o
9. -cyte
10. aden/o

Exercise 3
1. histology
2. exacerbation
3. somatic
4. lesion
5. chronic
6. idiopathic
7. acute
8. gene
9. necrosis
10. homeostasis

Exercise 4
1. group of organs with related structure or function
2. cytologic and chemical changes in tissue in response to an injury or disease
3. any virus, microorganism, or other substance that causes disease
4. lessening in severity of disease symptoms
5. pertaining to the internal organs
6. the study of cells
7. the study of cause of disease
8. a differentiated structure of similar tissues or cells with a specific function
9. sum of the normal chemical and physical changes occurring in tissue
10. excessive growth of tissue

Exercise 5
1. exacerbation
2. nucleus
3. systemic
4. tissue
5. idiopathic
6. cytoplasm
7. cytology
8. pathogen

Exercise 6
1. thorax, chest
2. neck
3. lumbar region, lower back
4. abdomen
5. pelvis

Exercise 7
1. abdominocentesis
2. thoracoplasty
3. pelvimeter
4. lumbar
5. cervicectomy
6. podalgia

Exercise 8
1. thorax
2. spinal cavity
3. umbilical region
4. abdomen
5. cranium

Exercise 9
1. limb
2. abdominal region above the umbilical region
3. hollow area within the chest occupied by the lungs, heart, and other organs
4. muscle between the abdominal and thoracic cavities
5. abdominal region to left or right of hypogastric region

Exercise 10
1. abdominal
2. hypochondriac
3. four
4. cranial
5. thoracic

Exercise 11
1. below, beneath
2. within
3. tail
4. back
5. front
6. on, following
7. side
8. head
9. around
10. back

Exercise 12
1. pertaining to between vertebrae
2. pertaining to around (surrounding) the heart
3. pertaining to behind the cecum
4. pertaining to the middle of the carpal bone
5. pertaining to a high number

Exercise 13
1. distal
2. supine
3. superior
4. superficial
5. lateral
6. anterior
7. anteroposterior
8. ventral
9. cephalad
10. Fowler position

Exercise 14
1. lying face up
2. below or downward
3. vertical plane dividing the body into anterior and posterior halves
4. nearer the trunk or point of origin
5. toward the tail
6. horizontal plane dividing the body into upper and lower halves
7. pertaining to both sides
8. body in standard reference position: standing erect, arms at the sides, palms facing forward
9. pertaining to the middle
10. pertaining to the back

Exercise 15
1. side
2. sagittal
3. deep
4. unilateral
5. posterior
6. distal
7. ventral
8. superior
9. decubitus
10. proximal

Exercise 16
1. black, dark
2. blue
3. yellow
4. green
5. white
6. red
7. color

Exercise 17
1. erythrocyte
2. xanthoderma
3. melanoma
4. chromaturia
5. leukocyte
6. blue discoloration of skin and other tissues

Exercise 18
1. surgical removal of lobe
2. after surgery
3. incision into the thorax
4. pertaining to above the clavicle (collar bone)
5. disease affecting lymph node (gland)
6. organ enlargement
7. condition of bluish discoloration of the skin and other tissues

Exercise 19
1. cranial cavity
2. spinal cavity
3. thoracic cavity
4. diaphragm
5. abdominal cavity
6. pelvic cavity
7. abdominopelvic cavity

Exercise 20
1. right hypochondriac region
2. epigastric region
3. left hypochondriac region
4. right lumbar region
5. umbilical region
6. left lumbar region
7. right iliac region
8. hypogastric (suprapubic) region
9. left iliac region

Exercise 21
1. fibr/o / -osis
   fiber / abnormal condition
   abnormal condition of fibrous tissue
2. path/o / -genic
   disease / producing
   causing or producing disease
3. hem/o / -stasis
   blood / stopped
   stopping of bleeding
4. neur/o / blast/o
   nerve / immature cell
   immature never cell

5. oste/o / necr/o / -osis
   bone / death / abnormal condition
   abnormal condition of death of bone tissue
6. cervic/o / brachi/o / -al
   neck / arm / pertaining to
   pertaining to the neck and arm
7. crani/o / cerebr/o / -al
   cranium, skull / brain, cerebrum / pertaining to
   pertaining to the skull and brain
8. super/o or super- / later/o / -al
   above / side / pertaining to
   pertaining to at the side and above
9. viscer/o / -megaly
   internal organs / enlargement
   enlargement of internal organs
10. hyper- / glyc/o / -emia
    above, excessive / glucose, sugar / blood (condition of)
    condition of above normal blood glucose

Exercise 22
1. hyperplasia
2. abnormal
3. study of form or shape
4. condition of lipids (fat) in the blood
5. remission
6. left lumbar
7. anteroposterior
8. Fowler
9. blue
10. exacerbation

Exercise 23
1. the edge nearest the trunk (in direction of shoulder)
2. standing erect, arms at the sides, palms facing forward
3. a group of organs with related structure or function
4. the nucleus
5. when it persists
6. the study of cause of a disease
7. a cavity is a hollow area (occupied by internal organs)
8. the back of the hand
9. having a yellow coloration of the skin
10. somatic (condition)

Exercise 24
1. B
2. A
3. D
4. C
5. A
6. B
7. D
8. C
9. D
10. B

Exercise 25
Practice until your pronunciation matches that heard in the Audio Glossary in the Student Resources.

Exercise 26
1. chromosome
2. diaphragm
3. homeostasis
4. cephalad
5. cytoplasm

6. erythrocyte
7. decubitus
8. umbilical
9. pathogen
10. leukocyte
11. inflammation
12. cytology
13. metabolism
14. cyanosis
15. nuclei
16. idiopathic
17. somatic
18. exacerbation
19. systemic
20. caudad
21. thoracic
22. etiology
23. necrosis
24. sagittal
25. superficial
26. proximal
27. hypochondriac
28. epigastric
29. visceral
30. chromaturia

Exercise 27
1. pulmonary
2. thoracotomy
3. lobectomy
4. lateral
5. proximally
6. distally

Exercise 28
1. bronchogenic
2. segmentectomy
3. lymphadenectomy
4. endotracheal
5. bronchoscopy
6. intercostal
7. subcutaneous

Chapter 4

Exercise 1
1. epidermis
2. sudoriferous glands
3. integumentary system
4. sebaceous glands
5. subcutaneous layer
6. arrector pili
7. dermis
8. epidermis
9. hair
10. sebum

Exercise 2
1. nail
2. hair follicle
3. sudoriferous glands
4. melanocytes
5. sebaceous glands
6. keratinocytes
7. keratin
8. adipocytes

Exercise 3
1. hair
2. wrinkle
3. nail
4. skin
5. fat

6. sebum
7. dry
8. skin
9. hard
10. red
11. sweat
12. cold

Exercise 4
1. xanth/o
2. seb/o
3. cyan/o
4. derm/o, dermat/o, cutane/o
5. electr/o
6. erythr/o
7. pachy/o
8. py/o
9. myc/o
10. melan/o
11. necr/o
12. hidr/o
13. kerat/o, scler/o

Exercise 5
1. softening
2. below, beneath
3. disease
4. inflammation
5. through
6. around, beside, near
7. instrument used to cut
8. to eat
9. within
10. flow, discharge
11. across, through
12. formation, growth
13. life

Exercise 6
1. inflammation of the skin
2. flow or discharge of pus
3. study of fungus
4. abnormal condition of sweating
5. excision or surgical removal of a nail

Exercise 7
1. xeroderma
2. dermatome
3. dermatologist
4. rhytidoplasty
5. necrosis
6. onychomalacia
7. melanocyte

Exercise 8
1. an-   / hidr/o / -osis
   without, not / sweat / abnormal
                          condition
   abnormal condition of not sweating
2. erythr/o / -derma
   red   / skin condition
   condition of reddening of the skin
3. scler/o / -derma
   hard   / skin condition
   condition of hardening of the skin
4. seb/o   / -rrhea
   sebum   / flow, discharge
   flow or discharge of oil or sebum
5. onych/o / -phagia
   nail   / to eat
   to eat (one's) nails (nail biting)

6. rhytid/o / -ectomy
   wrinkle / excision, surgical removal
   surgical removal of wrinkles
7. trans-   / derm/o / -al
   across, through / skin   / pertaining
                              to
   pertaining to across or through the skin
8. epi-   / derm/o / -al
   on, following / skin   / pertaining to
   pertaining to (the layer of skin) on top
   of the dermis
9. sub-   / cutane/o / -ous
   below, beneath / skin   / pertaining
                                  to
   pertaining to below or beneath the skin
10. myc/o   / -osis
    fungus / abnormal condition
    abnormal condition of fungus
11. kerat/o / -genic
    hard   / originating, producing
    producing hardness

Exercise 9
1. hyperplasia
2. atypical
3. purulent
4. indurated
5. integumentary
6. dysplasia
7. circumscribed
8. adipose

Exercise 10
1. erythematous
2. turgor
3. cyanosis
4. pallor
5. exfoliation
6. eschar
7. pruritic
8. diaphoresis

Exercise 11
1. full-thickness burn
2. papule
3. pustule
4. varicella
5. superficial burn
6. cellulitis
7. herpes zoster
8. psoriasis
9. eczema
10. herpes simplex
11. keloid
12. jaundice
13. lesion
14. abrasion

Exercise 12
1. wheal
2. nevus
3. decubitus ulcer
4. nodule
5. scabies
6. cicatrix
7. rosacea
8. gangrene
9. contusion
10. acne

Exercise 13
1. vesicle
2. macule

3. verruca
4. pediculosis
5. tinea pedis
6. comedo
7. urticaria
8. paronychia
9. cyst
10. impetigo
11. burn
12. abscess

Exercise 14
1. tuberculosis skin test
2. scratch test
3. biopsy
4. culture and sensitivity
5. frozen section

Exercise 15
1. surgical repair of the skin
2. the use of heat, cold, electric current, or caustic chemicals to destroy tissue
3. a graft transplanted using skin from a source other than the patient
4. the act of cutting out

Exercise 16
1. incision and drainage
2. incision
3. irrigation
4. sutured
5. débrided
6. dermatoautoplasty

Exercise 17
1. rhytid/o   wrinkle
2. derm/o   skin
3. cry/o   cold
4. electr/o   electric, electricity
5. rhytid/o   wrinkle
6. derm/o   skin

Exercise 18
1. steroid
2. antiinfective
3. antifungal
4. pediculicide
5. antiinflammatory
6. liquid nitrogen
7. antipruritic
8. intralesional injection
9. scabicide

Exercise 19
1. medical esthetician
2. dermatologist
3. dermatology

Exercise 20
1. purified protein derivative
2. culture and sensitivity
3. incision and drainage

Exercise 21
1. FS
2. bx
3. ED&C

Exercise 22
1. epidermis
2. dermis
3. subcutaneous layer
4. sebaceous gland
5. arrector pili muscle
6. hair follicle
7. sudoriferous (sweat) gland

Exercise 23
1. hidr/o   sweat
2. kerat/o   hard
3. cry/o   cold
4. dermat/o   skin
5. scler/o   hard
6. onych/o; myc/o nail; fungus
7. rhytid/o   wrinkle
8. py/o   pus
9. lip/o   fat
10. seb/o   sebum
11. dermat/o; myc/o skin; fungus
12. cutane/o   skin

Exercise 24
1. an-   / hidr/o / -osis
   without, not / sweat / abnormal
                          condition
   abnormal condition of not sweating
2. erythr/o / cyan/o / -osis
   red   / blue   / abnormal condition
   abnormal condition characterized by red and blue coloring
3. trich/o / -pathy
   hair   / disease
   disease of the hair
4. py/o / -derma
   pus / skin condition
   condition of pus in the skin
5. para- / onych/o / -ia
   beside / nail   / pertaining to
   pertaining to beside the nail (nail infection)
6. dermat/o / -logist
   skin   / one who specializes in
   physician who specializes in the skin
7. trans-   / derm/o / -al
   across, through/ skin   / pertaining to
   pertaining to across or through the skin
8. dermat/o / heter/o   / -plasty
   skin   / other, different / surgical
                                repair, reconstruction
   surgical repair or reconstruction of the skin using a source other than the patient
9. pachy/o / -derma
   thick   / skin condition
   condition of thick skin
10. onych/o / -malacia
    nail   / softening
    softening of the nail
11. cyan/o / -osis
    blue   / abnormal condition
    abnormal condition characterized by blue coloring
12. onych/o / -phagia
    nail   / to eat
    to eat one's nails (nail biting)
13. intra- / derm/o / -al
    within / skin   / pertaining to
    pertaining to within the skin
14. xer/o / -derma
    dry   / skin condition
    condition of dry skin

Exercise 25
1. epidermis, dermis, and subcutaneous layer (in any order)
2. arrector pili
3. comedo

4. sudoriferous
5. medical esthetician
6. abscess
7. rhytidoplasty
8. Adipocytes
9. indurated
10. vitiligo
11. Tinea
12. excoriation
13. furuncle
14. necrosis
15. tinea pedis
16. albinism
17. fissure

Exercise 26
1. B
2. C
3. B
4. C
5. D
6. D
7. A
8. C
9. B

Exercise 27
1. dermabrasion
2. circumscribed
3. débridement
4. carbuncle
5. tinea
6. impetigo
7. urticaria
8. paronychia
9. scratch
10. dermatome

Exercise 28
1. A
2. B
3. D
4. C
5. D
6. A
7. B
8. D

Exercise 29
1. C
2. D
3. A
4. the back of the foot

Exercise 30
1. B
2. A
3. C
4. pertaining to the nose and stomach

Exercise 31
Practice until your pronunciation matches that heard in the Audio Glossary in the Student Resources.

Exercise 32
1. anhidrosis
2. cicatrix
3. dermatomycosis
4. onychophagia
5. urticaria
6. psoriasis
7. gangrene
8. tinea

9. dysplasia
10. pruritic
11. keratogenic
12. xeroderma
13. jaundice
14. erythematous
15. arrector pili

Chapter 5

Exercise 1
1. jejunum
2. appendix
3. gallbladder
4. mouth, oral cavity
5. palate
6. pharynx
7. fundus
8. liver
9. ileum
10. anus
11. salivary glands
12. bile

Exercise 2
1. duodenum
2. pancreas
3. esophagus
4. sigmoid colon
5. pylorus
6. rectum
7. cecum
8. descending colon
9. uvula
10. rugae

Exercise 3
1. stomach
2. teeth
3. transverse
4. tongue
5. water
6. cardia
7. three
8. saliva
9. body
10. ascending

Exercise 4
1. duodenum
2. mouth
3. pancreas
4. small intestine
5. lip
6. saliva
7. liver
8. cheek
9. anus
10. digestion
11. pharynx
12. rectum and anus
13. pylorus
14. colon
15. sigmoid colon
16. tooth
17. abdomen

Exercise 5
1. jejun/o
2. appendic/o
3. phag/o
4. hemat/o, hem/o
5. gastr/o

6. esophag/o
7. bucc/o
8. rect/o
9. polyp/o
10. cholecyst/o
11. cec/o
12. lingu/o
13. ile/o
14. odont/o, dent/o
15. col/o, colon/o
16. lith/o
17. palat/o
18. bil/o, chol/e
19. herni/o
20. lapar/o, abdomin/o
21. aliment/o

Exercise 6
1. in, within
2. crushing
3. enzyme
4. around, surrounding
5. surgical opening
6. abnormal condition
7. one who specializes in
8. herniation, protrusion
9. origin, production
10. enlargement
11. backward, behind
12. prolapse, drooping, sagging
13. process of examining, examination
14. meal
15. after, behind
16. above, excessive
17. pain
18. softening
19. process of recording
20. vomiting
21. instrument for examination
22. puncture to aspirate
23. stricture, narrowing
24. record, recording
25. suture
26. pain
27. incision

Exercise 7
1. inflammation of the pancreas
2. instrument for examination of the sigmoid colon
3. pertaining to nutrition
4. surgical opening into the colon
5. surgical removal or excision of the gallbladder
6. inflammation of a diverticulum

Exercise 8
1. proctologist
2. hepatitis
3. buccal
4. lithotripsy
5. abdominocentesis
6. anoplasty
7. gastrectomy
8. colonoscopy

Exercise 9
1. esophagitis
2. appendectomy
3. gastroscopy
4. colostomy
5. cheilorrhaphy

6. laparotomy
7. cholecystogram
8. oral
9. alimentary
10. hepatitis
11. pancreatopathy

Exercise 10
1. gastr/o / enter/o / -logist
   stomach / small intestine / one who specializes in
   one who specializes in the treatment of the stomach and small intestine
2. dys- / peps/o / -ia
   painful, / digestion / pertaining to
   difficult,
   abnormal
   pertaining to painful digestion (heartburn)
3. hyper- / -emesis
   above, excessive / vomiting
   condition of excessive vomiting
4. col/o / -ectomy
   colon / surgical removal, excision
   surgical removal of the colon
5. herni/o / -rrhaphy
   hernia / suture
   suture of a hernia
6. dys- / phag/o / -ia / eat, swallow
   painful, / condition of / condition of
   difficult, / painful
   abnormal / swallowing
7. chol/e / lith/o / -iasis
   gall, bile / stone, calculus / abnormal condition
   abnormal condition of gallstones
8. hemat/o / -emesis
   blood / vomiting
   vomiting blood
9. rect/o / -cele
   rectum / herniation, protrusion
   herniation of the rectum
10. palat/o / -plasty
    palate / surgical repair, reconstruction
    surgical repair of the palate
11. ile/o / -stomy
    ileum / surgical opening
    surgical opening into the ileum
12. sub- / lingu/o / -al
    below, beneath / tongue / pertaining to
    pertaining to below or beneath the tongue

Exercise 11
1. eructation
2. occult
3. feces
4. peristalsis
5. mastication
6. halitosis
7. digestion
8. bolus
9. defecation
10. bloody stools

Exercise 12
1. deglutition
2. melena
3. inguinal
4. nausea

5. flatus
6. chyme
7. vomit
8. anorexia

Exercise 13
1. ascites
2. anorexia nervosa
3. volvulus
4. gastroesophageal reflux disease
5. Crohn disease
6. ileus
7. incontinence
8. pruritus ani
9. gastric ulcer
10. hiatal hernia

Exercise 14
1. diverticula
2. peritonitis
3. constipation
4. anorexia nervosa
5. dysentery
6. peptic ulcer disease
7. cirrhosis
8. irritable bowel syndrome
9. polyp
10. intussusception

Exercise 15
1. pancreatitis
2. gastralgia
3. polyposis
4. gastroenteritis
5. hepatomegaly
6. cholelithiasis
7. cholecystitis

Exercise 16
1. polyp/o — polyp
2. hepat/o — liver
3. diverticul/o — diverticulum
4. esophag/o — esophagus
5. cholecyst/o — gallbladder
6. stomat/o — mouth
7. hemat/o — blood
8. appendic/o — appendix
9. phag/o — eat, swallow
10. cheil/o — lip

Exercise 17
1. stool culture
2. barium swallow
3. endoscopy
4. paracentesis
5. Hemoccult test

Exercise 18
1. proctoscopy
2. flexible sigmoidoscopy
3. colonoscopy
4. abdominal ultrasound
5. barium enema
6. cholecystogram
7. esophagogastroduodenoscopy

Exercise 19
1. abdomin/o — abdomen
2. cholecyst/o — gallbladder
3. lapar/o — abdomen
4. sigmoid/o — sigmoid colon
5. colon/o — colon
6. proct/o — rectum and anus

Exercise 20
1. incision into the abdominal area
2. suturing of the tongue
3. removal of the stomach
4. process of feeding a patient through nasogastric intubation
5. surgical repair of the roof of the mouth
6. removal of a section of the stomach
7. an operative union of two hollow or tubular structures
8. crushing of gallstones
9. removal of the appendix
10. artificial opening into the ileum of the small intestine

Exercise 21
1. bariatric surgery
2. abdominoperineal resection
3. gavage
4. palatoplasty
5. anastomosis
6. cholecystectomy
7. gastric lavage
8. nasogastric intubation
9. TPN
10. gastric bypass

Exercise 22
1. col/o / -stomy
2. pancreat/o / -graphy
3. peri- / odont/o / -al
4. cheil/o / -rrhaphy
5. ile/o / -tomy
6. cholecyst/o / lith/o / -tripsy
7. polyp/o / -ectomy
8. hemi- / colon/o / -ectomy
9. abdomin/o / -plasty

Exercise 23
1. surgical repair of the palate
   palate
   surgical repair
2. surgical opening into the colon
   colon
   surgical opening
3. suture of a hernia
   hernia
   suture
4. incision into the ileum
   ileum
   incision
5. surgical removal of the appendix
   appendix
   surgical removal, excision
6. suturing of the tongue
   tongue
   suturing

Exercise 24
1. antidiarrheal
2. laxative, cathartic
3. antacid
4. emetic
5. antiemetic

Exercise 25
1. medical speciality concerned with diagnosis and treatment of disorders of the gastrointestinal tract
2. physician who specializes in proctology
3. medical speciality concerned with diagnosis and treatment of disorders of the anus and rectum.

4. physician who specializes in gastroenterology

Exercise 26
1. gastrointestinal
2. barium enema
3. total parenteral nutrition
4. esophagogastroduodenoscopy
5. nasogastric
6. upper gastrointestinal
7. gastroesophageal reflux disease

Exercise 27
1. IBS
2. BM
3. PUD
4. A&P resection
5. BE

Exercise 28
1. mouth
2. pharynx
3. liver
4. duodenum
5. gallbladder
6. ascending colon
7. cecum
8. appendix
9. salivary glands
10. esophagus
11. stomach
12. pancreas
13. transverse colon
14. descending colon
15. sigmoid colon
16. rectum
17. anus

Exercise 29
1. duodenum
2. jejunum
3. ascending colon
4. ileum
5. cecum
6. appendix
7. anal canal
8. anus
9. transverse colon
10. descending colon
11. sigmoid colon
12. rectum
13. anal sphincter

Exercise 30
1. surgical repair of the pylorus
   pylorus
   surgical repair
2. herniation of the esophagus
   esophagus
   herniation, protrusion
3. stomach pain
   stomach
   pain
4. softening of the mouth
   mouth
   softening
5. enlargement of the liver
   liver
   enlargement

6. process of examining through the abdominal wall into the stomach
   abdomen
   stomach
   process of examining
7. instrument used to examine the anus
   anus
   instrument to examine
8. eating (biting) the lip
   lip
   eat, swallow
9. surgical opening between the sigmoid colon and rectum
   sigmoid colon
   rectum
   surgical opening
10. inflammation of the small intestine and colon
    small intestine
    colon
    inflammation
11. narrowing of the rectum
    rectum
    stricture, narrowing
12. suturing of the lip
    lip
    suturing
13. teeth pain
    teeth
    pain
14. disease of the appendix
    appendix
    disease
15. incision into gallbladder to remove gall stones
    gall, bile
    stone, calculus
    incision
16. surgical opening into the jejunum
    jejunum
    surgical opening
17. surgical removal of the esophagus and stomach
    esophagus
    stomach
    surgical removal
18. drooping of the rectum
    rectum
    prolapse, drooping, sagging

Exercise 31
1. sial/o   saliva
2. aliment/o   nutrition
3. pylor/o   pylorus
4. pharyng/o   pharynx
5. duoden/o   duodenum
6. gastr/o; enter/o   stomach; small intestine
7. hepat/o   liver
8. palat/o   palate
9. bucc/o; pharyng/o   cheek; pharynx
10. dent/o   tooth
11. cec/o   cecum
12. proct/o   rectum and anus
13. polyp/o   polyp

Exercise 32
1. abdominocentesis
2. proctologist
3. Hemoccult test
4. gastroesophageal reflux disease
5. hyperemesis

6. pancreatolithectomy
7. gastroenterostomy

Exercise 33
1. B
2. A
3. C
4. A
5. C
6. B
7. A
8. C
9. C
10. A
11. D
12. A
13. C
14. C
15. D

Exercise 34
1. C
2. B
3. B
4. C
5. B
6. C

Exercise 35
1. gastrointestinal
2. diarrhea
3. constipation
4. bowel movement
5. nausea
6. anal
7. peptic ulcer
8. a deep furrow, cleft, slit or tear in the anus

Exercise 36
1. C
2. A
3. A
4. C
5. to decrease the reflux of acid from the stomach to the esophagus

Exercise 37
Practice until your pronunciation matches that heard in the Audio Glossary in the Student Resources.

Exercise 38
1. rugae
2. cecum
3. tongue
4. regurgitation
5. ileus
6. feces
7. occult
8. pylorus
9. uvula
10. gavage
11. nausea
12. mastication
13. polyposis
14. palate
15. incontinence

Chapter 6

Exercise 1
1. opening that carries urine from the urethra to the outside of the body
2. one of two narrow tubes that carry urine from the kidneys to the bladder

3. one of two bean-shaped organs that remove waste products from the blood and help maintain fluid and electrolyte balance in the body
4. microscopic urine-producing unit
5. a reservoir in each kidney that collects urine

Exercise 2
1. glomerulus
2. urinary meatus
3. kidney
4. urethra
5. urinary bladder
6. renal pelvis
7. urine

Exercise 3
1. meat/o
2. olig/o
3. ur/o, urin/o
4. nephr/o, ren/o
5. hydr/o
6. pyel/o
7. noct/i
8. lith/o
9. enur/o

Exercise 4
1. -stomy
2. -lith
3. -cele
4. -scopy
5. -ptosis
6. -emia
7. -iasis, esis
8. -stenosis

Exercise 5
1. nephr/o
2. py/o
3. urethr/o
4. son/o
5. vesic/o
6. ureter/o
7. hydr/o

Exercise 6
1. hematuria
2. ureterostenosis
3. lithotripsy
4. uremia
5. glomerulitis
6. ureterolith
7. sonogram
8. pyelography

Exercise 7
1. pyuria
2. hematuria
3. albuminuria
4. glycosuria
5. oliguria
6. bacteriuria
7. polyuria
8. dysuria

Exercise 8
1. nephr/o / -megaly
   kidney / enlargement
   enlargement of the kidney
2. cyst/o   / -scope
   fluid-filled sac / instrument for
   (urinary bladder) examination
   instrument for examining the bladder

3. noct/i / -uria
night / urine, urination
urination at night
4. ureter/o / -stomy
ureter / surgical opening
creation of a surgical opening into a
ureter
5. ren/o / -gram
kidney / record
recording of kidney (function)
6. nephr/o / -lysis
kidney / destruction, breakdown,
separation
separation of the kidney
7. vesicul/o / -ar
fluid-filled sac
(urinary bladder) / pertaining to
pertaining to the urinary bladder
8. nephr/o / -rrhaphy
kidney / suture
suturing of the kidney

Exercise 9
1. to release urine from the bladder
2. pertaining to the kidney
3. pertaining to the urinary bladder
4. to release urine from the bladder
5. pertaining to the urethra
6. pertaining to urine

Exercise 10
1. micturition
2. vesical
3. meatal
4. genitourinary
5. nephric
6. urinate
7. ureteral

Exercise 11
1 urin/o / -ary
urine, urinary system/tract / pertaining
to
pertaining to urine or the urinary
system/tract
2. ren/o / -al
kidney / pertaining to
pertaining to the kidney
3. cyst/o / -ic
fluid-filled sac
(urinary bladder) / pertaining to
pertaining to the urinary bladder
4. urethr/o / -al
urethra / pertaining to
pertaining to the urethra
5. ureter/o / -al
ureter / pertaining to
pertaining to the ureter

Exercise 12
1. stricture
2. enuresis
3. renal calculus, nephrolith
4. nephrolithiasis
5. renal failure
6. urethral stenosis
7. urinary tract infection
8. uremia
9. hypospadias
10. anuria
11. hydronephrosis
12. polyuria

Exercise 13
1. stress urinary incontinence
2. diuresis
3. hydroureter
4. nocturia
5. urinary suppression
6. polycystic kidney disease
7. urinary retention
8. nephroptosis
9. hematuria
10. urge incontinence
11. epispadias
12. urethral stenosis
13. renal hypertension
14. nocturnal enuresis
15. end-stage renal disease

Exercise 14
1. ureter/o / -lith
2. protein/o / -uria
3. albumin/o / -uria
4. ur/o / -emia
5. urethr/o / -itis
6. glycos/o / -uria
7. ureter/o / -itis
8. pyel/o / nephr/o / -itis
9. nephr/o / lith/o / -iasis
10. glomerul/o / nephr/o / -itis

Exercise 15
1. uretero<u>lith</u>
2. py<u>uria</u>
3. cyst<u>itis</u>
4. nephr<u>optosis</u>
5. <u>cyst</u>ocele
6. <u>dys</u>uria
7. poly<u>uria</u>
8. <u>pyel</u>itis
9. <u>olig</u>uria
10. uretero<u>cele</u>
11. <u>nephr</u>itis
12. cysto<u>lith</u>
13. <u>bacter</u>iuria
14. nephro<u>megaly</u>
15. uretero<u>stenosis</u>

Exercise 16
1. creatinine clearance test
2. cystoscope
3. kidneys, ureters, and bladder (KUB)
x-ray
4. renogram
5. urinalysis (UA)
6. specific gravity (SG)
7. urethroscopy
8. intravenous pyelography (IVP),
intravenous urography (IVU)
9. nephrogram
10. blood urea nitrogen (BUN)

Exercise 17
1. cystometrogram
2. retrograde pyelogram
3. urodynamics
4. nephrosonography
5. voiding cystourethrogram
6. nephrotomogram
7. urinometer
8. urinalysis

Exercise 18
1. nephroscopy
2. cystogram

3. nephrography
4. urethroscope
5. cystoscopy
6. renogram
7. cystography
8. nephroscope

Exercise 19
1. procedure of inserting a tube through
the urethra into the bladder to drain it
of urine
2. incision into the bladder to remove a stone
3. fixation of a floating kidney
4. creation of a surgical opening into the
bladder
5. incision into a renal pelvis to remove a
stone
6. excision of a ureter
7. repair of the urethra
8. excision of the bladder
9. breaking up of renal or ureteral calculi
by focused ultrasound energy

Exercise 20
1. hemodialysis
2. renal transplant, kidney transplant
3. Nephrolithotomy
4. Ureterostomy
5. peritoneal dialysis
6. Cystoplasty
7. vesicourethral suspension
8. nephrotomy

Exercise 21
1. lith/o / -tomy
stone, calculus / incision
incision (to remove a) stone or calculus
2. cyst/o / -rrhaphy
fluid-filled sac
(urinary bladder) / suture
suturing the urinary bladder
3. ureter/o / -tomy
ureter / incision
incision into the bladder
4. nephr/o / -ectomy
kidney / excision, surgical removal
excision or surgical removal of the
kidney
5. pyel/o / -plasty
renal pelvis / surgical repair,
reconstruction
repair of the renal pelvis
6. meat/o / -tomy
meatus / incision
incision into a meatus
7. lith/o / -tripsy
stone, calculus / crushing
crushing of a stone or calculus
8. nephr/o / -lysis
kidney / destruction, breakdown,
separation
separation of the kidney (from
adhesions)
9. urethr/o / -tomy
urethra / incision
incision into a urethra

Exercise 22
1. urinary analgesic
2. antibiotic
3. diuretic
4. antibacterial

Exercise 23
1. nephrologist
2. urology
3. urologist
4. nephrology

Exercise 24
1. creatinine
2. intravenous pyelogram, intravenous pyelography
3. end-stage renal disease
4. specific gravity
5. catheter, catheterize, catheterization
6. voiding cystourethrogram, voiding cystourethrography
7. blood urea nitrogen
8. acute renal failure
9. genitourinary
10. intravenous urogram, intravenous urography
11. urinary tract infection

Exercise 25
1. kidneys, ureters, and bladder (x-ray)
2. extracorporeal shock wave lithotripsy
3. chronic renal failure
4. urinalysis
5. stress urinary incontinence

Exercise 26
1. ureters
2. urinary bladder
3. left kidney
4. urethra
5. urinary meatus

Exercise 27
1. renal artery
2. renal vein
3. renal pelvis
4. ureter

Exercise 28
1. cyst/o   fluid-filled sac (urinary bladder)
2. meat/o   meatus
3. urethr/o   urethra
4. hemat/o   blood
5. cyst/o   fluid-filled sac (urinary bladder)
6. ren/o   kidney
7. ureter/o   ureter
8. py/o   pus
9. pyel/o   renal pelvis
10. urethr/o   urethra
11. glycos/o   glucose, sugar
12. nephr/o   kidney
13. vesic/o   bladder
14. noct/i   night
15. ur/o   urine, urinary system/tract
16. cyst/o   fluid-filled sac (urinary bladder)
17. nephr/o   kidney
18. urethr/o   urethra
19. olig/o   scanty, few
20. ureter/o   ureter

Exercise 29
1. ureter/o / -lith
   ureter   / stone, calculus
   stone or calculus in the ureter
2. glycos/o   / -uria
   glucose, sugar / urine, urination
   glucose or sugar in the urine

3. nephr/o / -ptosis
   kidney   / prolapse, drooping, sagging
   drooping of the kidney
4. ureter/o / -stenosis
   ureter   / stricture, narrowing
   narrowing of the ureter
5. nephr/o / -tomy
   kidney   / incision
   incision into the kidney
6. ur/o   / -emia
   urine, urinary system/tract / blood
                                  (condition of)
   condition of urine in the blood
7. pyel/o   / -itis
   renal pelvis / inflammation
   inflammation of the renal pelvis
8. glomerul/o / nephr/o / -itis
   glomerulus / kidney   / inflammation
   inflammation of the glomeruli of the kidney

Exercise 30
1. specific gravity
2. KUB
3. hydroureter
4. catheterization
5. proteinuria
6. hemodialysis
7. stress urinary incontinence
8. renal hypertension
9. vesicourethral suspension
10. nephroptosis
11. cystometrogram
12. urinalysis
13. urinary retention
14. nocturnal enuresis
15. hypospadias

Exercise 31
1. the amount of urea in the blood
2. a kidney
3. urine sample
4. the kidney stone may obstruct the flow of urine
5. to release waste products (urine) from the body
6. to surgically crush the stone in the bladder
7. the kidney
8. nephrologist
9. urinary analgesic
10. urine
11. urethra and bladder
12. catheterization
13. urology
14. make an incision to remove a stone from an organ
15. the kidney
16. a ureter
17. cystogram
18. urinometer
19. antibacterial and antibiotic
20. the kidney

Exercise 32
1. D
2. B
3. D
4. A
5. B
6. A
7. B

8. D
9. C
10. A
11. C
12. A
13. C
14. A
15. D

Exercise 33
1. B
2. A
3. C
4. D
5. C

Exercise 34
1. oliguria
2. nocturnal enuresis
3. pyelonephritis
4. hydronephrosis
5. urinalysis
6. catheterization
7. SG
8. urinary retention
9. hydroureter
10. KUB
11. a stone in the urinary tract

Exercise 35
1. C
2. B
3. D
4. A
5. C
6. B
7. B
8. pertaining to through the vagina

Exercise 36
Practice until your pronunciation matches that heard in the Audio Glossary in the Student Resources.

Exercise 37
1. glomerulus
2. meatus
3. cystic
4. correct
5. correct
6. nephromegaly
7. correct
8. cystocele
9. diuresis
10. correct
11. hydroureter
12. correct
13. correct
14. urinalysis
15. cystoscopy

Chapter 7

Exercise 1
1. atrium
2. venule
3. myocardium
4. aortic valve
5. septum
6. arteriole
7. superior vena cava and inferior vena cava
8. heart
9. endocardium
10. pericardium

Exercise 2
1. clear fluid consisting of fluctuating amounts of white blood cells and a few red blood cells that accumulates in tissue and is removed by the lymphatic capillaries
2. vessel carrying blood away from the heart
3. vessel carrying blood to the heart
4. microscopic thin-walled lymph vessels that pick up lymph, proteins, and waste from body tissues.
5. largest artery that carries oxygenated blood away from the heart
6. structures that carry or transport blood
7. vessels transporting lymph from body tissues to the venous system
8. the largest lymph vessels that transport lymph to the venous system
9. small bean-shaped masses of lymphatic tissue that filter bacteria and foreign material from the lymph
10. heart valve between the right atrium and right ventricle

Exercise 3
1. atria
2. outer
3. endocardium
4. bicuspid
5. aorta
6. artery
7. capillaries
8. vein
9. capillary
10. tricuspid
11. two
12. pericardium
13. arteriole
14. heart

Exercise 4
1. pulmonary valve
2. myocardium
3. lumen
4. lymph
5. septum
6. apex

Exercise 5
1. lymph nodes
2. ventricles
3. arteries
4. aortic valve
5. pericardium
6. lumen
7. capillary
8. ducts
9. lymph
10. inferior

Exercise 6
1. atrium
2. muscle
3. vessel, duct
4. vessel, duct
5. vein
6. electric, electricity
7. artery
8. heart
9. ventricle
10. lung
11. circle, crown
12. vein
13. vessel, duct

14. thorax, chest
15. valve

Exercise 7
1. scler/o
2. sphygm/o
3. varic/o
4. lymph/o
5. valv/o, valvul/o
6. aort/o
7. arteri/o
8. atri/o
9. cardi/o
10. steth/o, thorac/o

Exercise 8
1. stricture, narrowing
2. small
3. rapid, fast
4. across, through
5. within
6. between
7. in, within
8. instrument for recording
9. slow
10. on, following
11. around, surrounding
12. tissue, structure
13. pertaining to
14. three
15. away from, cessation, without
16. pertaining to destruction, breakdown, separation

Exercise 9
1. inflammation of a vein
2. study of the heart
3. heart muscle tissue
4. abnormal condition of blood clot
5. recording of a vein
6. surgical removal or excision of fatty paste
7. resembling lymph
8. process of recording the aorta

Exercise 10
1. angioplasty
2. thoracic
3. arteriole
4. venule
5. vascular
6. adenoid
7. lymphopathy
8. sonography

Exercise 11
1. above
2. paroxysmal
3. patent
4. narrowed
5. cyanotic
6. Systole
7. diastole

Exercise 12
1. constriction
2. cardiovascular
3. cyanotic
4. precordial
5. varicose
6. oxygenation
7. thoracic
8. ischemic
9. atrioventricular
10. deoxygenation

Exercise 13
1. sphygm/o — pulse
2. cardi/o; vascul/o — heart; vessel, duct
3. varic/o — swollen or twisted vein
4. arteri/o; ven/o — artery; vein
5. thromb/o — blood clot

Exercise 14
1. weakening
2. hardening
3. high
4. low
5. narrowing
6. death
7. valve
8. lack of
9. irregular
10. regular
11. early
12. abnormal
13. edema
14. chest pain
15. cramping
16. outside

Exercise 15
1. backward
2. fluid
3. narrowed
4. filariae
5. myocardial infarction
6. angina pectoris
7. cardiac arrest
8. cyanotic
9. circulation
10. tachycardia
11. phlebitis
12. decrease
13. embolus
14. blood clot
15. varicose
16. coronary occlusion

Exercise 16
1. angiostenosis
2. palpitation
3. arrhythmia
4. lymphedema
5. occlusion
6. plaque
7. mitral valve stenosis
8. lymphadenitis
9. dysrhythmia
10. cardiomegaly

Exercise 17
1. bradycardia
2. pericarditis
3. endocardium
4. interventricular
5. pericardium
6. tachycardia
7. polyarteritis

Exercise 18
1. lymph/o / angi/o / -itis
   lymph / vessel, duct / inflammation
   inflammation of a lymph vessel
2. lymph/o / aden/o / -pathy
   lymph / gland / disease
   disease of the lymph nodes

3. thromb/o / phleb/o / -itis
blood clot / vein / inflammation
inflammation of a vein (with formation of a) blood clot
4. cardi/o / my/o / -pathy
heart / muscle / disease
disease of the heart muscle
5. endo- / cardi/o / -itis
in, within / heart / inflammation
inflammation within the heart (inflammation of the endocardium)
6. cardi/o / valvul/o / -itis
heart / valve / inflammation
inflammation of the valves of the heart
7. my/o / cardi/o / -itis
muscle / heart / inflammation
inflammation of the heart muscle
8. tel- / angi/o / -ectasia
end / vessel, duct / dilation, stretching
dilation of end (or terminal) vessels

Exercise 19
1. Holter monitor
2. arteriography
3. lymphangiography
4. angioscopy
5. auscultation
6. electrocardiography
7. SPECT
8. sonography
9. percussion
10. magnetic resonance angiography

Exercise 20
1. graded exercise test (GXT), stress electrocardiogram, or exercise stress test
2. echocardiography
3. transesophageal echocardiography
4. multiple uptake gated acquisition (MUGA) scan or single photon emission computed tomography (SPECT) scan
5. coronary angiography or cardiac catheterization
6. exercise
7. heart ventricles
8. radiofrequency waves
9. sphygmomanometer
10. listen or auscultate

Exercise 21
1. electrolyte panel
2. cardiac enzyme tests
3. cardiac troponin
4. lipid panel
5. C-reactive protein

Exercise 22
1. sonography
2. venography
3. ventriculography
4. aortography
5. angiography

Exercise 23
1. adenectomy
2. percutaneous transluminal coronary angioplasty
3. embolectomy
4. valvuloplasty
5. atherectomy
6. lymphadenectomy
7. lymphadenotomy

Exercise 24
1. valve replacement
2. cardioversion
3. endarterectomy
4. cardiac pacemaker
5. PTCA
6. stent
7. CABG
8. aortocoronary bypass

Exercise 25
1. angioplasty
2. aneurysmectomy
3. pericardiocentesis
4. adenectomy
5. valvotomy

Exercise 26
1. valvul/o / -plasty
valve / surgical repair, reconstruction
surgical repair or reconstruction of a valve
2. angi/o / -plasty
vessel, duct / surgical repair, reconstruction
surgical repair reconstruction of a vessel
3. ather/o / -ectomy
fatty paste / excision, surgical removal
excision or surgical removal of fatty plaque
4. phleb/o / -ectomy
vein / excision, surgical removal
excision or surgical removal of vein
5. valv/o / -tomy
valve / incision
incision into a valve

Exercise 27
1. vasoconstrictor
2. anticoagulant
3. thrombolytic therapy
4. vasodilator
5. hemostatic agent
6. antiarrhythmic agent
7. nitroglycerin
8. hypolipidemic agent

Exercise 28
1. cardiology
2. lymphedema therapy
3. cardiologist
4. cardiac electrophysiology
5. lymphedema therapist
6. cardiac electrophysiologist

Exercise 29
1. congestive heart failure
2. aortocoronary bypass
3. single photon emission computed tomography
4. arteriosclerotic heart disease
5. deep venous thrombosis
6. premature ventricular contraction
7. blood pressure
8. acute coronary syndrome
9. hypertension
10. coronary artery bypass graft

Exercise 30
1. Holter monitor
2. percutaneous transluminal coronary angioplasty

3. magnetic resonance angiogram
4. atrioventricular
5. transesophageal echocardiogram
6. coronary artery disease
7. rheumatic heart disease
8. graded exercise test
9. myocardial infarction
10. peripheral arterial disease

Exercise 31
1. ECG
2. MRI
3. MRA
4. DS
5. MUGA

Exercise 32
1. superior vena cava
2. right atrium
3. endocardium
4. right ventricle
5. inferior vena cava
6. left atrium
7. epicardium
8. left ventricle
9. myocardium
10. apex

Exercise 33
1. cervical lymph node
2. mediastinal lymph node
3. axillary lymph node
4. inguinal lymph node

Exercise 34
1. angi/o / -stenosis
vessel / stricture, narrowing
narrowing of a blood vessel
2. phleb/o / -itis
vein / inflammation
inflammation of a vein
3. electr/o / cardi/o / -graphy
electric, electricity / heart / process of recording
process of recording the electrical conduction of the heart
4. atri/o / ventricul/o / -ar
atrium / ventricle / pertaining to
pertaining to the atrium and ventricle
5. tachy- / cardi/o / -ia
rapid, fast / heart / condition of
condition of fast heart (rate)
6. inter- / ventricul/o / -ar
between / ventricle / pertaining to
pertaining to between the ventricles
7. thromb/o / -osis
blood clot / abnormal condition
abnormal condition of a blood clot
8. poly- / arteri/o / -itis
many, much / artery / inflammation
inflammation of many arteries
9. thromb/o / phleb/o / -itis
blood clot / vein / inflammation
inflammation of a vein (related to) a blood clot
10. cardi/o / my/o / -pathy
heart / muscle / disease
disease of the heart muscle
11. arteri/o / scler/o / -osis
artery / hard / abnormal condition
abnormal condition of hardening of the arteries

12. sphygm/o / -ic
    pulse / pertaining to
    pertaining to the pulse
13. ven/o / -graphy
    vein / process of recording
    process of recording a vein
14. brady- / cardi/o / -ia
    slow / heart / condition of
    condition of slow heart (rate)
15. ather/o- / scler/o / -osis
    fatty paste / hard / abnormal
    condition
    abnormal condition of hardening due to
    fatty paste
16. my/o / cardi/o / -ium
    muscle / heart / tissue, structure
    heart muscle tissue
17. valvul/o / -tomy
    valve / incision
    incision into a valve
18. lymph/o / aden/o / -pathy
    lymph / gland / disease
    disease of a lymph gland
19. lymph/o / angi/o / -itis
    lymph / vessel, duct / inflammation
    inflammation of a lymph vessel
20. thromb/o / -lytic
    blood clot / pertaining to destruction,
                breakdown, separation
    pertaining to destruction of a blood clot

Exercise 35
1. myocardium
2. septum
3. cardiologist
4. pulmonary
5. aorta
6. diastole
7. telangiectasia
8. varicose
9. flutter
10. fibrillation
11. Elephantiasis
12. intermittent claudication
13. ischemia
14. myocardial infarction
15. cardiac
16. deep venous thrombosis
17. premature ventricular contraction
18. murmurs
19. open
20. inflammation

Exercise 36
1. hemostatic agent
2. the wrist or neck
3. within a blood vessel
4. cholesterol, high density lipoprotein
   (HDL), low density lipoprotein (LDL),
   and triglycerides
5. hypotension is below normal blood
   pressure and hypertension is
   persistently high blood pressure
6. stethoscope and sphygmomanometer
7. angina pectoris
8. pericardiocentesis
9. tapping over the body
10. to view an image of the beating heart
11. defibrillation and drug therapy
12. bradycardia
13. to stop a fibrillation or cardiac arrest

14. aortocoronary bypass graft and
    coronary artery bypass graft
15. it is inflated at the site of stenosis,
    thereby enlarging the lumen

Exercise 37
1. A
2. B
3. A
4. B
5. D
6. A
7. A
8. B
9. A
10. B
11. D
12. B
13. D
14. C
15. A
16. D
17. C
18. C
19. B
20. D

Exercise 38
1. B
2. C
3. A
4. A
5. D
6. C
7. D
8. D
9. D
10. B
11. C

Exercise 39
1. cardiovascular
2. echocardiogram
3. graded exercise test
4. myocardial infarction
5. ventricular
6. cyanosis
7. arteriosclerosis
8. atherosclerosis

Exercise 40
1. B
2. D
3. A
4. C
5. A
6. redness

Exercise 41
*Practice until your pronunciation matches
that heard in the Audio Glossary in the
Student Resources.*

Exercise 42
1. aneurysm
2. lymphangiitis
3. valvoplasty
4. telangiectasia
5. Doppler
6. sphygmomanometer
7. vasoconstrictor
8. diastole
9. auscultation
10. elephantiasis

11. paroxysmal
12. ischemic
13. dysrhythmia
14. arrhythmia
15. claudication

Chapter 8
Exercise 1
1. leukocyte, white blood cell
2. thrombocyte, platelet
3. blood
4. lymphocyte
5. plasma
6. spleen
7. granulocyte
8. agranulocyte
9. monocyte
10. eosinophil
11. basophil
12. erythrocyte, red blood cell
13. hemoglobin
14. bone marrow
15. serum

Exercise 2
1. essential trace element necessary for
   hemoglobin to transport oxygen on red
   blood cells
2. soldier-like cell that protects the body
   and inactivates antigens
3. agent or substance that provokes an
   immune response
4. any virus, microorganism, or other
   substance that causes disease
5. protection against disease
6. hormone released by kidneys that
   stimulates red blood cell production in
   bone marrow
7. formation of blood cells and other
   formed elements
8. type of granulocyte that fights against
   bacterial infections; stains a neutral pink
9. any of the various plasma components
   involved in the clotting process
10. protein substance present in the red
    blood cells of most people capable of
    inducing intense antigenic reactions

Exercise 3
1. erythrocyte
2. Hemoglobin
3. formed elements
4. Histamine
5. antibodies
6. antigens
7. bone marrow
8. spleen
9. erythropoietin
10. leukocyte
11. macrophage
12. serum

Exercise 4
1. Rh factor
2. coagulation
3. antibody
4. fibrin
5. leukocyte
6. hemoglobin
7. pathogen
8. thrombocyte
9. phagocytosis

Exercise 5
1. B
2. T
3. spleen
4. erythrocyte, red blood cell
5. fibrin
6. granulocyte
7. macrocyte
8. Fibrinogen
9. macrophage

Exercise 6
1. blood
2. disease
3. blood clot
4. immune, safe
5. white
6. red
7. eat, swallow
8. granules
9. vein
10. color
11. neutral
12. formation, growth

Exercise 7
1. thromb/o
2. plas/o
3. lymph/o
4. neutr/o
5. hem/o, hemat/o
6. erythr/o
7. leuk/o
8. phag/o
9. cyt/o
10. nucle/o

Exercise 8
1. self, same
2. flowing forth
3. one
4. base
5. many, much
6. attraction for
7. deficiency
8. destruction, breakdown, separation
9. production, formation
10. large, long
11. small
12. blood (condition of)
13. origin, production
14. abnormal condition

Exercise 9
1. study of veins
2. flowing forth of blood
3. blood clotting cell
4. red (blood) cell
5. attraction for neutral (stain)

Exercise 10
1. leukocyte
2. thrombolysis
3. mononucleosis
4. pancytopenia
5. polycythemia
6. erythropoiesis
7. phlebology

Exercise 11
1. hemorrhagic
2. systemic
3. Rejection
4. predisposition

5. Hemolytic
6. cytopathic
7. autoimmunity

Exercise 12
1. hemostasis
2. rejection
3. proliferative
4. inflammatory
5. virulent
6. hypersensitive
7. hematopoietic
8. systemic

Exercise 13
1. bleed
2. bleeding
3. platelets
4. transport
5. iron
6. produce
7. destruction
8. clotting
9. increase
10. low

Exercise 14
1. platelets
2. pernicious
3. Sjögren syndrome
4. lymph nodes
5. sickle cell anemia
6. autoimmune disease
7. coagulate
8. polycythemia
9. blood
10. autoimmune
11. joints

Exercise 15
1. deficiency in all types of (blood) cells
2. abnormal condition of (increase of white blood cells with) one nucleus
3. pertaining to without formation or growth
4. attraction for blood (tendency to bleed)
5. inflammation of a joint

Exercise 16
1. hemochromatosis
2. hemophilia
3. thrombocytopenia
4. thrombosis
5. hemorrhage

Exercise 17
1. Sjögren syndrome
2. EBV antibody test
3. cross-matching
4. prothrombin time
5. HGB
6. inflammation
7. WBC differential count
8. hematocrit
9. pathogen, antibiotic
10. ANA

Exercise 18
1. blood smear
2. red blood cell count
3. hemogram
4. platelet count
5. albumin
6. bilirubin
7. white blood cell count

Exercise 19
1. plasmapheresis
2. bone marrow transplant
3. splenectomy
4. blood transfusion
5. blood component therapy
6. autologous blood
7. homologous blood
8. apheresis

Exercise 20
1. splenectomy
2. immunizations
3. phlebotomy
4. blood transfusions
5. aspiration
6. vaccinations
7. immunosuppression

Exercise 21
1. anticoagulant
2. vaccine
3. antibiotic
4. immune serum
5. hemostatic agent, procoagulant
6. immunosuppressant
7. antihistamine
8. thrombolytic agent

Exercise 22
1. allergology
2. rheumatologist
3. hematologist
4. hematology
5. immunology
6. allergist
7. immunologist
8. rheumatology

Exercise 23
1. prothrombin time, von Willebrand disease
2. bone marrow aspiration, bone marrow transplant
3. complete blood count
4. erythrocyte sedimentation rate
5. hemoglobin, hematocrit
6. red blood cells, white blood cells
7. idiopathic thrombocytopenic purpura, blood transfusions
8. antibody, antigens
9. culture and sensitivity

Exercise 24
1. Fe
2. PLT
3. ESR
4. EPO
5. ANA
6. EBV
7. SLE
8. RA

Exercise 25
1. neutrophil
2. eosinophil
3. basophil
4. lymphocyte
5. monocyte

Exercise 26
1. hem/o / -stasis
   blood / stopped, standing still
   stopped bleeding

2. erythr/o / -cyte
   red / cell
   red (blood) cell
3. hemat/o / -poiesis
   blood / production, formation
   blood (cell) production or formation
4. thromb/o / cyt/o / -penia
   blood clot / cell / deficiency
   deficiency of blood clotting cells
5. path/o / -gen
   disease / origin, production
   disease-producing
6. cyt/o / path/o / -ic
   cell / disease / pertaining to
   pertaining to cell disease
7. a- / plas/o / -tic
   without / formation, / pertaining to
   growth
   pertaining to without formation or growth
8. chromat/o / -ic
   color / pertaining to
   pertaining to color
9. an- / -emia
   without / blood (condition of)
   condition of without blood cells
10. hem/o / chromat/o / -osis
    blood / color / abnormal
    condition
    abnormal condition of blood color
11. hem/o / -philia
    blood / attraction for
    attraction for blood
12. granul/o / -cyte
    granules / cell
    cell containing granules
13. lymph/o / cyt/o / -ic
    lymph / cell / pertaining to
    pertaining to a lymph cell
14. hem/o / -rrhage
    blood / flowing forth
    flowing forth of blood
15. mono- / nucle/o / -osis
    one / nucleus / abnormal condition
    abnormal condition of one nucleus

Exercise 27
1. antibodies
2. Antigens
3. immunization or vaccination
4. Hemorrhagic or Blood loss
5. Thrombocytopenia
6. Inflammation
7. erythrocyte sedimentation rate
8. white

Exercise 28
1. to decrease rejection of the donor organ
2. erythrocytes, leukocytes, thrombocytes, or white blood cells, red blood cells, platelets
3. anticoagulant
4. erythrocyte sedimentation rate
5. Antigens are agents or substances that produce an immune response; antibodies protect the body and inactivate antigens.
6. clotting or coagulation
7. leukocytes (macrophages)
8. mononuclear leukocytes
9. bone marrow
10. autologous blood transfusion

11. Rheumatoid arthritis is an autoimmune disease, and immunosuppressants reduce the normal immune response.
12. A vaccine is the preparation composed of a weakened or killed pathogen, and a vaccination is the administration of a vaccine.
13. "Systemic" is a term meaning affecting the body as a whole, and this disease can affect the entire body.
14. culture and sensitivity
15. in the bone marrow

Exercise 29
1. D
2. D
3. B
4. D
5. B
6. C
7. A
8. A
9. C
10. A
11. D
12. D

Exercise 30
1. B
2. D
3. C
4. A
5. D
6. A
7. C
8. B
9. D
10. B
11. C
12. A
13. C

Exercise 31
1. hemolytic
2. thrombocytopenia
3. NKA
4. as needed
5. anti- / bi/o / -tic
   opposing, / life / pertaining to
   against
   pertaining to against life

Exercise 32
1. B
2. C
3. D
4. A
5. A

Exercise 33
1. systemic lupus erythematosus
2. erythrocyte sedimentation rate
3. white blood count
4. Epstein-Barr virus test
5. antinuclear antibody test
6. hematuria

Exercise 34
Practice until your pronunciation matches that heard in the Audio Glossary in the Student Resources.

Exercise 35
1. erythrocyte
2. granulocyte

3. leukocyte
4. neutrophil
5. eosinophil
6. agranulocyte
7. erythropoietin
8. phagocytosis
9. hemoglobin
10. hemorrhagic
11. virulent
12. proliferation
13. immunosuppressant
14. thalassemia
15. thrombocytopenia

Chapter 9

Exercise 1
1. lobes
2. expiration, exhalation
3. epiglottis
4. eupnea
5. larynx
6. pharynx, throat
7. inspiration, inhalation
8. diaphragm
9. nose
10. external respiration, breathing
11. nasal septum
12. bronchi
13. alveoli
14. visceral layer
15. sputum

Exercise 2
1. nose and pharynx
2. cilia, nose
3. airway
4. larynx
5. epiglottis
6. trachea
7. bronchioles
8. diaphragm
9. paranasal sinuses
10. carina
11. parietal layer
12. pleural cavity
13. respiration

Exercise 3
1. internal respiration
2. glottis
3. adenoids
4. mediastinum
5. lungs
6. pleura
7. patent
8. thorax

Exercise 4
1. carbon dioxide
2. trachea
3. epiglottis
4. thorax, chest
5. to breathe in or suck in
6. septum
7. pleura
8. mediastinum
9. bronchus
10. mucus
11. tonsil
12. listening
13. lung, air

14. lung
15. incomplete

Exercise 5
1. pect/o, pector/o, thorac/o
2. tonsill/o
3. phon/o
4. thorac/o
5. pharyng/o
6. laryng/o
7. pleur/o
8. spir/o
9. lob/o
10. bronch/o, bronchi/o
11. sinus/o
12. nas/o, rhin/o
13. diaphragmat/o
14. ox/o, ox/a
15. capn/o, capn/i

Exercise 6
1. through
2. below, deficient
3. in
4. breathing
5. rapid, fast
6. flowing forth
7. all, entire
8. involuntary movement
9. paralysis
10. herniation, protrusion
11. excision, surgical removal
12. blood (condition of)
13. process of examining, examination
14. without, not
15. process of recording

Exercise 7
1. -metry
2. -al, -ar, -ary, -ic
3. -rrhea
4. -phonia
5. -emia
6. -centesis
7. -ectasis
8. dys-
9. -stomy
10. per-
11. eu-
12. -plasty
13. -itis
14. -cele
15. -tomy

Exercise 8
1. excision or surgical removal of the adenoids
2. inflammation of the alveoli
3. instrument for examination of the bronchus
4. herniation or protrusion of the diaphragm
5. inflammation of the epiglottis
6. instrument for examination of the larynx
7. pertaining to the lobes of the lung
8. pertaining to the nose
9. involuntary movement of the pharynx
10. inflammation of the pleura

Exercise 9
1. pneumonitis
2. septoplasty

3. tracheotomy
4. thoracostomy
5. tonsillitis
6. sinusitis
7. laryngitis
8. lobar
9. alveolar
10. pharyngitis

Exercise 10
1. pertaining to or suffering from apnea
2. pertaining to the trachea
3. pertaining to the diaphragm
4. pertaining to a low level of oxygen
5. pertaining to pleurisy
6. pertaining to respiration
7. pertaining to the tonsil
8. pertaining to within the trachea
9. pertaining to the mediastinum
10. pertaining to mucus or a mucous membrane

Exercise 11
1. thoracic
2. bronchial
3. pleural
4. alveolar
5. diaphragmatic
6. lobar
7. anoxic
8. pharyngeal
9. intercostal
10. pectoral

Exercise 12
1. pulmonary, lobar
2. thoracic
3. pharyngeal
4. mediastinal
5. lobar

Exercise 13
1. lob/o   lobe
2. phren/o   diaphragm
3. pleur/o   pleura
4. nas/o   nose
5. pulmon/o   lung

Exercise 14
1. hypoxemia
2. tonsillitis
3. upper respiratory infection (URI)
4. bronchiectasis
5. bronchitis
6. pleural effusion
7. rhinitis
8. tracheorrhagia
9. epistaxis
10. lobar pneumonia
11. pharyngitis
12. pansinusitis
13. atelectasis
14. pneumonitis
15. rhonchi
16. dyspnea
17. rubs
18. wheeze
19. chronic obstructive pulmonary disease (COPD)

Exercise 15
1. pulmonary edema
2. bronchopneumonia
3. influenza

4. hemothorax
5. empyema
6. pertussis
7. pansinusitis
8. adult respiratory distress syndrome
9. pleuritis
10. tuberculosis
11. pulmonary embolism

Exercise 16
1. croup
2. asthma
3. hypoxia
4. pneumococcal pneumonia
5. rales
6. interstitial lung disease
7. pulmonary embolism
8. bronchiolitis obliterans with organizing pneumonia
9. emphysema
10. reactive airway disease
11. Cheyne-Stokes respiration

Exercise 17
1. pneumon/o / -ia
    lung   / condition of
    condition of the lung
2. a-   / -phonia
    without, not / condition of the voice
    condition of without a voice
3. bronchi/o / -ectasis
    bronchus / dilation, stretching
    dilation of the bronchi
4. bronch/o / pneumon/o / -ia
    bronchus / lung   / condition
    condition of the bronchus and lung
5. laryng/o / -spasm
    larynx   / involuntary movement
    involuntary movement of the larynx
6. pleur/o / -itis
    pleura / inflammation
    inflammation of the pleura
7. a-   / -pnea
    without, not / breathing
    not breathing
8. laryng/o / -itis
    larynx   / inflammation
    inflammation of the larynx
9. pneumon/o / -itis
    lung   / inflammation
    inflammation of the lung
10. sinus/o / -itis
    sinus   / inflammation
    inflammation of the sinus(es)
11. trache/o / -itis
    trachea / inflammation
    inflammation of the trachea
12. diaphragmat/o / -cele
    diaphragm   / herniation, protrusion
    herniation of the diaphragm
13. nas/o / pharyng/o / -itis
    nose / pharynx   / inflammation
    inflammation of the nose and pharynx
14. dys-   / -phonia
    painful, difficult, / condition of the voice
    abnormal
    condition of vocal difficulty
15. pharyng/o / -itis
    pharynx   / inflammation
    inflammation of the pharynx

Exercise 18
1. Computed tomography
2. chest radiograph
3. V/Q scan
4. PPD test
5. Bronchoalveolar lavage
6. magnetic resonance imaging
7. VATS
8. spirometry

Exercise 19
1. pulse oximetry
2. arterial blood gases (ABGs)
3. percussion
4. acid-fast bacilli (AFB) smear
5. radiography
6. laryngoscopy
7. pulmonary function tests (PFTs)
8. polysomnography
9. auscultation
10. peak flow monitoring

Exercise 20
1. thoracoscopy
2. rhinoscopy
3. pharyngoscopy
4. bronchoscopy
5. laryngoscopy

Exercise 21
1. thoracotomy
2. adenoidectomy
3. tracheoplasty
4. hyperbaric medicine
5. mechanical ventilation
6. aspiration
7. continuous positive airway pressure (CPAP) therapy
8. tracheotomy
9. laryngotracheotomy
10. endotracheal intubation
11. bronchoplasty
12. tracheostomy
13. pneumonectomy
14. incentive spirometry

Exercise 22
1. tracheostomy
2. tonsillectomy
3. rhinoplasty
4. thoracentesis
5. CPR

Exercise 23
1. septoplasty
2. laryngectomy
3. thoracentesis
4. bronchoscopy
5. thoracotomy

Exercise 24
1. laryng/o / -scope
   larynx / instrument for examination
   instrument for examination of the larynx
2. rhin/o / -plasty
   nose / surgical repair, reconstruction
   surgical repair of the nose
3. laryng/o / -stomy
   larynx / surgical opening
   surgical opening in the larynx
4. pneumon/o / -ectomy
   lung / excision, surgical removal
   surgical removal of a lung

5. sinus/o / -tomy
   sinus / incision
   incision of the sinus
6. bronch/o / -plasty
   bronchus / surgical repair, reconstruction
   surgical repair of the bronchus
7. thorac/o / -centesis
   thorax / puncture to aspirate
   puncture to aspirate the thorax (pleural cavity)
8. trache/o / -tomy
   trachea / incision
   incision of the trachea
9. adenoid/o / -ectomy
   adenoids / excision, surgical removal
   excision of the adenoids
10. trache/o / -stomy
   trachea / surgical opening
   surgical opening of the trachea

Exercise 25
1. nebulizer
2. expectorant
3. corticosteroid
4. antitussive
5. antihistamine
6. bronchodilator
7. antibiotic
8. decongestant
9. antitubercular

Exercise 26
1. otorhinolaryngologist
2. pulmonologist
3. otorhinolaryngology
4. pulmonology

Exercise 27
1. reactive airway disease
2. computed tomography (scan)
3. upper respiratory infection
4. ventilation-perfusion (scan)
5. tuberculosis
6. cardiopulmonary resuscitation
7. magnetic resonance imaging
8. purified protein derivative
9. video-assisted thorascopic surgery
10. arterial blood gas
11. continuous positive airway pressure
12. bronchoalveolar lavage

Exercise 28
1. chronic obstructive pulmonary disease, interstitial lung disease
2. pulmonary function tests, respiratory failure
3. acute respiratory distress syndrome
4. acid-fast bacilli, bronchiolitis obliterans with organizing pneumonia
5. chest x-ray

Exercise 29
1. nasal cavity
2. nasal septum
3. nose
4. epiglottis
5. larynx
6. bronchi
7. bronchioles
8. paranasal sinuses
9. adenoids
10. tonsils
11. pharynx

12. glottis
13. trachea
14. mediastinum
15. lung
16. diaphragm

Exercise 30
1. frontal sinus
2. nasal cavity
3. nose
4. oral cavity
5. epiglottis
6. sphenoid sinus
7. nasopharynx
8. oropharynx
9. tonsils
10. laryngopharynx
11. esophagus

Exercise 31
1. laryng/o / -eal
   larynx / pertaining to
   pertaining to the larynx
2. rhin/o / -rrhea
   nose / flow, discharge
   discharge from the nose
3. pulmon/o / -ary
   lung / pertaining to
   pertaining to the lung
4. phren/o / -spasm
   diaphragm / involuntary movement
   involuntary movement of the diaphragm
5. thorac/o / -tomy
   thorax / surgical incision
   surgical incision of the thorax
6. tachy- / -pnea
   fast / breathing
   fast breathing (rate)
7. thorac/o / -ic
   thorax / pertaining to
   pertaining to the thorax
8. bronch/o / -spasm
   bronchus / involuntary movement
   involuntary movement of the bronchus
9. pulmon/o / -logy
   lung / study of
   study of the lungs
10. bronch/o / -scopy
   bronchus / process of examining, examination
   process of examining the bronchus

Exercise 32
1. visceral layer
2. alveoli
3. epiglottis
4. tachypnea
5. Hemothorax
6. asthma
7. laryngospasm
8. upper respiratory
9. Stridor
10. pharynx

Exercise 33
1. the larynx, trachea, bronchi, lungs, and diaphragm
2. glottis or vocal cords
3. the anatomic region formed by the sternum, the thoracic vertebrae, and the ribs, extending from the neck to the diaphragm

4. three on the right and two on the left
5. tracheostomy
6. pulmonary fibrosis
7. to aspirate fluid from the chest cavity
8. a mask is used to pump constant pressurized air through the nasal passages to keep the airway open
9. flow and volume of air inspired and expired by the lungs
10. windpipe

Exercise 34
1. B
2. A
3. D
4. B
5. D
6. B
7. B
8. B
9. C
10. D

Exercise 35
1. B
2. D
3. A
4. C
5. C
6. B
7. A
8. C
9. B
10. A

Exercise 36
1. erythema
2. tuberculosis
3. rhonchi
4. auscultation
5. wheezing
6. bilateral
7. to rule out active tuberculosis

Exercise 37
1. bronchitis
2. sputum
3. dyspnea
4. pulmonary embolism
5. pulmonary
6. pulmonologist

Exercise 38
Practice until your pronunciation matches that heard in the Audio Glossary in the Student Resources.

Exercise 39
1. alveolar
2. pulmonary
3. CORRECT
4. diaphragm
5. pneumopleuritis
6. pleuralgia
7. CORRECT
8. CORRECT
9. tonsillar
10. dyspnea

Chapter 10

Exercise 1
1. prepuce, foreskin
2. scrotum

3. seminal vesicles
4. sperm, spermatozoon
5. vas deferens
6. bulbourethral glands
7. penis
8. seminiferous tubules

Exercise 2
1. testosterone
2. glans penis
3. epididymis
4. semen
5. prostate gland
6. testis

Exercise 3
1. prostate
2. sperm, spermatozoon
3. male
4. fluid-filled sac (seminal vesicle)
5. testis, testicle
6. glans penis
7. epididymis
8. sperm, spermatozoon
9. duct, vessel, vas deferens
10. testis, testicle

Exercise 4
1. crypt-
2. -lysis
3. -ism
4. -cele
5. -tomy
6. an-
7. -pexy
8. -plasty
9. -stomy

Exercise 5
1. orchi/o, testicul/o
2. balan/o
3. vesicul/o
4. vas/o
5. prostat/o

Exercise 6
1. vasectomy
2. andropathy
3. prostatolith
4. vesiculitis
5. spermatogenesis
6. balanorrhea
7. orchiopexy

Exercise 7
1. prostatic
2. testicular
3. condom
4. ejaculation
5. epididymal
6. spermatic
7. balanic

Exercise 8
1. spermicide
2. testicular
3. balanic
4. prostatic
5. puberty
6. epididymal
7. condom

Exercise 9
1. testicul/o   testis, testicle
2. prostat/o   prostate

3. balan/o   glans penis
4. epididym/o   epididymis
5. sperm/o   sperm, spermatozoon

Exercise 10
1. inflammation of the prostate
2. abnormal persistent erection of the penis
3. absence of sperm; inability to produce sperm
4. abnormal discharge from the glans penis
5. inflammation of the epididymis
6. narrowing of the opening of the prepuce that prevents it from being drawn back over the glans penis
7. a wartlike lesion on the genitals

Exercise 11
1. chlamydia
2. genital herpes
3. varicocele
4. gonorrhea
5. acquired immunodeficiency syndrome
6. hydrocele
7. benign prostatic hypertrophy
8. erectile dysfunction

Exercise 12
1. human papillomavirus
2. benign prostatic hyperplasia, benign prostatic hypertrophy
3. human immunodeficiency virus
4. sexually transmitted disease
5. spermatocele
6. testicular torsion
7. syphilis
8. Peyronie disease

Exercise 13
1. spermat/o / -cele
2. prostat/o / -itis
3. balan/o / -rrhea
4. a- / sperm/o / -ia
5. orchid/o / -itis
   orch/o   / -itis
   test/o   / -itis
6. balan/o / -itis
7. crypt/o / orchid/o / -ism
8. epididym/o / -itis

Exercise 14
1. andr/o / -pathy
   male / disease
   disease found in males
2. prostat/o / -lith
   prostate / stone
   stone in the prostate
3. balan/o   / -itis
   glans penis / inflammation
   inflammation of the glans penis
4. olig/o   / sperm/o   / -ia
   few, scanty / sperm,   / condition
             spermatozoon of
   scanty production of sperm
5. an-   / orch/o   / -ism
   without, not / testis, testicle /
   condition of
   condition of being without a testis
6. prostat/o / -rrhea
   prostate / discharge
   discharge from the prostate

7. crypt- / orchid/o / -ism
hidden / testis, testicle / condition of
condition of hidden testes

Exercise 15
1. transrectal ultrasound
2. digital rectal examination
3. prostatic-specific antigen

Exercise 16
1. creation of a new opening using an
   incision between two pieces of vas
   deferens to reverse the effects of a
   vasectomy
2. excision of the prepuce (foreskin) from
   the penis
3. excision of a testis
4. incision to remove a stone from the
   prostate
5. removal of prostatic tissue through the
   urethra using a resectoscope; used for
   treatment of benign prostatic hyperplasia
6. surgical procedure to place a penile
   prosthesis for patients with erectile
   dysfunction

Exercise 17
1. orchioplasty
2. epididymectomy
3. prostatolithotomy
4. orchiectomy
5. vasectomy
6. prostatectomy

Exercise 18
1. epididymectomy
2. orchioplasty
3. vesiculectomy
4. orchidotomy
5. vasectomy

Exercise 19
1. orchi/o / -tomy
   testis, testicle / incision
   incision into a testis
2. balan/o / -plasty
   glans penis / surgical repair,
                 reconstruction
   surgical repair of the glans penis
3. prostat/o / -ectomy
   prostate / excision, surgical removal
   excision of the prostate
4. orchi/o / -pexy
   testis, testicle / surgical fixation
   surgical fixation of a testis
5. vas/o / -ectomy
   duct, vessel, / excision, surgical
   vas deferens   removal
   excision of the vas deferens

Exercise 20
1. impotence agent
2. antiretroviral
3. vasodilator
4. antiviral

Exercise 21
1. urology
2. urologist

Exercise 22
1. benign prostatic hyperplasia, benign
   prostatic hypertrophy
2. transurethral incision of the prostate
3. erectile dysfunction

4. human immunodeficiency virus
5. prostatic-specific antigen
6. venereal disease
7. transrectal ultrasound

Exercise 23
1. transurethral resection of the prostate
2. sexually transmitted disease
3. digital rectal examination
4. human papillomavirus
5. acquired immunodeficiency syndrome
6. benign prostatic hyperplasia or benign
   prostatic hypertrophy

Exercise 24
1. prostate gland
2. vas deferens
3. penis
4. glans penis
5. prepuce (foreskin)
6. epididymis
7. seminal vesicle
8. testicle
9. scrotum

Exercise 25
1. testicul/o   testis, testicle
2. prostat/o   prostate
3. balan/o   glans penis
4. orch/o   testis, testicle
5. epididym/o   epididymis
6. sperm/o   sperm, spermatozoon
7. vesicul/o   fluid-filled sac (seminal
                 vesicle)
8. andr/o   male

Exercise 26
1. excision of the vas deferens
   duct, vessel, vas deferens
   excision
2. discharge from the prostate
   prostate
   discharge
3. inflammation of the glans penis
   glans penis
   inflammation
4. pertaining to the epididymis
   epididymis
   pertaining to
5. surgical fixation of the testes
   testis, testicle
   surgical fixation
6. stone in the prostate
   prostate
   stone
7. repair of a testis
   testis, testicle
   surgical repair, reconstruction
8. excision of the seminal vesicle
   fluid-filled sac (seminal vesicle)
   excision, surgical removal

Exercise 27
1. through sexual contact
2. to reverse the effects of a vasectomy
   and reproduce
3. testosterone
4. secretions from the testes, seminal
   glands, prostate, and bulbourethral
   glands
5. spermatocele
6. human papillomavirus
7. prostate

8. prepuce or foreskin
9. cryptorchidism
10. vasectomy
11. in tissues inside the penis

Exercise 28
1. B
2. D
3. B
4. C
5. A
6. C
7. A
8. D
9. C
10. B
11. D
12. C
13. B
14. A
15. A
16. D
17. B
18. B

Exercise 29
1. D
2. B
3. C
4. B
5. D
6. A

Exercise 30
1. digital rectal examination
2. dysuria
3. hydrocele
4. orchiopexy
5. transrectal ultrasound

Exercise 31
1. D
2. B
3. A
4. D
5. D
6. transrectal ultrasound and needle
   biopsy

Exercise 32
1. orchialgia
2. balanorrhea
3. spermicide
4. condyloma
5. urethritis

Exercise 33
1. D
2. A
3. B
4. C
5. B
6. an accumulation of an excessive
   amount of watery fluid in cells, tissues,
   or serous cavities (exact answer will
   vary depending on dictionary used)

Exercise 34
*Practice until your pronunciation matches
that heard in the Audio Glossary in the
Student Resources.*

Exercise 35
1. scrotum
2. spermatozoon

3. semen
4. prostate
5. coitus
6. epididymis
7. balanorrhea
8. aspermia
9. phimosis
10. hydrocele
11. prostatitis
12. varicocele
13. chlamydia
14. condyloma
15. syphilis

Chapter 11

Exercise 1
1. placenta
2. lactiferous ducts
3. endometrium
4. breasts
5. genitalia
6. ovum
7. amnion
8. umbilical cord
9. mammary papilla
10. fundus
11. areola
12. corpus luteum
13. vesicular ovarian follicles, graafian follicles
14. greater vestibular glands, Bartholin glands
15. zygote

Exercise 2
1. outer layer of the uterus that covers the body of the uterus and part of the cervix
2. fluid that encases the fetus and provides a cushion for the fetus as the mother moves
3. tubular, lower portion of the uterus that opens into the vagina
4. hormone secreted by the fertilized ovum soon after conception
5. an immature ovum contained in a follicle
6. outermost membrane surrounding the fetus
7. tubular structures that carry the ovum from the ovary to the uterus
8. state of a female after conception and until delivery
9. glands in the breast that make breast milk
10. lactation-stimulating hormone
11. pear-shaped organ located in the middle of the pelvis that supports a growing fetus and is the site of menses
12. part of the labia that covers and protects the female external genital organs
13. fertilized ovum from the time of implantation in the uterus until about the eighth week of gestation

Exercise 3
1. corpus luteum
2. labia
3. Fimbriae
4. mons pubis
5. ovulation
6. introitus
7. labia minora
8. ovaries
9. vagina
10. zygote

Exercise 4
1. vulva
2. fetus
3. cervical os
4. lactation
5. effacement
6. gamete
7. lochia
8. vagina
9. lactiferous lobules
10. ovaries

Exercise 5
1. endometrium
2. clitoris
3. labia
4. perineum
5. mammary glands
6. genitalia
7. adnexa
8. myometrium

Exercise 6
1. fundus
2. pelvis, pelvic cavity
3. cervix, neck (neck of uterus)
4. breast, mammary gland
5. from conception to birth
6. pubis
7. salpinx, fallopian tube
8. vagina
9. pregnancy
10. scanty, few
11. uterus
12. milk
13. birth
14. chorion
15. perineum

Exercise 7
1. vagin/o, colp/o
2. gyn/o, gynec/o
3. my/o
4. salping/o
5. mamm/o, mast/o
6. cephal/o
7. gravid/o
8. perine/o
9. hydr/o
10. toc/o
11. men/o, menstru/o
12. cervic/o
13. galact/o, lact/o
14. vulv/o, episi/o
15. pub/o

Exercise 8
1. above
2. surgical repair, reconstruction
3. incision
4. none
5. herniation, protrusion
6. measurement of
7. flow, discharge
8. condition of
9. new
10. beginning
11. suture
12. puncture to aspirate
13. before
14. in, within
15. childbirth, labor

Exercise 9
1. flowing forth (of blood) from the uterus
2. study of woman
3. excision or surgical removal of the uterus
4. record of the breast
5. incision into the vulva
6. suture of the vagina
7. excision or surgical removal of (one or both) ovaries
8. inflammation of the cervix
9. surgical repair or reconstruction of the vagina
10. excision or surgical removal of the salpinges

Exercise 10
1. gynecologist
2. hysteroscopy
3. colporrhaphy
4. omphalocele
5. vaginitis
6. mammography
7. amniotomy
8. fetal
9. embryology
10. mastectomy

Exercise 11
1. suprapubic
2. intrauterine
3. menarche
4. estimated date of confinement
5. stillbirth
6. para
7. prenatal
8. meconium
9. primigravida

Exercise 12
1. chorionic
2. nullipara
3. transabdominal
4. neonate
5. congenital
6. cystic
7. gestational
8. gravida

Exercise 13
1. in vitro
2. ovarian
3. uterine
4. postpartum
5. neonatal
6. perineal
7. menses
8. date of birth
9. last menstrual period
10. nulligravida

Exercise 14
1. fet/o   fetus
2. vagin/o   vagina
3. pelv/i   pelvis
4. metri/o   uterus

5. abdomin/o, pelv/i   abdomen, pelvis
6. embry/o   embryo
7. abdomin/o   abdomen
8. ovari/o   ovary

Exercise 15
1. sexually transmitted disease
2. oligohydramnios
3. gastroschisis
4. cervical dysplasia
5. Turner syndrome
6. ectopic pregnancy
7. menopause
8. atrial septal defect
9. cleft lip
10. nuchal cord
11. abortion, spontaneous abortion
12. toxoplasmosis
13. rupture of membranes
14. patent ductus arteriosus
15. abruptio placenta
16. tetralogy of Fallot
17. bacterial vaginosis
18. pelvic inflammatory disease
19. atresia
20. breech pregnancy

Exercise 16
1. metrorrhagia
2. dyspareunia
3. infertility
4. polycystic ovary syndrome
5. ventricular septal defect
6. Braxton Hicks
7. gestational diabetes
8. eclampsia
9. postpartum depression
10. atrophic vaginitis
11. spina bifida
12. uterine prolapse
13. cleft palate
14. placenta previa
15. prolapsed cord
16. congenital
17. jaundice of newborn
18. incomplete abortion
19. adenomyosis

Exercise 17
1. a-   / men/o   / -rrhea
   without, not / menstruation / flow, discharge
   without (absence of) menstrual flow
2. salping/o   / -itis
   salpinx, fallopian tube / inflammation
   inflammation of the salpinx
3. mast/o / -itis
   breast / inflammation
   inflammation of the breast
4. endo-   / metri/o / -osis
   in, within / uterus / abnormal condition
   abnormal condition within the uterus (endometrium)
5. vulv/o / -dynia
   vulva / pain
   pain in the vulva
6. micro- / cephal/o / -y
   small / head / condition of
   condition of abnormally small head

7. my/o   / -oma
   muscle (uterus) / tumor
   tumor of the uterus
8. omphal/o   / -cele
   umbilicus, navel / herniation, protrusion
   herniation of the umbilical cord
9. mast/o / -dynia
   breast / pain
   pain in the breast
10. dys-   / men/o   / -rrhea
    painful, / menstruation / flow, discharge
    difficult
    painful or difficult menstrual flow

Exercise 18
1. fetoscope
2. transvaginal ultrasound
3. hysterosalpingography
4. Apgar
5. group B streptococcus
6. quad marker screen
7. Papanicolaou test

Exercise 19
1. pelvic ultrasound
2. colposcopy
3. pregnancy test
4. mammography
5. chorionic villus sampling
6. amniocentesis
7. TORCH panel

Exercise 20
1. puncture to aspirate (fluid) from the amnion
2. instrument for examination of the vagina
3. process of recording the uterus and salpinges
4. process of recording the breast
5. instrument for examining (listening to) the fetus
6. process of examining the vagina

Exercise 21
1. dilation and curettage
2. myomectomy
3. pessary
4. total abdominal hysterectomy
5. cerclage
6. vaginal hysterectomy
7. induction of labor
8. in vitro fertilization
9. loop electrosurgical excision procedure (LEEP)
10. amniotomy, artificial rupture of membranes

Exercise 22
1. tubal ligation
2. cryosurgery
3. salpingo-oophorectomy
4. salpingectomy
5. therapeutic abortion
6. cesarean section

Exercise 23
1. mammoplasty
2. amniotomy
3. mastopexy
4. hysteroplasty or uteroplasty
5. episiotomy

Exercise 24
1. salping/o   / oophor/o / -ectomy
   salpinx,
   fallopian tube / ovary   / excision, surgical removal
   excision of the ovary and salpinx
2. colp/o / -rrhaphy
   vagina / suture
   suture of the vagina
3. uter/o / -tomy
   uterus / incision
   incision of the uterus
4. mamm/o   / -plasty
   breast, mammary gland / surgical repair, reconstruction
   surgical repair of the breast
5. hyster/o / -ectomy
   uterus   / excision, surgical removal
   excision of the uterus
6. episi/o / -tomy
   vulva / incision
   incision of the vulva
7. salping/o   / -ectomy
   salpinx, fallopian tube / excision, surgical removal
   excision of a salpinx
8. oophor/o / -ectomy
   ovary   / excision, surgical removal
   excision of an ovary
9. mast/o   / -pexy
   breast, mammary gland / surgical fixation
   surgical fixation of the breast
10. vulv/o / -ectomy
    vulva   / excision, surgical removal
    excision of all or part of the vulva

Exercise 25
1. oxytocin
2. abortifacient
3. contraceptive
4. ovulation induction
5. tocolytic agent
6. hormone replacement therapy

Exercise 26
1. midwife
2. neonatal intensive care unit
3. reproductive endocrinology
4. neonatology
5. obstetrics
6. pediatrics
7. neonatologist
8. midwifery
9. reproductive endocrinologist
10. gynecology
11. obstetrician
12. pediatrician
13. gynecologist

Exercise 27
1. total abdominal hysterectomy
2. spontaneous abortion
3. abortion
4. pelvic inflammatory disease
5. sexually transmitted disease

Exercise 28
1. neonatal intensive care unit
2. obstetrician
3. hormone replacement therapy
4. total abdominal hysterectomy

5. therapeutic abortion
6. estimated date of delivery
7. last menstrual period
8. in vitro fertilization
9. dilation and curettage
10. loop electrosurgical excision procedure

Exercise 29
1. D&C
2. CVS
3. HSG
4. GYN
5. DOB
6. hCG

Exercise 30
1. peritoneal cavity
2. salpinx
3. ovary
4. uterus
5. clitoris
6. labium minora
7. labium majora
8. vagina
9. fimbriae
10. cervix
11. rectum

Exercise 31
1. hyster/o / salping/o / -graphy
   uterus / salpinx, / process of
   fallopian recording
   tube
   process of recording the uterus and
   salpinges
2. episi/o / -tomy
   vulva / incision
   incision of the vulva
3. colp/o / -rrhaphy
   vagina / suture
   suture of the vagina
5. endo- / cervic/o / -al
   in, within / cervix / pertaining to
   pertaining to within the cervix
6. pelv/i / metry
   pelvis / measurement of
   measurement of the pelvis
7. oophor/o / -ectomy
   ovary / excision, surgical removal
   excision of an ovary
8. mamm/o / -graphy
   breast, mammary gland / process of
   recording
   process of recording the breast
9. metr/o / -rrhagia
   uterus / flowing forth
   flowing forth (of blood) from the uterus
   between periods
10. olig/o / men/o / -rrhea
    scanty, few / menstruation / flow,
    discharge
    scanty discharge (of blood) during
    menstruation
11. mamm/o / -plasty
    breast / surgical repair, reconstruction
    surgical repair of the breast
12. salping/o / -ectomy
    salpinx, fallopian tube / excision,
    surgical removal
    surgical removal of a salpinx

13. colp/o / -scopy
    vagina / process of examining,
    examination
    process of examining the vagina (and cervix)
14. vagin/o / -itis
    vagina / inflammation
    inflammation of the vagina
15. cervic/o / -itis
    cervix / inflammation
    inflammation of the cervix

Exercise 32
1. ectopic
2. nulligravida
3. infertility
4. in vitro fertilization
5. cesarean section
6. nuchal cord

Exercise 33
1. salpingo-oophorectomy
2. embryo
3. salpinx or fallopian tube
4. Nulligravida refers to a woman who has
   had no pregnancies; primigravida refers
   to a woman who has had a single
   pregnancy; gravida refers to a woman
   who is pregnant.
5. perimetrium (outer layer); myometrium
   (muscular middle layer); endometrium
   (inner layer)
6. Gynecology deals with diseases of the
   female genital tract as well as
   endocrinology and reproductive health.
   Obstetrics deals with childbirth and the
   care of the mother.
7. anywhere other than the lining of the
   uterus
8. Rupture of membranes is a
   spontaneous rupture of the amniotic
   sac. An amniotomy is an artificial
   tearing of the amniotic sac.
9. to test for various problems in the fetus,
   such as genetic defects, fetal infections,
   or fetal lung immaturity

Exercise 34
1. D
2. A
3. B
4. A
5. C
6. B
7. B
8. D

Exercise 35
1. C
2. B
3. A
4. C
5. A
6. B
7. A
8. C
9. A
10. D
11. B
12. A
13. C
14. D
15. D

Exercise 36
1. sexually transmitted disease
2. endocervical curettage
3. colposcopy
4. stenosis
5. patient has been pregnant 3 times
6. Papanicolaou test

Exercise 37
1. prenatal
2. cervix
3. episiotomy
4. neonatologist
5. Apgar score
6. to enlarge the vagina and assist
   childbirth

Exercise 38
*Practice until your pronunciation matches
that heard in the Audio Glossary in the
Student Resources.*

Exercise 39
1. hysterectomy
2. suprapubic
3. cervicitis
4. cystic
5. laparotomy
6. mastectomy
7. endometrial
8. ovulation
9. perimetrium
10. mammography
11. placenta
12. clitoris
13. areola
14. colposcopy
15. zygote

Chapter 12
Exercise 1
1. pons
2. occipital lobe
3. cerebrum
4. central nervous system
5. cerebellum
6. ventricle
7. temporal lobe
8. parietal lobe
9. frontal lobe
10. brainstem

Exercise 2
1. portion of the central nervous system
   contained in the spinal or vertebral
   canal; responsible for nerve conduction
   to and from the brain and body
2. outer layer of the cerebrum; controls
   higher mental functions
3. whitish cordlike structure that
   transmits stimuli from the central
   nervous system to another area of the
   body or the reverse
4. groove or fissure on the surface of the brain
5. thin inner layer of the meninges that
   attaches directly to the brain and spinal
   cord
6. part of the nervous system external to
   the brain and spinal cord that consists
   of all other nerves throughout the body
7. part of the brainstem that connects the
   brainstem to the cerebellum; controls
   sensory processes

8. the 12 pairs of nerves that emerge from the cranium
9. part of the central nervous system contained within the cranium
10. membranous covering of the brain and spinal cord

Exercise 3
1. ganglion
2. spinal nerves
3. neuron
4. arachnoid
5. cerebrospinal fluid
6. gyrus
7. neuroglia
8. dura mater
9. diencephalon

Exercise 4
1. entire brain
2. glue, neuroglia
3. brain, cerebrum
4. nerve
5. hard, dura mater
6. meninges
7. cerebellum (little brain)
8. nerve root
9. sleep
10. mind, mental
11. ganglion
12. thalamus
13. cranium, skull
14. sensation, perception
15. speech
16. vertebra
17. bone marrow, spinal cord
18. spine
19. mind, mental
20. gray

Exercise 5
1. gli/o
2. ventricul/o
3. encephal/o
4. anxi/o
5. myel/o
6. cerebell/o
7. cortic/o
8. gangli/o
9. thalam/o
10. schiz/o
11. spin/o
12. thym/i, thym/o
13. cerebr/o
14. psych/o, phren/o, ment/o
15. spondyl/o, vertebr/o
16. esthesi/o
17. dur/o
18. hallucin/o
19. narc/o

Exercise 6
1. one who specializes in
2. half
3. attraction for
4. excited state, obsession
5. abnormal fear, aversion to, sensitivity to
6. many, much
7. four
8. condition of
9. incision
10. above, excessive
11. partial or incomplete paralysis

12. below, deficient
13. paralysis
14. on, following
15. seizure

Exercise 7
1. inflammation of the entire brain
2. incision into the skull
3. record of the spinal cord
4. pertaining to neuroglia
5. condition of painful or difficult speech
6. pertaining to the spine
7. pertaining to the cerebellum
8. one who specializes in the mind
9. splitting of the mind
10. condition of without sensation
11. disease of the (spinal) nerve roots
12. disease involving many nerves

Exercise 8
1. myelitis
2. craniotomy
3. neuropathy
4. glioma
5. cranial
6. dysesthesia
7. meningitis
8. subdural
9. meningioma
10. encephalopathy

Exercise 9
1. pertaining to the meninges
2. pertaining to the cranium or skull
3. pertaining to on or outside the dura mater
4. pertaining to the cerebrum
5. pertaining to a lack of blood flow
6. pertaining to a root (nerve)
7. pertaining to the mind

Exercise 10
1. bipolar
2. dural
3. neural
4. glial
5. ictal
6. postictal
7. cerebellar
8. ischemic
9. subdural

Exercise 11
1. cerebr/o   cerebrum
2. radicul/o   nerve root
3. ment/o   mind
4. dur/o   dura mater
5. spin/o   spine
6. cerebell/o   cerebellum (little brain)

Exercise 12
1. concussion
2. stupor
3. coma
4. parkinsonism, Parkinson disease
5. disorientation
6. stroke
7. multiple sclerosis
8. cerebral aneurysm
9. cerebral embolism
10. amnesia
11. amyotrophic lateral sclerosis, Lou Gehrig disease
12. paraplegia

Exercise 13
1. obsessive-compulsive disorder
2. anxiety
3. attention deficit hyperactivity disorder
4. posttraumatic stress disorder
5. paranoia
6. delusions
7. compulsion
8. depression
9. catatonia
10. agoraphobia
11. autism
12. delirium

Exercise 14
1. poly- / neur/o / -itis
   many, much / nerve / inflammation
   inflammation of many nerves
2. radicul/o / -pathy
   nerve roots / disease
   disease of the nerve roots
3. a- / phas/o / -ia
   without, not / speech / condition of
   condition of without speech
4. mening/o / myel/o / -cele
   meninges / spinal bone / herniation, marrow, cord protrusion
   herniation or protrusion of the meninges and spinal cord
5. encephal/o / -itis
   entire brain / inflammation of
   inflammation of the entire brain
6. hemi- / -paresis
   half / partial or incomplete paralysis
   partial paralysis of half of the body
7. neur/o / -algia
   nerve / pain
   pain in a nerve
8. schiz/o / -phrenia
   split / the mind
   splitting of the mind
9. sub- / dur/o / -al
   below, / hard, dura / pertaining to
   beneath matter
   pertaining to below the dura matter
10. poli/o / myel/o / -itis
    gray / bone marrow, / inflammation of
    spinal cord
    inflammation of the gray matter of the spinal cord

Exercise 15
1. Glasgow coma scale
2. evoked potential studies
3. Babinski sign
4. positron emission tomography
5. cerebral angiography

Exercise 16
1. lumbar puncture
2. polysomnography
3. magnetic resonance imaging
4. deep tendon reflex
5. electroencephalogram
6. myelogram

Exercise 17
1. neuroplasty
2. craniectomy
3. laminectomy
4. craniotomy
5. radicotomy
6. neurolysis

7. ganglionectomy
8. psychotherapy

Exercise 18
1. neuroplasty
2. ganglionectomy
3. radicotomy, rhizotomy
4. craniectomy

Exercise 19
1. anticonvulsant
2. antidepressant
3. antianxiety agent, anxiolytic
4. antiinflammatory
5. sedative
6. analgesic
7. neuroleptic
8. epidural injection

Exercise 20
1. drug that breaks down anxiety
2. drug used to turn the mind (treat mental illnesses)
3. drug that pertains to a loss of sensation
4. drug that pertains to (promotes) sleep

Exercise 21
1. psychologist
2. neurology
3. psychiatry
4. psychiatrist
5. EEG technician
6. psychology
7. neurologist

Exercise 22
1. cerebral palsy
2. transient ischemic attack
3. lumbar puncture
4. multiple sclerosis
5. cerebral spinal fluid
6. obsessive-compulsive disorder
7. magnetic resonance imaging
8. cerebrovascular accident

Exercise 23
1. EEG
2. CVA
3. ALS
4. PTSD
5. ADHD
6. PET
7. CNS
8. DTR

Exercise 24
1. frontal lobe
2. cerebral cortex
3. parietal lobe
4. occipital lobe
5. cerebellum
6. brain stem
7. temporal lobe

Exercise 25
1. pia mater
2. arachnoid
3. dura mater

Exercise 26
1. meningi/o / -cyte
   meninges / cell
   cell of the meninges
2. neur/o / -pathy
   nerve / disease
   disease of a nerve

3. crani/o / cerebr/o / -al
   cranium, skull / brain, / pertaining
                              to cerebrum
   pertaining to the skull and brain
4. quadri- / -paresis
   four / partial or incomplete paralysis
   partial paralysis in four limbs
5. radicul/o / myel/o / -pathy
   nerve root / bone marrow, / disease
                   spinal cord
   disease involving the spinal cord and the nerve roots
6. electr/o / encephal/o / -graphy
   electric, / entire / process of
   electricity brain recording
   electrical recording of activity of the brain
7. encephal/o / -scopy
   brain / process of examining, examination
   process of examining the brain
8. poli/o / dys- / -trophy
   gray / painful, / development,
           difficult, nourishment
           abnormal
   wasting of the gray matter of the nervous system
9. spondyl/o / -osis
   vertebra / abnormal condition
   abnormal condition of the vertebra
10. ganglion/o / -ectomy
    ganglion / excision, surgical removal
    excision of a ganglion

Exercise 27
1. hallucinations
2. Lethargy
3. ataxia
4. Bell palsy
5. sleep apnea
6. Alzheimer disease
7. anesthesia
8. electroencephalogram
9. shingles
10. paranoia
11. cerebral palsy
12. meningitis
13. radiculopathy
14. migraine
15. cerebral thrombosis
16. cerebrum
17. gyri (gyrus)
18. brain stem
19. syncope
20. epilepsy

Exercise 28
1. D
2. C
3. A
4. B
5. B
6. B
7. C
8. D
9. C
10. B
11. B
12. B
13. C
14. C

Exercise 29
1. C
2. C
3. D
4. A
5. D
6. C
7. D
8. B

Exercise 30
1. B
2. C
3. B
4. B
5. C

Exercise 31
1. aphasia
2. cerebrovascular accident
3. transient ischemic attack
4. electroencephalogram
5. seizure
6. Lamictal and Dilantin
7. carotid endarterectomy

Exercise 32
Practice until your pronunciation matches that heard in the Audio Glossary in the Student Resources.

Exercise 33
1. cerebrum
2. encephalopathy
3. temporal
4. delusion
5. Alzheimer
6. schizophrenia
7. radiculopathy
8. catatonia
9. cerebellum
10. myelopathy
11. anesthesia
12. neuropathy
13. parietal
14. hallucination
15. seizure

Chapter 13

Exercise 1
1. lens
2. vitreous humor
3. choroid
4. orbit
5. iris
6. conjunctiva
7. pupil
8. cornea
9. optic nerve
10. nasolacrimal ducts

Exercise 2
1. retina
2. sclera
3. lacrimal ducts
4. choroid
5. tarsal glands, meibomian glands
6. lens
7. conjunctiva
8. lacrimal glands
9. pupil
10. aqueous humor

Exercise 3
1. tarsal glands
2. retina
3. aqueous humor
4. optic nerve
5. cornea
6. vitreous humor
7. lacrimal glands
8. iris
9. sclera

Exercise 4
1. eye
2. tears or tear ducts
3. iris
4. pupil
5. tears or tear ducts
6. cornea
7. eye
8. pupil
9. cornea
10. eyelid

Exercise 5
1. conjunctiv/o
2. scler/o
3. phot/o
4. blephar/o
5. ton/o
6. presby/o
7. dipl/o
8. opt/o
9. ir/o or irid/o
10. retin/o

Exercise 6
1. paralysis
2. vision
3. prolapse, drooping, sagging
4. two, twice
5. destruction, breakdown, separation
6. flow, discharge
7. surgical fixation
8. softening
9. surgical repair, reconstruction
10. process of examining, examination
11. dilation, stretching
12. abnormal fear, aversion to, sensitivity to

Exercise 7
1. ir/o
2. retin/o
3. pupill/o
4. conjunctiv/o
5. scler/o
6. corne/o

Exercise 8
1. conjunctivitis
2. diplopia
3. blepharoptosis
4. pupillometer
5. photophobia
6. retinopathy
7. iridoplegia
8. keratoplasty
9. sclerotomy
10. ophthalmologist

Exercise 9
1. instrument for examining the eye
   eye
   instrument for examining

2. measurement of vision
   vision, eye
   measurement of
3. involuntary movement of the eyelid
   eyelid
   involuntary movement
4. discharge of tears
   tears or tear ducts
   flow, discharge
5. vision loss that is age-related
   related to aging
   vision
6. surgical fixation of the retina
   retina
   surgical fixation
7. dilation of the pupil
   pupil
   dilation, stretching
8. inflammation of the iris
   iris
   inflammation
9. instrument for measuring pressure
   tension, pressure
   instrument for measuring
10. disease of the cornea
    cornea
    disease

Exercise 10
1. pertaining to the eye
2. pertaining to tears
3. pertaining to vision
4. within or inside the eye
5. pertaining to the iris
6. pertaining to the conjunctiva
7. pertaining to the eye
8. pertaining to the sclera
9. ability of the eye to adjust focus on near objects

Exercise 11
1. intraocular
2. binocular
3. blepharal
4. pupillary
5. retinal
6. optic
7. corneal
8. iridial

Exercise 12
1. ophthalmic
2. conjunctival
3. optic
4. intraocular
5. corneal
6. blepharal
7. binocular

Exercise 13
1. involuntary rhythmic movements of the eye
2. any disease of the retina
3. softening of the iris
4. inflammation of the eyelid
5. clouding of the lens of the eye, which causes poor vision
6. abnormal protrusion of one or both eyeballs
7. stone in the lacrimal sac or ducts
8. condition involving dry eye(s)

9. group of diseases of the eye characterized by increased intraocular pressure that damages the optic nerve
10. disease of the eye(s)

Exercise 14
1. astigmatism
2. hyperopia
3. color blindness
4. amblyopia
5. diplopia
6. presbyopia
7. nyctalopia
8. myopia
9. macular degeneration
10. photophobia
11. ophthalmia

Exercise 15
1. diabetic retinopathy
2. ophthalmoplegia
3. dacryoadenitis
4. chalazion
5. dacryocystitis
6. hordeolum
7. pterygium
8. retinitis pigmentosa
9. strabismus
10. detached retina

Exercise 16
1. scler/o / -malacia
   hard, sclera / softening
   softening of the sclera
2. kerat/o / -itis
   cornea / inflammation
   inflammation of the cornea
3. irid/o / -plegia
   iris / paralysis
   paralysis of the iris
4. dacry/o / -rrhea
   tears or tear ducts / flow, discharge
   discharge of tears
5. blephar/o / -spasm
   eyelid / involuntary movement
   involuntary movement of the eyelid
6. scler/o / -itis
   hard, sclera / inflammation
   inflammation of the sclera
7. conjunctiv/o / -itis
   conjunctiva / inflammation
   inflammation of the conjunctiva
8. ophthalm/o / -algia
   eye / pain
   pain in the eye
9. blephar/o / -ptosis
   eyelid / prolapse, drooping, sagging
   sagging eyelid
10. kerat/o / -malacia
    cornea / softening
    softening of the cornea

Exercise 17
1. instrument for measuring pressure within the eye
2. instrument used for examining the interior of the eye through the pupil
3. examination of the retina
4. instrument for measuring the curvature of the cornea
5. measurement of the pupil

Exercise 18
1. visual field assessment
2. Snellen chart
3. pupillometry
4. fluorescein angiography
5. refraction
6. extraocular movement assessment

Exercise 19
1. fluorescein angiography
2. retinoscopy
3. Snellen chart
4. refraction
5. tonometer
6. visual acuity

Exercise 20
1. pupill/o / -meter
   pupil / instrument for measuring
   instrument for measuring the pupil
2. ton/o / -metry
   tension, pressure / measurement of
   measurement of pressure (within the eye)
3. ophthalm/o / -scopy
   eye / process of examining,
   examination
   examination of the eye
4. kerat/o / -meter
   cornea / instrument for measuring
   instrument for measuring (the
   curvature of) the cornea
5. retin/o / -scopy
   retina / process of examining,
   examination
   examination of the retina
6. ophthalm/o / -scope
   eye / instrument for examining
   instrument for examining (the interior of)
   the eye

Exercise 21
1. enucleation
2. cryoretinopexy
3. vitrectomy
4. photorefractive keratectomy (PRK)
5. cataract extraction
6. retinal photocoagulation
7. laser-assisted in situ keratomileusis
   (LASIK)

Exercise 22
1. phacoemulsification
2. trabeculectomy
3. dacryocystotomy
4. scleral buckling
5. keratoplasty
6. blepharoplasty
7. intraocular lens implant

Exercise 23
1. tomy
2. blepharo
3. ectomy
4. kerato
5. ectomy
6. irido

Exercise 24
1. mydriatic
2. corticosteroid
3. prostaglandin
4. miotic
5. hypotonic

Exercise 25
1. optometry
2. ophthalmology
3. optician
4. ophthalmologist
5. optometrist

Exercise 26
1. each eye or both eyes (oculus uterque)
2. extraocular movement
3. intraocular lens
4. left eye (oculus sinister)
5. visual field

Exercise 27
1. visual acuity
2. laser-assisted in situ keratomileusis
3. right eye (oculus dexter)
4. photorefractive keratectomy
5. intraocular pressure

Exercise 28
1. auditory ossicle shaped like a stirrup
2. receptor for hearing located inside the
   cochlea; the organ of hearing
3. canal that extends from the auricle to
   the tympanic membrane
4. auditory ossicle shaped like an anvil
5. external portion of the ear
6. auditory ossicle shaped like a hammer
   or club
7. middle ear bones contained in the
   tympanic cavity that transmit sound
   vibrations
8. waxy substance created by glands of
   the external auditory meatus; earwax
9. inner ear, which is made up of a series
   of semicircular canals, the vestibule,
   and the cochlea

Exercise 29
1. vestibule
2. semicircular canals
3. auditory ossicles
4. tympanic membrane
5. pharyngotympanic tube
6. mastoid bone
7. auricle
8. cochlea
9. external auditory canal

Exercise 30
1. auditory ossicles
2. mastoid bone
3. labyrinth
4. cerumen
5. spiral organ
6. semicircular canals
7. vestibule
8. pharyngotympanic tube
9. tympanic membrane

Exercise 31
1. hearing
2. pain
3. vestibule
4. ear
5. hearing, sound
6. hard, sclera
7. painful, difficult, abnormal
8. cochlea

Exercise 32
1. labyrinth/o

2. -ectomy
3. -stomy
4. scler/o
5. dys-
6. ot/o

Exercise 33
1. inflammation of the labyrinth or inner
   ear
2. surgical opening into the middle ear
3. inflammation of the mastoid bone
4. flow or discharge from the ear
5. instrument for measuring hearing
6. incision into the tympanic membrane
   (eardrum)
7. excision of the stapes

Exercise 34
1. vestibulotomy
2. aural
3. acoustic
4. cochleitis
5. sclerosis
6. otalgia
7. myringitis

Exercise 35
1. pertaining to the ear
2. pertaining to hearing or sound
3. pertaining to the ear
4. pertaining to the tympanic
   membrane
5. pertaining to a vestibule
6. pertaining to hearing
7. pertaining to the cochlea

Exercise 36
1. aural
2. vestibular
3. tympanic
4. acoustic
5. labyrinthine
6. mastoid

Exercise 37
1. aural
2. labyrinthine
3. auditory
4. otic
5. mastoid
6. tympanic

Exercise 38
1. otomycosis
2. otosclerosis
3. tinnitus
4. cholesteatoma
5. cerumen impaction
6. presbycusis
7. vertigo
8. acoustic neuroma

Exercise 39
1. otitis media
2. sensorineural hearing loss
3. presbycusis
4. otitis externa
5. conductive hearing loss
6. dysacousia

Exercise 40
1. sensorineural hearing loss
2. otitis externa
3. conductive hearing loss
4. otopyorrhea

5. Ménière disease
6. tympanic membrane perforation
7. otitis media

Exercise 41
1. ot/o / -algia
2. labyrinth/o / -itis
3. ot/o / -rrhea
4. mastoid/o / -itis
5. myring/o / -itis

Exercise 42
1. unit of measure of frequency or pitch of sound
2. record of hearing (presented in graph form)
3. use of an otoscope to examine the external auditory canal and tympanic membrane
4. measurement of middle ear function
5. unit for expressing the intensity of sound
6. record of middle ear function (presented in graph form)

Exercise 43
1. audiometer
2. audiometry
3. audiogram
4. tympanometer

Exercise 44
1. otoscope
2. tympanogram
3. audiometer
4. otoscopy
5. tympanometry
6. audiogram

Exercise 45
1. labyrinthectomy
2. mastoidotomy
3. stapedectomy
4. ear lavage
5. otoplasty

Exercise 46
1. cochlear implant
2. myringotomy or tympanostomy
3. myringotomy; tympanostomy tube placement
4. tympanoplasty
5. mastoidectomy

Exercise 47
1. mastoidotomy
2. stapedectomy
3. tympanostomy
4. tympanoplasty

Exercise 48
1. otic
2. antibiotic
3. ceruminolytic

Exercise 49
1. otology
2. audiologist
3. otorhinolaryngology
4. audiology
5. otologist
6. otorhinolaryngologist

Exercise 50
1. eyes, ears, nose, and throat
2. each ear, both ears (auris utraque)

3. hertz
4. otitis media
5. decibel
6. right ear (auris dexter)

Exercise 51
1. ears, nose, and throat
2. otitis externa
3. left ear (auris sinister)
4. electronystagmography
5. tympanic membrane

Exercise 52
1. cornea
2. iris
3. pupil
4. lens
5. anterior chamber
6. posterior chamber
7. sclera
8. choroid
9. retina
10. optic nerve

Exercise 53
1. auricle
2. tympanic membrane
3. external auditory canal
4. ossicles
5. semicircular canals
6. cochlea
7. vestibule
8. pharyngotympanic or auditory tube

Exercise 54
1. ophthalm/o / -ic
   eye / pertaining to
   pertaining to the eye
2. audi/o / -meter
   hearing / instrument for measuring
   instrument for measuring hearing
3. blephar/o / -itis
   eyelid / inflammation
   inflammation of the eyelid
4. tympan/o / -stomy
   tympanic membrane, / surgical opening
   eardrum
   surgical opening into the tympanic membrane
5. irid/o / -malacia
   iris / softening
   softening of the iris
6. labyrinth/o / -itis
   labyrinth, inner ear / inflammation
   inflammation of the labyrinth
7. retin/o / -pathy
   retina / disease
   disease of the retina
8. acous/o / -tic
   hearing, sound / pertaining to
   pertaining to hearing or sound
9. pupill/o / -meter
   pupil / instrument for measuring
   instrument for measuring the pupil
10. staped/o / -ectomy
    stapes / excision, surgical removal
    excision of the stapes
11. ton/o / -meter
    tension, pressure / instrument for measuring
    instrument for measuring pressure

12. vestibul/o / -ar
    vestibule / pertaining to
    pertaining to a vestibule
13. scler/o / -tomy
    hard, sclera / incision
    incision into the sclera
14. ot/o / -scopy
    ear / process of examining, examination
    examination of the ear

Exercise 55
1. discharge from the ear
   ear
   flow, discharge
2. examination of the eye
   eye
   process of examining, examination
3. measurement of vision
   vision
   measurement of
4. inflammation of the tympanic membrane
   tympanic membrane, eardrum
   inflammation
5. discharge of pus from the ear
   ear
   pus
   flow, discharge
6. discharge of tears
   tears
   flow, discharge
7. pertaining to the ear
   ear
   pertaining to
8. vision (loss) that is related to aging
   related to aging
   vision
9. recording of hearing
   hearing
   record, recording
10. excision of (part of) the mastoid bone
    mastoid
    excision, surgical removal
11. inflammation of the conjunctiva
    conjunctiva
    inflammation
12. measurement of middle ear (function)
    middle ear
    measurement of
13. surgical repair of the cornea
    cornea
    surgical repair, reconstruction
14. hearing loss that is related to aging
    related to aging
    hearing

Exercise 56
1. otorhinolaryngologist
2. optometrist
3. audiologist
4. otologist
5. ophthalmologist

Exercise 57
1. cochlea
2. ossicles
3. retina
4. cerumen impaction
5. lacrimal glands
6. Ménière disease
7. otitis externa

8. astigmatism
9. presbycusis
10. mydriatic
11. hypotonic
12. retinal detachment
13. laser-assisted in situ keratomileusis (LASIK)
14. xerophthalmia
15. fluorescein angiography
16. ear lavage
17. Snellen test
18. stapedectomy
19. Prostaglandins
20. Cryoretinopexy

Exercise 58
1. myopia
2. a spinning sensation; commonly used to mean dizziness
3. impaired vision
4. diplopia
5. photophobia
6. hyperopia is farsightedness, myopia is nearsightedness
7. to soften earwax
8. myringotomy

Exercise 59
1. C
2. A
3. D
4. C
5. D
6. A
7. B
8. A
9. C
10. D
11. B
12. B
13. D
14. D
15. A
16. B
17. D
18. B
19. B
20. A

Exercise 60
1. B
2. D
3. D
4. C
5. A
6. B
7. A
8. C
9. B
10. D

Exercise 61
1. C
2. A
3. B

Exercise 62
1. corneal
2. intraocular
3. microkeratome
4. keratography
5. speculum

Exercise 63
1. audiometry
2. otorrhea
3. otic
4. tympanoplasty
5. dysacousia
6. tympanic membrane perforation
7. tympanic
8. tinnitus
9. tympanostomies
10. conductive hearing loss
11. toward the front of the body and above or upward
12. a significant conductive hearing loss in the right ear

Exercise 64
Practice until your pronunciation matches that heard in the Audio Glossary in the Student Resources.

Exercise 65
1. tarsal
2. choroid
3. vitreous
4. corneal
5. ophthalmology
6. chalazion
7. diplopia
8. glaucoma
9. nystagmus
10. presbyopia
11. pterygium
12. strabismus
13. fluorescein
14. refraction
15. Snellen
16. pupillometry
17. acuity
18. cataract
19. mydriatic
20. optician

Chapter 14

Exercise 1
1. humerus
2. metacarpal bones
3. scapula
4. sternum
5. diaphysis
6. tendon
7. fascicle
8. calcaneus
9. axial skeleton
10. vertebrae

Exercise 2
1. moving away from the midline
2. band of strong connective tissue joining bones
3. the site where bones come together
4. bending foot upward
5. the socket of the pelvic bone where the femur articulates
6. the skull
7. lower bone of the jaw
8. a joint that moves freely; the joint cavity contains synovial fluid
9. upper bone of the jaw
10. dense connective tissue attached to bone in many joints

11. the growth area of a long bone
12. bony

Exercise 3
1. patella
2. meniscus
3. unstriated
4. Fascia
5. fibula
6. ilium
7. lamina
8. clavicle
9. metaphysis
10. tibia
11. bursa
12. ischium, pubis
13. vertebrae
14. tarsal
15. flexion

Exercise 4
1. endosteum
2. compact bone
3. radius
4. carpal bones
5. cancellous bone
6. sacrum
7. intervertebral disk
8. ulna
9. ossa
10. osteocyte

Exercise 5
1. clavicle
2. humerus
3. cancellous
4. ligament
5. insertion
6. antagonist
7. striated, unstriated
8. synovial
9. eversion
10. suture
11. ligaments
12. sacrum

Exercise 6
1. cranium, skull
2. lumbar region, lower back
3. crooked, twisted
4. bone
5. sternum
6. maxilla
7. cartilage
8. carpals
9. tendon
10. vertebra
11. fascia, band
12. muscle
13. mandible
14. sacrum
15. femur

Exercise 7
1. cost/o
2. tars/o
3. lei/o
4. fibul/o
5. burs/o
6. arthr/o, articul/o
7. pelv/i, pelv/o
8. thorac/o

9. ischi/o
10. clavic/o, clavicul/o
11. lamin/o
12. cervic/o
13. menisc/o
14. phalang/o

Exercise 8
1. surgical repair, reconstruction
2. weakness
3. below, beneath
4. surgical fixation, binding
5. excision, surgical removal
6. growth
7. suture
8. together, with
9. to split
10. to break

Exercise 9
1. inflammation of bone
2. condition of bent forward
3. muscle pain
4. inflammation of a bursa
5. inflammation of the maxilla
6. below the scapula
7. relating to the pelvis
8. inflammation of a tendon
9. between vertebrae
10. surgical repair of a joint

Exercise 10
1. myositis
2. cranioplasty
3. patellectomy
4. tenorrhaphy
5. arthralgia
6. intracranial
7. tarsectomy
8. meniscitis
9. diskectomy
10. chondroplasty

Exercise 11
1. intercostal
2. femoral
3. intervertebral
4. ischiofemoral
5. synovial
6. pelvic
7. subscapular
8. carpal

Exercise 12
1. humeral
2. intercostal
3. substernal
4. suprapatellar
5. cranial
6. sacral
7. intervertebral
8. intracranial
9. lumbar
10. costovertebral
11. submandibular
12. lumbosacral

Exercise 13
1. scoliosis
2. tendonitis or tendinitis
3. fracture
4. chondromalacia
5. bursitis

6. osteoporosis
7. rickets
8. tenodynia
9. spondylarthritis
10. ankylosing spondylitis
11. kyphosis
12. arthralgia
13. arthritis
14. osteomalacia

Exercise 14
1. myasthenia
2. polymyositis
3. gout
4. strain, sprain
5. rheumatoid arthritis
6. Fibromyalgia
7. bursolith
8. atrophy
9. carpal
10. Dyskinesia
11. tenosynovitis

Exercise 15
1. arthritis
2. arthralgia
3. rachischisis
4. maxillitis
5. tenodynia
6. bursitis
7. myalgia
8. arthrochondritis
9. osteomalacia

Exercise 16
1. hyper-   / -trophy
   above, excessive / development
   excessive development
   (of a part or organ)
2. scoli/o   / -osis
   crooked, twisted / abnormal condition
   abnormal condition of crooked or
   twisted (spine)
3. crani/o   / -schisis
   cranium, skull / split
   split skull
4. carp/o   / -ptosis
   carpal bones / dropping
   dropping of the carpal bones
5. ankyl/o / -osis
   stiff   / abnormal condition
   abnormal condition of stiffening
   (of a joint)
6. burs/o / -lith
   bursa / stone
   calculus (stone) in a bursa
7. a-   / -trophy
   not, without / development
   without (absence of) development
8. oste/o / -itis
   bone   / inflammation
   inflammation of bone
9. brady- / kines/o   / -ia
   slow   / movement / condition of
   condition of slow movement
10. poly-   / myos/o / -itis
    many, much / muscle / inflammation
    inflammation of many muscles

Exercise 17
1. computed tomography
2. electromyogram

3. arthrography
4. nuclear medicine imaging
5. radiography
6. creatine kinase
7. uric acid
8. rheumatoid factor

Exercise 18
1. bone densitometry
2. range of motion testing
3. bone scan
4. arthroscopy
5. magnetic resonance imaging
6. erythrocyte sedimentation rate
7. synovial fluid analysis

Exercise 19
1. synovectomy
2. reduction
3. myorrhaphy
4. chondrectomy
5. arthroclasia
6. diskectomy
7. traction
8. cranioplasty
9. spondylosyndesis
10. osteoclasis
11. patellectomy
12. osteoclast
13. chondroplasty
14. meniscectomy
15. maxillotomy
16. arthroplasty

Exercise 20
1. ostectomy
2. bursectomy
3. craniotomy
4. myoplasty
5. orthosis
6. open reduction, internal
   fixation
7. laminectomy
8. tenorrhaphy
9. arthrocentesis
10. prosthesis

Exercise 21
1. myoplasty
2. chondrectomy
3. arthrodesis
4. tenorrhaphy
5. craniotomy

Exercise 22
1. oste/o / -clasis
   bone / to break
   intentional fracture of bone
   (to correct deformity)
2. my/o   / -rrhaphy
   muscle / suture
   suture of a muscle
3. arthr/o / -plasty
   joint   / surgical repair,
   reconstruction
   surgical repair of a joint
4. phalang/o / -ectomy
   phalanges / excision, surgical
   removal
   excision of a phalanges
5. rachi/o / -tomy
   spine   / incision
   incision into the spine

6. disk/o / -ectomy
vertebral disk / excision, surgical
removal
excision of (part or all) of a vertebral disk

7. chondr/o / -plasty
cartilage / surgical repair,
reconstruction
surgical repair of cartilage

8. arthr/o / -centesis
joint / puncture to aspirate
puncture to aspirate (fluid) from a joint

9. synov(i)/o / -ectomy
synovial joint / excision, surgical
or fluid removal
excision of (part or all of) a synovial
membrane

10. oste/o / -ectomy
bone / excision, surgical removal
excision of bone

Exercise 23
1. skeletal muscle relaxant
2. analgesic
3. corticosteroid
4. NSAID

Exercise 24
1. chiropractor
2. podiatrist
3. orthotist
4. osteopath
5. rheumatologist
6. orthopedist

Exercise 25
1. magnetic resonance imaging
2. myasthenia gravis
3. 2nd cervical vertebra
4. Muscular dystrophy
5. range of motion
6. open reduction, internal fixation
7. electromyogram
8. carpal tunnel syndrome
9. rheumatoid arthritis
10. nonsteroidal anti-inflammatory drug
11. deep tendon reflex
12. erythrocyte sedimentation rate,
rheumatoid factor, creatine kinase

Exercise 26
1. T4
2. fx
3. CT
4. L3
5. MRI
6. OA

Exercise 27
1. vertebrae
2. carpal bones
3. phalanges
4. tarsal bones
5. cranium
6. mandible
7. clavicle
8. acromion
9. scapula
10. ribs
11. sternum
12. femur
13. patella

Exercise 28
1. tendon(s)

2. biceps brachii
3. origins
4. insertion
5. humer/o
6. ten/o, tend/o, tendin/o

Exercise 29
1. ankyl/o / -osis
stiff / abnormal condition
abnormal condition of stiffening
(of a joint)

2. carp/o / -ptosis
carpal bones / dropping
dropping of the carpal bones

3. electr/o / my/o / -gram
electricity / muscle / record, recording
recording of a muscle's electrical
activity

4. myos/o / -itis
muscle / inflammation
inflammation of muscle

5. kyph/o / -osis
humpback / abnormal condition
abnormal condition of humpback

6. intra- / crani/o / -al
within / skull / pertaining to
pertaining to within the skull

7. poly- / my/o / -itis
many, much / muscle / inflammation
inflammation of many muscles

8. supra- / patell/o / -ar
above / patella / pertaining to
pertaining to above the patella

9. ten/o / -dynia
tendon / pain
pain in a tendon

10. arthr/o / -centesis
joint / puncture to aspirate
puncture to aspirate (fluid) from
a joint

11. chondr/o / -ectomy
cartilage / excision, surgical removal
excision of cartilage

12. cost/o / vertebr/o / -al
rib / vertebra / pertaining to
pertaining to the ribs and vertebrae

13. sub- / mandibul/o / -ar
below, / mandible / pertaining to
beneath
pertaining to below the mandible

14. oste/o / arthr/o / -itis
bone / joint / inflammation
inflammation of bone and joint

15. my/o / -rrhaphy
muscle / suture
suture of a muscle

16. oste/o / -malacia
bone / softening
softening of bones

17. arthr/o / -scopy
joint / process of examining,
examination
process of examining (the interior of) a
joint

18. my/o / -algia
muscle / pain
muscle pain

19. spondyl/o / arthr/o / -itis
vertebra / joint / inflammation
inflammation of a vertebral joint

Exercise 30
1. adduction
2. orthotics
3. arthroplasty
4. podiatrist or chiropodist
5. prosthesis
6. carpal tunnel syndrome
7. compact
8. dystrophy
9. fibromyalgia
10. extension
11. bone scan
12. dystrophy
13. rheumatoid arthritis
14. range of motion (ROM)
15. hyperkinesia
16. chiropractic
17. dorsiflexion
18. orthopedics

Exercise 31
1. an immovable joint, such as joins skull
bones
2. bones
3. the hand
4. composed of bone (or bony)
tissue
5. Osteopathy is school of medicine
emphasizing manipulative
measures in addition to techniques of
conventional medicine
6. when a tendon is partly or completely
separated (torn)
7. vitamin D
8. Arthrodesis surgically stiffens the joint
9. crystals
10. x-ray image of a joint using a contrast
agent (arthrogram)
11. the end of the muscle attached to bone
that moves with contraction
12. the lower section of the sternum
13. cardiac muscle
14. chiropodist

Exercise 32
1. C
2. D
3. A
4. D
5. A
6. D
7. B
8. A
9. B
10. D
11. A
12. A
13. C
14. A

Exercise 33
1. A
2. D
3. B
4. C
5. B
6. C
7. D
8. A
9. D
10. B
11. A

Exercise 34
1. paraspinal
2. sacral
3. myofascial
4. range of motion
5. the knees – "bilateral total knee replacement"

Exercise 35
1. arthralgia
2. myalgia
3. arthritis
4. range of motion
5. rheumatoid arthritis
6. inflammation in many joints

Exercise 36
1. B
2. C
3. D
4. A
5. A
6. bursal

Exercise 37
Practice until your pronunciation matches that heard in the Audio Glossary in the Student Resources.

Exercise 38
1. laminotomy
2. osteoarthritis
3. rheumatology
4. tenodynia
5. osseous
6. clavicle
7. myorrhaphy
8. vertebrae
9. fibromyalgia
10. dorsiflexion
11. ankylosis
12. polymyositis
13. fascia
14. osteoporosis
15. intervertebral
16. dyskinesia
17. cranioschisis
18. kyphosis
19. acetabulum
20. bursolith

Chapter 15

Exercise 1
1. pituitary gland
2. adrenal glands, suprarenal glands
3. islets of Langerhans
4. thyroid gland
5. parathyroid glands
6. pineal gland, pineal body
7. hypothalamus
8. thymus gland
9. ovaries

Exercise 2
1. growth hormone
2. thyroxine
3. follicle-stimulating hormone
4. parathyroid hormone
5. prolactin
6. oxytocin
7. aldosterone
8. melatonin
9. insulin

Exercise 3
1. parathyroid hormone (PTH)
2. Thymosin
3. adrenocorticotrophic
4. luteinizing hormone
5. thyroid-stimulating hormone
6. Thyroxine, triiodothyronine
7. antidiuretic hormone
8. testes
9. ovaries
10. cortisol

Exercise 4
1. glucose, sugar
2. cortex
3. thyroid gland
4. potassium
5. to secrete
6. thirst
7. glucose, sugar
8. sodium

Exercise 5
1. excision or surgical removal of an adrenal gland
2. deficiency of calcium
3. pertaining to a hormone
4. enlargement of the extremities
5. incision into the thyroid gland
6. inflammation of the thymus gland
7. excision or surgical removal of a parathyroid gland
8. one who specializes in the endocrine system

Exercise 6
1. condition of a deficient thyroid gland below, deficient thyroid gland condition of
2. pertaining to the pancreas pancreas pertaining to
3. resembling a normal thyroid gland good, normal thyroid gland resembling
4. glucose or sugar in the urine glucose, sugar urine, urination
5. condition of excessive glucose in the blood above, excessive glucose, sugar blood (condition of)
6. disease of an adrenal gland adrenal gland disease
7. condition of much thirst many, much thirst condition of
8. abnormal condition of a gland gland abnormal condition

Exercise 7
1. cortical
2. exogenous
3. pancreatic
4. thymic
5. endogenous

Exercise 8
1. euthyroid
2. pancreatic
3. metabolism
4. thymic
5. exogenous

Exercise 9
1. thym/o   thymus gland
2. cortic/o   cortex
3. adren/o   adrenal glands
4. thyroid/o   thyroid gland
5. pancreat/o   pancreas
6. hormon/o   hormone

Exercise 10
1. polydipsia
2. Hashimoto thyroiditis, Hashimoto disease
3. exophthalmos
4. acidosis
5. thyrotoxicosis
6. hirsutism
7. ketosis
8. Type 1 diabetes mellitus
9. myxedema
10. polyuria
11. adenomegaly
12. hyperthyroidism
13. Type 2 diabetes mellitus

Exercise 11
1. gigantism
2. Addison disease
3. congenital hypothyroidism
4. acromegaly
5. hypothyroidism
6. Graves disease
7. diabetes insipidus
8. Diabetic ketoacidosis
9. Cushing syndrome
10. adrenalitis
11. Goiter
12. tetany

Exercise 12
1. hyponatremia
2. hyperkalemia
3. hypercalcemia
4. polyuria
5. glycosuria
6. hyperglycemia
7. calcipenia
8. polydipsia
9. hypocalcemia

Exercise 13
1. glucosuria, glycosuria
2. endocrinopathy
3. adenalgia
4. adrenomegaly
5. thyroiditis
6. adenitis
7. pancreatitis
8. calcipenia
9. adrenopathy
10. thyromegaly

Exercise 14
1. above,   / parathyroid / condition of excessive   glands
2. below,   / parathyroid / condition of deficient   glands

3. above,   / calcium / blood
   excessive   (condition of)
4. below,   / calcium / blood
   deficient   (condition of)
5. above,   / glucose, / blood
   excessive   sugar   (condition of)
6. below,   / glucose, / blood
   deficient   sugar   (condition of)
7. above,   / sodium / blood
   excessive   (condition of)
8. below,   / sodium / blood
   deficient   (condition of)
9. above,   / potassium / blood
   excessive   (condition of)
10. below,   / potassium / blood
    deficient   (condition of)

Exercise 15
1. glucometer
2. thyroid function tests
3. glucose tolerance test (GTT)
4. radioactive iodine uptake test
5. thyroid scan
6. thyroid-stimulating hormone level

Exercise 16
1. thyroxine level
2. glucose tolerance test
3. blood glucose
4. fasting blood glucose
5. electrolyte panel
6. glycosylated hemoglobin

Exercise 17
1. excision of the thyroid gland
2. excision of an adrenal gland
3. excision of the thymus gland
4. excision of the thyroid and parathyroid glands

Exercise 18
1. thyroid
2. adrenalectomy
3. incision
4. thyroid

Exercise 19
1. pancreat/o   pancreas
2. thyroid/o   thyroid gland
3. aden/o   gland
4. parathyroid/o   parathyroid gland
5. thym/o   thymus gland

Exercise 20
1. insulin therapy
2. antithyroid
3. hormone replacement therapy
4. antidiabetic
5. continuous subcutaneous insulin infusion, insulin pump

Exercise 21
1. endocrinology
2. endocrinologist

Exercise 22
1. diabetes insipidus
2. thyroid-stimulating hormone
3. fasting blood glucose
4. antidiuretic hormone
5. parathyroid hormone
6. glucose tolerance test
7. radioactive iodine uptake
8. triiodothyronine

Exercise 23
1. ACTH
2. DM
3. FSH
4. T_4
5. DKA
6. CSII
7. DI
8. GH
9. LH

Exercise 24
1. pituitary gland
2. thyroid
3. adrenal gland
4. testis
5. pineal gland
6. parathyroid gland
7. thymus gland
8. pancreas
9. ovary

Exercise 25
1. pancreat/o / -ic
   pancreas   / pertaining to
   pertaining to the pancreas
2. adrenal /o   / -itis
   adrenal gland / inflammation
   inflammation of an adrenal gland
3. glucos/o   / -uria
   glucose, sugar / urine, urination
   glucose in the urine
4. acr/o   / -megaly
   extremity, tip / enlargement
   enlargement of the extremities
5. cortic/o / -al
   cortex   / pertaining to
   pertaining to the cortex
6. calc/i   / -penia
   calcium / deficiency
   deficiency of calcium
7. thyroid/o   / -tomy
   thyroid gland / incision
   incision into the thyroid gland

Exercise 26
1. thym/o   thymus gland
2. thyr/o   thyroid gland
3. kal/i   potassium
4. adrenal/o   adrenal gland
5. natr/i   sodium
6. endocrin/o *or* crin/o   endocrine *or* to secrete
7. aden/o   gland
8. dips/o   thirst

Exercise 27
1. hyperthyroidism
2. glucose tolerance test
3. adrenalectomy
4. antidiuretic hormone
5. Islets of Langerhans
6. polyuria
7. euthyroid
8. congenital hypothyroidism
9. diabetes insipidus
10. endocrinologist

Exercise 28
1. A
2. D
3. B
4. D
5. A
6. B
7. B
8. B
9. C
10. B

Exercise 29
1. C
2. B
3. B
4. A
5. C
6. B
7. D
8. B

Exercise 30
1. endogenous
2. polyuria
3. blood glucose
4. pancreatitis
5. glycosuria

Exercise 31
1. C
2. B
3. A
4. C
5. B

Exercise 32
1. hyperthyroidism
2. thyromegaly or goiter
3. exophthalmos
4. thyroid scan
5. thyroidectomy
6. hemostasis
7. lying face up

Exercise 33
Practice until your pronunciation matches that heard in the Audio Glossary in the Student Resources.

Exercise 34
1. pituitary
2. pancreas
3. CORRECT
4. CORRECT
5. euthyroid
6. diabetes
7. exophthalmos
8. hirsutism
9. CORRECT
10. CORRECT
11. myxedema
12. CORRECT
13. CORRECT
14. glycosylated
15. CORRECT

Chapter 16

Exercise 1
1. disease
2. cancer
3. tumor
4. cancer
5. cold
6. black, dark
7. white

8. flesh
9. x-rays, radiation
10. abdomen

Exercise 2
1. cyt/o
2. kary/o
3. chem/o
4. lei/o
5. rhabd/o
6. squam/o
7. plas/o
8. bi/o
9. ablat/o
10. sarc/o

Exercise 3
1. change, beyond
2. process of examining, examination
3. tumor
4. origin, production
5. within
6. bad, poor
7. process of viewing
8. new
9. painful, difficult, abnormal
10. originating, producing
11. beside
12. across, through

Exercise 4
1. tumor of the bone
2. tumor of cartilage
3. tumor of smooth muscle
4. cancerous tumor
5. condition of white blood cells (type of cancer)
6. process of viewing life
7. tumor of the muscle
8. pertaining to a duct

Exercise 5
1. cytology
2. squamous
3. leiomyoma
4. sarcoma
5. adenoma
6. lymphoma
7. myeloma
8. nephroma
9. angioma
10. neuroma

Exercise 6
1. benign
2. malignant
3. myelomas
4. melanoma
5. glandular tissue
6. oncogenic
7. recurrence
8. neuroma
9. malignant
10. lipoma
11. malignant neoplasm

Exercise 7
1. carcinoma
2. benign
3. lesion
4. dysplasia
5. tumor
6. cancer
7. in situ

8. invasion
9. metastasis

Exercise 8
1. adenoma
2. fibroma
3. biopsy
4. lipoma
5. sarcoma
6. myeloma
7. cancerous
8. fibrosarcoma

Exercise 9
1. lymphoma
2. bronchogenic carcinoma
3. leiomyoma
4. chondroma
5. osteosarcoma
6. liposarcoma
7. lymphangioma
8. Wilms tumor
9. melanoma
10. glioma
11. osteofibroma
12. giant cell tumor
13. rhabdomyoma
14. mesothelioma
15. glomus tumor

Exercise 10
1. Leukemia
2. GIST
3. Wilms
4. Hodgkin
5. pheochromocytoma
6. bone
7. chondrosarcoma
8. giant cell tumor
9. retinoblastoma
10. meningioma

Exercise 11
1. medulloblastoma
2. stromal cell tumor
3. oat cell carcinoma
4. squamous cell carcinoma
5. basal cell carcinoma
6. neuroblastoma
7. Kaposi sarcoma

Exercise 12
1. nephroma
2. lymphoma
3. leukemia
4. glioma
5. adenoma
6. leiomyoma
7. leiomyosarcoma
8. astrocytoma
9. carcinoma
10. rhabdomyosarcoma

Exercise 13
1. radionuclide scan
2. Endoscopic retrograde cholangiopancreatography
3. cholescintigraphy
4. fine needle aspiration
5. lumbar puncture
6. Pap test
7. tumor markers
8. thoracoscopy

9. single photon emission computed tomography scan
10. hCG

Exercise 14
1. sentinel lymph node biopsy
2. alpha-fetoprotein (AFP)
3. prostate-specific antigen (PSA)
4. estrogen receptors
5. shave biopsy
6. punch biopsy
7. endoscopic ultrasound
8. mammography
9. transrectal ultrasound
10. colposcopy

Exercise 15
1. colposcopy
2. biopsy
3. thoracoscopy
4. mammography

Exercise 16
1. radiofrequency ablation
2. radiation therapy
3. mastectomy
4. bone marrow transplant (BMT)
5. loop electrosurgical excision procedure (LEEP)
6. amputation
7. fulguration
8. Mohs surgery
9. debulking surgery
10. peripheral stem cell transplant

Exercise 17
1. TURB
2. palliative
3. colectomy
4. Whipple
5. limb salvage surgery
6. transsphenoidal resection
7. wedge resection
8. radical
9. stereotactic radiosurgery
10. brachytherapy

Exercise 18
1. esophagectomy
2. thyroidectomy
3. gastrectomy
4. mastectomy
5. nephrectomy
6. lymphadenectomy
7. myomectomy
8. lobectomy

Exercise 19
1. pneumon/o / -ectomy
   lung   / excision, surgical removal
   excision of the lung
2. col/o / -ectomy
   colon / excision, surgical removal
   excision of (all or part of) the colon
3. cyst/o   / -ectomy
   bladder / excision, surgical removal
   excision of the bladder
4. thyroid/o   / -ectomy
   thyroid gland / excision, surgical removal
   excision of the thyroid gland
5. laryng/o / -ectomy, surgical removal
   larynx   / excision
   excision of (all or part of) the larynx

6. irid/o / -ectomy, surgical removal
   iris / excision
   excision of (part of) the iris
7. crani/o / -ectomy, surgical removal
   skull, / excision
   cranium
   excision of (part of) the cranium
8. gastr/o / -ectomy
   stomach / excision, surgical removal
   excision of (all or part of) the stomach

Exercise 20
1. adjuvant chemotherapy
2. hormonal therapy
3. intrathecal chemotherapy
4. aromatase inhibitors
5. immunotherapy, biologic therapy
6. palliative chemotherapy
7. chemotherapy
8. chemoprevention
9. epidermal growth factor receptor
   (EGFR) inhibitor therapy
10. interstitial chemotherapy

Exercise 21
1. gynecologic oncology
2. radiation oncology
3. surgical oncology
4. pediatric oncology
5. gynecologic oncologist
6. medical oncologist
7. medical oncology
8. pediatric oncologist
9. radiation oncologist
10. surgical oncologist

Exercise 22
1. gastrointestinal stromal tumor
2. ductal carcinoma in situ
3. transurethral resection of prostate
4. hepatobiliary iminodiacetic acid
5. bone marrow transplant
6. radiofrequency ablation
7. transrectal ultrasound
8. epidermal growth factor
   receptors
9. magnetic resonance
   cholangiopancreatography
10. endoscopic ultrasound
11. single photon emission computed
    tomography
12. alpha fetoprotein

Exercise 23
1. LP
2. FNA
3. CA
4. TURB
5. ERCP
6. LEEP
7. PSA
8. BCC
9. hCG
10. MEN
11. NHL
12. SCC

Exercise 24
1. rhabd/o / my/o / sarc/o / -oma
   striated / muscle / connective / tumor
                           tissue
   (malignant) tumor of connective tissue
   of striated muscle

2. my/o / -oma
   muscle / tumor
   (benign) tumor of muscle
3. nephr/o / -oma
   kidney / tumor
   tumor of the kidney
4. bronch/o / -scopy
   bronchus / process of examining,
              examination
   process of examining the bronchus
5. meningi/o / -oma
   meninges / tumor
   (benign) tumor of the meninges
6. endo- / -scopy
   in, within / process of examining,
               examination
   process of examining within
7. oste/o / sarc/o / -oma
   bone / connective tissue / tumor
   (malignant) connective tissue tumor of
   bone
8. neur/o / -oma
   nerve / tumor
   tumor of a nerve
9. irid/o / -ectomy
   iris / excision, surgical removal
   excision or surgical removal of the iris
10. lapar/o / -scopy
    abdomen / process of examining,
              examination
    process of examining the abdomen

Exercise 25
1. colorectal
2. cryotherapy
3. cystoscopy
4. benign
5. melanoma
6. Whipple procedure
7. fulguration
8. shave biopsy
9. mammogram
10. osteosarcoma

Exercise 26
1. A simple mastectomy is the removal of
   a breast in which the underlying
   muscles and the lymph nodes are left
   intact. A radical mastectomy is the
   removal of the breast as well as the
   underlying muscles and lymph nodes in
   the adjacent armpit.
2. Hodgkin lymphoma is indicated by the
   presence of Reed-Sternberg cells.
   Non-Hodgkin lymphomas are
   lymphomas other than the Hodgkin
   type.
3. debulking
4. to relieve pain and other symptoms but
   not to cure cancer
5. astrocytoma
6. A chondroma is benign and a
   chondrosarcoma is malignant.
7. Oncogenes are mutated forms of genes
   that cause normal cells to grow out of
   control and become cancer cells.
8. A beam of high-energy radiation is
   applied externally directly to the
   tumor while minimizing damage to
   other tissues.

9. They reduce estrogen levels in a
   woman's body and stop the growth of
   cancer cells that depend on estrogen to
   live and grow.
10. malignant

Exercise 27
1. C
2. B
3. D
4. C
5. C
6. A
7. B
8. B
9. A
10. C

Exercise 28
1. B
2. C
3. A
4. D
5. C
6. B
7. C
8. B
9. A
10. D

Exercise 29
1. stenosis
2. ulceration
3. rhinoscopy
4. carcinoma
5. rhinectomy

Exercise 30
1. B
2. B
3. B
4. C
5. C
6. B
7. Ductal carcinoma in situ (DCIS) is
   breast cancer that is confined to the
   ducts and has not spread into the
   tissue of the breast. This patient's
   cancer has become invasive so has
   obviously spread into the tissues of the
   breast.

Exercise 31
*Practice until your pronunciation matches
that heard in the Audio Glossary in the
Student Resources.*

Exercise 32
1. craniectomy
2. fulguration
3. rhabdomyoma
4. thyroidectomy
5. chondrosarcoma
6. cryosurgery
7. glioma
8. leiomyosarcoma
9. mammography
10. pheochromocytoma
11. brachytherapy
12. cholescintigraphy
13. lipoma
14. nephrectomy
15. palliative

■ FIGURE CREDITS

Figure 2-3. Copyright © Jochen Sand/Digital Vision/GettyImages.

Figure 3-1. Nath JL. *Using Medical Terminology: A Practical Approach.* Baltimore: Lippincott Williams & Wilkins, 2005.

Figure 3-2. Modified from Nath JL. *Using Medical Terminology: A Practical Approach.* Baltimore: Lippincott Williams & Wilkins, 2005.

Figure 3-3. Anatomical Chart Company.

Figure 3-4. Nath JL. *Using Medical Terminology: A Practical Approach.* Baltimore: Lippincott Williams & Wilkins, 2005.

Figure 3-5. Nath JL. *Using Medical Terminology: A Practical Approach.* Baltimore: Lippincott Williams & Wilkins, 2005.

Figure 3-6. Nath JL. *Using Medical Terminology: A Practical Approach.* Baltimore: Lippincott Williams & Wilkins, 2005.

Figure 3-7. Anatomical Chart Company.
Figure Labeling 1. Modified from Nath JL. *Using Medical Terminology: A Practical Approach.* Baltimore: Lippincott Williams & Wilkins, 2005.
Figure Labeling 2. Anatomical Chart Company.
Photo of nurse practitioner with patient. Copyright © Martin Barraud/ OJO Images/GettyImages

Figure 4-1. Anatomical Chart Company.

Figure 4-2. Image provided by Stedman's (Dr. Barankin Collection).

Figure 4-3. Ills: Anatomical Chart Company. Photos: From Riordan CL, McDonough M, Davidson JM, et al. Noncontact laser Doppler imaging in burn depth analysis of the extremities. *J Burn Care Rehabil.* 2003,24: 177-86.

Figure 4-4. Fleisher GR, Ludwig W, Baskin MN. Atlas of Pediatric Emergency Medicine. Philadelphia: Lippincott Williams & Wilkins, 2003:fig 11-37.

Figure 4-5. From Weber J RN, EdD and Kelley J RN, PhD. Health Assessment in Nursing, 2nd edition. Philadelphia: Lippincott Williams & Wilkins, 2003.

Figure 4-6. Bickley LS. Bates' Guide to Physical Examination and History Taking, 8th ed. Philadelphia: Lippincott Williams & Wilkins, 2003.

Figure 4-7. From Goodheart HP, MD. Goodheart's Photoguide of Common Skin Disorders, 2nd Edition. Philadelphia: Lippincott Williams & Wilkins, 2003.

Figure 4-8. From Weber J RN, EdD and Kelley J RN, PhD. Health Assessment in Nursing, 2nd edition. Philadelphia: Lippincott Williams & Wilkins, 2003.

Figure 4-9. From Smeltzer SC, Bare BG. Textbook of Medical-Surgical Nursing, 9th Ed. Philadelphia: Lippincott Williams & Wilkins, 2000.

Figure 4-10. Fleisher GR, Ludwig S, Henretig FM. Textbook of Pediatric Emergency Medicine, 5th ed. Philadelphia: Lippincott Williams & Wilkins, 2005.

Figure 4-11. From Tasman W, Jaeger E. The Wills Eye Hospital Atlas of Clinical Ophthalmology, 2e. Lippincott Williams & Wilkins, 2001.

Figure 4-12. From Goodheart HP, MD. Goodheart's Photoguide of Common Skin Disorders, 2nd Edition. Philadelphia: Lippincott Williams & Wilkins, 2003.

Figure 4-13. From Willis MC. Medical Terminology A Programmed Learning Approach to the Language of Health Care, 2nd ed. Baltimore: Lippincott Williams & Wilkins, 2007.

Figure 4-14. Bickley LS. Bates' Guide to Physical Examination and History Taking, 8th ed. Philadelphia: Lippincott Williams & Wilkins, 2003.

Figure 4-15. Hall JC. Sauer's Manual of Skin Diseases, 9th Edition. Philadelphia: Lippincott Williams & Wilkins, 2006.

Figure 4-16. Ill: Anatomical Chart Company. Photo: Image provided by Stedman's (Dr. Barankin Collection).

Figure 4-17. Berg D, Worzala K. Atlas of Adult Physical Diagnosis. Philadelphia: Lippincott Williams & Wilkins, 2006.

Figure 4-18. From Neville B et al: Color Atlas of Clinical Oral Pathology. Philadelphia: Lea & Febiger, 1991. Used with permission.

Figure 4-19. Image provided by Stedman's (Dr. Barankin Collection).

Figure 4-20. Berg D, Worzala K. Atlas of Adult Physical Diagnosis. Philadelphia: Lippincott Williams & Wilkins, 2006.

Figure 4-21. From Goodheart HP, MD. Goodheart's Photoguide of Common Skin Disorders, 2nd Edition. Philadelphia: Lippincott Williams & Wilkins, 2003.

Figure 4-23. F. Malzieu / Photo Researchers, Inc.

Figure 4-25. Image provided by Stedman's (Dr. Barankin Collection)

Figure 4-26. From Goodheart HP, MD. Goodheart's Photoguide of Common Skin Disorders, 2nd Edition. Philadelphia: Lippincott Williams & Wilkins, 2003.
Figure Labeling 1. Anatomical Chart Company.
Photo of pharmacist. Copyright © sozaijiten/Datacraft/GettyImages

Figure 5-1. Nath JL. Using Medical Terminology: A Practical Approach. Baltimore: Lippincott Williams & Wilkins, 2005.

Figure 5-2. Nath JL. Using Medical Terminology: A Practical Approach. Baltimore: Lippincott Williams & Wilkins, 2005.

Figure 5-3. Nath JL. Using Medical Terminology: A Practical Approach. Baltimore: Lippincott Williams & Wilkins, 2005.

Figure 5-4. Modified from Anatomical Chart Company.

Figure 5-5. Anatomical Chart Company.

Figure 5-6. Willis MC. Medical Terminology A Programmed Learning Approach to the Language of Health Care, 2nd ed. Baltimore: Lippincott Williams & Wilkins, 2007.

Figure 5-7. Rubin R, Strayer DS, Rubin E. Rubin's Pathology: Clinicopathologic Foundations of Medicine, 5th Edition. Baltimore: Lippincott Williams & Wilkins, 2008.

Figure 5-8. Willis MC. Medical Terminology A Programmed Learning Approach to the Language of Health Care, 2nd ed. Baltimore: Lippincott Williams & Wilkins, 2007.

Figure 5-9. Willis MC. Medical Terminology A Programmed Learning Approach to the Language of Health Care, 2nd ed. Baltimore: Lippincott Williams & Wilkins, 2007.

Figure 5-10. Modified from LifeART image copyright © 2011 Lippincott Williams & Wilkins. All rights reserved.

Figure 5-11. Michael W. Mulholland, Ronald V. Maier etal. Greenfield's Surgery Scientific Principles And Practice, Fourth Edition. Philadelphia: Lippincott Williams & Wilkins, 2006.

Figure 5-12. From Cohen BJ. Medical Terminology, 5th Edition. Philadelphia. Lippincott Williams & Wilkins 2007.

Figure 5-13. MIXA/Punchstock

Figure 5-14. Snell RS. Clinical Anatomy By Regions, Eighth Edition. Philadelphia: Lippincott Williams & Wilkins, 2008.

Figure 5-15. From Cohen BJ. Medical Terminology, 5th Edition. Philadelphia. Lippincott Williams & Wilkins 2007.

Figure 5-16a. Kronenberger J, Durham LS, Woodson D. Lippincott Williams & Wilkins' Comprehensive Medical Assisting, 3rd Edition. Baltimore: Lippincott Williams & Wilkins, 1008.

Figure 5-16b. Smeltzer SC, Bare BG, Hinkle J, Cheever KH. Brunner and Suddarth's Textbook of Medical Surgical Nursing, 12th Edition. Philadelphia: Lippincott Williams & Wilkins, 2009.

Figure 5-18. Smeltzer SC, Bare BG, Hinkle J, Cheever KH. Brunner and Suddarth's Textbook of Medical Surgical Nursing, 12th Edition. Philadelphia: Lippincott Williams & Wilkins, 2009.

Figure 5-19. Smeltzer SC, Bare BG, Hinkle J, Cheever KH. Brunner and Suddarth's Textbook of Medical Surgical Nursing, 12th Edition. Philadelphia: Lippincott Williams & Wilkins, 2009.

Figure 5-20. Willis MC. Medical Terminology A Programmed Learning Approach to the Language of Health Care, 2nd ed. Baltimore: Lippincott Williams & Wilkins, 2007.
Figure Labeling 1. Nath JL. Using Medical Terminology: A Practical Approach. Baltimore: Lippincott Williams & Wilkins, 2005.
Figure Labeling 2. Nath JL. Using Medical Terminology: A Practical Approach. Baltimore: Lippincott Williams & Wilkins, 2005.

Figure 6-1. Anatomical Chart Company and Nath JL. Using Medical Terminology: A Practical Approach. Baltimore: Lippincott Williams & Wilkins, 2005.

Figure 6-2. A. From Premkumar K. The Massage Connection Anatomy and Physiology. Baltimore: Lippincott Williams & Wilkins 2004. **B.** Anatomical Chart Company.

Figure 6-3. Anatomical Chart Company.

Figure 6-4. Nath JL. Using Medical Terminology: A Practical Approach. Baltimore: Lippincott Williams & Wilkins, 2005.

Figure 6-5. Anatomical Chart Company.

Figure 6-6. McConnell TH. The Nature Of Disease Pathology for the Health Professions, Philadelphia: Lippincott Williams & Wilkins, 2007.

Figure 6-8. Mulholland MW, Maier RV, et al. Greenfield's Surgery Scientific Principles And Practice, Fourth Edition. Philadelphia: Lippincott Williams & Wilkins, 2006.

Figure 6-10. From Snell, MD, PhD, Clinical Anatomy, 7th ed. Lippincott, Williams & Wilkins, 2003.

Figure 6-11. From Harwood-Nuss A, MD FACEP, Wolfson AB, MD, FACEP, FACP, et al. The Clinical Practice of Emergency Medicine, 3rd Edition. Philadelphia: Lippincott Williams & Wilkins, 2001.

Figure 6-13. Nath JL. Using Medical Terminology: A Practical Approach. Baltimore: Lippincott Williams & Wilkins, 2005.

Figure 6-14. From Premkumar K. The Massage Connection Anatomy and Physiology. Baltimore: Lippincott Williams & Wilkins 2004.

Figure 6-16. McClatchey KD M.D., D.D.S. Clinical Laboratory Medicine, 2nd Edition. Philadelphia: Lippincott Williams & Wilkins, 2002.
Urine dipstick. Saturn Stills / Photo Researchers, Inc.
Figure Labeling 1. Anatomical Chart Company and Nath JL. Using Medical Terminology: A Practical Approach. Baltimore: Lippincott Williams & Wilkins, 2005.
Figure Labeling 2. From Premkumar K. The Massage Connection Anatomy and Physiology. Baltimore: Lippincott Williams & Wilkins 2004.

Figure 7-2. McArdle WD, Katch KI, Katch VL. Exercise Physiology, 7th Edition. Baltimore: Lippincott Williams & Wilkins, 2009.

Figure 7-3. From Premkumar K. The Massage Connection Anatomy and Physiology. Baltimore: Lippincott Williams & Wilkins 2004.

Figure 7-4. Anatomical Chart Company.

Figure 7-5. McArdle WD, Katch KI, Katch VL. Exercise Physiology, 7th Edition. Baltimore: Lippincott Williams & Wilkins, 2009.

Figure 7-6. Anatomical Chart Company.

Figure 7-7. From Premkumar K. The Massage Connection Anatomy and Physiology. Baltimore: Lippincott Williams & Wilkins 2004.

Figure 7-8. Nath JL. Using Medical Terminology: A Practical Approach. Baltimore: Lippincott Williams & Wilkins, 2005.

Figure 7-9. Brant WE, Helms CA. Fundamentals of Diagnostic Radiology, 3rd Edition. Philadelphia: Lippincott Williams & Wilkins, 2007.

Figure 7-10. Anatomical Chart Company.

Figure 7-11. Anatomical Chart Company.

Figure 7-12. Anatomical Chart Company.

Figure 7-13. Image from Rubin E MD and Farber JL MD. Pathology, 3rd Edition. Philadelphia: Lippincott Williams & Wilkins, 1999.

Figure 7-14. From Willis MC. Medical Terminology A Programmed Learning Approach to the Language of Health Care, 2nd ed. Baltimore: Lippincott, Williams & Wilkins, 2007.

Figure 7-15. Bickley LS. Bates' Guide to Physical Examination and History Taking, 8th ed. Philadelphia: Lippincott Williams & Wilkins, 2003.

Figure 7-16. Sherwood L. Gorbach, John G. Bartlett, etal. Infectious Diseases. Philadelphia: Lippincott Williams & Wilkins, 2004.

Figure 7-17. From Cohen BJ. Medical Terminology, 5th Edition. Philadelphia. Lippincott Williams & Wilkins 2007.

Figure 7-19. From Willis MC. Medical Terminology A Programmed Learning Approach to the Language of Health Care, 2nd ed. Baltimore: Lippincott Williams & Wilkins, 2007.

Figure 7-20. Copyright © Comstock Images/GettyImages

Figure 7-21. Smeltzer SC, Bare BG, Hinkle J, Cheever KH. Brunner and Suddarth's Textbook of Medical Surgical Nursing, 12th Edition. Philadelphia: Lippincott Williams & Wilkins, 2009.

Figure 7-22. Smeltzer SC, Bare BG, Hinkle J, Cheever KH. Brunner and Suddarth's Textbook of Medical Surgical Nursing, 12th Edition. Philadelphia: Lippincott Williams & Wilkins, 2009.

Figure 7-23. LifeART image copyright © 2011 Lippincott Williams & Wilkins. All rights reserved.

Figure 7-24. LifeART image copyright © 2011 Lippincott Williams & Wilkins. All rights reserved.

Figure 7-26. Anatomical Chart Company.
Figure Labeling 1. McArdle WD, Katch KI, Katch VL. Exercise Physiology, 7th Edition. Baltimore: Lippincott Williams & Wilkins, 2009.
Figure Labeling 2. From Premkumar K. The Massage Connection Anatomy and Physiology. Baltimore: Lippincott Williams & Wilkins 2004.
Photo of Massage Therapist. Braun MB, Simonson SJ. Introduction to Massage Therapy, 2nd Edition. Baltimore: Lippincott Williams & Wilkins, 2007.

Figure 8-1. From Cohen BJ. Medical Terminology, 5th Edition. Philadelphia. Lippincott Williams & Wilkins 2007.

Figure 8-2. From Willis MC. Medical Terminology A Programmed Learning to the Language of Health Care, 2nd ed. Baltimore: Lippincott Williams & Wilkins, 2007.

Figure 8-3. From Cohen BJ. Medical Terminology, 5th Edition. Philadelphia. Lippincott Williams & Wilkins 2007.

Figure 8-4. From Cohen BJ. Medical Terminology, 5th Edition. Philadelphia. Lippincott Williams & Wilkins 2007.

Figure 8-5. From Cohen BJ. Medical Terminology, 5th Edition. Philadelphia. Lippincott Williams & Wilkins 2007.

Figure 8-6. From Cohen BJ. Medical Terminology, 5th Edition. Philadelphia. Lippincott Williams & Wilkins 2007.

Figure 8-7. From Cohen BJ. Medical Terminology, 5th Edition. Philadelphia. Lippincott Williams & Wilkins 2007.

Figure 8-8. From Cohen BJ. Memmler's The Human Body in Health and Disease, 11th Edition. Baltimore: Lippincott Williams & Wilkins, 2008.

Figure 8-9. From Willis MC. Medical Terminology A Programmed Learning to the Language of Health Care, 2nd ed. Baltimore: Lippincott Williams & Wilkins, 2007.

Figure 8-10. From Willis MC. Medical Terminology A Programmed Learning to the Language of Health Care, 2nd ed. Baltimore: Lippincott Williams & Wilkins, 2007.

Figure 8-11. A. From Cohen BJ. Medical Terminology, 5th Edition. Philadelphia. Lippincott Williams & Wilkins 2007.

Figure 8-12. From Cohen BJ. Medical Terminology, 5th Edition. Philadelphia. Lippincott Williams & Wilkins 2007.

Figure 8-15. From Cohen BJ. Medical Terminology, 5th Edition. Philadelphia. Lippincott Williams & Wilkins 2007.

Figure 8-17. Springhouse. Lippincott's Visual Encyclopedia of Clinical Skills. Philadelphia: Wolters Kluwer Health, 2009.

Figure 8-18. A. Russ Curtis / Photo Researchers, Inc. **B.** Aaron Haupt / Photo Researchers, Inc.

Figure 8-19. Dr P. Marazzi / Photo Researchers, Inc

Figure 8-20. Anatomical Chart Company.

Figure Labeling 1. From Cohen BJ. Medical Terminology, 5th Edition. Philadelphia. Lippincott Williams & Wilkins 2007.

Photo of emergency medical technicians. Copyright © Valueline/ Punchstock.

Figure 9-1. Anatomical Chart Company.

Figure 9-2. Nath JL. Using Medical Terminology: A Practical Approach. Baltimore: Lippincott Williams & Wilkins, 2005.

Figure 9-3. Anatomical Chart Company.

Figure 9-4. Anatomical Chart Company.

Figure 9-5. Anatomical Chart Company.

Figure 9-6. Anatomical Chart Company.

Figure 9-7. Terry R. Yochum, Lindsay J. Rowe, Yochum And Rowe's Essentials of Skeletal Radiology, Third Edition. Philadelphia: Lippincott Williams & Wilkins, 2004.

Figure 9-8. A. Brant WE, Helms CA. Fundamentals of Diagnostic Radiology, 3rd Edition. Philadelphia: Lippincott Williams & Wilkins, 2007. **B.** Fleisher GR, et al. Textbook of Pediatric Emergency Medicine, 5th Edition. Philadelphia: Lippincott Williams & Wilkins, 2005.

Figure 9-9. Smeltzer SC, Bare BG, Hinkle J, Cheever KH. Brunner and Suddarth's Textbook of Medical Surgical Nursing, 12th Edition. Philadelphia: Lippincott Williams & Wilkins, 2009.

Figure 9-10. Anatomical Chart Company.

Figure 9-11. McConnell TH. The Nature Of Disease Pathology for the Health Professions, Philadelphia: Lippincott Williams & Wilkins, 2007.

Figure 9-12. A. Southern Illinois University / Photo Researchers, Inc. **B.** From Crapo JD, MD, Glassroth J, MD, Karlinsky JB, MD, MBA, and King TE, Jr., MD. Baum's Textbook of Pulmonary Diseases, 7th Edition. Philadelphia: Lippincott Williams & Wilkins, 2004.

Figure 9-13. Copyright © Lifesize/Monica Rodriguez/GettyImages

Figure 9-14. Willis MC. Medical Terminology: The Language of Health Care, 2nd Edition. Baltimore: Lippincott Williams & Wilkins, 2005.

Figure 9-15. From Cohen BJ. Medical Terminology, 5th Edition. Philadelphia. Lippincott Williams & Wilkins 2007.

Figure 9-17. Photo courtesy of Respironics, Inc. Murrysville, PA (from Willis Programmed, 2e).

Figure 9-19. Smeltzer SC, Bare BG, Hinkle J, Cheever KH. Brunner and Suddarth's Textbook of Medical Surgical Nursing, 12th Edition. Philadelphia: Lippincott Williams & Wilkins, 2009.

Figure 9-20. A. Courtesy of Tyco Healthcare/Nelicor Puritan Bennett, Pleasanton, CA. **B.** Smeltzer SC, Bare BG, Hinkle J, Cheever KH. Brunner and Suddarth's Textbook of Medical Surgical Nursing, 12th Edition. Philadelphia: Lippincott Williams & Wilkins, 2009.

Figure 9-21. Moore KL, Agur AM, Dalley AF. Essential Clinical Anatomy, 4th Edition. Baltimore: Lippincott Williams & Wilkins, 2010.

Figure 9-22. Pillitteri A. Maternal & Child Health Nursing: Care of the Childbearing & Childrearing Family, 6th Edition. Philadelphia: Lippincott Williams & Wilkins, 2010.

Figure 9-23. Stern EJ, Swensen SJ, Kanne JP. High-Resolution CT of the Chest: Comprehensive Atlas, 3rd Edition. Philadelphia: Lippincott Williams & Wilkins, 2010.

Figure Labeling 1. Anatomical Chart Company.

Figure Labeling 2. Nath JL. Using Medical Terminology: A Practical Approach. Baltimore: Lippincott Williams & Wilkins, 2005.

Figure 10-1. Modified from Anatomical Chart Company.

Figure 10-2. Anatomical Chart Company.

Figure 10-4. Modified from Anatomical Chart Company.

Figure 10-6. From Goodheart HP, MD. Goodheart's Photoguide of Common Skin Disorders, 2nd Edition. Philadelphia: Lippincott Williams & Wilkins, 2003.

Figure 10-7. Image from Rubin E MD and Farber JL MD. Pathology, 3rd Edition. Philadelphia: Lippincott Williams & Wilkins, 1999.

Figure 10-8. Nath JL. Using Medical Terminology: A Practical Approach. Baltimore: Lippincott Williams & Wilkins, 2005.

Figure 10-11. Nath JL. Using Medical Terminology: A Practical Approach. Baltimore: Lippincott Williams & Wilkins, 2005.

Figure 10-12. © 2010 Intuitive Surgical, Inc.

Figure Labeling 1. Modified from Anatomical Chart Company.

Figure 11-1. Anatomical Chart Company.

Figure 11-2. Anatomical Chart Company.

Figure 11-3. Anatomical Chart Company.

Figure 11-4. Anatomical Chart Company.

Figure 11-5. From Cohen BJ. Memmler's The Human Body in Health and Disease, 11th Edition. Baltimore: Lippincott Williams & Wilkins, 2008. Courtesy of Dana Morse Bittus and BJ Cohen.

Figure 11-6. Anatomical Chart Company.

Figure 11-7. Reprinted with permission from Pillitteri A. Maternal and Child Health Nursing. 4th ed. Philadelphia: Lippincott Williams & Wilkins, 2003.

Figure 11-9. Baggish MS, Valle RF, Guedj H. Hysteroscopy: Visual Perspectives of Uterine Anatomy, Physiology and Pathology. Philadelphia: Lippincott Williams & Wilkins, 2007.

Figure 11-10. Anatomical Chart Company.

Figure 11-11. Anatomical Chart Company.

Figure 11-12. From Pillitteri A. Maternal and Child Nursing, 4th Ed., Philadelphia: Lippincott, Williams & Wilkins, 2003.

Figure 11-14. Anatomical Chart Company.

Figure 11-15. Used with permission from Moore KL, Dalley AF. Clinical oriented anatomy. 4th ed. Baltimore: Lippincott Williams & Wilkins; 1999.

Figure 11-16. Nettina SM. Lippincott Manual of Nursing Practice, 9th Edition. Philadelphia: Wolters Kluwer Health, 2010.

Figure 11-17. Ills: Anatomical Chart Company. Photo: From O'Doherty N. Atlas of the Newborn. Philadelphia: JB Lippincott, 1979:254, with permission.

Figure 11-19. Anatomical Chart Company.

Figure 11-20. Deep Light Productions / Photo Researchers, Inc

Figure 11-21. Sonograms: Willis MC. Medical Terminology A Programmed Learning Approach to the Language of Health Care, 2nd ed. Baltimore: Lippincott Williams & Wilkins, 2007.

Figure 11-24. Klossner NJ, Hatfield N. Introductory Maternity and Pediatric Nursing. Philadelphia: Lippincott Williams & Wilkins, 2005.

Figure Labeling 1. Anatomical Chart Company.

Photo of nurse midwife. PHANIE / Photo Researchers, Inc.

Figure 12-1. Modified from Bear MF, Connors BW, and Parasido, MA. Neuroscience—Exploring the Brain, 3rd ed. Philadelphia: Lippincott Williams & Wilkins. 2006.

Figure 12-2. Modified from Bear MF, Connors BW, and Parasido, MA. Neuroscience—Exploring the Brain, 3rd ed. Philadelphia: Lippincott Williams & Wilkins. 2006.

Figure 12-3. Anatomical Chart Company.

Figure 12-4. Copyright © Hulton Archive/Stringer/GettyImages.

Figure 12-5. Modified from Anatomical Chart Company.

Figure 12-6. Living Art Enterprises, LLC / Photo Researchers, Inc.

Figure 12-7. Modified from Anatomical Chart Company.

Figure 12-8. Rubin R, Strayer DS. Rubin's Pathology: Clinicopathologic Foundations of Medicine, Fifth Edition. Philadelphia: Lippincott Williams & Wilkins, 2008.

Figure 12-9. From O'Doherty N. Atlas of the Newborn. Philadelphia: JB Lippincott, 1979:254, with permission.

Figure 12-10. Daffner RH. Clinical Radiology The Essentials, 3rd Edition. Philadelphia: Lippincott Williams & Wilkins, 2007.

Figure 12-12. Anatomical Chart Company.

Figure 12-13. From Bickley, LS and Szilagyi, P. Bates' Guide to Physical Examination and History Taking, 8th Ed. Philadelphia: Lippincott Williams & Wilkins 2003.

Figure 12-14. From the National Institute of Mental Health website.

Figure 12-15. Simon Fraser/RVI, Newcastle upon Tyne / Photo Researchers, Inc.

Figure 12-16. Normal: From Snell, MD, PhD, Clinical Anatomy, 7th ed. Lippincott, Williams & Wilkins, 2003. Multiple sclerosis: Ronald L. Eisenberg, an atlas of differential diagnosis Fourth Edition. Philadelphia: Lippincott Williams & Wilkins, 2003.

Figure 12-17. From Willis MC. Medical Terminology A Programmed Learning Approach to the Language of Health Care, 2nd ed. Baltimore: Lippincott Williams & Wilkins, 2007.

Figure 12-19. From Fleisher GR, MD, Ludwig S, MD, Baskin MN, MD. Atlas of Pediatric Emergency Medicine. Philadelphia: Lippincott Williams & Wilkins, 2004.
Figure Labeling 1. From Bear MF, Connors BW, and Parasido, MA. Neuroscience—Exploring the Brain, 3rd ed. Philadelphia: Lippincott Williams & Wilkins. 2006.
Figure Labeling 2. Anatomical Chart Company.

Figure 13-1. Modified from Anatomical Chart Company.

Figure 13-2. Modified from Tank PW, Gest TR. Lippincott Williams & Wilkins Atlas of Anatomy. Baltimore: Lippincott Williams & Wilkins, 2008.

Figure 13-3. From Tasman W, Jaeger E. The Wills Eye Hospital Atlas of Clinical Ophthalmology, 2e. Lippincott Williams & Wilkins, 2001.

Figure 13-4. Rubin E, Farber JL. Pathology. 4th ed. Philadelphia: Lippincott Williams & Wilkins, 2005.

Figure 13-5. From Tasman W, Jaeger E. The Wills Eye Hospital Atlas of Clinical Ophthalmology, 2e. Lippincott Williams & Wilkins, 2001.

Figure 13-6. Anatomical Chart Company.

Figure 13-7. Nath JL. Using Medical Terminology: A Practical Approach. Baltimore: Lippincott Williams & Wilkins, 2005.

Figure 13-9. Image provided by Stedman's.

Figure 13-10. A. From Bickley, LS and Szilagyi, P. Bates' Guide to Physical Examination and History Taking, 8th Ed. Philadelphia: Lippincott Williams & Wilkins 2003. **B.** McConnell TH. The Nature Of Disease Pathology for the Health Professions, Philadelphia: Lippincott Williams & Wilkins, 2007. **C** and **D.** From Tasman W, Jaeger E. The Wills Eye Hospital Atlas of Clinical Ophthalmology, 2e. Lippincott Williams & Wilkins, 2001.

Figure 13-11. Bill Bachmann / Photo Researchers, Inc.

Figure 13-12. LifeART image copyright © [current year] Lippincott Williams & Wilkins. All rights reserved.

Figure 13-13. A. Anatomical Chart Company.

Figure 13-14. Anatomical Chart Company.

Figure 13-15. Anatomical Chart Company.

Figure 13-16. From Moore KL, PhD, FRSM, FIAC & Dalley AF II, PhD. Clinical Oriented Anatomy (4th ed.). Baltimore, Lippincott Williams & Wilkins 1999.

Figure 13-17. © Barbara Sauder/iStockphoto

Figure 13-18. A. From Moore KL, PhD, FRSM, FIAC & Dalley AF II, PhD. Clinical Oriented Anatomy (4th ed.). Baltimore, Lippincott Williams & Wilkins 1999. **B.** From Taylor C, Lillis C, LeMone P. Fundamentals of Nursing: The Art and Science of Nursing Care. 4th Ed. Philadelphia: Lippincott Williams & Wilkins, 2001.

Figure 13-20. Anatomical Chart Company.

Figure 13-21. Courtesy of Larry E. Humes, PhD.
Figure Labeling 1. Modified from Anatomical Chart Company.
Figure Labeling 2. Anatomical Chart Company.
Photo of LASIK surgery: Copyright © Collection Mix—Subjects/ Photodisc.

Figure 14-1. Nath JL. Using Medical Terminology: A Practical Approach. Baltimore: Lippincott Williams & Wilkins, 2005.

Figure 14-2. Cohen BJ. Medical Terminology: An Illustrated Guide, 5th Edition. Baltimore: Lippincott Williams & Wilkins, 2007.

Figure 14-3. Nath JL. Using Medical Terminology: A Practical Approach. Baltimore: Lippincott Williams & Wilkins, 2005.

Figure 14-4. Tank PW, Gest TR. Lippincott Williams & Wilkins Atlas of Anatomy. Baltimore: Lippincott Williams & Wilkins, 2008.

Figure 14-6. Stedman's Medical Dictionary, 28th Edition. Baltimore: Lippincott Williams & Wilkins, 2006.

Figure 14-8. Premkumar K. The Massage Connection, Anatomy and Physiology, 2nd Ed. Baltimore: Lippincott Williams and Wilkins, 2004.

Figure 14-9. Braun MB, Simonson SJ. Introduction to Massage Therapy, 2nd Edition. Baltimore: Lippincott Williams & Wilkins, 2007.

Figure 14-10. Nath JL. Using Medical Terminology: A Practical Approach. Baltimore: Lippincott Williams & Wilkins, 2005.

Figure 14-12. Granger, Neuromuscular Therapy Manual. Baltimore: Lippincott Williams & Wilkins, 2010, and Anatomical Chart Company.

Figure 14-13. Nath JL. Using Medical Terminology: A Practical Approach. Baltimore: Lippincott Williams & Wilkins, 2005.

Figure 14-14. Yochum TR, Rowe LJ. Yochum and Rowe's Essentials of Skeletal Radiology, Third Edition. Philadelphia: Lippincott Williams & Wilkins, 2004.

Figure 14-15. B. Nath JL. Using Medical Terminology: A Practical Approach. Baltimore: Lippincott Williams & Wilkins, 2005.

Figure 14-16. Image from Rubin E MD and Farber JL MD. Pathology, 3rd Edition. Philadelphia: Lippincott Williams & Wilkins, 1999.

Figure 14-17. A. Copyright © Photodisc/Jim Wehtje/GettyImages. **B.** From Strickland JW, Graham TJ. Master Techniques in Orthopeadic Surgery: The Hand, 2nd Edition. Philadelphia: Lippincott Williams & Wilkins, 2005.

Figure 14-18. A. From Cohen BJ. Medical Terminology, 4th ed. Philadelphia. Lippincott Williams & Wilkins 2003. **B.** From Koval KJ, MD and Zuckerman, JD, MD. Atlas of Orthopaedic Surgery: A Multimeidal Reference. Philadelphia: Lippincott Williams & Wilkins, 2004.

Figure 14-19. Daffner RH. Clinical Radiology The Essentials, 3rd Edition. Philadelphia: Lippincott Williams & Wilkins, 2007.

Figure 14-20. A, C, and **E.** From Bucholz RW, MD and Heckman JD, MD. Rockwood & Green's Fractures in Adults, 5th ed. Lippincott, Williams & Wilkins, 2001. **B** and **D.** Daffner RH. Clinical Radiology The Essentials, 3rd Edition. Philadelphia: Lippincott Williams & Wilkins, 2007.

Figure 14-21. Deep Light Productions / Photo Researchers, Inc.

Figure 14-22. From Cohen BJ. Medical Terminology, 4th ed. Philadelphia. Lippincott Williams & Wilkins 2003.

Figure 14-25. From Koval KJ, MD and Zuckerman, JD, MD. Atlas of Orthopaedic Surgery: A Multimedia Reference. Philadelphia: Lippincott Williams & Wilkins, 2004.

Figure 14-26. From Strickland JW, Graham TJ. Master Techniques in Orthopaedic Surgery: The Hand, 2nd Edition. Philadelphia: Lippincott Williams & Wilkins, 2005.

Figure 14-27. Photo courtesy of Drive Medical Design & Manufacturing, Port Washington, NY.

Figure 14-28. Photos courtesy of U.S. Orthotics, Tampa, FL.

Figure 14-29. Anatomical Chart Company.

Figure 14-30. Jackson DW. Master Techniques in Orthopaedic Surgery: Reconstructive Knee Surgery. Philadelphia: Lippincott Williams & Wilkins, 2007.
Figure Labeling 1. Nath JL. Using Medical Terminology: A Practical Approach. Baltimore: Lippincott Williams & Wilkins, 2005.
Figure Labeling 2. Braun MB, Simonson SJ. Introduction to Massage Therapy, 2nd Edition. Baltimore: Lippincott Williams & Wilkins, 2007.

Figure 15-1. From Westheimer R, Lopater S. 2002. Human Sexuality-A Psychosocial Perspective. Baltimore: Lippincott Williams & Wilkins.

Figure 15-2. Anatomical Chart Company.

Figure 15-3. Anatomical Chart Company.

Figure 15-4. McConnell TH. The Nature Of Disease Pathology for the Health Professions, Philadelphia: Lippincott Williams & Wilkins, 2007.

Figure 15-5. From Rubin E. Essential Pathology, 3rd Ed. Philadelphia: Lippincott Williams & Wilkins, 2000.

Figure 15-6. From Goodheart HP. Photoguide of Common Skin Disorders. 2nd Ed. Philadelphia: Lippincott Williams & Wilkins, 2003.

Figure 15-7. Anatomical Chart Company.

Figure 15-8. Klossner NJ, Hatfield N. Introductory Maternity and Pediatric Nursing. Philadelphia: Lippincott Williams & Wilkins, 2005.

Figure 15-9. From Smeltzer SC, Bare BG. Textbook of Medical-Surgical Nursing, 12th Ed. Philadelphia: Lippincott Williams & Wilkins, 2010. (Courtesy of Medtronic Diabetes.)

Figure 15-10. Southern Illinois University / Photo Researchers, Inc

Figure 15-11. Olivier Voisin / Photo Researchers, Inc.

Figure 15-12. Spencer Grant / Photo Researchers, Inc.

Figure 15-13. Eisenberg RL. An Atlas of Differential Diagnosis, 4th Edition. Philadelphia: Lippincott Williams & Wilkins, 2003. *Figure Labeling 1.* From Westheimer R, Lopater S. 2002. Human Sexuality— A Psychosocial Perspective. Baltimore: Lippincott Williams & Wilkins.

Figure 16-1. McConnell TH. The Nature Of Disease Pathology for the Health Professions, Philadelphia: Lippincott Williams & Wilkins, 2007.

Figure 16-2. McConnell TH. The Nature Of Disease Pathology for the Health Professions, Philadelphia: Lippincott Williams & Wilkins, 2007.

Figure 16-3. Neuroma figure: CNRI / Photo Researchers, Inc. All other figs: From Cagle PT, MD. Color Atlas and Text of Pulmonary Pathology. Philadelphia: Lippincott Williams & Wilkins, 2005.

Figure 16-4. Mulholland MW, Maier RV, et al. Greenfield's Surgery Scientific Principles And Practice, Fourth Edition. Philadelphia: Lippincott Williams & Wilkins, 2006.

Figure 16-5. A. From Goodheart HP, MD. Goodheart's Photoguide of Common Skin Disorders, 2nd Edition. Philadelphia: Lippincott Williams & Wilkins, 2003. **B.** Image provided by Stedman's (Dr. Barankin Collection). **C.** DeVita VT, Lawrence TS, Rosenberg SA. DeVita, Hellman, and Rosenberg's Cancer Principles & Practice of Oncology, 8th Edition. Philadelphia: Wolters Kluwer Health, 2008.

Figure 16-6. Rubin R, Strayer DS, Rubin E. Rubin's Pathology: Clinicopathologic Foundations of Medicine, 5th Edition. Baltimore: Lippincott Williams & Wilkins, 2008.

Figure 16-7. Rubin R, Strayer DS, Rubin E. Rubin's Pathology: Clinicopathologic Foundations of Medicine, 5th Edition. Baltimore: Lippincott Williams & Wilkins, 2008.

Figure 16-8. Anatomical Chart Company.

Figure 16-9. Anatomical Chart Company.

Figure 16-10. Fleisher GR, et al. Textbook of Pediatric Emergency Medicine, 5th Edition. Philadelphia: Lippincott Williams & Wilkins, 2005.

Figure 16-11. Rubin R, Strayer DS, Rubin E: Rubin's Pathology: Clinicopathologic Foundations of Medicine, 5th Edition. Baltimore: Lippincott Williams & Wilkins, 2008.

Figure 16-12. John Bavosi / Photo Researchers, Inc.

Figure 16-13. Harris JR, et al. Diseases of the Breast, 3rd Edition. Philadelphia: Lippincott Williams & Wilkins, 2004.

Figure 16-14. Modified from Anatomical Chart Company.

Figure 16-16. Véronique Burger / Photo Researchers, Inc.

Figure 16-17. From Varian Medical Systems, Palo Alto, CA, with permission.
Photo of physician's assistant with patient: Copyright © Image Source/ GettyImages.

■ INDEX

Note: Page numbers followed by f refer to figures.

⭒ STEDMAN'S
Anatomy Atlas

Digestive System, Anterior View

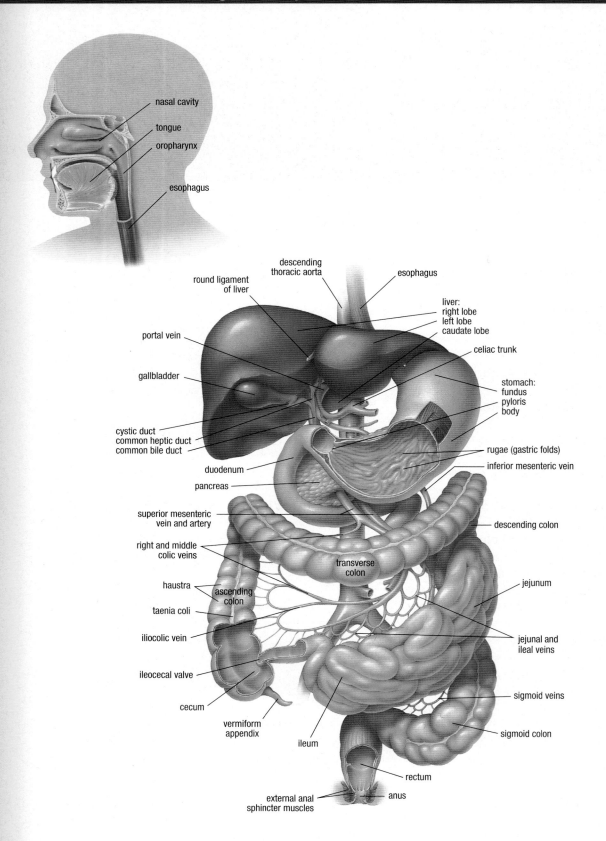

nasal cavity
tongue
oropharynx
esophagus

descending thoracic aorta
round ligament of liver
esophagus
liver:
right lobe
left lobe
caudate lobe
portal vein
celiac trunk
gallbladder
stomach:
fundus
pyloris
body
cystic duct
common heptic duct
common bile duct
rugae (gastric folds)
inferior mesenteric vein
duodenum
pancreas
superior mesenteric vein and artery
descending colon
right and middle colic veins
transverse colon
haustra
ascending colon
jejunum
taenia coli
iliocolic vein
jejunal and ileal veins
ileocecal valve
cecum
sigmoid veins
vermiform appendix
sigmoid colon
ileum
rectum
external anal sphincter muscles
anus

Imagery © Anatomical Chart Company

Urinary System, Anterior View

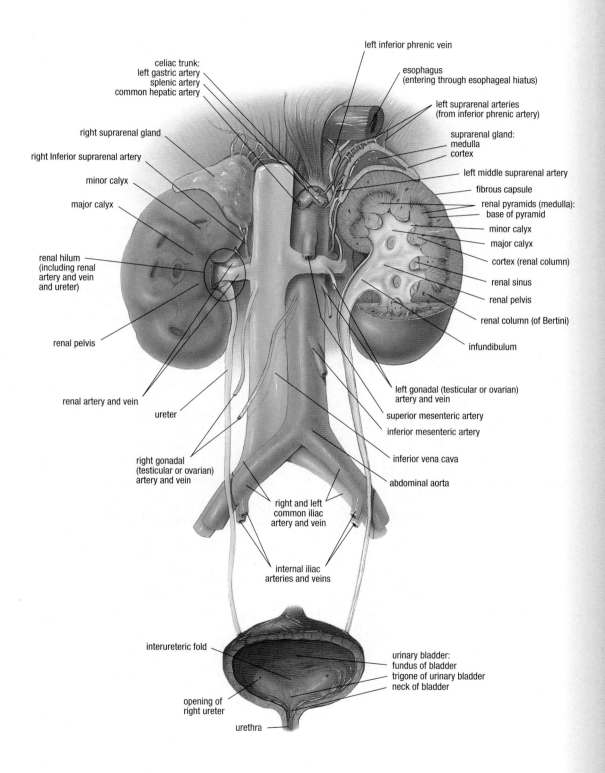

left inferior phrenic vein

celiac trunk:
left gastric artery
splenic artery
common hepatic artery

esophagus
(entering through esophageal hiatus)

left suprarenal arteries
(from inferior phrenic artery)

right suprarenal gland

suprarenal gland:
medulla
cortex

right Inferior suprarenal artery

left middle suprarenal artery

minor calyx

fibrous capsule

major calyx

renal pyramids (medulla):
base of pyramid

minor calyx

major calyx

renal hilum
(including
renal
artery and vein
and ureter)

cortex (renal column)

renal sinus

renal pelvis

renal column (of Bertini)

renal pelvis

infundibulum

renal artery and vein

left gonadal (testicular or ovarian)
artery and vein

ureter

superior mesenteric artery

inferior mesenteric artery

right gonadal
(testicular or ovarian)
artery and vein

inferior vena cava

abdominal aorta

right and left
common iliac
artery and vein

internal iliac
arteries and veins

interureteric fold

urinary bladder:
fundus of bladder
trigone of urinary bladder
neck of bladder

opening of
right ureter

urethra

Imagery © Anatomical Chart Company

Anatomy of the Heart, Anterior View

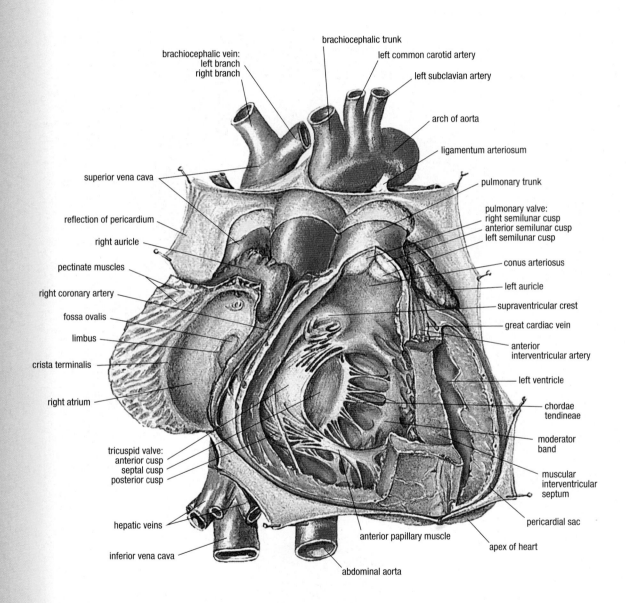

brachiocephalic trunk

brachiocephalic vein:
left branch
right branch

left common carotid artery

left subclavian artery

arch of aorta

ligamentum arteriosum

superior vena cava

pulmonary trunk

reflection of pericardium

pulmonary valve:
right semilunar cusp
anterior semilunar cusp
left semilunar cusp

right auricle

conus arteriosus

pectinate muscles

left auricle

right coronary artery

supraventricular crest

fossa ovalis

great cardiac vein

limbus

anterior
interventricular artery

crista terminalis

left ventricle

right atrium

chordae
tendineae

moderator
band

tricuspid valve:
anterior cusp
septal cusp
posterior cusp

muscular
interventricular
septum

hepatic veins

pericardial sac

inferior vena cava

anterior papillary muscle

apex of heart

abdominal aorta

Imagery © Anatomical Chart Company

Arterial System, Anterior View

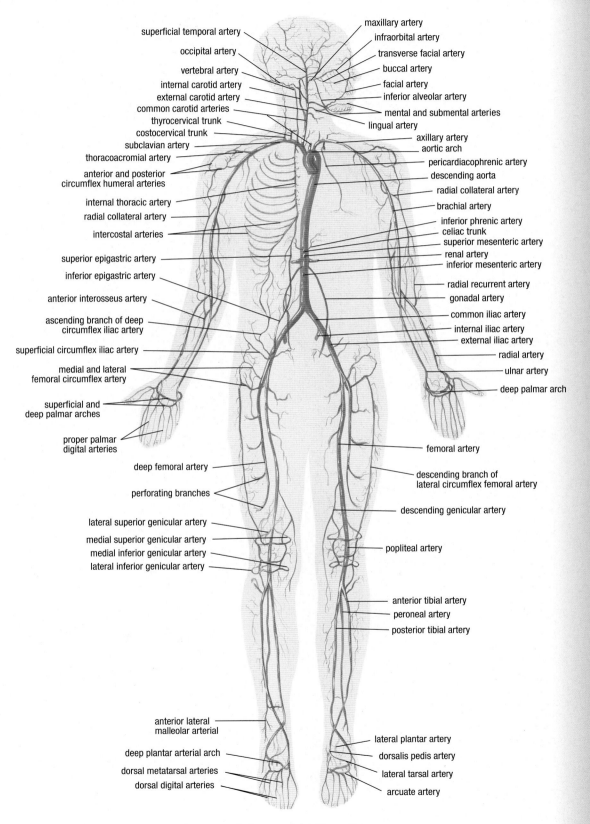

superficial temporal artery
occipital artery
vertebral artery
internal carotid artery
external carotid artery
common carotid arteries
thyrocervical trunk
costocervical trunk
subclavian artery
thoracoacromial artery
anterior and posterior
circumflex humeral arteries
internal thoracic artery
radial collateral artery
intercostal arteries
superior epigastric artery
inferior epigastric artery
anterior interosseus artery
ascending branch of deep
circumflex iliac artery
superficial circumflex iliac artery
medial and lateral
femoral circumflex artery
superficial and
deep palmar arches
proper palmar
digital arteries
deep femoral artery
perforating branches
lateral superior genicular artery
medial superior genicular artery
medial inferior genicular artery
lateral inferior genicular artery
anterior lateral
malleolar arterial
deep plantar arterial arch
dorsal metatarsal arteries
dorsal digital arteries

maxillary artery
infraorbital artery
transverse facial artery
buccal artery
facial artery
inferior alveolar artery
mental and submental arteries
lingual artery
axillary artery
aortic arch
pericardiacophrenic artery
descending aorta
radial collateral artery
brachial artery
inferior phrenic artery
celiac trunk
superior mesenteric artery
renal artery
inferior mesenteric artery
radial recurrent artery
gonadal artery
common iliac artery
internal iliac artery
external iliac artery
radial artery
ulnar artery
deep palmar arch
femoral artery
descending branch of
lateral circumflex femoral artery
descending genicular artery
popliteal artery
anterior tibial artery
peroneal artery
posterior tibial artery
lateral plantar artery
dorsalis pedis artery
lateral tarsal artery
arcuate artery

Imagery © Anatomical Chart Company

Venous System, Anterior View

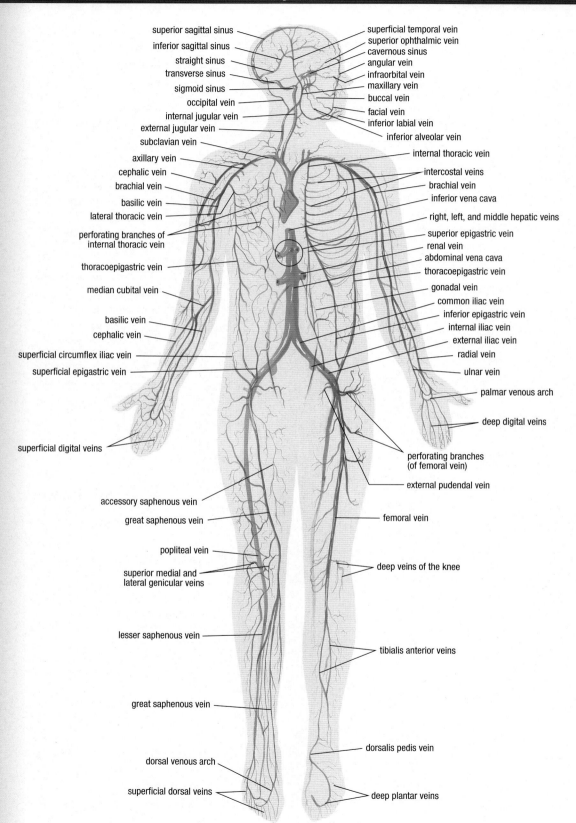

superior sagittal sinus
inferior sagittal sinus
straight sinus
transverse sinus
sigmoid sinus
occipital vein
internal jugular vein
external jugular vein
subclavian vein
axillary vein
cephalic vein
brachial vein
basilic vein
lateral thoracic vein
perforating branches of
internal thoracic vein
thoracoepigastric vein
median cubital vein
basilic vein
cephalic vein
superficial circumflex iliac vein
superficial epigastric vein
superficial digital veins
accessory saphenous vein
great saphenous vein
popliteal vein
superior medial and
lateral genicular veins
lesser saphenous vein
great saphenous vein
dorsal venous arch
superficial dorsal veins

superficial temporal vein
superior ophthalmic vein
cavernous sinus
angular vein
infraorbital vein
maxillary vein
buccal vein
facial vein
inferior labial vein
inferior alveolar vein
internal thoracic vein
intercostal veins
brachial vein
inferior vena cava
right, left, and middle hepatic veins
superior epigastric vein
renal vein
abdominal vena cava
thoracoepigastric vein
gonadal vein
common iliac vein
inferior epigastric vein
internal iliac vein
external iliac vein
radial vein
ulnar vein
palmar venous arch
deep digital veins
perforating branches
(of femoral vein)
external pudendal vein
femoral vein
deep veins of the knee
tibialis anterior veins
dorsalis pedis vein
deep plantar veins

Imagery © Anatomical Chart Company

Lymphatic System, Anterior View

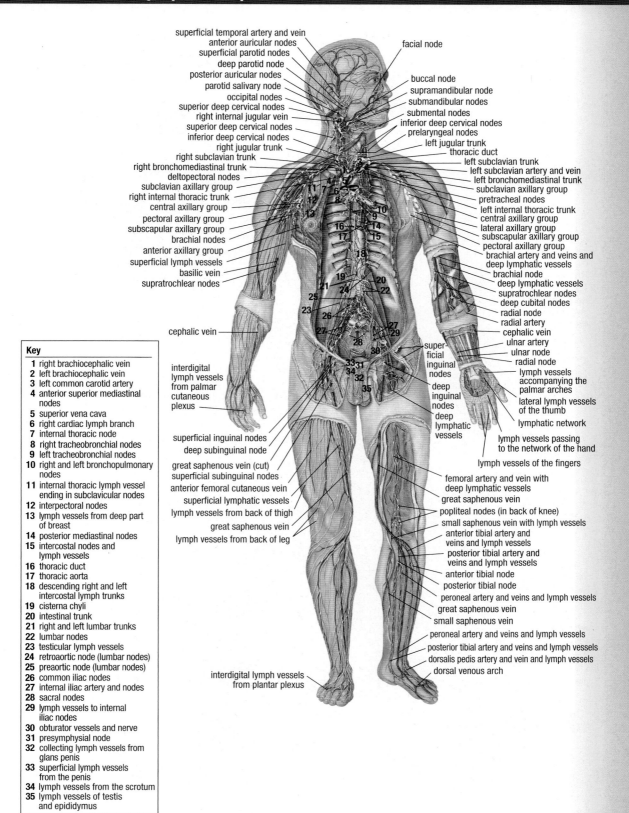

superficial temporal artery and vein
anterior auricular nodes
superficial parotid nodes
deep parotid node
posterior auricular nodes
parotid salivary node
occipital nodes
superior deep cervical nodes
right internal jugular vein
superior deep cervical nodes
inferior deep cervical nodes
right jugular trunk
right subclavian trunk
right bronchomediastinal trunk
deltopectoral nodes
subclavian axillary group
right internal thoracic trunk
central axillary group
pectoral axillary group
subscapular axillary group
brachial nodes
anterior axillary group
superficial lymphatic vessels
basilic vein
supratrochlear nodes

facial node
buccal node
supramandibular node
submandibular nodes
submental nodes
inferior deep cervical nodes
prelaryngeal nodes
left jugular trunk
thoracic duct
left subclavian trunk
left subclavian artery and vein
left bronchomediastinal trunk
subclavian axillary group
pretracheal nodes
left internal thoracic trunk
central axillary group
lateral axillary group
subscapular axillary group
pectoral axillary group
brachial artery and veins and
deep lymphatic vessels
brachial node
deep lymphatic vessels
supratrochlear nodes
deep cubital nodes
radial node
radial artery
cephalic vein
ulnar artery
ulnar node
radial node
lymph vessels
accompanying the
palmar arches
lateral lymph vessels
of the thumb
lymphatic network

cephalic vein

super-
ficial
inguinal
nodes
deep
inguinal
nodes
deep
lymphatic
vessels

lymph vessels passing
to the network of the hand
lymph vessels of the fingers

interdigital
lymph vessels
from palmar
cutaneous
plexus

superficial inguinal nodes
deep subinguinal node
great saphenous vein (cut)
superficial subinguinal nodes
anterior femoral cutaneous vein
superficial lymphatic vessels
lymph vessels from deep part of breast
great saphenous vein
lymph vessels from back of leg

femoral artery and vein with
deep lymphatic vessels
great saphenous vein
popliteal nodes (in back of knee)
small saphenous vein with lymph vessels
anterior tibial artery and
veins and lymph vessels
posterior tibial artery and
veins and lymph vessels
anterior tibial node
posterior tibial node
peroneal artery and veins and lymph vessels
great saphenous vein
small saphenous vein
peroneal artery and veins and lymph vessels
posterior tibial artery and veins and lymph vessels
dorsalis pedis artery and vein and lymph vessels
dorsal venous arch

interdigital lymph vessels
from plantar plexus

Key

1 right brachiocephalic vein
2 left brachiocephalic vein
3 left common carotid artery
4 anterior superior mediastinal nodes
5 superior vena cava
6 right cardiac lymph branch
7 internal thoracic node
8 right tracheobronchial nodes
9 left tracheobronchial nodes
10 right and left bronchopulmonary nodes
11 internal thoracic lymph vessel ending in subclavicular nodes
12 interpectoral nodes
13 lymph vessels from deep part of breast
14 posterior mediastinal nodes
15 intercostal nodes and lymph vessels
16 thoracic duct
17 thoracic aorta
18 descending right and left intercostal lymph trunks
19 cisterna chyli
20 intestinal trunk
21 right and left lumbar trunks
22 lumbar nodes
23 testicular lymph vessels
24 retroaortic node (lumbar nodes)
25 preaortic node (lumbar nodes)
26 common iliac nodes
27 internal iliac artery and nodes
28 sacral nodes
29 lymph vessels to internal iliac nodes
30 obturator vessels and nerve
31 presymphysial node
32 collecting lymph vessels from glans penis
33 superficial lymph vessels from the penis
34 lymph vessels from the scrotum
35 lymph vessels of testis and epididymus

Imagery © Anatomical Chart Company

Respiratory System, Anterior View

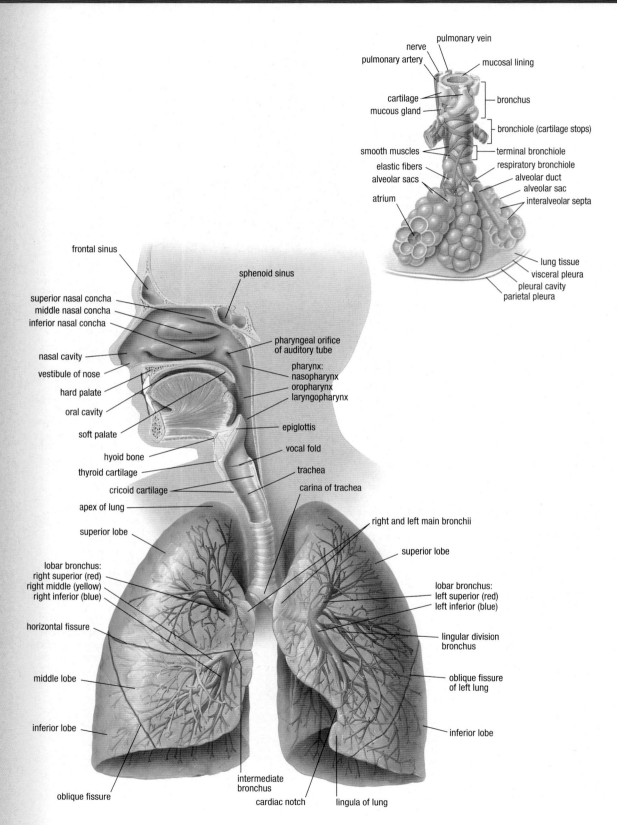

pulmonary vein

nerve

pulmonary artery

mucosal lining

cartilage

bronchus

mucous gland

bronchiole (cartilage stops)

smooth muscles

terminal bronchiole

elastic fibers

respiratory bronchiole

alveolar sacs

alveolar duct

atrium

alveolar sac

interalveolar septa

lung tissue

visceral pleura

pleural cavity

parietal pleura

frontal sinus

sphenoid sinus

superior nasal concha

middle nasal concha

inferior nasal concha

pharyngeal orifice
of auditory tube

nasal cavity

pharynx:
nasopharynx
oropharynx
laryngopharynx

vestibule of nose

hard palate

oral cavity

soft palate

epiglottis

hyoid bone

vocal fold

thyroid cartilage

trachea

cricoid cartilage

carina of trachea

apex of lung

right and left main bronchii

superior lobe

superior lobe

lobar bronchus:
right superior (red)
right middle (yellow)
right inferior (blue)

lobar bronchus:
left superior (red)
left inferior (blue)

horizontal fissure

lingular division
bronchus

middle lobe

oblique fissure
of left lung

inferior lobe

inferior lobe

oblique fissure

intermediate
bronchus

cardiac notch

lingula of lung

Imagery © Anatomical Chart Company

Male and Female Urogenital Systems, Midsagittal View

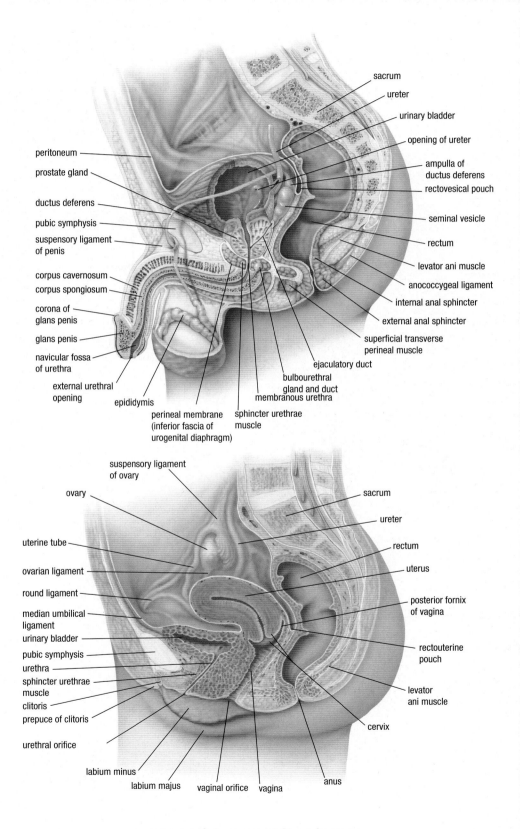

sacrum

ureter

urinary bladder

opening of ureter

ampulla of
ductus deferens

rectovesical pouch

seminal vesicle

rectum

levator ani muscle

anococcygeal ligament

internal anal sphincter

external anal sphincter

superficial transverse
perineal muscle

ejaculatory duct

bulbourethral
gland and duct

membranous urethra

sphincter urethrae
muscle

perineal membrane
(inferior fascia of
urogenital diaphragm)

epididymis

external urethral
opening

navicular fossa
of urethra

glans penis

corona of
glans penis

corpus spongiosum

corpus cavernosum

suspensory ligament
of penis

pubic symphysis

ductus deferens

prostate gland

peritoneum

suspensory ligament
of ovary

ovary

uterine tube

ovarian ligament

round ligament

median umbilical
ligament

urinary bladder

pubic symphysis

urethra

sphincter urethrae
muscle

clitoris

prepuce of clitoris

urethral orifice

labium minus

labium majus

vaginal orifice

vagina

anus

cervix

levator
ani muscle

rectouterine
pouch

posterior fornix
of vagina

uterus

rectum

ureter

sacrum

Imagery © Anatomical Chart Company

Spinal and Cranial Nerves

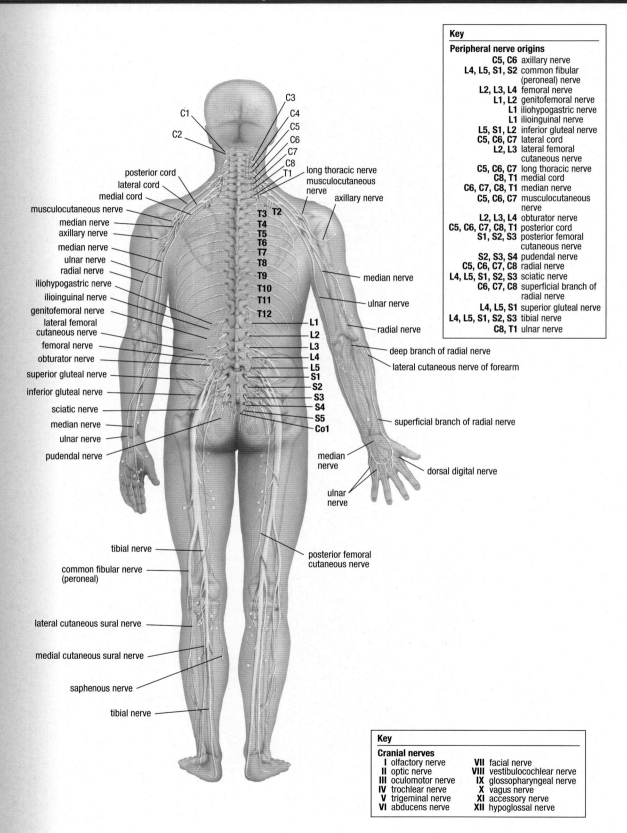

Key

Peripheral nerve origins

C5, C6	axillary nerve
L4, L5, S1, S2	common fibular (peroneal) nerve
L2, L3, L4	femoral nerve
L1, L2	genitofemoral nerve
L1	iliohypogastric nerve
L1	ilioinguinal nerve
L5, S1, L2	inferior gluteal nerve
C5, C6, C7	lateral cord
L2, L3	lateral femoral cutaneous nerve
C5, C6, C7	long thoracic nerve
C8, T1	medial cord
C6, C7, C8, T1	median nerve
C5, C6, C7	musculocutaneous nerve
L2, L3, L4	obturator nerve
C5, C6, C7, C8, T1	posterior cord
S1, S2, S3	posterior femoral cutaneous nerve
S2, S3, S4	pudendal nerve
C5, C6, C7, C8	radial nerve
L4, L5, S1, S2, S3	sciatic nerve
C6, C7, C8	superficial branch of radial nerve
L4, L5, S1	superior gluteal nerve
L4, L5, S1, S2, S3	tibial nerve
C8, T1	ulnar nerve

Key

Cranial nerves

I	olfactory nerve	**VII**	facial nerve
II	optic nerve	**VIII**	vestibulocochlear nerve
III	oculomotor nerve	**IX**	glossopharyngeal nerve
IV	trochlear nerve	**X**	vagus nerve
V	trigeminal nerve	**XI**	accessory nerve
VI	abducens nerve	**XII**	hypoglossal nerve

Labels on figure:

C1, C2, C3, C4, C5, C6, C7, C8, T1
posterior cord
lateral cord
medial cord
musculocutaneous nerve
median nerve
axillary nerve
median nerve
ulnar nerve
radial nerve
iliohypogastric nerve
ilioinguinal nerve
genitofemoral nerve
lateral femoral cutaneous nerve
femoral nerve
obturator nerve
superior gluteal nerve
inferior gluteal nerve
sciatic nerve
median nerve
ulnar nerve
pudendal nerve
tibial nerve
common fibular nerve (peroneal)
lateral cutaneous sural nerve
medial cutaneous sural nerve
saphenous nerve
tibial nerve

T2, T3, T4, T5, T6, T7, T8, T9, T10, T11, T12
L1, L2, L3, L4, L5
S1, S2, S3, S4, S5
Co1

long thoracic nerve
musculocutaneous nerve
axillary nerve
median nerve
ulnar nerve
radial nerve
deep branch of radial nerve
lateral cutaneous nerve of forearm
superficial branch of radial nerve
median nerve
dorsal digital nerve
ulnar nerve
posterior femoral cutaneous nerve

Imagery © Anatomical Chart Company

Cerebral Hemispheres

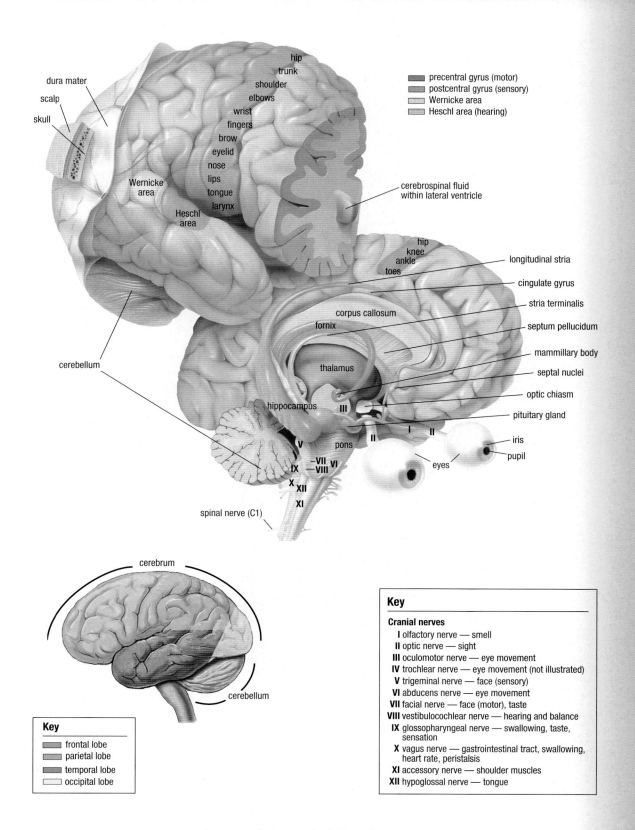

dura mater

scalp

skull

hip
trunk
shoulder
elbows
wrist
fingers
brow
eyelid
nose
lips
tongue
larynx

precentral gyrus (motor)
postcentral gyrus (sensory)
Wernicke area
Heschl area (hearing)

Wernicke
area

Heschl
area

cerebrospinal fluid
within lateral ventricle

hip
knee
ankle
toes

longitudinal stria

cingulate gyrus

stria terminalis

corpus callosum

septum pellucidum

fornix

mammillary body

thalamus

septal nuclei

optic chiasm

hippocampus

III

pituitary gland

cerebellum

I

II

iris

II

pupil

V

pons

eyes

—VII VI
IX —VIII
X XII
XI

spinal nerve (C1)

cerebrum

cerebellum

Key

frontal lobe
parietal lobe
temporal lobe
occipital lobe

Key

Cranial nerves

I olfactory nerve — smell
II optic nerve — sight
III oculomotor nerve — eye movement
IV trochlear nerve — eye movement (not illustrated)
V trigeminal nerve — face (sensory)
VI abducens nerve — eye movement
VII facial nerve — face (motor), taste
VIII vestibulocochlear nerve — hearing and balance
IX glossopharyngeal nerve — swallowing, taste,
sensation
X vagus nerve — gastrointestinal tract, swallowing,
heart rate, peristalsis
XI accessory nerve — shoulder muscles
XII hypoglossal nerve — tongue

Imagery © Anatomical Chart Company

Muscular System, Anterior View

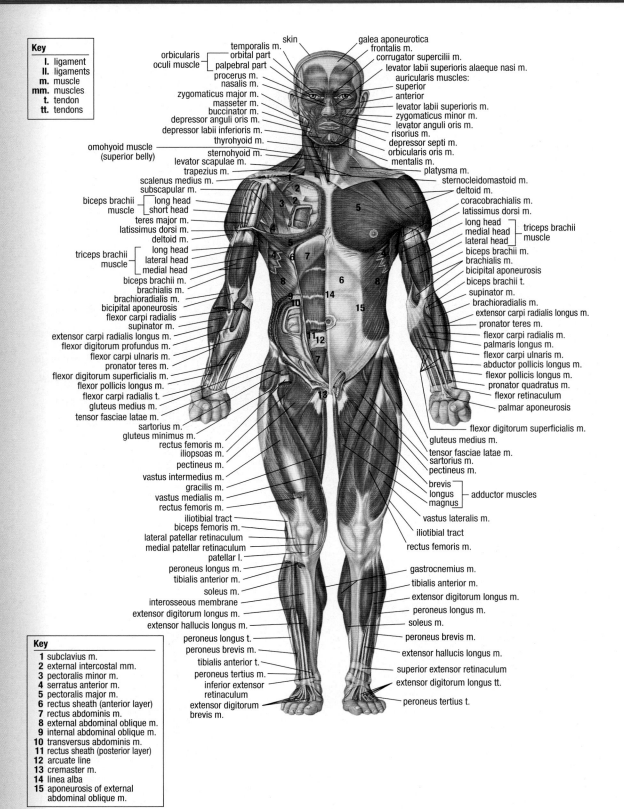

Key
- **l.** ligament
- **ll.** ligaments
- **m.** muscle
- **mm.** muscles
- **t.** tendon
- **tt.** tendons

skin
temporalis m.
orbicularis oculi muscle — orbital part / palpebral part
procerus m.
nasalis m.
zygomaticus major m.
masseter m.
buccinator m.
depressor anguli oris m.
depressor labii inferioris m.
thyrohyoid m.
omohyoid muscle (superior belly)
sternohyoid m.
levator scapulae m.
trapezius m.
scalenus medius m.
subscapular m.
biceps brachii muscle — long head / short head
teres major m.
latissimus dorsi m.
deltoid m.
triceps brachii muscle — long head / lateral head / medial head
biceps brachii m.
brachialis m.
brachioradialis m.
bicipital aponeurosis
flexor carpi radialis
supinator m.
extensor carpi radialis longus m.
flexor digitorum profundus m.
flexor carpi ulnaris m.
pronator teres m.
flexor digitorum superficialis m.
flexor pollicis longus m.
flexor carpi radialis t.
gluteus medius m.
tensor fasciae latae m.
sartorius m.
gluteus minimus m.
rectus femoris m.
iliopsoas m.
pectineus m.
vastus intermedius m.
gracilis m.
vastus medialis m.
rectus femoris m.
iliotibial tract
biceps femoris m.
lateral patellar retinaculum
medial patellar retinaculum
patellar l.
peroneus longus m.
tibialis anterior m.
soleus m.
interosseous membrane
extensor digitorum longus m.
extensor hallucis longus m.
peroneus longus t.
peroneus brevis m.
tibialis anterior t.
peroneus tertius m.
inferior extensor retinaculum
extensor digitorum brevis m.

galea aponeurotica
frontalis m.
corrugator supercilii m.
levator labii superioris alaeque nasi m.
auricularis muscles: superior / anterior
levator labii superioris m.
zygomaticus minor m.
levator anguli oris m.
risorius m.
depressor septi m.
orbicularis oris m.
mentalis m.
platysma m.
sternocleidomastoid m.
deltoid m.
coracobrachialis m.
latissimus dorsi m.
triceps brachii muscle — long head / medial head / lateral head
biceps brachii m.
brachialis m.
bicipital aponeurosis
biceps brachii t.
supinator m.
brachioradialis m.
extensor carpi radialis longus m.
pronator teres m.
flexor carpi radialis m.
palmaris longus m.
flexor carpi ulnaris m.
abductor pollicis longus m.
flexor pollicis longus m.
pronator quadratus m.
flexor retinaculum
palmar aponeurosis
flexor digitorum superficialis m.
gluteus medius m.
tensor fasciae latae m.
sartorius m.
pectineus m.
adductor muscles — brevis / longus / magnus
vastus lateralis m.
iliotibial tract
rectus femoris m.
gastrocnemius m.
tibialis anterior m.
extensor digitorum longus m.
peroneus longus m.
soleus m.
peroneus brevis m.
extensor hallucis longus m.
superior extensor retinaculum
extensor digitorum longus tt.
peroneus tertius t.

Key
1. subclavius m.
2. external intercostal mm.
3. pectoralis minor m.
4. serratus anterior m.
5. pectoralis major m.
6. rectus sheath (anterior layer)
7. rectus abdominis m.
8. external abdominal oblique m.
9. internal abdominal oblique m.
10. transversus abdominis m.
11. rectus sheath (posterior layer)
12. arcuate line
13. cremaster m.
14. linea alba
15. aponeurosis of external abdominal oblique m.

Imagery © Anatomical Chart Company

Muscular System, Posterior View

Key
- **l.** ligament
- **ll.** ligaments
- **m.** muscle
- **mm.** muscles
- **t.** tendon
- **tt.** tendons

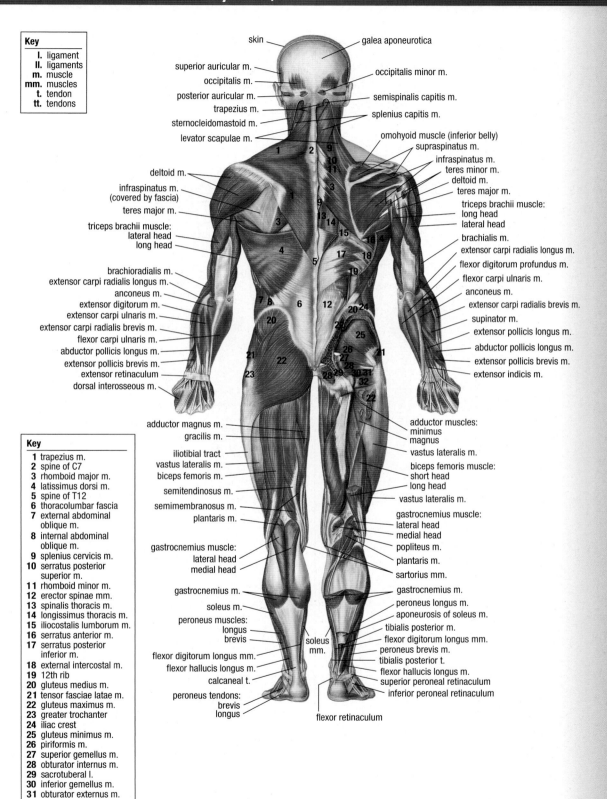

skin
galea aponeurotica
superior auricular m.
occipitalis m.
occipitalis minor m.
posterior auricular m.
semispinalis capitis m.
trapezius m.
splenius capitis m.
sternocleidomastoid m.
omohyoid muscle (inferior belly)
levator scapulae m.
supraspinatus m.
infraspinatus m.
teres minor m.
deltoid m.
deltoid m.
infraspinatus m.
(covered by fascia)
teres major m.
teres major m.
triceps brachii muscle:
long head
lateral head
triceps brachii muscle:
lateral head
long head
brachialis m.
extensor carpi radialis longus m.
flexor digitorum profundus m.
brachioradialis m.
flexor carpi ulnaris m.
extensor carpi radialis longus m.
anconeus m.
anconeus m.
extensor carpi radialis brevis m.
extensor digitorum m.
extensor carpi ulnaris m.
supinator m.
extensor carpi radialis brevis m.
extensor pollicis longus m.
flexor carpi ulnaris m.
abductor pollicis longus m.
abductor pollicis longus m.
extensor pollicis brevis m.
extensor pollicis brevis m.
extensor retinaculum
extensor indicis m.
dorsal interosseous m.

adductor magnus m.
adductor muscles:
gracilis m.
minimus
magnus
iliotibial tract
vastus lateralis m.
vastus lateralis m.
biceps femoris m.
biceps femoris muscle:
semitendinosus m.
short head
long head
semimembranosus m.
vastus lateralis m.
plantaris m.
gastrocnemius muscle:
lateral head
medial head
popliteus m.
gastrocnemius muscle:
plantaris m.
lateral head
sartorius mm.
medial head
gastrocnemius m.
gastrocnemius m.
soleus m.
peroneus longus m.
peroneus muscles:
aponeurosis of soleus m.
longus
tibialis posterior m.
brevis
flexor digitorum longus mm.
soleus
peroneus brevis m.
flexor digitorum longus mm.
mm.
tibialis posterior t.
flexor hallucis longus m.
flexor hallucis longus m.
calcaneal t.
superior peroneal retinaculum
peroneus tendons:
inferior peroneal retinaculum
brevis
longus
flexor retinaculum

Key
1. trapezius m.
2. spine of C7
3. rhomboid major m.
4. latissimus dorsi m.
5. spine of T12
6. thoracolumbar fascia
7. external abdominal oblique m.
8. internal abdominal oblique m.
9. splenius cervicis m.
10. serratus posterior superior m.
11. rhomboid minor m.
12. erector spinae mm.
13. spinalis thoracis m.
14. longissimus thoracis m.
15. iliocostalis lumborum m.
16. serratus anterior m.
17. serratus posterior inferior m.
18. external intercostal m.
19. 12th rib
20. gluteus medius m.
21. tensor fasciae latae m.
22. gluteus maximus m.
23. greater trochanter
24. iliac crest
25. gluteus minimus m.
26. piriformis m.
27. superior gemellus m.
28. obturator internus m.
29. sacrotuberal l.
30. inferior gemellus m.
31. obturator externus m.
32. quadratus femoris m.

Imagery © Anatomical Chart Company

Skeletal Anatomy, Anterior View

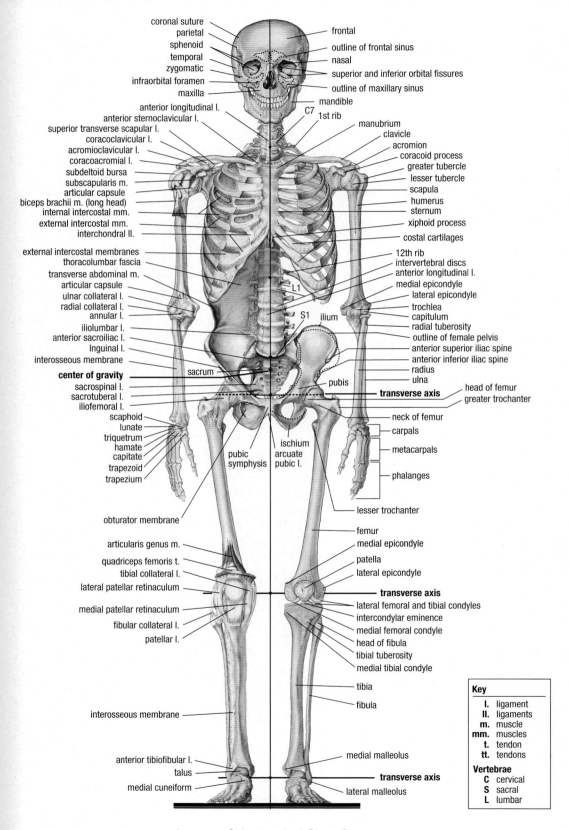

coronal suture
parietal
sphenoid
temporal
zygomatic
infraorbital foramen
maxilla
anterior longitudinal l.
anterior sternoclavicular l.
superior transverse scapular l.
coracoclavicular l.
acromioclavicular l.
coracoacromial l.
subdeltoid bursa
subscapularis m.
articular capsule
biceps brachii m. (long head)
internal intercostal mm.
external intercostal mm.
interchondral ll.
external intercostal membranes
thoracolumbar fascia
transverse abdominal m.
articular capsule
ulnar collateral l.
radial collateral l.
annular l.
iliolumbar l.
anterior sacroiliac l.
Inguinal l.
interosseous membrane
center of gravity
sacrospinal l.
sacrotuberal l.
iliofemoral l.
scaphoid
lunate
triquetrum
hamate
capitate
trapezoid
trapezium

obturator membrane

articularis genus m.
quadriceps femoris t.
tibial collateral l.
lateral patellar retinaculum
medial patellar retinaculum
fibular collateral l.
patellar l.

interosseous membrane

anterior tibiofibular l.
talus
medial cuneiform

frontal
outline of frontal sinus
nasal
superior and inferior orbital fissures
outline of maxillary sinus
mandible
C7 1st rib
manubrium
clavicle
acromion
coracoid process
greater tubercle
lesser tubercle
scapula
humerus
sternum
xiphoid process
costal cartilages
12th rib
intervertebral discs
anterior longitudinal l.
medial epicondyle
lateral epicondyle
trochlea
capitulum
radial tuberosity
outline of female pelvis
anterior superior iliac spine
anterior inferior iliac spine
radius
ulna
head of femur
greater trochanter
transverse axis
neck of femur
carpals
metacarpals
phalanges
lesser trochanter
femur
medial epicondyle
patella
lateral epicondyle
transverse axis
lateral femoral and tibial condyles
intercondylar eminence
medial femoral condyle
head of fibula
tibial tuberosity
medial tibial condyle
tibia
fibula
medial malleolus
transverse axis
lateral malleolus

L1
S1 ilium
sacrum
pubis
ischium
arcuate
pubic l.
pubic
symphysis

Key

l.	ligament
ll.	ligaments
m.	muscle
mm.	muscles
t.	tendon
tt.	tendons

Vertebrae
C	cervical
S	sacral
L	lumbar

Imagery © Anatomical Chart Company

Skeletal Anatomy, Posterior View

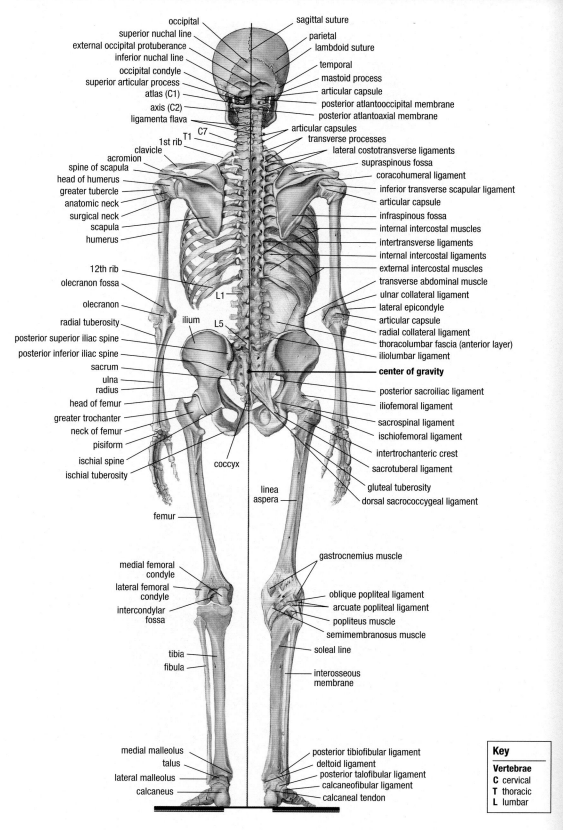

occipital
superior nuchal line
external occipital protuberance
inferior nuchal line
occipital condyle
superior articular process
atlas (C1)
axis (C2)
ligamenta flava
1st rib
clavicle
acromion
spine of scapula
head of humerus
greater tubercle
anatomic neck
surgical neck
scapula
humerus
12th rib
olecranon fossa
olecranon
radial tuberosity
posterior superior iliac spine
posterior inferior iliac spine
sacrum
ulna
radius
head of femur
greater trochanter
neck of femur
pisiform
ischial spine
ischial tuberosity
femur

medial femoral condyle
lateral femoral condyle
intercondylar fossa
tibia
fibula

medial malleolus
talus
lateral malleolus
calcaneus

C7
T1
ilium
L1
L5
coccyx
linea aspera

sagittal suture
parietal
lambdoid suture
temporal
mastoid process
articular capsule
posterior atlantooccipital membrane
posterior atlantoaxial membrane
articular capsules
transverse processes
lateral costotransverse ligaments
supraspinous fossa
coracohumeral ligament
inferior transverse scapular ligament
articular capsule
infraspinous fossa
internal intercostal muscles
intertransverse ligaments
internal intercostal ligaments
external intercostal muscles
transverse abdominal muscle
ulnar collateral ligament
lateral epicondyle
articular capsule
radial collateral ligament
thoracolumbar fascia (anterior layer)
iliolumbar ligament
center of gravity
posterior sacroiliac ligament
iliofemoral ligament
sacrospinal ligament
ischiofemoral ligament
intertrochanteric crest
sacrotuberal ligament
gluteal tuberosity
dorsal sacrococcygeal ligament

gastrocnemius muscle
oblique popliteal ligament
arcuate popliteal ligament
popliteus muscle
semimembranosus muscle
soleal line
interosseous membrane

posterior tibiofibular ligament
deltoid ligament
posterior talofibular ligament
calcaneofibular ligament
calcaneal tendon

Key

Vertebrae
C cervical
T thoracic
L lumbar

Imagery © Anatomical Chart Company

The Skull, Anterior and Posterior Views

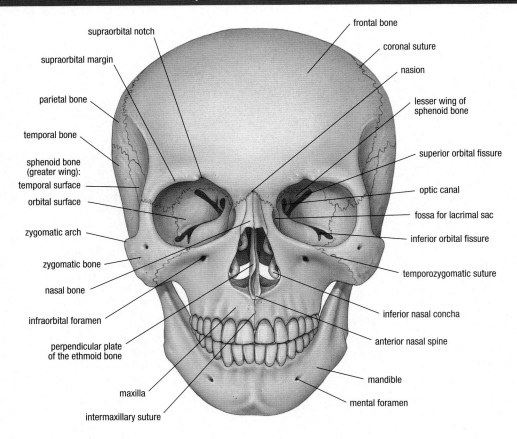

supraorbital notch

supraorbital margin

parietal bone

temporal bone

sphenoid bone
(greater wing):

temporal surface

orbital surface

zygomatic arch

zygomatic bone

nasal bone

infraorbital foramen

perpendicular plate
of the ethmoid bone

maxilla

intermaxillary suture

frontal bone

coronal suture

nasion

lesser wing of
sphenoid bone

superior orbital fissure

optic canal

fossa for lacrimal sac

inferior orbital fissure

temporozygomatic suture

inferior nasal concha

anterior nasal spine

mandible

mental foramen

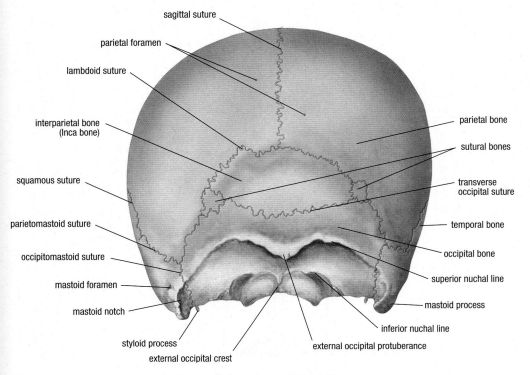

sagittal suture

parietal foramen

lambdoid suture

interparietal bone
(Inca bone)

squamous suture

parietomastoid suture

occipitomastoid suture

mastoid foramen

mastoid notch

styloid process

external occipital crest

parietal bone

sutural bones

transverse
occipital suture

temporal bone

occipital bone

superior nuchal line

mastoid process

inferior nuchal line

external occipital protuberance

Imagery © Anatomical Chart Company

Meaning	Meaning
blood clot	striated muscle
Meaning	Meaning
tension, pressure	flesh
Meaning	Meaning
nourishment	sound, sound waves
Meaning	Meaning
belly	above
Meaning	Meaning
internal organs	thorax, chest

Combining Form	Combining Form
rhabd/o	thromb/o
Combining Form	Combining Form
sarc/o	ton/o
Combining Form	Combining Form
son/o	troph/o
Combining Form	Combining Form
super/o	ventr/o
Combining Form	Combining Form
thorac/o	viscer/o

Meaning	Meaning
formation, growth	pancreas
Meaning	Meaning
near point of origin	disease
Meaning	Meaning
pubis	foot
Meaning	Meaning
lung	eat, swallow
Meaning	Meaning
pus	pharynx

Combining Form

pancreat/o

Combining Form

plas/o

Combining Form

path/o

Combining Form

proxim/o

Combining Form

ped/o, pod/o

Combining Form

pub/o

Combining Form

phag/o

Combining Form

pulmon/o

Combining Form

pharyng/o

Combining Form

py/o

Meaning

kidney

Meaning

black, dark

Meaning

nerve

Meaning

form, shape

Meaning

nucleus

Meaning

muscle

Meaning

scanty, few

Meaning

bone marrow,
spinal cord

Meaning

bone

Meaning

death

Combining Form

melan/o

Combining Form

nephr/o, ren/o

Combining Form

morph/o

Combining Form

neur/o

Combining Form

my/o, myos/o

Combining Form

nucle/o

Combining Form

myel/o

Combining Form

olig/o

Combining Form

necr/o

Combining Form

oste/o

Meaning	Meaning
fat	water, fluid
Meaning	Meaning
stone, calculus	below
Meaning	Meaning
lumbar region, lower back	side
Meaning	Meaning
lymph	smooth
Meaning	Meaning
middle	white

Combining Form	Combining Form
hydr/o	lip/o
Combining Form	Combining Form
infer/o	lith/o
Combining Form	Combining Form
later/o	lumb/o
Combining Form	Combining Form
lei/o	lymph/o
Combining Form	Combining Form
leuk/o	medi/o

Meaning	Meaning
fiber	disk (as in disk of spine)
Meaning	Meaning
stomach	back
Meaning	Meaning
glucose, sugar	electric, electricity
Meaning	Meaning
blood	epithelium (type of tissue)
Meaning	Meaning
tissue	red

Combining Form	Combining Form
disk/o	fibr/o

Combining Form	Combining Form
dors/o, poster/o	gastr/o

Combining Form	Combining Form
electr/o	gluc/o, glyc/o

Combining Form	Combining Form
epitheli/o	hem/o, hemat/o

Combining Form	Combining Form
erythr/o	hist/o

Meaning cranium, skull	Meaning neck
Meaning cold	Meaning green
Meaning blue	Meaning color
Meaning cell	Meaning colon (section of large intestine)
Meaning skin	Meaning rib

Combining Form

cervic/o

Combining Form

crani/o

Combining Form

chlor/o

Combining Form

cry/o

Combining Form

chrom/o

Combining Form

cyan/o

Combining Form

col/o, colon/o

Combining Form

cyt/o

Combining Form

cost/o

Combining Form

dermat/o

Meaning

arm

Meaning

abdomen

Meaning

heart

Meaning

extremity, tip

Meaning

tail

Meaning

gland

Meaning

head

Meaning

front

Meaning

brain, cerebrum

Meaning

immature cell

Combining Form	Combining Form
abdomin/o	**brachi/o**
Combining Form	Combining Form
acr/o	**cardi/o**
Combining Form	Combining Form
aden/o	**caud/o**
Combining Form	Combining Form
anter/o	**cephal/o**
Combining Form	Combining Form
blast/o	**cerebr/o**

Meaning

condition, process

Meaning

prolapse, drooping, sagging

Meaning

stopped, standing still

Meaning

suture

Meaning

stricture, narrowing

Meaning

flow, discharge

Meaning

surgical opening

Meaning

instrument for examination

Meaning

incision

Meaning

process of examining, examination

-ptosis

-sis

-rrhaphy

-stasis

-rrhea

-stenosis

-scope

-stomy

-scopy

-tomy

Meaning

surgical fixation

Meaning

resembling

Meaning

abnormal fear, aversion to, sensitivity to

Meaning

small

Meaning

formation, growth

Meaning

tumor

Meaning

surgical repair, recon-struction

Meaning

abnormal condition

Meaning

paralysis

Meaning

disease

-oid

-pexy

-ole

-phobia

-oma

-plasia

-osis

-plasty

-pathy

-plegia

Meaning

destruction, breakdown, separation

Meaning

condition of

Meaning

softening

Meaning

inflammation

Meaning

enlargement

Meaning

tissue, structure

Meaning

instrument for measuring

Meaning

one who specializes in

Meaning

measurement of

Meaning

study of

Suffix	Suffix
-ia, -ism, -y	-lysis

Suffix	Suffix
-itis	-malacia

Suffix	Suffix
-ium	-megaly

Suffix	Suffix
-logist, -ist	-meter

Suffix	Suffix
-logy	-metry

Meaning

excision, surgical removal

Meaning

pertaining to

Meaning

blood (condition of)

Meaning

pain

Meaning

originating, producing

Meaning

herniation, protrusion

Meaning

record, recording

Meaning

puncture to aspirate

Meaning

process of recording

Meaning

cell

Suffix

-ac, -al, -ary, -ic, -ous

Suffix

-ectomy

Suffix

-algia

Suffix

-emia

Suffix

-cele

Suffix

-genic, -genesis

Suffix

-centesis

Suffix

-gram

Suffix

-cyte

Suffix

-graphy

Meaning

together, with

Meaning

four

Meaning

rapid, fast

Meaning

again, backward

Meaning

across, through

Meaning

backward, behind

Meaning

three

Meaning

below, beneath

Meaning

excess, beyond

Meaning

above

Prefix

quad-, quadri-

Prefix

sym-, syn-

Prefix

re-

Prefix

tachy-

Prefix

retro-

Prefix

trans-

Prefix

sub-, infra-

Prefix

tri-

Prefix

supra-, super-

Prefix

ultra-

Meaning

around, surrounding

Meaning

new

Meaning

many, much

Meaning

normal

Meaning

after, behind

Meaning

all, entire

Meaning

before (in time or space)

Meaning

beside

Meaning

false

Meaning

through

Prefix

neo-

Prefix

peri-

Prefix

normo-

Prefix

poly-

Prefix

pan-

Prefix

post-

Prefix

para-

Prefix

pre-

Prefix

per-

Prefix

pseudo-

Meaning	Meaning
large, long	below, deficient

Meaning	Meaning
large, oversize	not

Meaning	Meaning
small	between

Meaning	Meaning
one	within

Meaning	Meaning
many	equal, alike

Prefix

hypo-

Prefix

macro-

Prefix

in-, im-, non-

Prefix

mega-, megalo-

Prefix

inter-

Prefix

micro-

Prefix

intra-

Prefix

mono-, uni-

Prefix

iso-

Prefix

multi-

Meaning

good, normal

Meaning

painful, difficult, abnormal

Meaning

half

Meaning

out of, away from

Meaning

other, different

Meaning

outer, outside

Meaning

same, alike

Meaning

in, within

Meaning

above, excessive

Meaning

on, following

Prefix

dys-

Prefix

eu-

Prefix

ec-, ex-

Prefix

hemi-, semi-

Prefix

ecto-, exo-

Prefix

hetero-

Prefix

en-, end-, endo-

Prefix

homo-, homeo-

Prefix

epi-

Prefix

hyper-

Meaning

two, twice

Meaning

without, not

Meaning

slow

Meaning

away from

Meaning

around

Meaning

to, toward

Meaning

away from, cessation, without

Meaning

opposing, against

Meaning

separate, remove

Meaning

self, same

Prefix

a-, an-

Prefix

bi-, di-

Prefix

ab-

Prefix

brady-

Prefix

ad-

Prefix

circum-

Prefix

anti-, contra-

Prefix

de-

Prefix

auto-

Prefix

dis-

⚡ STEDMAN'S MEDICAL TERMINOLOGY
Steps to Success in Medical Language

Discover the language of health care with **STEDMAN'S** – the trusted source for medical language for 100 years. *Stedman's Medical Terminology: Steps to Success in Medical Language* is a medical terminology work text that will prepare you to speak and understand medical language. When you have completed the course, you will have the skills needed to advance your education and the confidence to effectively communicate with patients, clients, and other medical professionals.

The hands-on work text approach in *Stedman's Medical Terminology* alternates term presentation with engaging exercises, allowing you to immediately apply what you've learned. Special features throughout the text will help you develop a firm knowledge of the language you'll need to succeed in your health care career, including:

- **Comprehensive coverage of terms within a logical organization**: Each chapter follows a consistent and cohesive organization to present the terms used for anatomical structures, symptoms and conditions, tests and procedures, surgical and therapeutic interventions, medications, and more.

- **Progressive exercises**: The progressive exercises are the heart of *Stedman's Medical Terminology*. Advancing from simple recall to application, the exercises have been engineered to help you learn, retain, and apply word parts, terminology, definitions, and abbreviations.

SIMPLE RECALL   ADVANCED RECALL   TERM CONSTRUCTION   COMPREHENSION   APPLICATION

- **A robust art program**: Especially helpful for the visual learner, the vivid illustrations and realistic photographs throughout *Stedman's Medical Terminology* bring concepts into focus.

- **Real-world application**: Make real-life connections with illustrated **Case Reports** and **Medical Record Analysis** exercises within each chapter.

- **Media Connection**: The electronic Student Resources for *Stedman's Medical Terminology* include hundreds of additional exercises, games, audio pronunciations, flashcards, animations, and more to help you master the language of health care.

- *LiveAdvise Medical Terminology*: Students have exclusive access to *LiveAdvise Medical Terminology*, an online tutoring service. View the inside back cover for more details!

Attention Instructors! A full suite of Instructor Resources have been designed with your needs in mind. Teach more effectively and save time with:

- Lesson Plans
- Image Bank
- Test Generator
- PowerPoint Slides
- Classroom Hand-outs
- Medical Record Library
- And more!

Trust Stedman's 100 years of experience to help you master the language of health care!

LWW.com

⬛ Wolters Kluwer | Lippincott Williams & Wilkins
Health

ISBN-13: 978-1-58255-816-5
ISBN-10: 1-58255-816-7

90000

9 781582 558165